Temporomandibular Joint Dysfunction and Occlusal Equilibration

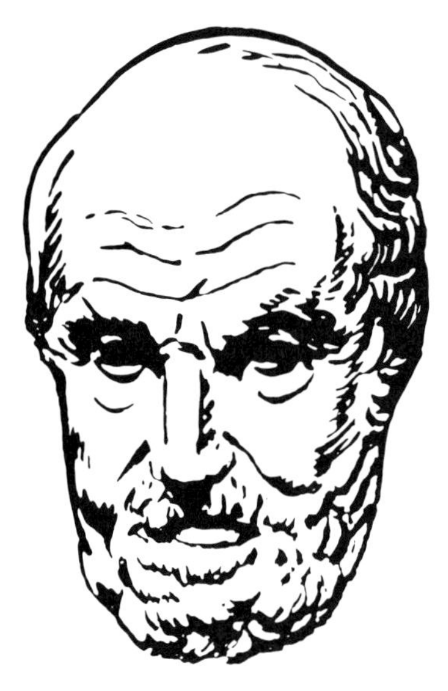

"Divine is the work to relieve pain."

Temporomandibular Joint Dysfunction and Occlusal Equilibration

NATHAN ALLEN SHORE
D.D.S., F.A.C.D., F.I.C.D.

Postgraduate Instructor, New York University College of Dentistry;
Fellow, Academy of General Dentistry;
Past President and Founder, Society of Oral Physiology and Occlusion

Second Edition

346 Illustrations

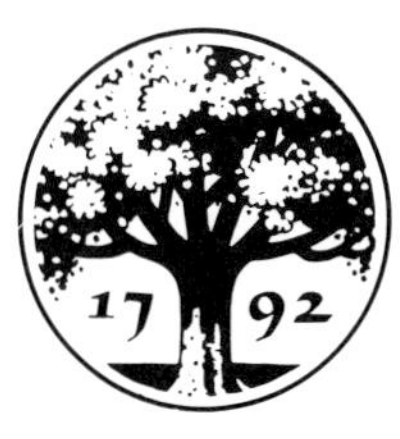

J. B. LIPPINCOTT COMPANY
Philadelphia • Toronto

SECOND EDITION

Library of Congress Catalog Card Number 76-2443

ISBN 0-397-50353-9

Printed in the United States of America

5

Library of Congress Cataloging in Publication Data

Shore, Nathan Allen.
Temporomandibular joint dysfunction and occlusal equilibration.

First ed. published in 1959 under title: Occlusal equilibration and temporomandibular joint dysfunction.
Bibliography: p.
Includes index.
1. Malocclusion. 2. Temporomandibular joint—Diseases. 3. Occlusion (Dentistry) I. Title.
[DNLM: 1. Dental occlusion, Balanced. 2. Temporomandibular joint. WU440 S559o]
RK523.S5 1976 617.6'43 76-2443
ISBN 0-397-50353-9

To
MIMI and ELIZABETH

Foreword

One of the most basic and important studies in the practice of dentistry is that of the occlusion of the natural dentition. Despite the fact that it is fundamental to the maintenance of normal oral physiology and is an integral part of every branch of dental practice, this essential principle has received woefully inadequate consideration in the teaching programs of most dental colleges. Too often, conflicting concepts of occlusion are taught in the departments of fixed prosthodontics, removable prosthodontics, periodontics, orthodontics and operative dentistry. These concepts should be resolved and coordinated in the curriculum. Otherwise, the student is likely to graduate with a confused impression of the problems of occlusion as they relate to the various divisions of dentistry that he will encounter in practice. This book enunciates a basic set of principles that can be applied to every branch of dentistry and to every age group.

The sequelae to occlusal anomalies of the dentition are extensive and manifold. Those most frequently encountered include abnormal postural relationship between the mandible and the maxilla, pathological changes, a widespread pain syndrome of the face, the head and the neck associated with malfunction of the temporomandibular joint, and generalized deterioration of the oral physiology. Consequently, the ultimate success of every oral rehabilitation is directly dependent upon the dentist's concept of both the static and the dynamic relationships of the occluding tooth surfaces. His knowledge of the factors that influence and control the functional and the nonfunctional movements of the mandible will determine in large measure the success of his corrective procedures. His skill in establishing a favorable postural relation between the mandible and the maxilla and his technical ability in creating a functional harmony of the guiding inclines of the teeth will contribute to the establishment of an equitable distribution of occlusal stress in both the centric and the eccentric mandibular relationships.

The correction of occlusal disharmonies of the natural dentition can be accomplished effectively by selective and judicious spot grinding. If it is done injudiciously, without a careful preliminary study of the interfering occlusal contacts, it may not only fail to relieve the trauma but may in turn contribute to additional oral discomfort.

The pain syndromes and the muscle spasms associated with temporomandibular joint dysfunction and its wide range of associated symptomatology frequently present a complex diagnostic problem to both physician and dentist. Even when the underlying causative factors are clearly recognized by the dentist, too often he is inadequately prepared to administer the necessary therapeutic measures.

This book deals with the problems of joint dysfunction and occlusal equilibration in a comprehensive and detailed fashion. The complex is viewed as a diagnostic and therapeutic entity. The book develops in logical and sequential steps from theory and etiology to examination, diagnosis and practical procedure. It is amply illustrated with figures and roentgenograms.

Dr. Shore is to be commended for the clear and detailed manner with which he has dealt with the subject in conformity with our present-day knowledge. His book is filled with basic and fundamental tenets that are indispensable to the success of every dentist's practice. It will provide impetus to those interested in dental research.

The study of the pain syndromes associated with temporomandibular joint dysfunction should be a project for research by medical and dental teams. It is worthy of being liberally supported by federal and private research funds in an effort to restore many pathetic sufferers to health, happiness and employability.

CLYDE H. SCHUYLER, D.D.S.
Formerly Professor of
Prosthetic Dentistry
New York University
College of Dentistry

Preface

In the seventeen years that have elapsed since the first edition of this book appeared, an ever-increasing interest in temporomandibular joint dysfunction and occlusal equilibration has been evident. To meet the growing awareness of the subject, I have made a special effort to bridge the gap between theory and clinical application. All too frequently, we learn and then forget theories before we have the opportunity to implement them. Those returning to the theoretical aspects in this book will find that extensive revisions have been made in the original text: five new chapters have been added.

There are many individuals to whom I am deeply indebted for the roles they played in helping to make this book possible. My heartfelt thanks go to each of them. To Clyde H. Schuyler, D.D.S., who inspired me many years ago to undertake further study in the field of temporomandibular joint dysfunction. For assistance and encouragement during early research, my thanks to Samuel D. Shapiro, M.D. To Janet G. Travell, M.D. my appreciation for her assistance in studies on pain and muscle spasm. My gratitude to L. D. Pankey, D.D.S., who has served as an inspiration of the best in dentistry. To E. Lloyd DuBrul, Ph.D., my thanks for permission to utilize his many original ideas from his treatise on the evolution of the jaw joints. To Seymour Diamond, M.D., who forged a link between the medical and dental professions through his erudite study of headaches, my appreciation. My thanks also, to Stanley Hoppenfeld, M.D., orthopaedist, who enhanced my knowledge of similarities between the temporomandibular joint and other joints of the body. For his unfailing friendship, help and encouragement, my thanks to Herman S. Harris, D.D.S. To my very good friend, Abraham I. Irvings, and to Manheim S. Shapiro my appreciation. Thanks also to Michael Hoffman, D.M.D., and to my associate, Merlin Schaefer, D.D.S., for their help, and to Edwin Felder for his encouragement.

Great appreciation to Barbara Lambert, my assistant, and thanks to her husband, James Lambert, for his help with electronics and photography. Further assistance with photography was provided by Gordon Emont, D.D.S., and Rosalind and David Greenspan.

My deep gratitude to a wonderful office staff and to Louise Donohue, the embodiment of a perfect secretary.

To Robert V. Andrews, Jane B. Asselin and Frances Thomas, my appreciation for their incisive editorial abilities.

Special thanks to my daughter, Elizabeth A. Shore for her unwavering faith.

And to my devoted wife, Mimi, my deepest gratitude for her exceptional moral support and help in the countless ways that enabled me to write this book.

NATHAN ALLEN SHORE, D.D.S.

Contents

Temporomandibular Joint Dysfunction and Occlusal Equilibration

1 The Role of Occlusion in Dentistry

Concepts of dental occlusion have been undergoing a radical change in the past few years. The former emphasis of the dental colleges on mechanical training and digital dexterity colored the thinking of an entire generation of practitioners. In treating the teeth as individual and independent entities, dentists overlooked the important fact that the teeth are but part of a whole masticatory organ, and that the masticatory organ, in turn, is a unit in the entire human organism. The older view of occlusion saw merely the physical mechanism of the teeth in their occluding positions. Because of this limited outlook, many dentists failed to correlate the mechanical operative procedures they performed on the teeth with the anatomy and the physiology of the total masticatory organ. Based upon a more scientific approach to the entire practice of dentistry, the newer concept of occlusion considers the teeth as part of but one organ in the entire stomatognathic system. In this light, the purpose of the dentist is more far-reaching than the mere care of the teeth and their supporting structures. The objective of modern dentistry is to achieve and maintain as much control as possible of the entire masticatory organ. The modern practitioner hopes to keep the stomatognathic system at the same age level as the rest of the body. To attain this objective, care of the masticatory organ must begin as early in life as possible and must be maintained throughout the life span.

As the masticatory organ functions throughout life, nature attempts to make compensatory adjustments to assure equal wear of the occlusal surfaces of the teeth. Occlusal equilibration is both a method for providing conditions under which nature can make these adjustments and a technique for assisting nature in her attempts to make these adjustments. A study of occlusion involves more than a mere examination of tooth-to-tooth and cusp-to-fossa relationships. It is concerned with the function of the entire stomatognathic system and the form of the masticatory organ that is integrated with this function. Based upon this concept of the intimate relationship between the form of the masticatory organ and the function of the stomatognathic system, the method of occlusal equilibration enables the dentist to distribute the forces delivered to and through the teeth to the maximum number of teeth, thus reducing the forces on individual teeth and other components of the masticatory organ to their physiological limits.

During deglutition, mastication and other bodily functions involving occlusal contacts, the forces delivered to and through the teeth to the supporting structures sometimes reach 100 pounds.[8] When there are so-called premature contacts, more accurately termed interfering occlusal contacts, during the static or dynamic ranges of occlusion, those teeth receiving the initial contact bear the brunt of this load. This may result in destruction of the teeth themselves, breakdown of the supporting tissues, dysfunction of the temporomandibular joints, temporomandibular joint arthrosis and general disease of the entire stomatognathic system. Orban[9] stated,

> A patient does not have to have periodontal disease, loose teeth, or a cracking or sore temporomandibular joint to be eligible for occlusal adjustment. A harmonious relation between teeth, temporomandibular joint and masticatory muscles is the basic objective of a biologic, functional approach to dentistry. If periodontal disease is present, establishment of a harmony is more than a theoretically sound biologic objective. It is an absolute basic clinical or practical requirement. . . . There are three questions which come up again and again—First: Is occlusal trauma a primary etiologic factor in periodontal disease? Second: Is it an aggravating or predisposing factor? Third: What is the biologic basis for correction of occlusal disharmonies?
>
> The first question has to be answered in the affirmative. Occlusal trauma is the primary etiologic factor for one form of periodontal disease, namely, periodontal disease traumatism.
>
> Is occlusal trauma a predisposing or aggravating factor in periodontal disease? This question again has to be answered affirmatively. If an inflammatory process such as a gingivitis or periodontitis involves a tooth or teeth that are also in traumatic occlusion, we can expect a more severe and a less favorable tissue reaction, especially a spreading of the inflammation into damaged areas of the supporting tissues. Under such aggravated conditions, the response to treatment cannot be expected to be favorable. However, we have to understand, without any doubt, that gingivitis, periodontitis, periodontosis, atrophy and hyperplasia are not to be confused with traumatic tissue changes. More often, diseases like gingivitis, periodontitis, periodontosis and hyperplastic changes will displace a tooth or teeth and thus expose them to secondary occlusal trauma. The described tissue changes of traumatism will aggravate and complicate the primary periodontal condition.
>
> An understanding and appreciation of a non-traumatic or better, a harmonious occlusion has to be based upon the general law of closest correlation of structure and function in any organism, organ, part of an organ or tissue. We have to regard structure and function as two aspects of living things. Thus, we see the beautiful functional adaption of the supporting dental tissues in alveolar bone, cementum, periodontal membrane and dentogingival junction, fibrous as well as epithelial attachment.
>
> It is also a general biologic law that almost all tissues and organs have a range of adaptability, without which they could not survive under the necessarily changing functional demands.
>
> With an understanding of this basic principle, we approach the problem of occlusion not only from the mechanical aspect, but from the point of view of biology. The fact that the teeth are not fixed in the jaw as if set in concrete, but rather are suspended in their sockets, attached to them by ligaments, permits a certain, slight mobility. The teeth are in a delicately balanced functional relation to each other, within the maxilla and mandible as well as in their occlusal and articular relations.

Starting from the identification of occlusal trauma caused by interfering occlusal contacts, the sections of this book on examination, clinical analysis, diagnosis, prognosis, planning of treatment, operative procedure and maintenance furnish the practicing dentist with a specific and detailed guide and handbook which should enable him to treat the occlusions of the vast majority of his patients. Specific reference is made to the Shore Mandibular Autorepositioning Appliance, which is recommended for use before any corrective procedures are begun.

The relationship between pathologic occlusion, temporomandibular joint dysfunction and temporomandibular joint arthrosis is discussed in detail. The importance of temporomandibular joint arthrosis is established by the fact that approximately 90 per cent of all temporomandibular joint dysfunctions may be attributed to this disease. The diagnosis of temporomandibular joint arthrosis is sometimes quite difficult unless every avenue is explored. White, Campbell and

Anderson[14] reported that in many cases of trigeminal nerve resection or evulsion, patients continued to have head pain which was relieved by adjustment of the occlusion.

Because pain symptoms and other manifestations of temporomandibular joint dysfunction and arthrosis occur in many areas of the head, the neck and the body, the patient tends to visit the physician, the radiologist, the neurologist, the otologist and the psychiatrist in that order. Careful inquiry, evaluation and correlation of the seemingly unrelated symptoms from the masticatory organ will make evident a diagnosis of disease of dental origin rather than a diagnosis of psychosomatic pain. It is because of the pathological physiology of muscular incoordination, muscle spasm and referred pain that these symptoms are related to malfunction of the masticatory organ.

From many studies[2,3,11] that have been made, it is generally agreed that roughly 20 per cent of the population have one or more symptoms of temporomandibular joint dysfunction. The severity of the symptoms may vary from a simple noise in the joint to extreme head pain, tenderness of the joints and limited mandibular movement accompanied by muscle spasm.

The basis for diagnosis and treatment of temporomandibular joint dysfunction and arthrosis is clearly outlined in this book, and the disease entities with similar symptoms are classified under differential diagnosis.

Furthermore, this book should enable the general practitioner to learn the technique of occlusal equilibration without too much difficulty and without devoting an inordinate amount of time to study. It is true that occlusal equilibration, like all procedures in dentistry, must be performed judiciously and carefully, and that injudicious selective reshaping of interfering tooth surfaces can destroy a patient's dentition. Nevertheless, the dentist who understands the scientific basis of occlusal equilibration and painstakingly follows the clinically tested operative procedures based upon these foundations that are described in this book can successfully incorporate in his daily practice the principles and the methods of this important technique.

Three basic methods, or a combination of these methods, may be employed to equilibrate the occlusion. The first is orthodontic, the second is occlusal rehabilitation, and the third is equilibration of the occlusion of the natural dentition by selective reshaping. While the first two methods require highly specialized training, the last method is within the scope of the general practitioner. Carried out by the careful and conscientious dentist, occlusal equilibration will help the patient to achieve and maintain a healthily functioning masticatory organ and stomatognathic system.

Although occlusal equilibration is a relatively recent development in dentistry, some of the principles and even the techniques of this procedure were known to the ancients. In the first century of the Christian Era, Pliny the Elder,[10] in his *Natural History,* discussed the correction of the teeth by filing irregularities. Galen[6] went into more detail, writing: "When one or more teeth, in consequence of a trauma, or from any other cause, become loose and projected above the level of the others, the part is removed by means of a small file." This is probably the first actual mention of occlusal trauma and equilibration in dental literature.

Until 1850, dentistry floundered along without much foundation in science. When Bonwill invented the first anatomical articulator in the middle of the last century, a new era of dentistry opened. It was during this period that the significance of mandibular movement was first recognized. Following Bonwill, Walker presented his studies on the movements of the mandible, and then, in rapid succession, men such as Balkwill, Bennet,

Black, Christensen, Constant, Gritman, Gysi, Hall, Hanau, Kerr, Luce, Monson, Miller, Needles, Parfitt, Schwarz, Snow, Spee and Wilson made their contributions to the science of dentistry.

A new approach to dentistry was heralded in 1925 when Washburn[13] wrote:

> Possibly the fact that individual tooth operations called for the remarkable technical ability that was displayed and the concentration of observing minute detail in such operations, may have been the reason for so many of our well-trained men overlooking the larger problem, made up of all the teeth, their relation to each other in the arch, one arch to the other, mandible to the rest of the bones of the skull, and the significance of all this in its influence upon physiologic action.

So far, the impetus for the study of occlusion came primarily from prosthodontists and orthodontists. However, it was soon recognized that the principles of occlusion and articulation form the basis for every aspect of dentistry. Occlusion and articulation are based upon the principle of function, and the purpose of all dentistry is the maintenance or the restoration of function.

Although Ferrein[5] published an article on mandibular movement and occlusion as long ago as 1748, not much more was heard on the relationship of these factors to occlusal equilibration and general dentistry until Karolyi gave his lectures in England in 1901. Karolyi,[7] Warnekros,[12] Arkovy[1] and Farrar[4] were among the first who actually dealt with occlusal equilibration as such. As one explores the history, one is struck by the fact that each writer places the stamp of his own specialty on the general field of occlusion. Orthodontists, prosthodontists, periodontists and general practitioners all contributed to the study of occlusion, but all of them concentrated on the problem primarily as it affected their own specialties. Nevertheless, once the principle of function as the basis for all dentistry is accepted and established, all the contributions can be tied together to make a useful and intelligible whole upon which the entire practice of dentistry may be based. To function, teeth must occlude and articulate; therefore, the principles of occlusion and articulation must be considered in every specialty as well as in the general practice of dentistry. Regardless of how clever a technician a dentist is, his work will be successful only if he understands and applies the principles of occlusion and articulation in his general practice.

There is a logical relationship between the cause of a pathological condition, the diagnosis, the prognosis, the development of a plan of treatment and the actual operative procedures of treatment. To study a case thoroughly and to analyze it critically, the dentist must have a thorough knowledge and understanding of the physiology and the pathology of all the related structures of the masticatory organ. In studying a case, the dentist must consider the dentition not as a static entity but as a part of a dynamically functioning organ. As the masticatory organ functions, many different stresses and strains will act upon it in many different ways. When the dentist understands that teeth function and must satisfy certain fundamental demands, he sees that this is the basic principle underlying dentistry in general and occlusal equilibration in particular. Every other aspect of the dentition is subordinate to the criterion of proper function.

With this background, the dentist must conceive of the teeth and the mouth as a part of the entire stomatognathic system and must treat this system as a single functioning unit in the body. Since he must analyze and treat the masticatory organ as a whole, it is most important for him to utilize a technique that will enable him to visualize the entire dentition of his patient, plan the treatment and test the plan.

Usually, occlusal equilibration and temporomandibular joint dysfunction are discussed in texts on periodontia and prosthetics. However, from the points of view of prevention of temporomandibular joint dysfunction and integrated restorative dentistry, the basic treatment of occlusal equilibration properly belongs in the field of the general practitioner.

REFERENCES

1. Arkovy, F.: A discussion on the premature loss of teeth by destruction of their alveoli. Tr. Int. Med. Cong. (London), *3*:575, 1881.
2. Boman, K.: Temporomandibular joint arthrosis and its treatment by extirpation of the disk. Acta Chir. Scand., *95*(Suppl. 118):21, 1947.
3. Brussels, J.: Temporomandibular joint diseases: differential diagnosis and treatment. JADA, *39:*532, 1949.
4. Farrar, J. N.: Irregularities of the Teeth. New York, 1888.
5. Ferrein, M.: Sur les movements de la machoire inferrieure. p. 427, Hist. de l'acad. royale des sciences, 1748.
6. Galen: De Compositione, Bk. 5.
7. Karolyi, M.: Beobachtungen über pyorrhea alveolaris. (Observations concerning the theory of pyorrhea alveolaris.) O.U.V.f.Z., *17:*279, 1901.
8. Langley, L. L., and Cheraskin, E.: The Physiological Foundation of Dental Practice. p. 421. St. Louis, C. V. Mosby, 1951.
9. Orban, B.: Biologic basis for correcting occlusal disharmonies. J. Periodont., *25:*257, 1954.
10. Pliny the Elder: Naturalis Historia. Bk. 28, ch. 178.
11. Staplemohr, V.: Sur les craquements de l'articulation temporomaxillaire et les luxations habituelles de la machoire. Acta Chir. Scand., *65:*1, 1929.
12. Warnekros, L.: Über die ursachen des fruhzeigigen verlustes der zahne. (The causes of early loss of the teeth.) Berl. Klin. Wchnschr., *43:*832, 1906.
13. Washburn, H. B.: History and evolution of the study of occlusion. D. Cosmos, *67:*331, 1925.
14. White, T. C., Campbell, J., and Anderson, H.: An investigation into temporomandibular joint dysfunction. D. Record, *72:*49, 1952.

Additional Basic Reference

Reynolds, J. M.: The organization of occlusion for natural teeth. J. Pros. Dent., *26:*56, 1971.

2 The Evolution of the Temporomandibular Joint

The jaw joint is significant in being the first true diarthrodial joint, and an examination of its origin reveals not only its unique role in vertebrate evolution but also the close relationship between it and the ear. In his excellent article on the evolution of the temporomandibular joint, Du Brul[1] describes the complex sequence of events involved in the development of the mammalian jaw joint, discusses the intimate relationships between form and function characterizing the evolutionary process, and examines some of the structural adaptations found in extant primates. The following introduction to this fascinating subject is based on his work.

The earliest vertebrates, the agnatha, had no jaws. Instead, there was a simple mouth opening directly anterior to a series of cartilaginous gill arches (Fig. 2-1*a*). The first simple jaw arose in the gnathostomes, as the first gill arch gradually came to function in concert with the mouth opening. The joint was a synarthrosis (i.e., the jaws were formed by connective tissue). The entire structure was pushed against the second gill arch (Fig. 2-1*b*). Meckel's cartilage is the vestige of the early cartilaginous lower jaw now found in the embryo. In the third stage of evolution, that of the osteichthyes, a truly diarthrodial joint appeared (Fig. 2-1*c*). At this point, the second gill arch came to serve as a brace for the jaw structure. The jaws were strengthened as well by the addition to their outer surfaces of tooth-bearing bony plates, known as secondary jaws.

The joint itself was an articulation between the quadrate bone, which was covered by three layers of cartilage (calcified, hyaline and fibrocartilage) and the ossified end of Meckel's cartilage. Between the two articulating surfaces was a large joint cavity lined with synovial membrane. Thus, at this stage the jaw joint comprised all the fundamental elements eventually found in vertebrates; yet "it took the evolutionary process something on the order of 130 million years to stabilize this composite, basic, vertebrate head skeleton with its built-in pincers called jaws."[2]

At the amphibian stage the upper jaw complex consisted of a premaxilla, jugal, quadratojugal, and quadrate bone. Above and in contact with the last three lay the squamosal. The lower jaw, like the upper, consisted of a cartilaginous core covered with bony plates. The most important of these was the dentary bone at the anterior end, opposed to the maxilla. The articular bone (the ossified end of Meckel's cartilage) contacted the quadrate bone to form the joint.

It is interesting to note that at this point the skull became kinetic—there were many movable parts in the jaw complex. The importance of this development to the amphibians was that it facilitated the swallowing of prey. While part of the complex clamped down rigidly to prevent escape, other parts could maneuver the

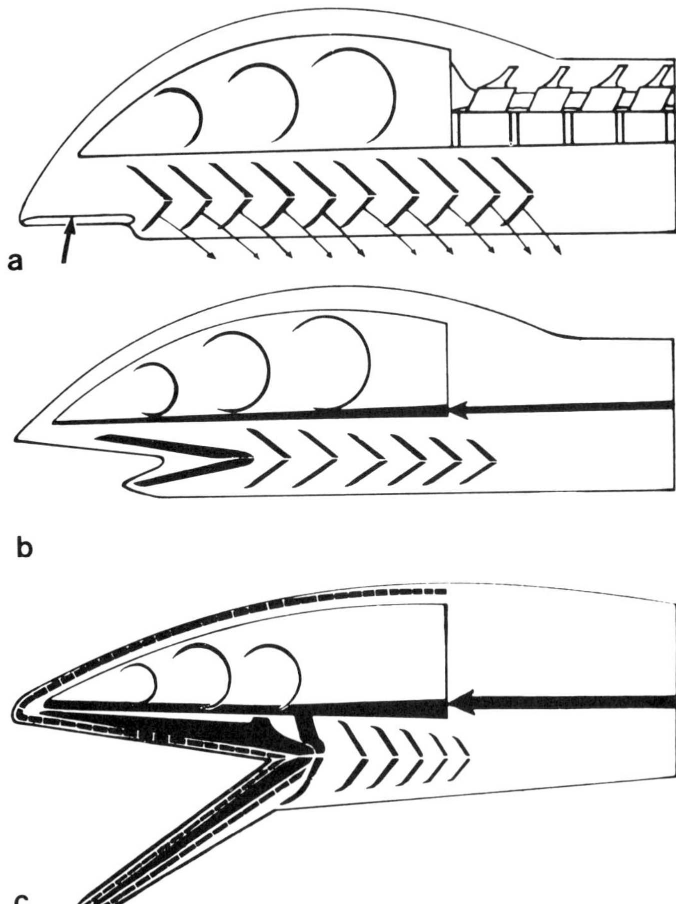

FIG. 2-1. A model of the origin of the oral apparatus: In the sedentary sucking animal, the early cranium is emphasized in heavy outline (*a*). The oral opening below takes in water and food and expels water through the gills. The foremost gill arches have begun to modify as active swimming begins, indicated as thrust against the skull by the arrow (*b*). In the swift-swimming predatory fish, the first gill arch forms the core of the jaws braced to the skull by the second arch as swimming thrust increases (*c*). The skull is consolidated as a unit encased in dermal bone plates indicated by the heavy interrupted line under the skin. (Modified from Du Brul)

prey back toward the gullet. The result of this adaptation in modern amphibians is that the jaw-closing muscles are often weaker than the muscles of the kinetic system.

The beginnings of the development of the ear from the primary jaw appeared for the first time with the amphibians. The tympanic membrane moved back toward the hyomandibular bone, which served to carry vibrations from the membrane to the inner ear. The other important evolutionary development at this stage was the decrease in number of bones forming the jaws, accompanied by greater differentiation of the teeth. The trend of the quadratoarticular joint toward the function of sound conduction continued in the mammallike reptiles. Parallel to this shift was the continued and now very marked backward and upward expansion of the dentary bone—a development that is part of the tendency toward fewer bones in the jaw complex. (This trend means a stronger jaw as the number of synarthroses is reduced.) The jaw-closing muscles attached to the dentary bone as it extended backward and finally contacted the upper jaw at the squamosal. This dentary-squamosal contact formed the new joint, and at this point in vertebrate evolution there existed animals with two jaw joints.

With the development of mammals, the new dentary-squamosal, or temporomandibular joint totally took over the function of jaw support; the old primary joint was no longer needed. Instead, it became very small and joined the old hyomandibular bone, now called the stapes, as part of the ear complex. The quadrato-articular joint thus became the joint between the incus and the malleus. This close relationship between the ear and jaw complexes

immediately makes sense of a well-known neurological detail. The tensor tympani muscle which moves the malleus—the proximal end of Meckel's cartilage—is innervated by a branch of the nerve to the medial pterygoid muscle, which, in turn, is a branch of the mandibular nerve. The muscle is a remnant of the old muscles that moved the jaws at the reptilian stage and it maintains its identity with the fifth cranial nerve, the basic nerve of the jaw apparatus. This suggests that early in embryonic development, neural patterns are established within the brainstem in which jaw bone and ear bone movements are integrated. Herein lies the key to the relationship between jaw and ear dysfunctions sometimes plaguing modern man along with deterioration of other parts of the jaw and dental apparatus. One need not invoke some impossible mechanical impingement of the joint on a nerve. One must look to disturbances in neuromuscular-joint coordination, which leads us at last, into the central nervous system.[3]

In brief, then, the evolution of the temporomandibular joint entailed the reduction in the number of bones comprising the jaw and the increase in size and eventual dominance of the dentary bone, resulting in a new, stronger articulation between the lower jaw and skull.

At all stages of jaw evolution, form follows function. As the requirements for mastication became more specialized, so did the jaw and the dentition. For example, in the amphibians, in which there is no mastication, a kinetic system is a necessity. As evolution progressed, some of the burden of killing prey shifted away from the mouth, and at the same time the diverse demands and options in terrestrial life made some form of mastication a necessity for survival. It was thus that the rigid bone structure and strong diarthrodial jaw articulation arose.

One final adaptation, which applies only to man, deserves mention. Because of man's vertical posture, a simple hinge joint in the jaw would be impossible—such a joint would, on opening, squeeze the soft structures between the mastoid and mandible. Hence, the initial hinge action is followed by a downward and forward movement of the condyles against the articular eminence, thereby enabling the jaws to open widely while avoiding any damage to deeper structures.

Curiously enough, we begin life with two temporomandibular joints and no teeth. Usually, although not necessarily, we end life the same way.

REFERENCES

1. Du Brul, E. L.: Evolution of the temporomandibular joint. *In* Sarnat, B. G. (ed.): The Temporomandibular Joint. pp. 3–27. Springfield (Ill.), Charles C Thomas, 1964.
2. Ibid.
3. Ibid.

Additional Basic References

Brekke, C. A.: Jaw function: Part I. Hinge rotation. J. Pros. Dent., 9:600, 1959.

Du Brul, E. L.: Personal communication.

Sicher, H., and Du Brul, E. L.: Oral Anatomy. ed. 5. St. Louis, C. V. Mosby, 1970.

3 *The Biomechanics of Tooth Movement*

There is some confusion in dentistry between mechanics and biology because most of the remedies applied by the profession are mechanical, whereas body reactions are biological. The dentist must learn to distinguish between the mechanical and the biological stresses of the stomatognathic system. Whether the results of mechanical overstress are confined to one or two teeth or whether temporomandibular joint dysfunction, with its attendant problems and complications, is set in motion, the tissue reactions are biological. To control mechanical force, it is essential to understand both its nature and the biological effects of stress upon the periodontium.

The true interrelationships of mechanics and biology in dentistry are clarified through an understanding of the tooth and its investing structures as a set of living tissues in a constant state of flux (i.e., in constant anabolic and catabolic change caused by mechanical and biological forces). The only factor that is relatively controllable by the dentist is the dentition. Wear of the teeth is one of nature's methods of making adjustments and compensations in this intricately operating masticatory organ. Often, however, nature's plans for adjustment go awry. When this happens unusual forces are set up in the masticatory organ. The most destructive of these and the one that is the chief cause of degeneration of the masticatory organ is overload resulting in unphysiological torque. Therefore, all mechanical treatment and intervention must be based on a thorough evaluation of the forces operating in the patient's masticatory organ.

MECHANICAL FORCE AND BIOLOGICAL STRESS

Through an analysis and understanding of the physical principles involved in the body, the dentist may be able to predict the results of combinations of forces that operate on the masticatory organ. The basic physical concept that he must constantly bear in mind is that of balance. Nature strives to maintain an equilibrium or balance of all the forces within and without the body. All forces and stresses that operate upon the human organism must be considered in terms of action and reaction. The state of balance between action and reaction determines the health of the body. All stresses that are exerted upon the organism or upon any part thereof must be kept within certain tolerable physiological limits if the tissues are not to degenerate or break down. It is this critical relationship between mechanical forces and physiological tolerance limits that makes it necessary to consider many of the problems of dentistry from the viewpoint of biomechanics.

The factor that determines whether or not trauma will result from stress is the resistive capacity of the individual. A high resistive capacity will cause the deposition of bone when the periodontal fibers are subjected to stress. However, in a patient with low resistive capacity, overstress of the periodontal fibers will cause breakdown of the bone. The dentition will usually maintain itself in the highest state of health when the biomechanical forces of the masticatory organ are harmoniously balanced.

METABOLISM, RESISTIVE CAPACITY AND FORCE

The body's response to stress is the determining principle of prognosis in any individual case. To a great degree, the mobility of the teeth depends on the periodontal fibers and the height and the quality of the alveolar process. As long as the force on any one tooth does not exceed normal limits and no other pathological processes exist, the bone around that tooth will maintain its proper level. However, if the force exceeds the normal limits for the patient, abnormal reactions result. Under these conditions tissue exhaustion, degeneration and breakdown occur. It is the resistive capacity of the bone that determines its ability to withstand excessive force. The maxilla and the mandible have the highest rate of calcium metabolism in the body. The ability of the bone to resist excessive force varies from individual to individual. A human being's adaptive capacity or level of resistance is determined by his systemic condition. The consequences of overstress vary widely, depending upon the stamina of the traumatized tissues. The evidences of tissue exhaustion or breakdown also vary among individuals. One case may react with accompanying inflammation but no pain, while another will react with great pain but no clinical symptoms other than the demonstrable occlusal interference.

The metabolism of the bone and the resistive capacity of the periodontium determine the rate of degeneration of the tissues under excessive force. As the body ages, resistance is lowered, and, indirectly, periodontal lesions tend to develop because occlusal forces may remain constant or even increase.

Roentgenography will reveal three different reactions of the bone to stress: condensation, rarefaction and absorption. The particular reaction that occurs in an individual as a result of stress depends on his or her resistive capacity. When the practitioner identifies these three reactions of the bone to stress, he is in a position not only to treat the patient rationally but also to prevent the symptoms from recurring.

By applying the laws of mechanics to dentistry, it is possible to explain many of the effects of force on the masticatory organ, and also it may be possible to predict what will happen when forces are applied and when they are removed or balanced. A review of these principles will help the dentist to understand more clearly the mechanics involved in mastication. When he equilibrates the occlusion, the practitioner is actually adjusting and balancing a biomechanical force machine to within the physiological metabolic limits of the patient.

The emotions of the patient can directly influence metabolism via the nervous system. Cannon[5] showed that the salivary and the adrenal glands are controlled by the autonomic nervous system, which also regulates the nutrient blood supply to the body. Selye's[16] concept of stress elaborately explains its results on emotions, which in turn cause pathological effects upon the body tissues (see Chap. 7). In this manner metabolism is disturbed, resistive capacity impaired and a formerly physiological state of the tissues becomes pathological.

An accompanying reaction to emotional stress may be neuromuscular dysfunction. Many investigators[4,15,17] maintain that bruxism is the result of stress. Bruxism coupled with emotional stress can and does cause pathological forces on the metabolically disturbed periodontium, exceeding the resistive capacity of the tissues. Since the purpose of dentistry is prevention as well as repair, the practitioner must understand all the forces that cause pathological conditions of the masticatory organ. Therefore, he must understand the pathological effects of poor nutrition and of emotions upon the body defense mechanism and the masticatory organ, and he must try to control these factors as well as any others that may be involved.

MECHANICS AND THE MASTICATORY ORGAN

It is a fundamental law of mechanics that every force has a reciprocal which is equal and opposite. The reciprocal to the occlusal force is the resistance furnished by the cementum, the periodontal fibers and the bone. These tissues either adapt themselves successfully to the stress of occlusal forces or they succumb and degenerate.

It is a generally accepted principle that form and function are interrelated. Nature adapts her structures to the tasks they are required to perform. As functions change because of metabolic processes or for other reasons, their forms will undergo adaptive changes. The physical forces of occlusion are transmitted through the occlusal surfaces of the teeth and are finally expended on the alveolar bone. The teeth are intermediaries and exert force on the periodontal tissues, which exert an equal and opposite force against the teeth. Actually, the maxillary and the mandibular teeth and the periodontium are in a state of stress and thus offer resistance to the force of the musculature during the acts of deglutition and mastication. During the act of swallowing, the upper and lower teeth attempt to come together in centric relation. Mastication, deglutition, oral habits and stomatognathic muscle spasms are the sources of occlusal forces on the teeth. Of the first two, the physiological act of swallowing is the more important, because while approximately one hour a day is spent on mastication, swallowing takes place about 1,500 times daily, and the teeth tap each other at each act of swallowing. Oral habits and stomatognathic muscle spasm are not physiological processes.

The tooth is a three-dimensional structure that is suspended in a well of alveolar bone process in a sling of periodontal fibers. The upper teeth are the fixed anvils; the lower teeth are the hammers which transmit their forces upward to the occlusal surfaces of the upper teeth. This arrangement must be borne in mind whenever the engineering problems and the mechanical laws involved in dentistry are considered.

Ideally, force should be equally distributed among as many teeth as possible in centric-relation occlusion as well as in the eccentric* ranges of articulation. The basic physical principles involved indicate that the direction of force should coincide as closely as possible with the long axes of the teeth if maximum function and efficiency are to be achieved with no damage to the periodontium. All loads placed upon the teeth are transmitted to the lamina dura through the fibers of the periodontal ligament. In the condition that Box refers to as individual overloading,[3] one or two pairs of teeth carry the entire load of closure. Because of the conical shape of the roots and the inclined planes of the cusps, a mechanical action known as torque is produced, and the teeth are actually twisted and tipped in the alveoli.

What Box calls impact loading[2] is found in a locked occlusion. In attempting to move into the lateral ranges

* The term "eccentric" describes an out-of-centric or incorrect sagittal relationship of the mandible to the maxilla.

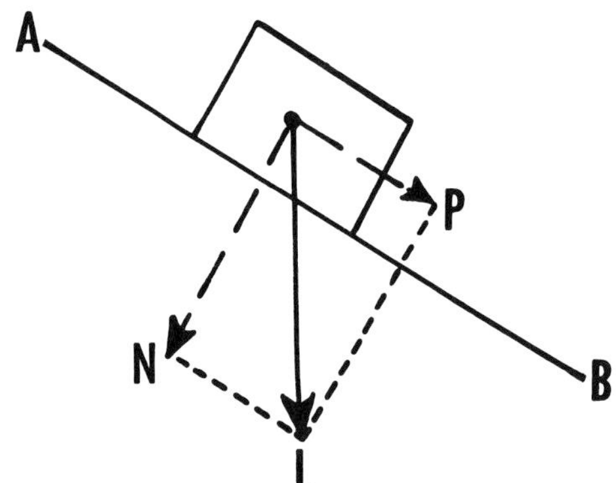

FIG. 3-1. The composition and resolution of forces on an inclined plane.

of articulation, the mandible tends to jar the teeth suddenly. This sudden load on the teeth is transmitted to the periodontal fibers so quickly that they do not cushion the blow, and therefore the stress is placed on the lamina dura, where it causes damage to this structure as well as to the nerve, the lymph and the blood vessels of the tooth involved.

STATICS AND DYNAMICS

To understand the operations of the masticatory organ, it is important to study the laws of those branches of physics that are most applicable (i.e., statics and dynamics). Statics deals with forces in equilibrium or bodies at rest. In the masticatory organ the laws of statics apply, for example, when the teeth are in contact during the act of swallowing. At this stage of the act of deglutition there are forces operating on the teeth, but there is no movement. In terms of physics, equilibrium is that state in which a body is acted upon by several counteracting forces in such a manner that it has no tendency to move and therefore remains in a fixed position. At each phase of function, a tooth should be in functional equilibrium and should perform its share of work without receiving more force than it is designed to bear.

Dynamics is that branch of physics which deals with forces that are created by bodies in variable motion. In the masticatory organ the laws of dynamics apply when, for example, mandibular movement creates forces during the act of mastication. Kinetics, a branch of dynamics, deals with motion. There are two types of motion: rotation (i.e., the movement of a wheel on its axle) and translation (i.e., the movement of a body from one place to another along a straight line). As the motion of a wheel on a moving vehicle exhibits both rotation and translation, so the motion of a tooth in its socket is both rotatory and translatory. Since the cusps of the teeth are actually inclined planes, it is also important to understand the composition and the resolution of forces on an inclined plane. The weight of an object which rests on an inclined plane is represented by a force vector. In Figure 3-1 this vector is L (load). This vector may be resolved into two component forces: N (perpendicular to the inclined plane AB) and P (parallel to the inclined plane AB). The purpose of resolving a single force into its components is to re-

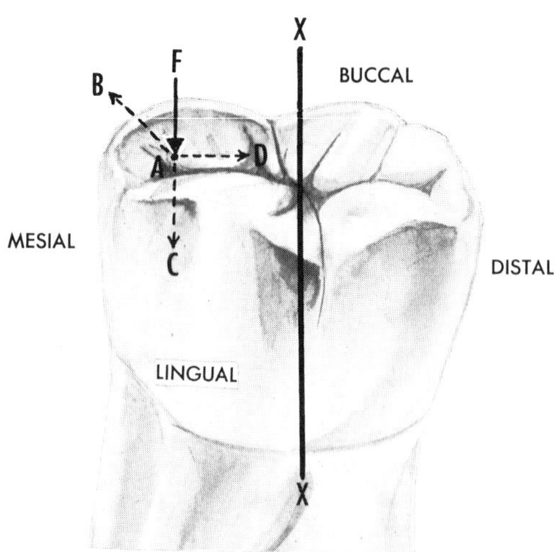

FIG. 3-2. The three directions B, D and C in which a tooth tends to move as a result of the force F on the mesiolingual inclined plane of the mesiobuccal cusp at A.

place the original force by some system that may be handled and studied more conveniently. The inverse process, whereby the component parts are resolved into the original single force, is referred to as composition of forces. This figure demonstrates how vector L may be determined if its component forces N and P are known.

CUSPS AND INCLINED PLANES

The occlusal anatomy of a tooth is not, however, a simple inclined plane. It ranges in complexity from a single inclined plane in an incisor to possibly eighteen inclined planes in a lower first molar. It is important to conceive of these planes in three dimensions. A force applied to any one of them will result in component forces operating in three directions because of the three dimensions. These component forces will extend mesiodistally, buccolingually and occlusoapically. Consider, for example, the mesiobuccal cusp of the lower right first molar and specifically its mesiolingual incline. This plane articulates with the distobuccal incline of the lingual cusp of the upper second bicuspid. A force F on the mesiolingual inclined plane of the mesiobuccal cusp of the lower right first molar (Fig. 3-2) will result in component forces which tend to move the tooth in three directions: buccally in the direction of arrow AB; distally in the direction of arrow AD; apically in the direction of arrow AC. The first two components, AB and AD, are horizontal and are resolved into one force that tends to produce twisting torque or rotation of the tooth about its long axis, X. The third component, AC, is a vertical force that tends to produce translatory movement or intrusion of the tooth vertically into the socket. These motions, of course, pull and compress the various periodontal fibers.

The lower first molar, as has been pointed out above, has eighteen possible occluding planes. To predict the movements of this tooth caused by the forces applied to it would require a complete mathematical study of all forces applied to the lower first molar by the opposing occluding teeth. This exhaustive study would have to consider both the direction of these forces and their magnitude as well as the torque-resisting factors. However, basically the movements of the teeth will be in three directions: buccolingual, mesiodistal and apical. The first two movements will cause rotation, and the third translation.

For purposes of explanation and sim-

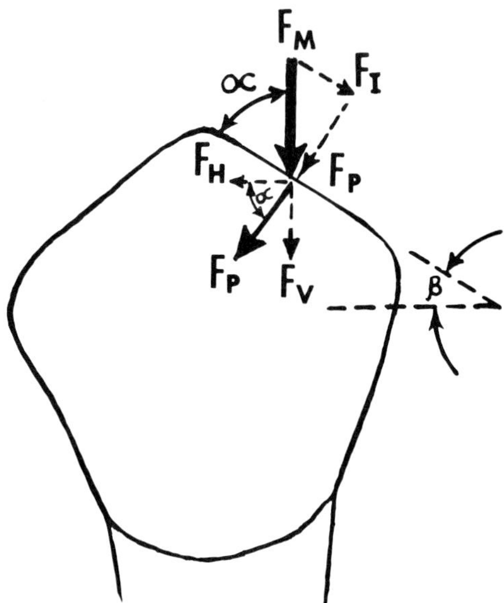

FIG. 3-3. The components of forces are seen on a two-dimensional diagram of a natural three-dimensional tooth.

F_M = vertical force of mastication

F_I = force tending to slide down the inclined plane

F_P = force perpendicular to the incline tending to move the tooth

F_H = the actual horizontal force moving the tooth

F_V = the vertical component of F_P intruding the tooth

α = angle between F_M and incline of the cusp

β = angulation of cusp measured from the horizontal

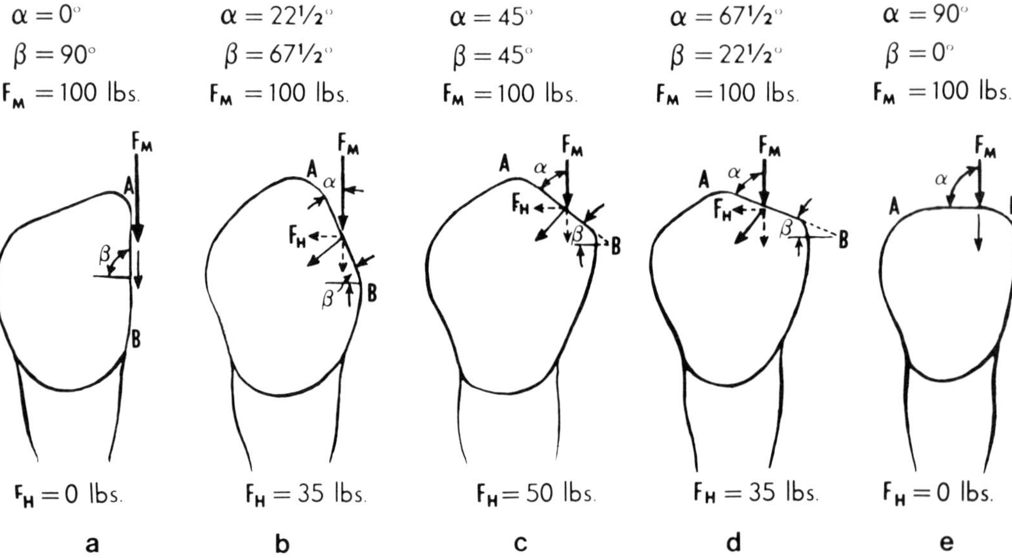

FIG. 3-4. The effects of cuspal angles from 0° to 90° on the direction and the intensity of forces acting upon a tooth.

plification let us consider a two-dimensional study of this mathematical problem. According to Langley and Cheraskin[11] the average person can exert 100 pounds of force in the molar region and, if needed, use it in mastication. In the simplified two-dimensional study of a case of interfering occlusal contact in which the inclined planes of the cusps are at an angle of 45°, it will be found that this force of 100 pounds functioning along an interfering inclined plane of 45° will produce a secondary horizontal displacement force of 50 pounds (Fig. 3-3).

As the teeth approach each other, all masticatory forces are essentially vertical, F_M. As an interfering occlusal contact is met, the vertical force, F_M, is broken into two components: F_I, parallel and tending to slide the opposing tooth down the incline of the cusp; F_P, perpendicular to the incline and therefore tending to move the teeth horizontally. This second force, F_P, contains the force, F_H, which actually tends to move the tooth horizontally. Breaking force F_P into its components, F_V and F_H, delivers the value of these forces. The following equation can be applied to Figure 3-3.

$$F_P = F_M \sin \alpha$$
$$F_H = F_P \cos \alpha$$

Substituting for F_P:

$$F_H = (F_M)(\sin \alpha)(\cos \alpha)$$

Trigonometrically:

$$2 \sin \alpha \cos \alpha = \sin 2\alpha$$
$$\therefore \sin \alpha \cos \alpha = \tfrac{1}{2} \sin 2\alpha$$

Substituting in the above:

$$F_H = F_M \left(\tfrac{1}{2} \sin 2\alpha\right)$$
$$F_H = \frac{F_M}{2} \sin 2\alpha$$

For example, if it is assumed that the average masticatory force is 100 pounds and the angle between the incline and the applied force is 45°, the problem is solved as follows:

$$F_H = \frac{F_M}{2} \sin 2\alpha$$
$$F_H = \frac{100}{2} \sin 2(45°)$$
$$F_H = 50 \sin 90°$$
$$F_H = 50\ (1)$$
$$F_H = 50 \text{ pounds}$$

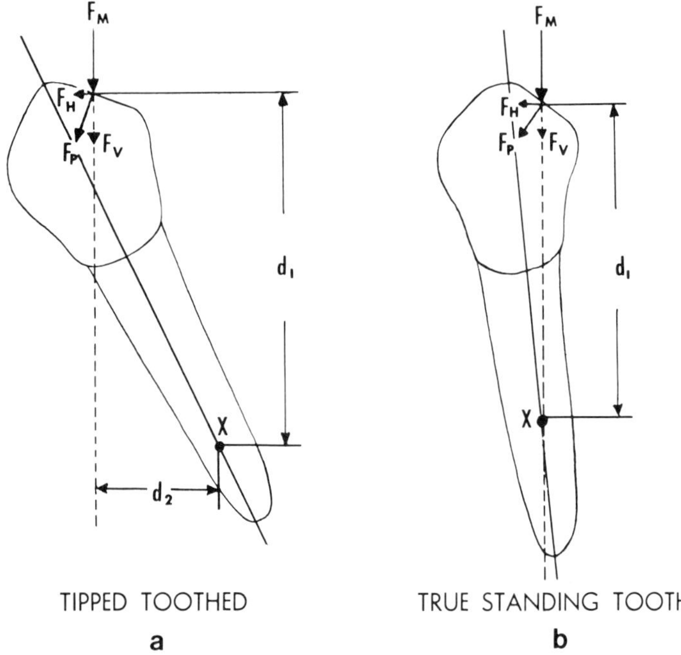

FIG. 3-5. The influence of excessive tipping on the forces acting upon the cuspal inclines of a tooth.

Figure 3-4 diagrams not only the condition of the above example but also with values from 0° to 90°. From (*a*) it can be seen that the force, F_M, is parallel with the incline, AB, at the point at which it is being applied, and that no horizontal force is possible. From (*b*) with an α of 22½° and a β of 67½° (the incline of the cusp) the F_H is 35 pounds. The fact that there is an incline automatically sets up a horizontal force. From (*c*) with α of 45° and β also of 45°, the maximum horizontal force that can be created with any given force F_M is attained. In this case, F_H is 50 pounds. At first glance, diagram (*b*) would lead one to expect force F_H to be greater than that found in diagram (*c*). This is not true because, due to the steep cuspal angulation, β, most of F_M tends to slide down the planes as F_I (Fig. 3-3). This F_P is small compared with F_M. Therefore, F_H, which is a component of F_P, must be smaller than F_P.

Figure 3-4*d* shows a cuspal angulation of 22½° that is flatter than that in (*c*). In this case, F_P is the greater component of F_M and almost equal to it. But of the components of F_P, F_V is much greater than F_H, and, mathematically, F_H equals 35 pounds. Figure 3-4*e* shows no cuspal inclination. Therefore, all of F_M (100-pound force of mastication) is taken as F_V (the intruding force along the long axis), and there is no F_H (horizontal force) to produce torque. While torque is not produced in Figure 3-4*e*, the full force of mastication is taken along the vertical axis of one interfering occlusal contact. Note that this dissertation is based on true standing teeth, with force F_M being directed parallel with the axial inclination of the tooth. It should also be noted that this is a two-dimensional representation for purposes of illustration and simplification.

The greatest horizontal forces of true standing teeth come from cuspal inclinations of 45°. Therefore, whenever the cusps are present, it is imperative that interfering occlusal contacts be removed and that as many teeth as possible be brought into contact in the centric and eccentric ranges of occlusion and articulation so that the horizontal forces may be

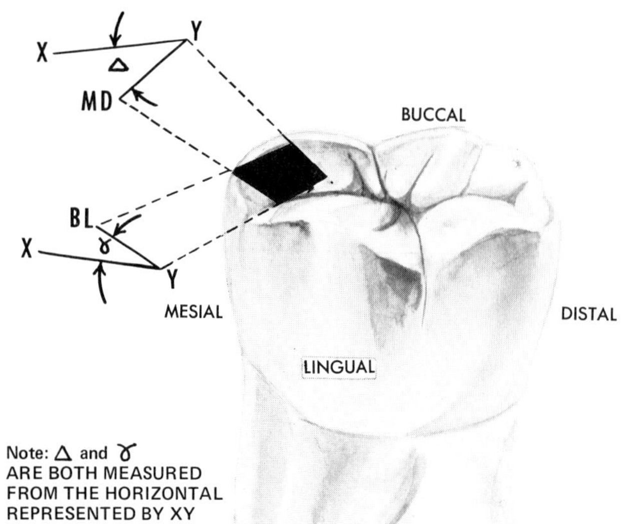

FIG. 3-6. A three-dimensional concept of all cuspal inclines is necessary because each cuspal incline has two angulations: a mesiodistal, XYMD and a buccolingual, BLYX.

reduced. This is true when the cuspal inclinations approach the critical 45° point.

Some investigators[1,13,14] have suggested a return to the flat-cusped teeth that are seen in some anthropological remains. This suggestion is based on the theory that the periodontal ligament absorbs vertical forces best because of its structural design. This hypothesis is fallacious because even though the periodontal ligament is designed to bear vertical forces, flat-cusped teeth require tremendous forces to triturate food and absorb the total masticatory force F_M in an axial direction. Evidence of this is seen in the width and the density of the mandibles in these anthropological remains. They show bone response to the enormous forces. In modern civilization, whenever a person exhibits flat cusps, he usually exhibits a corresponding increase of mandibular width and density as well as massive muscular development about the jaws. Such people have been able to flatten their cusps. However, most people are unable to do this. The cusped tooth, on the other hand, can shear and triturate food with greater efficiency and still develop no more than one-half the masticatory load per tooth (Fig. 3-4*c*). In the modern nonabrasive diets, cusps are rarely flattened, and the dentist must deal with cusped teeth. With interfering occlusal contact more likely to occur on cusped teeth, it is important that such contacts be removed and the load of mastication be distributed to as many teeth as possible in order to avoid excessive horizontal forces which the periodontal ligament is not designed to bear.

In the more common case, where the tooth axis is tilted (Fig. 3-5*a*), it can be seen that F_M is applied in the same manner as in Figure 3-3, and that F_P also remains a force perpendicular to the cuspal incline. X represents the tipping fulcrum of the tooth somewhere in the root along the center line. In the true standing tooth (Fig. 3-5*b*), F_H was the only force of consequence tending to tip the tooth (F_V force passes through the center of moments or tipping fulcrum). Now there are two tipping forces, F_H and F_V (Fig. 3-5*a*). F_H acts through a distance d_1, and F_V acts through a distance d_2. They are both significantly large moments and are additive so that they increase the tipping tendency. Thus, both an originally tipped tooth that becomes part of an interfering occlusal contact and one that has been tipped by a continuing interfering contact have their situations aggravated to the point where the tipping moments constantly become greater with each microtrauma.

The resultant force in any direction depends upon the angulation of the planes of the cusps. Observation of a natural tooth (Fig. 3-6), will show that the mesiodistal angulation, MD, of a cuspal plane is different from the buccolingual angulation, BL, of the same plane. To demonstrate the importance of these angles in relation to the forces produced by them, consider a plane whose buccolingual angle is 30° and whose mesiodistal angle is 45°. If an average occlusal force of 100 pounds is applied to this plane, the resultant buccolingual force produced will be 43 pounds whereas the resultant mesiodistal force will be 50 pounds.

If the natural three-dimensional tooth can be visualized diagrammatically, it will be seen that F_P (Fig. 3-3) does not lie parallel with the plane of the paper as in the two-dimensional representation. An incline of a cusp will transform the F_M force into an F_P component of F_I, the F_P of which moves into or out of the plane of the paper at right angles to the double incline of the cusps, depending upon which plane of a cusp of a tooth is in interfering contact. Therefore, the force F_M has the three components discussed previously. Thus with an interfering occlusal contact, the tooth is intruded, rotated about its neutral axis and moved off in some direction horizontally.

It is the angulations of the cuspal planes of the teeth that are responsible for the components—both in magnitude and in direction—which produce the resultant forces that tend to move the teeth. In Figure 3-7 an interfering contact at point 1 would produce a rotational movement around the axis of the tooth, X, in a direction from distal to lingual. The proximal contacting teeth and investing structures resist this rotation. Forces applied at other points will cause rotation, depending upon the direction of the resultants, R_1, R_2, R_3, R_4. All forces in the vertical direction tend to cause intrusion of the tooth.

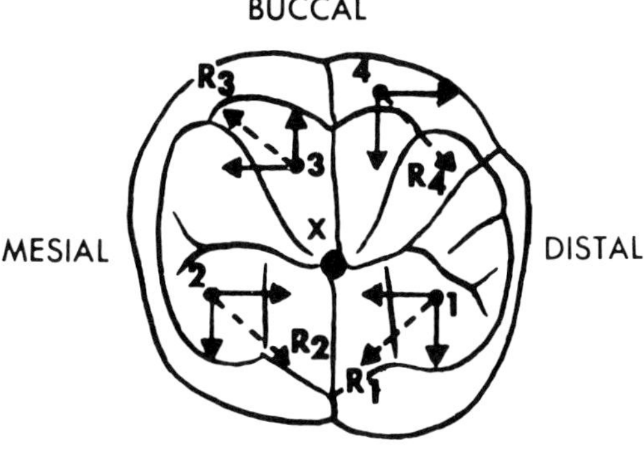

Fig. 3-7. The angulations of the cuspal planes of the teeth are responsible for the components producing the resultant forces that tend to move the teeth. The forces applied by interfering occlusal contacts at 1, 2, 3 and 4 will cause rotations of the teeth, depending upon the direction of the resultants R_1, R_2, R_3 and R_4.

The forces of occlusion are transmitted perpendicularly to the occlusal plane of the teeth. However, since the long axis of a tooth generally tilts toward the mesial, a tilting movement occurs around the fulcrum. Thus, the tooth has a tendency to move mesially.

The forces operating on the teeth are highly complex; therefore, the movements of the teeth are correspondingly complex. As viewed from the occlusal, the teeth tend to twist about their long axes. The buccal view shows a translatory movement into the alveoli and a tipping movement in which the teeth move in a direction determined by the inclination of the contacting plane.

FACTORS PRODUCING TORQUE

A number of factors determine the degree of torque on the teeth. The first of these is the height and the angulation of the cusps. In centric-relation occlusion, if

TABLE 3-1. RELATIVE HARDNESS OF DENTAL MATERIALS.

MATERIAL	BRINELL HARDNESS NUMBER
Tooth enamel	267
Dentin	65
Porcelain	415
Amalgam	90
24 k. Gold	29
22 k. Gold	54
Abutment Gold	150
Silicate	70*
Acrylic resins	22–29

* Skinner, E. W.: The Science of Dental Materials. p. 193. Philadelphia, W. B. Saunders, 1954. (Silver, M., Klein, G., and Howard, M. C.: Platinum porcelain restorations. J. Pros. Dent., 6:694, 1956.)

the teeth close and all the cusps and the fossae make contact, the forces are in equilibrium regardless of the height and the inclination of the cusps. If, on the other hand, the teeth close in centric relation and there is an interfering occlusal contact, the closer the inclines approach the critical 45° angle the greater will be the force of torque on the teeth. The importance of mastication as a producer of force on the teeth has been overstressed, while the importance of deglutition as a cause of force has not been fully recognized. In the act of swallowing, the teeth close in centric relation and tend, furthermore, to close on an interfering occlusal contact if one is present. Since the act of swallowing takes place about 1,500 times daily, the minute traumata caused by an occlusal interference cumulate into a serious hazard to the health and the function of the entire masticatory organ. The most dangerous of the effects produced is torque on the masticatory organ.

Another important torque-producing factor is improper crown-root relationships. If there is a large crown and a small root, there is a tendency toward tipping. In the case of a small crown and a large root, however, there is great resistance both to tipping and to twisting torque. When there is loss of bone height around a tooth, the crown-root ratio is altered, and the crown portion can be considered to extend to the bone as an extra-alveolar lever while the portion of the root that is in the bone acts as an intra-alveolar lever. This condition predisposes the tooth to tipping torque as in the case of the naturally large crown and short root.

Still another factor that tends to produce torque is uneven wearing of the cusps of a tooth. In such a case, the unworn cusps become relatively higher and the angles of inclination greater because of the wearing of the other portions of the occlusal surfaces of the tooth. The differences in rate of wear of enamel and such restorative materials as gold, amalgam and porcelain tend to exacerbate this factor of uneven wear. The relative hardness of tooth enamel and restorative materials is shown in Table 3-1. It is the relative hardness that determines the relative rate of wear for each material.

Improper restorative dentistry is another factor that tends to produce torque. When the anatomical form of a restoration is out of harmony with the normal function of a tooth, abnormal forces are produced on the restored teeth as well as on neighboring teeth. When teeth that have naturally flat cusps are restored with high cusps or when teeth that have naturally high cusps are restored with flat cusps, deleterious forces are set in motion. Malposition of the inclines caused by malposition of the teeth also tends to produce torque. Finally, a factor that tends to produce excessive torque is an abnormal force produced upon the teeth by abnormally strong masticatory muscles.

FACTORS RESISTING TORQUE

A number of factors tend to resist the effects of torque. An equitable distribution of forces in the masticatory organ so that no single tooth or component bears a load in excess of its physiological limit is one of the most important of these factors. Although the general health and resistance of the periodontium do not affect torque itself, they do resist the deleterious influences. In certain cases torque may produce degenerative effects on the periodontium, but in others in which general health is good and resistance is strong the force of the torque may be adequately resisted and compensated. The character, the quality and the amount of periodontal fibers and bone will also affect the influence of torque upon the dentition. Proper crown-root ratio and proper size and shape of the roots will also help to resist the effects of torque, as will physiological wear of the teeth. Finally, the dentist can remove the factors causing torque by equitably distributing the forces in the centric relation and the eccentric ranges of articulation.

VERTICAL AND HORIZONTAL FORCE

The teeth are subjected to two forces, singly or simultaneously: *vertical force,* transmitted along the long axis of the teeth; and *horizontal force,* transmitted at right angles to the teeth. Both are opposed by the shape of the teeth, the bone and the periodontium. The latter force is the more dangerous of the two because it produces the greater twisting and tipping torque effect on the periodontal ligament and alveolus.

VERTICAL AND HORIZONTAL INTERFERING OCCLUSAL CONTACTS

There are two types of interfering occlusal contacts: *vertical interfering occlusal contacts,* which occur when there is an interfering contact in centric relation; and *horizontal interfering occlusal contacts,* which occur in the lateral or protrusive ranges of articulation. The vertical and the horizontal interfering occlusal contacts can and do drive the teeth mesially, distally, buccally, lingually or apically, or they can drive the teeth in any combination of these directions.

Interfering occlusal contacts usually result in an acquired eccentric occlusal relationship, or what McLean[12] called a convenience relationship. This is the relationship in which the teeth occlude, but in which one or both of the condyles are out of their normal positions. The occlusal relationships of the teeth have determined the position of the mandible and of the heads of the condyles in the temporomandibular joints. In such cases, the teeth have usurped the function of the neuromuscular system that normally determines mandibular position.

PHYSICAL STRESS AND BONE

Any roentgenogram of bone is a diagram or graph of the reaction to the stresses that have been placed upon that bone. As one analyzes the relation of the periodontal fibers to the structure of the alveolar bone, this fact is demonstrated. Bone trabecularization is a diagram of lines of stress or directions of compression and tension in a structure under load. The structure of the lamina dura is a response to the forces on the teeth that have been transmitted through the periodontal fibers to the lamina dura. The story of stress can be read from the trabecularization of bone and the thickness of the lamina dura. The cellular connective tissue that forms the periodontal ligament does not furnish such a graph because it is radiolucent, but the roentgenogram of the bone does.

Normal, functional, intermittent pressures on the teeth, such as are produced by a normal occlusion during the acts of mastication and deglutition, produce forces on the teeth which, when they are transmitted to the alveolar bone through

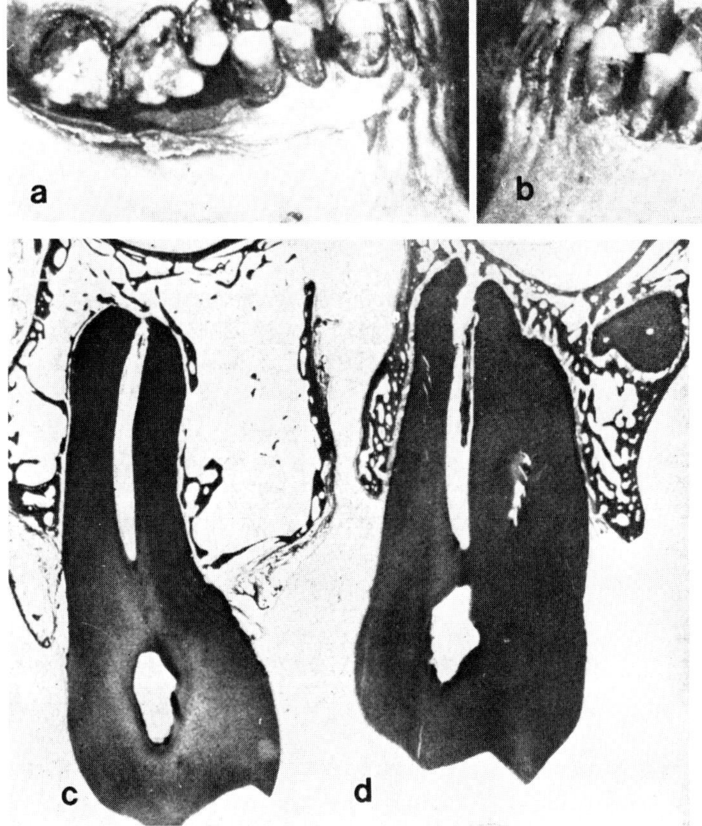

FIG. 3-8. Nonfunctioning upper molars (*a*); functioning upper molars (*b*); section (*c*) through (*a*), showing rarefaction of supporting bone and narrow periodontal ligament (nonfunctional atrophy); section (*d*) through (*b*), showing normal bone support and normal width of the periodontal ligament. (Kellner, E.: Histologische befunde an antagonistenlosen zahnen. Ztschr. Stomatol., *26*:271, 1928)

the periodontal fibers, stimulate bone formation.

Nonfunction results in a lack of physiological stimulation to the supporting bone; this in turn results in degeneration and rarefaction of the supporting bone (Fig. 3-8).

However, should an occlusal force become excessive, as occurs in the case of an interfering occlusal contact, the result may be the resorption of the lamina dura. Bone is living and highly plastic. The lamina dura and the trabeculae are constantly being formed, deformed and demolished and then formed anew. This process is directed by function and depends upon the metabolism of the tissues.

The role of normal axial and lateral stress as a means of developing proper bone support for the teeth is becoming more and more important. In the past, a hard and rough diet provided sufficient exercise and stimulation to assure proper trabecularization of the bone.

Teeth with hard enamel are relatively free from caries and exhibit little wear. However, a dentition that does not wear physiologically develops a convenience relationship caused by the efforts of the masticatory organ to compensate for interfering occlusal contacts.

Oral tissue fatigue results from the constant building up and breaking down of bone tissue, lowering tissue resistance. With high tissue resistance and hard enamel, there is bone thickening and condensation to offset the excessive forces. Bone degenerates when the tissue resistance is low and the enamel is hard and does not wear.

In summarizing the principles of mechanical adaptation as they apply to the problems of dentistry, it is important to emphasize the interrelationships of forces and structures in the functioning masticatory organ. This organ is one in which complex stresses of tension and compression are absorbed by structures that are admirably suited for their purposes. The important point is that all of the forces and structures must act in balanced correlation if the entire stomatognathic system is to function properly. No component of the masticatory organ functions alone, nor is it possible to evaluate the function of the entire organ, nor to treat dysfunction by viewing or correcting any single component. First, the dentist can control the occlusal anatomy of the teeth. Second, he can control other components of the stomatognathic system. Normally, it is the neuromuscular system that determines the position of the mandible and the condyles within the temporomandibular joints. The occlusal surfaces of the teeth must be harmonious with centric relation as it is determined by the neuromuscular system. Occlusal equilibration should reshape the teeth so that they are in harmony with the unique centric relation of the individual patient. In the convenience relationship, the neuromuscular system is in dysfunction because it attempts to avoid the trauma that is being caused by the interfering contact. The dentist can do very little to restore the neuromuscular system to its proper function, but he can do much to correct the interfering occlusal contact which is the cause of the neuromuscular dysfunction.

THE TOOTH AND THE PERIODONTIUM

Too frequently, the tooth is visualized as a two-dimensional object. This misconception leads to a distorted view of the relationship of the tooth to the periodontium. To achieve a proper view of this relationship, the tooth and its surrounding structures must be considered in their true three-dimensional nature. The tooth may be likened to a post embedded in the earth. When such a post is wiggled, it produces an hourglass-shaped hole[6] (Fig. 3-9). Similarly, when a tooth is subjected to excessive forces, the periodontal ligament and the bone eventually acquire the same hourglass shape, with the stricture appearing at some point between the alveolar crest and the apex.[7,10] Figure 3-10 shows this hourglass effect in both mesiodistal and buccolingual views. When torque and translation are produced on a tooth, its center of rotation is at the stricture of the hourglass. When a tooth is tested for mobility, it is luxated in a buc-

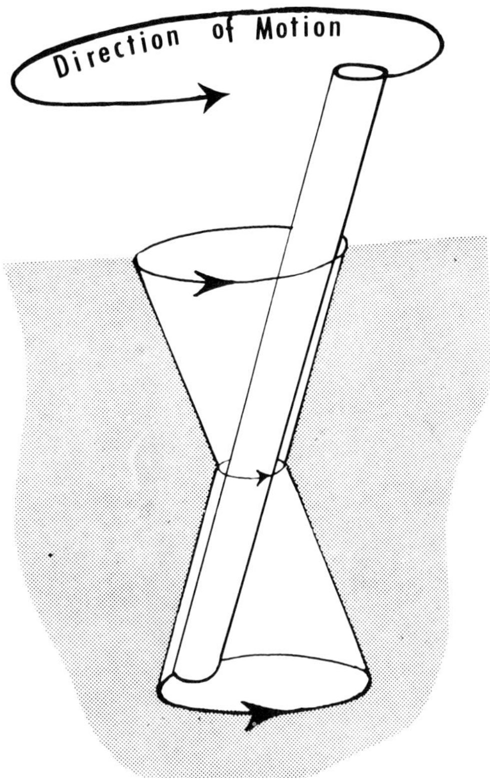

FIG. 3-9. A post in the ground producing an hourglass-shaped hole when tipped and rotated.

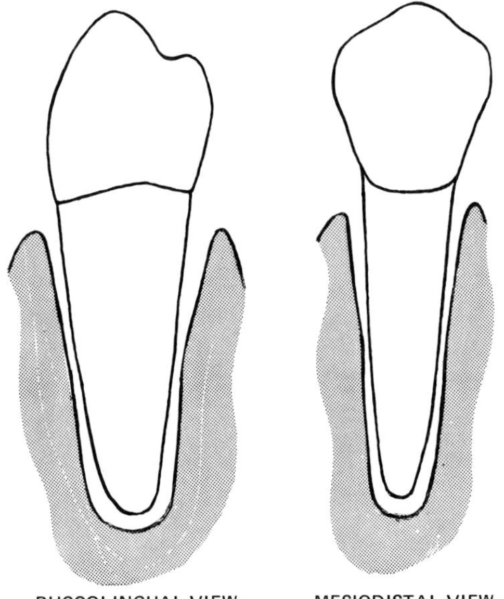

FIG. 3-10. Buccolingual and mesiodistal views of the hourglass effect produced in the periodontal space resulting from forces on a tooth.

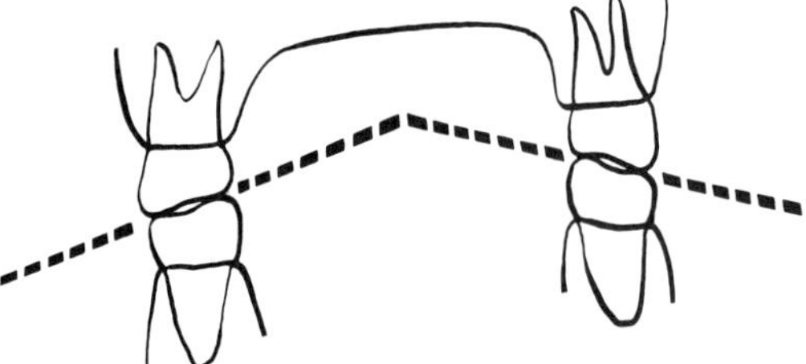

FIG. 3-11. Ruminant type of occlusion.

colingual direction. But when the roentgenogram is examined and a wide periodontal space noted, it is predicted that the tooth is probably mobile; one fails to realize that it had been observed mesiodistally. This is an interesting example of the way routinized thinking tends to interfere with accurate observation and how conclusions are sometimes drawn that are at variance with actually observed facts. As Figure 3-10 shows, such a tooth is actually mobile not in a simple buccolingual direction but in a circular manner. When such a tooth is in interfering occlusal contact, it actually undergoes a modified corkscrew action and both rotates and translates or intrudes into the socket.

To visualize the biomechanical problems involved in the transmission of forces, it is important to consider the histology of a tooth both in its passive and active states. This will be discussed in Chapter 4.

OCCLUSAL TOPOGRAPHY

Nature has designed the molar so that its occlusal surface over its greatest buccolingual diameter is one-half as great as

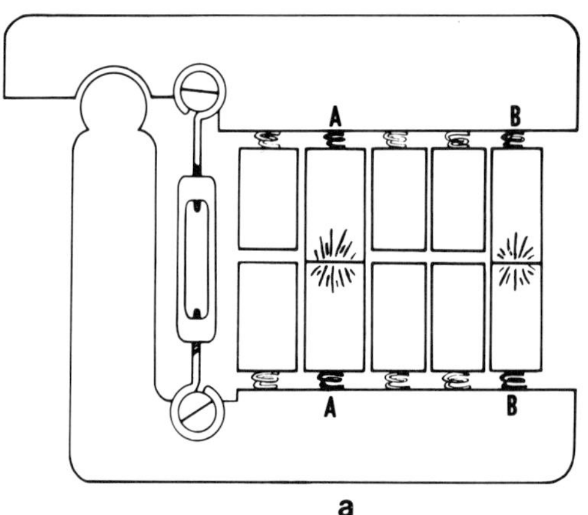

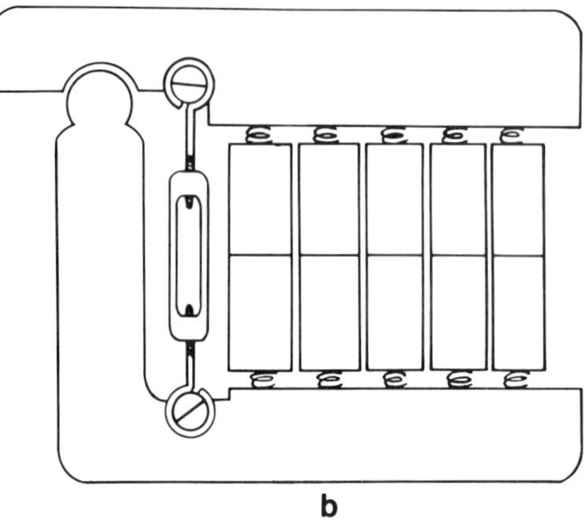

FIG. 3-12. Diagram of inequitable distribution of forces on the teeth (*a*); equitable distribution of forces on the teeth (*b*). (After Maxwell)

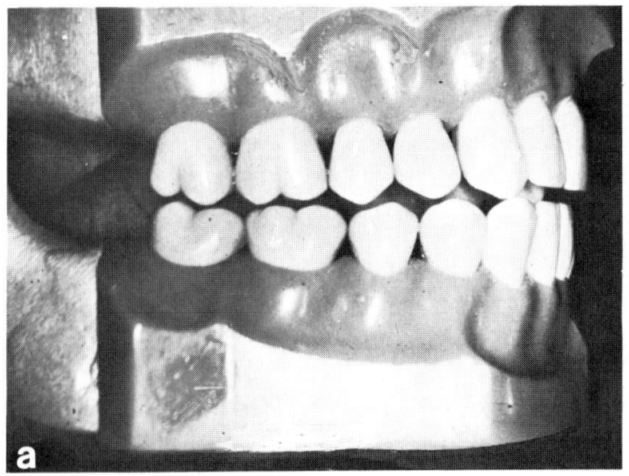

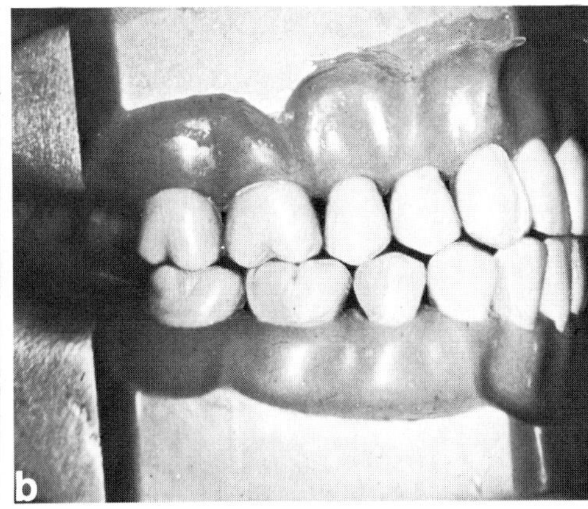

FIG. 3-13. The mandible is in the right functioning range of articulation, and only the cuspids contact (*a*). After occlusal equilibration has been performed, the cuspid, bicuspids and molars are in contact (*b*).

it is through the greatest buccolingual diameter. This engineering accomplishment limits the leverage that can be brought to bear on the tooth. In undertaking occlusal rehabilitation, this natural limitation of leverage must be understood and considered. The occlusal topography of restored bridgework should follow the same engineering principle by providing that the occlusal buccolingual diameter be narrower than the greatest buccolingual diameter.

As a person ages, his occlusal topography changes; the cusps become flatter and the buccolingual occlusal tables increase in size. This increase in buccolingual diameter must be reduced. The horizontal angulation of the flattened occlusal surfaces may vary and even take on a ruminant type of occlusion (Fig. 3-11). In such cases, the centric-relation forces will not be borne along the long axes of the teeth during mastication and deglutition. Such teeth should be reshaped so as to return the stresses as much as possible to the long axes. Furthermore, to increase masticatory efficiency, the flattened surfaces must be reshaped to provide for point-to-plane contact during mastication. While nature usually builds up a strong alveolar process under physiological stress, the abnormal stress set up by flattened "masher" types of occlusion will result in degeneration and breakdown when resistance is low.

FORCE DISTRIBUTION ON THE TEETH

One of the fundamental principles of occlusal equilibration is the division of the forces of function (mastication, deglutition, etc.) to as many teeth as possible during centric relation and the functioning ranges and positions.

If in centric relation or any functioning range or position only one pair of teeth make contact, each tooth bears 100 per cent of the load. This load is untenable physiologically and must be reduced on the involved teeth and distributed to as many teeth as possible. When, however, as in Figure 3-12*a* abnormal stresses are created at A and B because the forces of occlusion are not distributed properly, a 40 per cent efficient system in centric relation is set up leading to a progressive pattern of degeneration and collapse. An equitable distribution of forces is made possible by the coordination of all the occlusal surfaces (Fig. 3-12*b*). Under this condition there is maximal contact in centric-relation occlusion.

Similarly, these conditions and conclu-

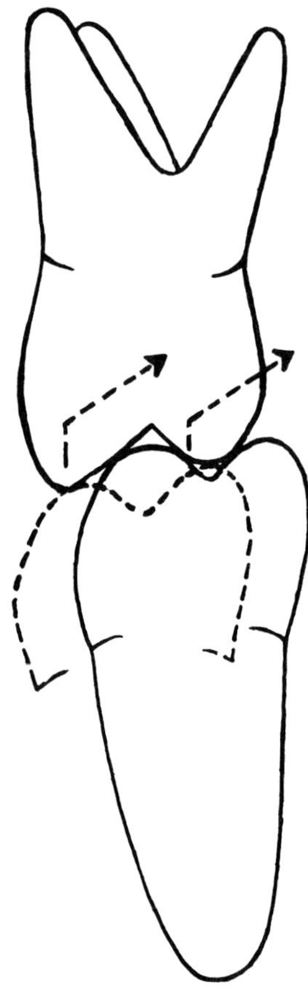

FIG. 3-14. Final absorption of force by the upper lingual and the lower buccal cusps in the Bennett movement.

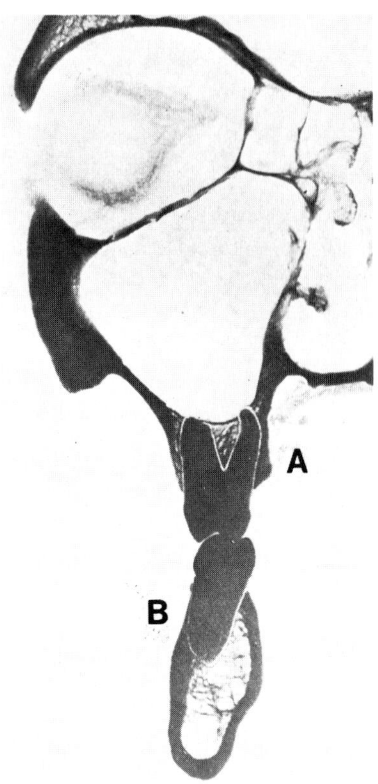

FIG. 3-15. Section through the skull in the first molar region, depicting the axial relationship of the teeth to the skull. (Diamond, M.: Dental Anatomy. p. 268. New York, Macmillan, 1929)

sions may exist in the functioning and protrusive ranges and positions. Figure 3-13*a* illustrates the functioning range and position in which the cuspids must bear 100 per cent of the load. If ten teeth, as in (*b*)—five maxillary and five mandibular—are brought into contact during the functioning range and position, each tooth now bears only 20 per cent of the load and each cuspid bears only one-fifth of its original load.

AXIAL INCLINATION

As there are variations in the cuspal inclined planes of anterior and posterior teeth, so are there differences in axial inclinations of these teeth. The mathematical proof of Figure 3-5 illustrates the importance of this fact. As the functioning side of the mandible moves upward, it shifts toward the lingual, and the force is finally taken by the upper lingual and the lower buccal cusps of the molars in the Bennett movement, as illustrated by the dotted lines and arrows in Figure 3-14.

Diamond's anatomical section (Fig. 3-15) shows the correct axial inclinations of the molars as well as their relationships to the skull. It is also worthwhile to note the design and the density of the bone at A and B. This fact must be considered in the technique of extracting molars. The lingual cusp of the upper first molar is sometimes called the pestle, while the central fossa of the lower first molar is called the mortar. The buccal cusps of the lower bicuspids and molars should act the same way as the fossae and the ridges of the upper bicuspids and molars. The pestle is thought of as grinding some substance in the mortar. However, here the relationship is entirely different. The upper lingual cusp actually remains stationary whereas the lower fossa is in active motion. Since the first molar is the first permanent tooth and frequently sets the entire pattern of the occlusion, the mesiolingual cusp of the upper molar is the most important cusp in the mouth. It is important to retain this cusp whenever possible, reshaping it only as a last resort.

STRESS-RESISTANT FORMS AND TISSUES

Nature, in her attempts to protect the masticatory organ from the effects of excessive forces, has designed the roots of the different teeth in such a manner as to provide the maximal periodontal ligamentous support in those areas which will have to tolerate the greatest forces. All root forms are basically conical, a shape that affords the maximal amount of periodontal attachment to take the applied forces. The periodontal ligament consists of many fibers which absorb and transmit the various components of all masticatory forces. For example, the upper central incisor receives its greatest stress from the lingual and the distal. Consequently, the cone is modified to a pyramidal shape with the greatest area of periodontal support on the lingual and the proximal surfaces. The cusped teeth have their greatest areas of fiber support on the proximal surfaces. Because the greatest amount of force is generated in the molar areas, the amount of periodontal support for these teeth is considerably greater than is generally realized. The upper molar has two buccal roots with flattened mesial and distal surfaces designed to resist mesial and distal forces. The lingual root has greater periodontal attachment on the buccal and the lingual to resist the buccal and the lingual forces.

The resultant thrusts of forces on the inclined planes of a tooth are received in a torquelike movement of the tooth or, if the tooth is firm, a shift of the mandible itself. If the supporting structures are weak, the tooth is twisted in its socket. If the supporting periodontal fibers and the lamina dura are strong, the forces of the inclined plane must be taken up by the mandible, and so torque is produced within that structure, resulting in malposition of the condyle heads within the temporomandibular joints.

The teeth, the periodontium, the bone, the neuromuscular system, the temporomandibular joint and all the other components of the stomatognathic system function as a coordinated whole and must be analyzed as such. The masticatory organ is a complex functioning structure. Its components have been designed to meet the conditions of force and stress to which they are subjected in normal use.

REFERENCES

1. Beyeler, K.: Über paradentose und artikulationsstorungen. (Paradentosis and disturbances of articulation.) Paradontologie, *2:*130, 1948.
2. Box, H. K.: Discussion of traumatic occlusion. New York State D. J., *15:*514, 1949.
3. ———: Studies in periodontal pathology. Toronto, Canadian Research Foundation, No. 7, 1927.
4. Boyens, P. J.: Value of autosuggestion in the therapy of "bruxism" and other biting habits. JADA, *27:*1773, 1940.
5. Cannon, W. B.: The Mechanical Factors of Digestion. p. 8. New York, Longmans, 1911.
6. Case, C. S.: Dental Orthopedia. Chicago, Case, 1908.
7. Coolidge, E. D., and Hine, M. K.: Periodontia, Clinical Pathology and Treat-

ment of the Periodontal Tissues. Philadelphia, Lea & Febiger, 1954.

8. Drum, W.: Abgestimmte gussklammern und parafunction (Surveying clasps and parafunction), Berlin, Quintessenz, 1956.
9. Fernex, E.: Quelques notes sur l'équilibre occluso-articulaire. (Equilibration of the occlusion.) Rev. Mens. Suisse Odont., *58:*459, 1948.
10. Kellner, E.: Histologische befunde an antagonistenlosen zahnen. (Histologic findings on teeth without antagonists.) Z. Stomatol., *26:*271, 1928.
11. Langley, L. L., and Cheraskin, E.: The Physiological Foundation of Dental Practice. p. 421. St. Louis, C. V. Mosby, 1956.
12. McLean, D. W.: Diagnosis and correction of occlusal deformities prior to restorative procedures, JADA, *26:*928, 1939.
13. Moses, C. H.: Studies of wear, arrangement and occlusion of the dentition of humans and animals and their relationship to orthodontia, periodontia and prosthodontia, D. Items Interest, *68:*953, 1946.
14. Parma, C.: Research on prehistoric jaws, Paradontologie, *2:*123, 1948.
15. Radusch, D. F.: Grinding for relief of occlusal trauma associated with periodontoclasia, JADA, *30:*384, 1943.
16. Selye, H.: Role of stress and adaptive hormones in dental medicine. Oral Surg., Oral Med., Oral Path., *7:*365, 1954.
17. Tishler, B.: Occlusal habit neurosis. D. Cosmos, *70:*690, 1928.

Additional Basic Reference

Ramfjord, S. P.: Bruxism: a clinical and electromyographic study. JADA *62:*21, 1961.

4 *Histological Reactions to Force*

The interaction of occlusal stresses and metabolic processes that are constantly going on in the periodontium may be studied in histological sections of periodontal tissue. Forces upon the teeth are reflected as stresses on, and strains within, the periodontium. The periodontium is constantly subjected to forces during mastication, deglutition and speech. Various mechanisms compensate for these forces and permit normal metabolic processes to repair the damage they cause. However, when force is excessive, these mechanisms can neither compensate for nor provide those conditions that make self-repair possible. The study of the histology of the periodontium is actually the study of the physiological efficiency of the tissues involved in relation to forces. Frequently, the dentist will observe the presence of abnormal force in the masticatory organ but will note that the resultant strain and stress to the periodontium are negligible. In such cases he should not dismiss the possibility that future changes in the physiological resistance or the resistive capacity of the periodontium may result in a condition in which the abnormal force can cause serious and extensive damage. Traumatized tissues undergo constant degeneration, no matter how slight. If the trauma is permitted to continue, the physiological defenses of the cells are finally breached, damage occurs, and trophic degeneration and neuromuscular dysfunction result.

In more primitive cultures, nature's mechanism for adjusting forces on the teeth is to provide a diet which is sufficiently hard and gritty to ensure a naturally "ground-in" occlusion. The elimination of fibrous and bulky foods from modern diets has tended to cause hypofunction, lack of resistive capacity and degeneration of the periodontal tissues. The stress-and-strain pattern that is established by function is graphically recorded in histological sections of the teeth, the periodontal ligament, the alveolar process and the skull.

REACTIONS OF ENAMEL TO FORCE

Enamel is the hard substance that nature provides for use against the wear of mastication and deglutition. Once it has been formed, it neither repairs nor resorbs, and the only histological evidences of the effects of force on the enamel will be abrasion and horizontally and vertically fractured rods. Some investigators[7] claim that enamel can be "work-hardened" under extreme occlusal forces. This relation to our present-day function has yet to be proved adequately.

REACTIONS OF DENTIN TO FORCE

Histologically, the normal dentin of a recently erupted tooth exhibits dental tubules which converge toward the pulp in

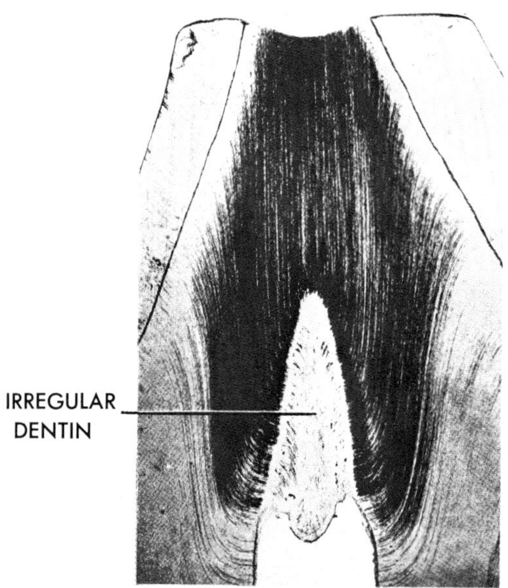

FIG. 4-1. Formation of reparative dentin as a protective mechanism against abrasion. (Orban, B.: Oral Histology and Embryology. ed. 4, p. 127. St. Louis, C. V. Mosby, 1957)

a regular arrangement. The tubules of secondary dentin show an abrupt change in direction but are parallel with each other. The term "irregular dentin" describes the condition not only in which the number of tubules is greatly reduced but also in which those that are present run an irregular course (Fig. 4-1). Both secondary and irregular dentin formations are protective mechanisms. Teeth that have been severely abraded occlusally or incisally, or injured in any other way, form secondary or irregular dentin to prevent exposure of the pulp. This secondary dentin is not evenly deposited on the pulpal surface of the primary dentin. In molars and premolars, more secondary dentin is laid down on the roof and the floor of the pulp chamber than on the side walls. Occlusal or incisal abrasion affects the formation of both the secondary and the primary dentin. The constant trauma to the primary dentin causes sclerotic dentin, which is characterized by additional calcification of the dental tubules and their ultimate obliteration.

REACTION OF PULP TO FORCE

Excessive wear reduces the occlusal surfaces of the teeth. Compensating secondary dentin is thus deposited, reducing the size of the pulp chamber. The primary function of the pulp is to produce dentin. The blood vessels of pulpal tissue supply nourishment to the dentin. The pulp also contains nerves which give sensation to the structures of the teeth and innervate the blood vessels of the pulp. Since these nerve endings cannot dif-

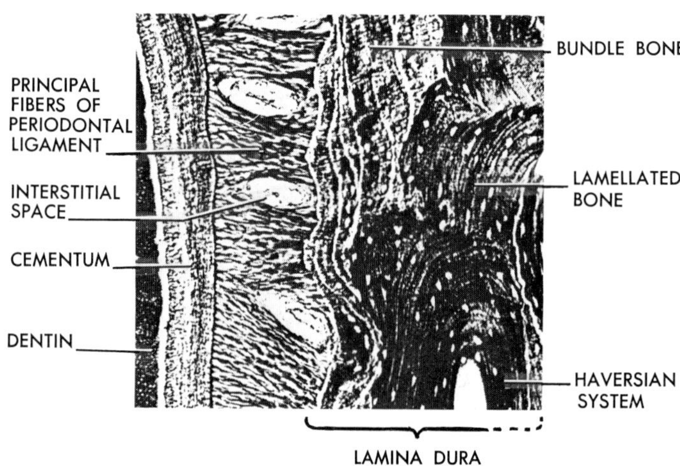

FIG. 4-2. Relationship of periodontal fibers to the cementum, bundle bone and lamellated bone. (Orban, B.: Oral Histology and Embryology. ed. 4, p. 212. St. Louis, C. V. Mosby, 1957)

ferentiate among causes, they always register heat, cold, pressure or any other stimuli as pain.

Normal force stimulates the pulp and enables it to function properly. Hyperemia of the pulp is found in teeth that are under excessive occlusal forces. The hyperemia and pain are reversible reactions if the force on the tooth is decreased within physiological limits. Pulp stones are often found in the pulp. It has been suggested[15] that these stones, which are sometimes so large that they block the chamber, are traumatic in origin.

THE DENTOALVEOLAR JOINT

A joint is a more or less movable place of union between two or more bones.[12] It is a relatively new concept to consider the tooth, the periodontal ligament, the cementum and the alveolar bone proper as a joint.

Since bone can be built up in response to stress, the lamina dura thickens in response to force on the tooth and the rest of the dentoalveolar joint. The fact that bone is deposited as a result of tension set up by the muscles is borne out by an examination of the relationship between the long bones and their muscle insertions. MacKenzie[5] states:

> Bone is dominated by muscular function: for that it is called into being. With the disappearance of that necessity, so also disappears the bone. It is the length, size, and tenacity of the muscle that maintains the normal length and size of the bone, and not the reverse, as is so often erroneously thought.

Whenever a muscle or a tendon is inserted into a bone, the bone is lamellated or compacted so that it can resist the stress set up by the muscle.

The dentoalveolar joint consists of the following: the tooth, which is set in motion under force; the fibers of the periodontal ligament, which act as the connecting link; and the lamina dura of the alveolar process. When force is applied to the teeth, torque is produced, and there is consequent stress and strain on the periodontal fibers. This stress and strain, in turn, create tension on the lamina dura. The periodontal fibers are inserted into the bundle bone of the lamina dura. The bundle bone is deposited or formed under applied tension. This intermittent tension on the periodontal fibers is responsible for the deposition of bone and the thickening of the lamina dura. When the bundle bone that is laid down is thick enough, it is converted into lamellated bone. The histological sections of the alveolar process, the lamina dura, and the bundle bone and lamellated bone (Fig. 4-2) demonstrate the processes discussed above.

THE ALVEOLAR PROCESS AND THE LAMINA DURA

Because of the confusion concerning the classification and the nomenclature of the bone surrounding the teeth, it is worthwhile to define and classify terms on the basis of function so that they may be clearly considered.[10]

Alveolar process: that part of the maxilla and the mandible which forms and supports the sockets of the teeth

Lamina dura, or alveolar bone proper, or cribriform plate (Fig. 4-1):

1. *Bundle bone:* that part of the lamina dura to which the principal fibers of the periodontal ligament are anchored. Bundle bone is not lamellated. The bundle bone is nearer to the periodontal fibers.

2. *Lamellated bone:* that part of the lamina dura which is composed of lamellae of bone

Supporting bone (Fig. 4-3): the bone which surrounds the lamina dura and gives support to the socket

1. *Cortical plate or compact bone:* the bone forming the vestibular and oral plates of the alveolar processes

2. *Spongy or trabeculated bone:* the

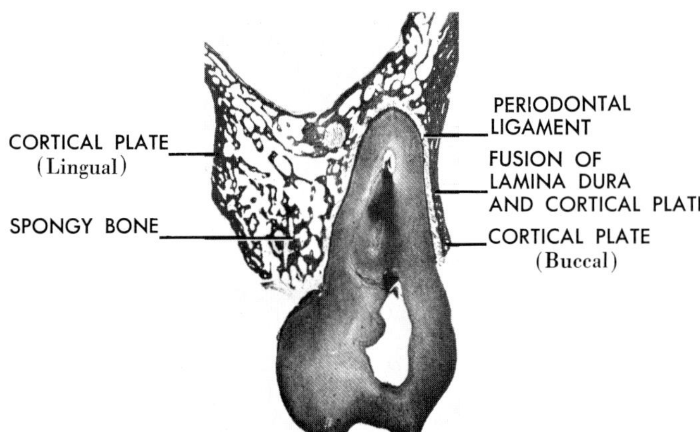

FIG. 4-3. Supporting bone consists of cortical plate or compact bone, spongy or trabeculated bone. Note fusion of the lamina dura and cortical bone. (Gordon, S.: Dental Science and Dental Art. Philadelphia, Lea & Febiger, 1938)

bone between the cortical plate and the lamina dura

Histologically, the lamina dura is composed of bundle bone and lamellated bone. The former is the more recently formed of the two and is adjacent to the periodontal ligament. The principal fibers of the periodontal ligament are attached to the bundle bone and extend into it as Sharpey's fibers. Adjacent to the bundle bone is lamellated bone. This is formed when the bundle bone achieves proper thickness. When this point is reached, the osteoclasts of adjacent marrow space resorb part of the bundle bone and then lamellated bone is deposited. The lamina dura is perforated by many small apertures which transmit branches of the intraalveolar nerves and blood vessels to the periodontal ligament. The thickness of the lamina dura varies with function and with the resistive capacity of the individual to force. For this reason, no exact dimension for the thickness of the normal lamina dura can be given. It is thinner on the mesial aspect of the teeth than it is on the distal because the teeth are inclined mesially and torque is produced by means of the mesially inclined planes of the teeth. This torque causes tension distally and therefore produces a thicker lamina dura on that aspect. The histological sections of lamina dura are usually mesiodistal. Because torque produces rotation and translation, it will have an effect on the buccal and lingual aspects as well. Only by histological studies that include these, will it be possible to understand the true nature of the lamina dura.

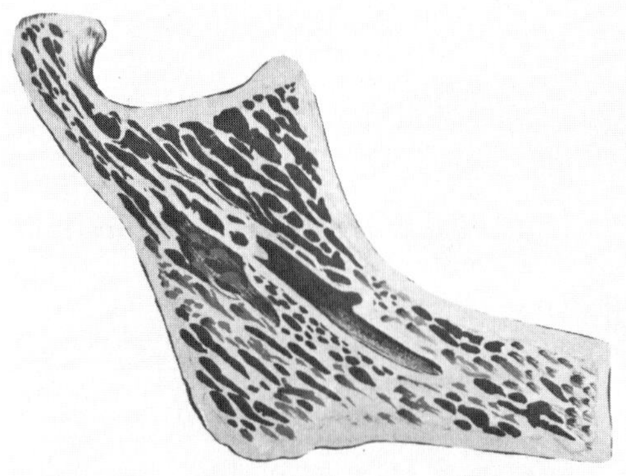

FIG. 4-4. Mandibular trabeculae are arranged into trajectories to withstand stress best. (After Sicher)

Histologically, spongy bone is composed of trabeculae interspersed with rich blood and lymph supplies. Architecturally, the trabeculae tend to arrange themselves in a direction that is best suited to withstand the stresses and strains imposed upon them. This arrangement provides not only for the intensity of these stresses and strains but also for their directions. Mandibular trabeculae arrange themselves into trajec-

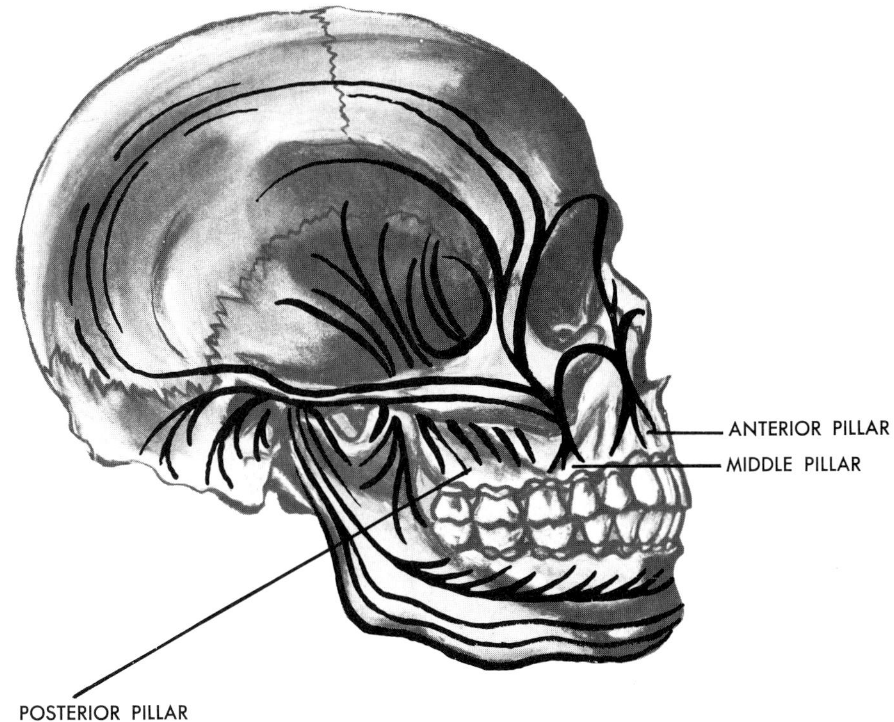

FIG. 4-5. Radiation of the trajectories of stress from forces on the teeth through the pillars of the maxilla and the condyles of the mandible to the skull. (After Sicher and Tandler, Benninghoff, Thouren)

tories such as are depicted in the cross sections of Figures 4-4 and 4-5. Force travels along these trajectories to and through the head of the condyle and thence to the temporal, auricular, parietal and occipital regions. The maxillary trabeculae arrange themselves into trajectories such as those illustrated in Figure 4-5. These trabeculated trajectories form three pillars: anterior, middle and posterior. This may also be seen in the cross section illustrated in Figure 4-6. Forces travel along these trajectories to the frontal, orbital, nasal and zygomatic areas. The arrangement of the trabeculae in the manner described assures maximal tissue resistance to stresses and strains with minimal structural material.[3,16]

The cortical bone is usually much thinner in the maxilla than it is in the mandible. The thickest section is found in the molar and premolar region of the mandible, especially on the buccal aspect. In the maxillary cortical bone, there are many small apertures through which blood and lymph vessels pass. Since this

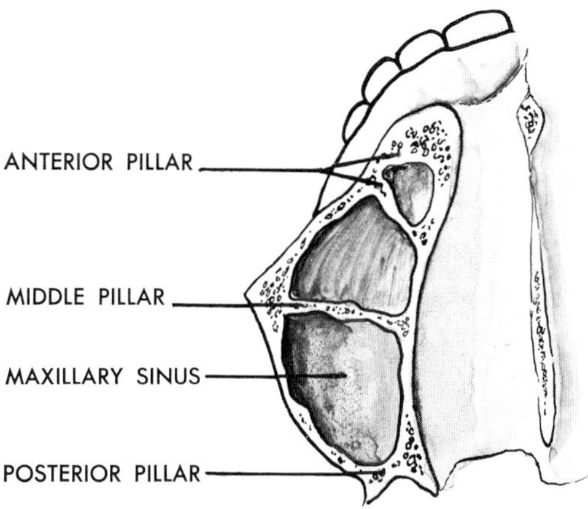

FIG. 4-6. A horizontal section through the facial skeleton above the nasal floor. Note the pillars. (After Sicher and Tandler)

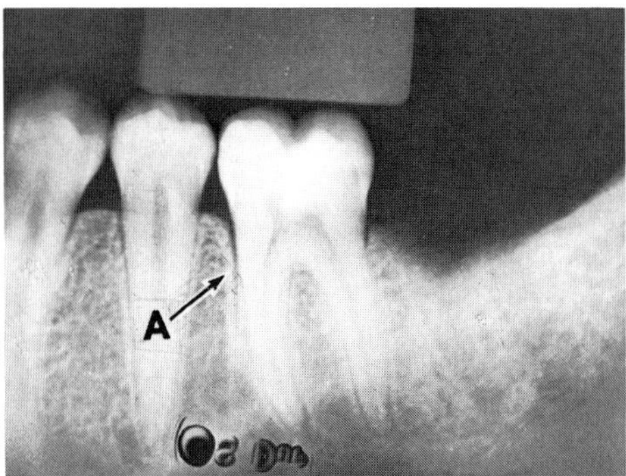

FIG. 4-7. A roentgenogram demonstrates the heavy lamina dura around a molar under heavy load but within the resistive capacity of the patient.

bone is denser in the mandible, there are fewer such apertures. In the labial and buccal regions of both jaws, thc supporting bone is very thin, and since there is no spongy bone, the cortical bone is fused with the lamina dura or the alveolar bone proper (Fig. 4-3). Histologically, the cortical bone is composed of longitudinal lamellae and haversian systems (Fig. 4-2).

REACTION OF BONE TO FORCE

Structural modifications of bone occur as a result of either diminished or increased external forces. The resistance of the person (the resistive capacity or the bone factor) determines the results of these forces. Abnormal forces occurring early in life when resistance is high may cause no visible damage. However, if similar forces occur later in life when resistance is lower, they may cause degeneration and breakdown of tissue. The dentist must be able to recognize the existence of excessive forces before their deleterious effects become visible in the bone structure.

Bone growth and transformation must be differentiated. Bone transformation of the lamina dura is a result of force transmitted to the bone through the dentoalveolar joint. Bone growth is an embryological phenomenon dictated by the genetic configuration of the individual. Because of the ability of the bone to be transformed as a result of forces exerted upon it, the investigator has an opportunity to study mechanical forces and their effects by tracing the results of such forces and their resultant stresses in the bone. It is the rich vascular supply to the bone that is responsible for the plasticity of bone in response to force. The fact that bone may be deformed by small forces demonstrates its plasticity. Muscles, tendons and blood vessels, which are soft tissues, can actually reshape bone, and the forces produced by the periodontal fibers can act similarly on the alveolar bone. It has been shown[5] that constant pressure can result in bone resorption. On the other hand, intermittent pressure will result in bone formation.

From a diagnostic standpoint, it is well to remember that when the resistance or the resistive capacity of an individual is great, excessive forces will be manifested in a heavy lamina dura. Histologically, the force is transmitted through the tooth by way of the periodontal ligament to the

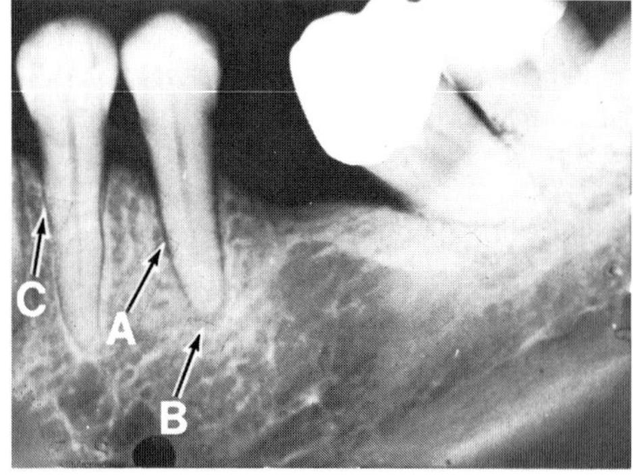

FIG. 4-8. A roentgenogram of the mandibular bicuspid area illustrates the effect of heavy force beyond the patient's resistive capacity. Note the absence of lamina dura and wide periodontal space around the root of the second bicuspid at A and B, and the loss of the lamina dura on part of the mesial aspect of the first bicuspid at C.

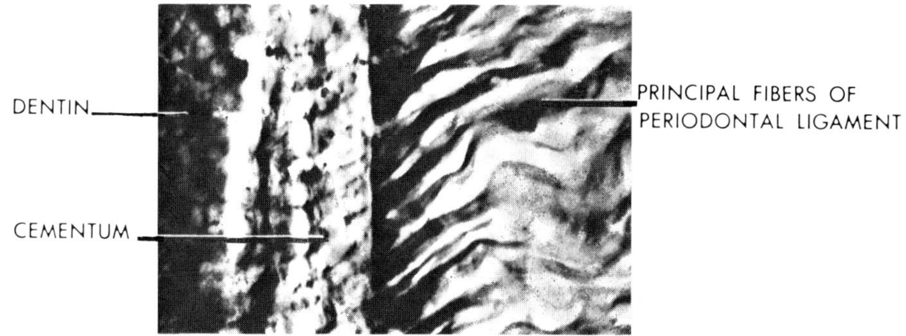

FIG. 4-9. The principal fibers of the periodontal ligament continue into the surface of the cementum. (Orban, B.: Oral Histology and Embryology. ed. 4, p. 168. St. Louis, C. V. Mosby, 1957)

bundle bone. Therefore, it can be seen that a heavy lamina dura is an indication of heavy forces on the tooth, as shown roentgenographically (Fig. 4-7). However, when the resistive capacity of the individual is great, the excessive forces that built up a heavy lamina dura in the situation discussed above will eventually cause its resorption. When the tooth is constantly forced against the lamina dura in cases of extreme pressure, its resorption on the pressure side will result. The constancy

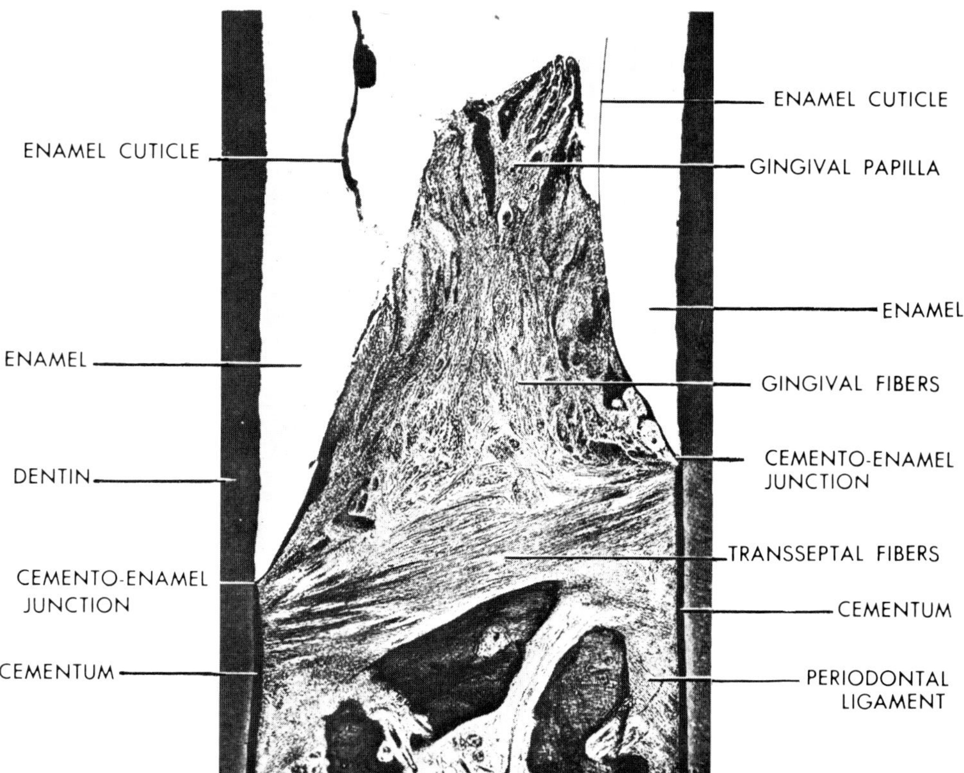

FIG. 4-10. Gingival and transseptal fibers. (Orban, B.: Oral Histology and Embryology. ed. 4, p. 188. St. Louis, C. V. Mosby, 1957)

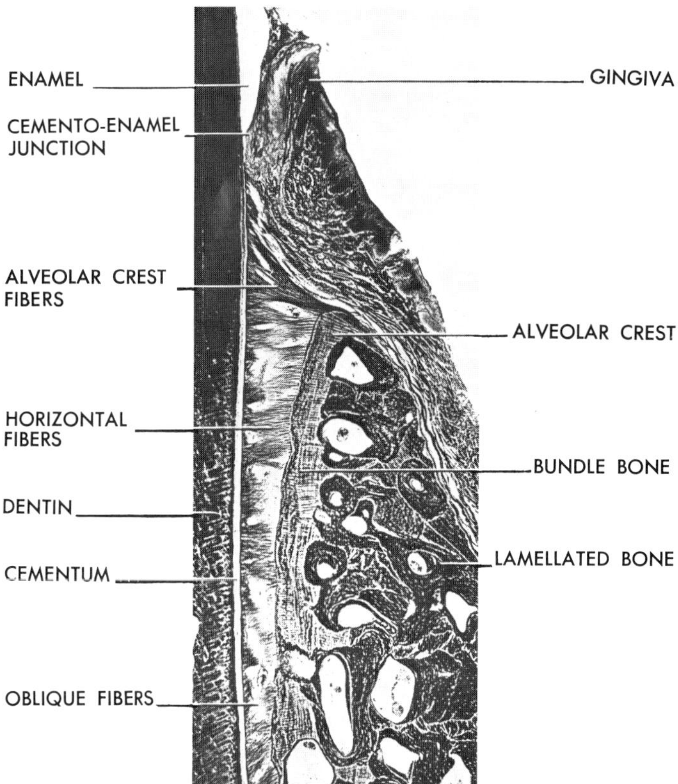

FIG. 4-11. Alveolar fibers of the periodontal ligament. (Orban, B.: Oral Histology and Embryology. ed. 4, p. 189. St. Louis, C. V. Mosby, 1957)

of this force does not allow for repair. The result of this process is an extremely wide periodontal space and a markedly mobile tooth (Fig. 4-8). A physiological force exerted on the tooth of a patient with a markedly low resistance or resistive capacity will have the same degenerative effect as an excessive force on a tooth of a patient with normal resistance and will produce the same pathological picture.

THE PERIODONTAL LIGAMENT

The periodontal ligament is a structure of connective tissue surrounding the tooth and joining it to the bone. It is most important to understand the structure of the periodontal ligament before analyzing its functions and relationship to the dentoalveolar joint.

Structure

The periodontal ligament is composed of fibers, blood vessels, lymphatics, nerves and cellular elements. Histologically, the fibers are white, collagenous connective tissue which cannot be lengthened and are inelastic. The apparent elasticity that gives the fibers their shock-absorbing effect is caused by the arrangement of the fiber bundles and by their wavy or crinkled course from their point of origin to their point of insertion (Fig. 4-9). The fibers of the periodontal ligament are attached to the cementum from bone, from cementum of other teeth and from the gingiva. These fibers may be classified under the following three categories:

Gingival fibers (Fig. 4-10): fibers which run from the cementum to the free and attached gingiva

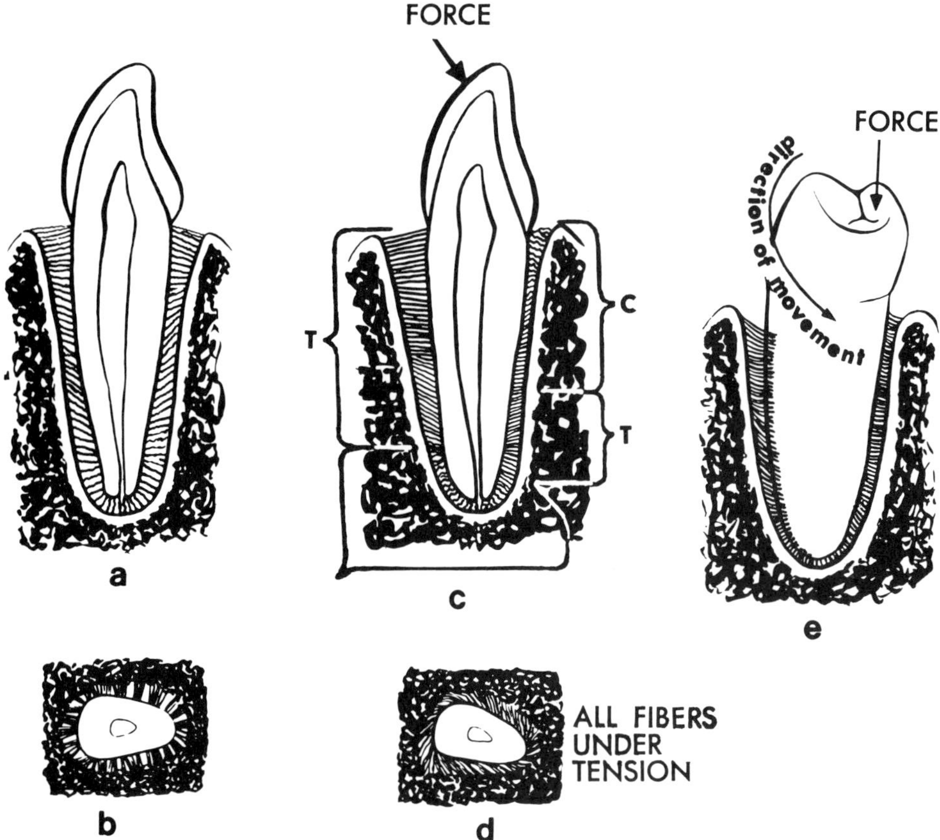

FIG. 4-12. The distribution and the direction of the unstrained periodontal fibers are illustrated in (*a*) and (*b*) and strained fibers in (*c*) and (*d*). The vertical section (*c*) depicts tipping torque which causes compression at C and tension at T in the areas so marked. The horizontal section (*d*) depicts twisting torque which causes tension on the fibers. The original force includes a vertical component which intrudes the tooth, causing tension on all the fibers except the apical fibers, which are compressed. The composite movement of (*c*) and (*d*) plus tooth intrusion results in (*e*), which is an attempt at three-dimensional portrayal of the vector summation of these movements. Most of the fibers in (*e*) are under tension.

Transseptal fibers (Fig. 4-10): fibers which run mesiodistally over the crest of the alveolus and connect adjacent teeth. These fibers also run around the tooth in a band and give support to the marginal gingiva.

Alveolar fibers (Fig. 4-11): fibers which run from the teeth to the lamina dura

1. *Alveolar crest:* fibers which run from the cervical cementum to the lamina dura
2. *Horizontal:* fibers which run at right angles to the long axis of the tooth from cementum to bone
3. *Oblique:* the most important and numerous of the periodontal fibers, which are attached to the cementum apically and run upward to the bone attachment in a hammocklike fashion
4. *Apical:* fibers which run from the apical region of the teeth to the bone
5. *Inter-radicular:* fibers which run from the crest of the inter-radicular septum to the bifurcation of the roots

Interspersed throughout the ligament are differentiated and undifferentiated cellular elements; at regular intervals there are interstitial spaces which contain the blood vessels, the lymphatics and the nerves (Fig. 4-2).

The blood supply of the periodontal ligament is derived from three sources. The most important of these are the vessels that branch from the interalveolar arteries and enter the periodontal ligament through openings in the lamina dura. A second source are the vessels that enter the apical foramen from the periapical area and branch off to the periodontal ligament before they enter the tooth. The third source are the gingival vessels that anastomose with those of the periodontal ligament. The lymphatics run from the periodontal ligament to the adjacent alveolar bone and then to the nodes. The nerve supply of the periodontal ligament follows the blood vessels. Both pain receptors and nerve endings for proprioception are present.

Function

The periodontal ligament has four basic functions: supportive, formative, sensory and nutritional. The supportive function can be subdivided into attachment of teeth to bone, transmission of force to the bone in the manner of a shock absorber and maintenance of teeth in proper relationship to the gingival tissues, the alveolar bone and the other teeth. It is important to understand the function of the fibers as a vehicle for the transmission of a force produced upon a tooth which, in turn, produces stress within the fibers. The distribution and the direction of the periodontal fibers around a tooth without a load are illustrated in Figure 4-12*a* and *b*. Under the forces of deglutition and mastication, the wavy or crinkled periodontal fibers straighten out during the split second of tension on the fibers as the teeth are moved by the applied force. This straightening action produces the shock-absorbing effect.

When force with its resultant torque is placed on a tooth, all of the fibers are brought into play. To visualize what happens when a tooth moves, it is important to bear in mind the position and the direction of the fibers, both in the vertical (Fig. 4-12*c*) and in the horizontal sections (*d*). As the teeth move axially, the fibers tend to straighten out and to extend to their full length in an action compatible with the torquelike movement of the teeth. The blood and the lymph in the periodontal ligament are displaced to make room for the rootward movement of the tooth.

When the force on a tooth is removed, the blood and the lymph rush back into the periodontal ligament. This is demonstrated in Figure 4-13, which illustrates the application of the principles of hydraulics to the action of teeth in the periodontal ligament. Note the wavy fibers in (*a*) before the force is applied to A and the stretched fibers in (*b*) as the full force is applied. As the force is removed from piston A, the fluid rushes back and restores the piston (teeth) and the fibers to their original positions.

The formative function of the periodontal ligament is to replace tissue that has been lost either through natural or pathological processes. In normal function, old tissue is constantly being replaced by new. The undifferentiated connective tissue cells of the periodontal ligament are the source of osteoblasts, which form bone; cementoblasts, which form cementum; fibroblasts, which form fibers; osteoclasts, which resorb bone; and phage cells to aid repair. Any pathological destruction of tissue is repaired by the same mechanism that provides for normal replacement, unless the pathological process is so severe that the mechanism cannot operate.

The nerve supply of the periodontal

ligament consists of pain receptors and proprioceptors. The function of the proprioceptors is most important. These nerve endings provide the ability to localize tooth position, and they are so exquisitely sensitive that a piece of the thinnest tissue paper is immediately perceived when it is placed between the teeth. It is through these proprioceptors that the patient perceives interfering occlusal contacts, and because of this mechanism the mandible assumes a convenience occlusal relationship to avoid constant trauma to the pair of opposing teeth in interfering contact. This is a most important concept in understanding the relationship of occlusal trauma to the abnormal convenience relationships which are observed in many patients. The pain receptors warn of impending or actual danger to the periodontium.

The function of the blood supply is to provide the nutritional needs for the metabolic processes of the periodontal ligament as well as the other plasma elements that are necessary for tissue resistance. The lymphatics aid the venous system to drain metabolic by-products and dead tissue from the area.

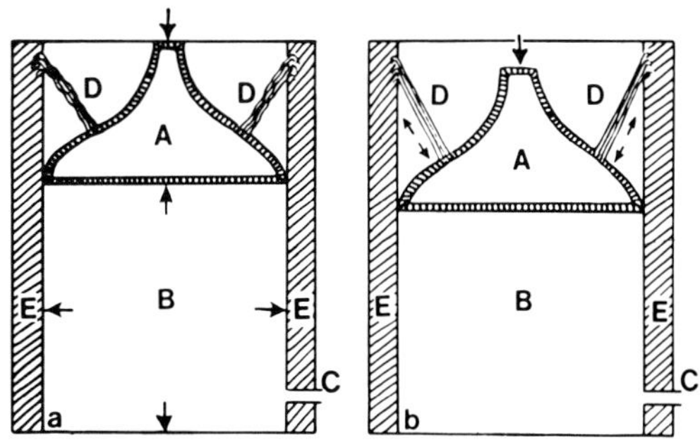

FIG. 4-13. The function of periodontal tissues during occlusion of the teeth. In (*a*) at first application of force, tooth (Piston A) distributes forces by way of periodontal ligament (hydraulic chamber B). There is no tension on periodontal fibers (D). Movement of tooth into alveolus is possible only as fluid escapes by way of vessel draining the periodontal ligament (C). In (*b*) movement of tooth into alveolus is checked by periodontal fibers (D). At this time full force of occlusion is transmitted as tension to alveolar bone (E) (Kronfeld, R., and Boyle, P. E.: Histopathology of the Teeth and Their Surrounding Structures. ed. 3. Philadelphia, Lea & Febiger, 1949)

REACTIONS OF THE PERIODONTAL LIGAMENT TO FORCE

The width of the periodontal ligament varies among individuals. The most important factor determining width is function. Other secondary factors are age, the specific tooth in question and hypofunction. It is within the periodontal space that the tooth moves. Normally, the width of this space ranges from .09 to .33 mm.[10] To visualize what this width really means, depress the thumbnail until the nail bed blanches. The distance that the thumbnail has been depressed is about .33 mm. A tooth that moves this slight distance can and actually does produce ischemia in the periodontal ligament. The narrowest area is at the middle or slightly apical to the middle of the ligament. The ligament is slightly thicker gingivally and apically. This variation in thickness in different areas gives us the typical hourglass effect of the periodontal ligament when viewed either in a buccolingual or a mesiodistal section (Fig. 3-10). Figure 4-14 is a roentgenogram illustrating the hourglass effect.

The resistive capacity or resistance of the patient determines the reaction of the periodontal ligament to force. When resistance is high, excessive forces produce a picture of functional hypertrophy and thickening of the periodontal ligament. Function probably toughens the fibers, and proper diet probably assists this process. The principal fibers are denser and more regular in arrangement. The nerve and blood vessel spaces are mark-

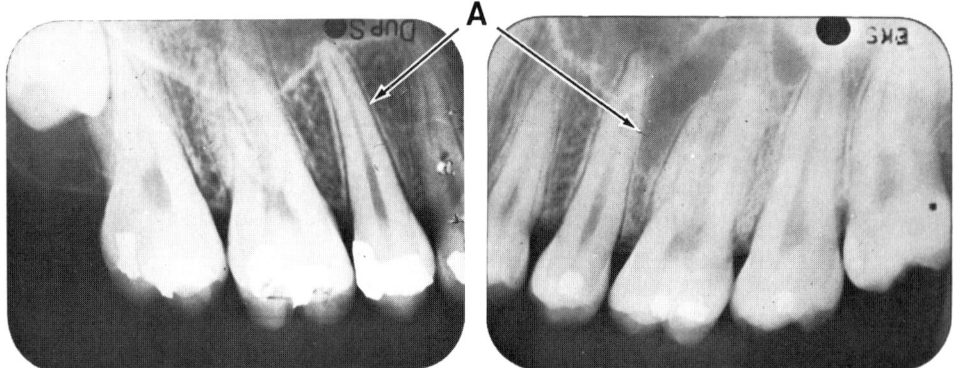

FIG. 4-14. Roentgenograms of the upper molar area illustrate the hourglass effect (mesiodistal view), with the strictures at A.

edly decreased, and the cellular elements are less distinct. The periodontal space is shaped like an hourglass with a relatively narrower area than normal. However, when resistance and resistive capacity are low, excessive forces produce the following conditions. The tooth, under excessive force, crushes part of the periodontal ligament against the lamina dura. The principal fibers are crushed; lymphatics and blood vessels are ruptured, and hemorrhage results; nerve endings are destroyed; and the cellular elements degenerate. Figure 4-15 is a histological section illustrating a hemorrhagic periodontal ligament. The tissues undergo general degeneration, and necrosis finally results. In those parts of the periodontal ligament that are not crushed between the teeth and the lamina dura, the fibers are under abnormal tension and are finally torn because their tensile strength has been exceeded. Blood and lymph vessels are distorted and eventually ruptured. In the crushed areas, the pain receptors are stimulated. Continuous trauma of the periodontal ligament produces tissue degeneration in the form of hyalinization of the fibers. When the periodontal ligament is compressed abnormally and repeatedly, it is injured and finally brought into a state of lowered resistance. The repaired tissue of the injured periodontal ligament is not firm and healthy but weak and improperly formed. It seems to be normal, but actually it is not. This is borne out by the fact that even though the teeth are loose, roentgenograms show the alveolar crest to be high. Under continued tension and stress, the periodontal ligament becomes

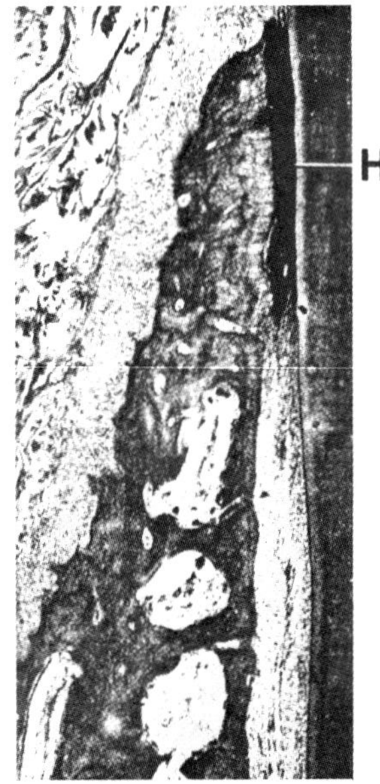

FIG. 4-15. Periodontal ligament is narrow and hemorrhagic (bloodstained), as seen in dark area at H. Normal periodontal ligament is seen immediately below the hemorrhagic area. (Gottlieb, B., and Orban, B.: Die Veraenderung der Gewebe bei uebermaesser Beanspruchung der Zaehne. Leipzig, Thieme)

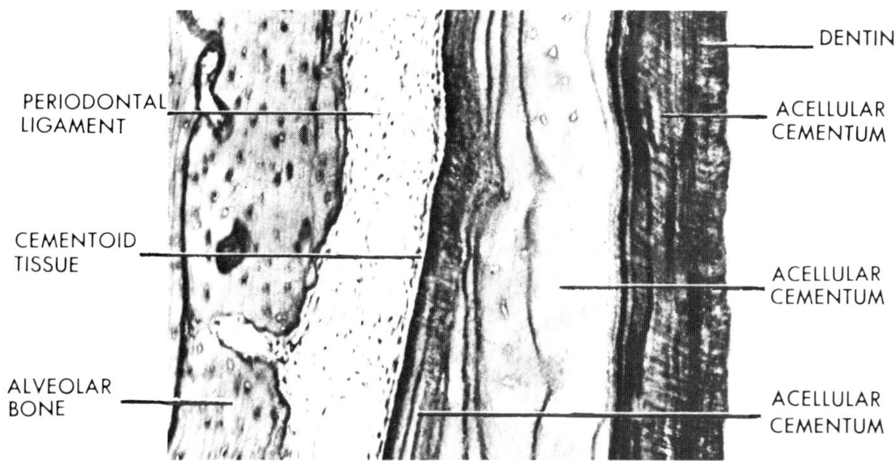

FIG. 4-16. Cellular cementum is seen on the surface of acellular cementum, and again as it is covered by acellular cementum (incremental lines). (Orban, B.: Oral Histology and Embryology. ed. 4, p. 169. St. Louis, C. V. Mosby, 1957)

disorganized and finally degenerates to the point where it is at the mercy of the forces on the crown of the tooth. In some cases, injuries to the periodontal ligament may not be expressed until years later when its resistance is low.

Under decreased physiological stress, the periodontal ligament reacts like other nonfunctional body tissues. That is, it exhibits a type of disuse or nonfunctional atrophy. The principal fibers lose their normal tone, are irregular and fewer in number. Since the metabolic level of the tissues is lowered, the blood circulation is reduced. As a result of decreased function, the periodontal ligament will be about one-third its normal width (Fig. 3-8).

REACTIONS OF CEMENTUM TO FORCE

Considered histologically, there are two kinds of cementum: cellular and acellular. From a functional viewpoint, however, these must be considered as being identical. Both cellular and acellular cementum are differentiated into layers by the incremental lines which indicate periodic formation (Fig. 4-16). Principal or Sharpey's fibers are embedded in the cementum throughout its thickness, but those in the deep layers are obscure (Fig. 4-9). Because its only source of blood supply is the periodontal ligament, the cementum does not resorb or build up in response to forces as quickly as does bone. Cementum may be considered as specialized bone.

Hypercementosis is an abnormal thickening of the cementum. If this thickening improves the functional qualities of the cementum, it is called cemental hypertrophy. If, on the other hand, the thickening occurs in nonfunctional teeth or if it is not associated with increased function, it is called cemental hyperplasia. Teeth that are exposed to great forces exhibit pronglike extensions of cementum into the periodontal ligament (Fig. 4-17). This is a functional adaptation designed to give the tooth a greater area of periodontal attachment with a resultingly firmer anchorage. Thickening of the cementum is often found on teeth that are not in function. This hyperplasia may encircle the entire root or it may occur in small areas. When this condition exists, Sharpey's fibers are absent.

The fact that cementum is more resis-

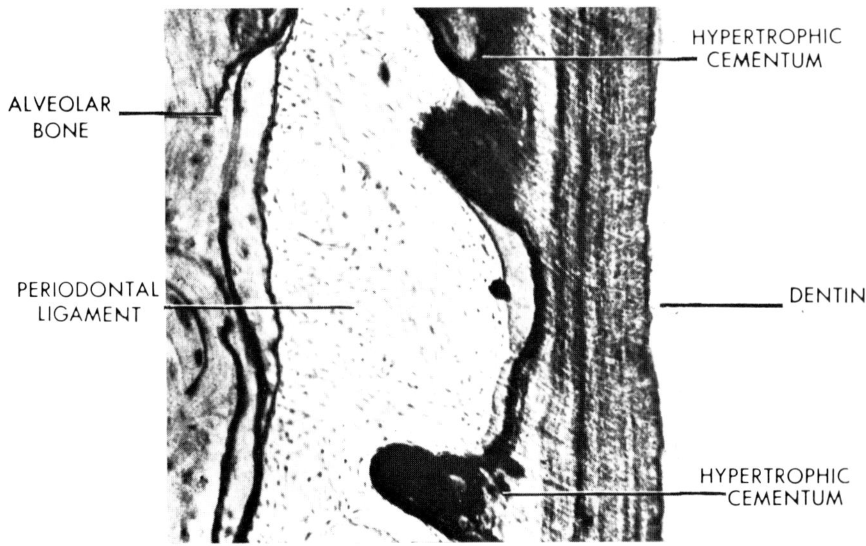

FIG. 4-17. Pronglike extensions of the cementum into the periodontal ligament. (Orban, B.: Oral Histology and Embryology. ed. 4, p. 176. St. Louis, C. V. Mosby, 1957)

tant to resorption than bone makes possible orthodontic treatment with gentle forces. Excessive force transmitted to the bone will cause it to resorb. If the force is great enough and is applied for a sufficiently long time, resorption of the cementum of the root of the tooth will also take place. If the intensity of the force is reduced and the surrounding connective tissue is still intact, the cementum will be repaired, but at a slower rate than the bone. The process of cemental repair varies among individuals. In some cases it occurs rapidly, while in others, in which apparently similar conditions exist, it does not occur at all. Poor cemental repair seems to occur in individuals who also react poorly to trauma and other irritations and readily develop periodontal disease. These differences in cemental formation and repair may be attributed to constitutional factors. Variations in the location and the shape of the apical foramina have been observed to result from forces on the teeth. It should be borne in mind constantly that resorption of the cementum in the permanent dentition is a pathological process.

Occlusal forces may be so excessive that they cause an actual fracture of the root tip, or they may merely tear off a piece of cementum. The latter condition (Fig. 4-18) is called a cemental tear. When the excessive occlusal forces are removed, both these conditions are repaired by a growth of the connective tissue of the periodontal ligament in which differentiating cementoblasts join the fragments by laying down osteocementum.

REACTIONS OF THE GINGIVA TO FORCE

The effect of occlusal force on the gingival crevice will vary with the individual's resistive capacity to stress. The patient with a lowered resistance is likely to exhibit recession. Since traumatogenic occlusion produces an injury, it increases the susceptibility of the crevicular tissues to bacterial invasion. Excessive force results in torque of the teeth which, in turn, causes trauma and in turn may lead to tearing or degeneration of the epithelial attachment. This will deepen the gingival crevice.

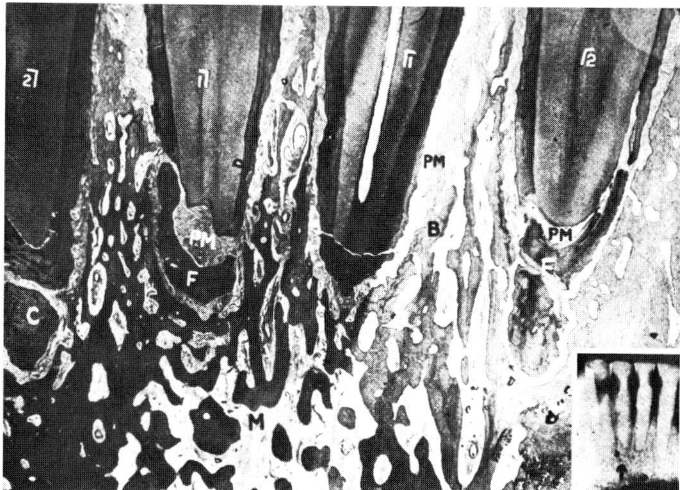

FIG. 4-18. A roentgenogram and photomicrograph of the apical and periapical region of the four incisors which were affected by abnormal occlusal trauma. The central incisors show fracture of the roots. The lower right lateral incisor presents a cementoma which is not found attached to the root in any serial section. The lower left lateral has a complete and incomplete cemental tear. Repair of the tears has begun, connective tissue from the periodontal ligament has invaded the tear, and osteocementum is being laid down. B, bone; M, marrow; F, fracture; PM, periodontal ligament; C, cementum. (Goldman, H. M.: Periodontia. ed. 2. St. Louis, C. V. Mosby, 1949)

DURABILITY OF THE TEMPOROMANDIBULAR JOINT

The histological explanation for the durability of the temporomandibular joint may be found in the nature of the tissues that compose its structure. The glenoid fossa is composed of a thin layer of compact bone, and the articular tubercle is composed of spongy bone covered by a thin layer of compact bone. Similarly, the condyle is composed of spongy bone covered by a thin layer of compact bone (Fig. 4-19). Both bony components—the head of the condyle and the glenoid fossa—are covered with fibrocartilage which does not have any blood supply and is not resorbed but wears when it is subjected to abnormal stresses. The fibrocartilage increases in thickness as it continues from the glenoid fossa to the posterior wall of the articular eminence. Evidence of inherent resistance to stress is found in the characteristic arrangement of the fiber bundles in the fibrous coverings. The surface fibers are parallel with the surface; the deep fibers are perpendicular to the surface. This arrangement is similar to that found in other articular cartilages. The surface layers are adapted to gliding, while the deep ones are adapted to the resistance of force. However, the bony components of the joint may change slowly under excessive stress. Cartilage acts as a shock absorber. This fibrous tissue does not cover the posterior part of the articular fossa. Instead, there is a thickened periosteum and loose connective tissue (as revealed in the sagittal section, Fig. 4-19).

Interposed between the two bones and dividing the joint into upper and lower compartments is the articular disc, which is composed mainly of fibrocartilage with a small amount of elastic fibers throughout. The fibrocartilaginous char-

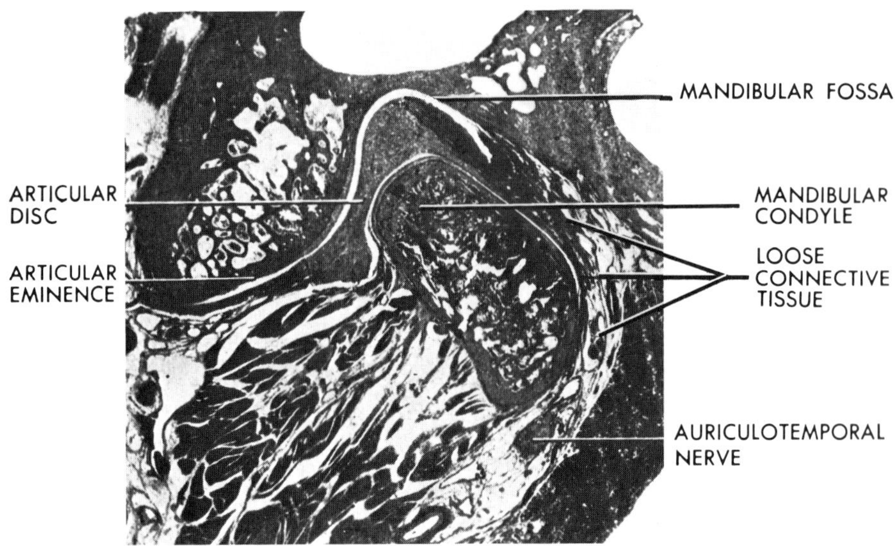

FIG. 4-19. Sagittal section through the temporomandibular articulation. (From S. W. Chase)

acter of the articular disc differs from the articular discs of other joints, as evidenced by its high degree of mobility and plasticity during function. It divides the joint into two compartments: the upper meniscotemporal is a sliding joint, and the lower meniscocondylar is a rotating joint with a hingelike motion (Fig. 4-19). In the posterior region, the disc is attached to a thick layer of vascularized connective tissue, which is attached to the posterior portion of the capsule and the glenoid fossa.

The fibrous capsule extending from the temporal bone to the articular disc is very loose, permitting extensive sliding movements of the upper joint compartment. However, the capsule between the disc and the condyle is quite tight; therefore, only hinge movements can take place. The degree of looseness of the capsule varies among individuals and is an important limiting factor in jaw movements.

The inner surface of the capsule, in the areas of the articular spaces, is composed of thin layers of special tissue called the synovial layer. It is composed of connective tissue with numerous capillary networks formed by the blood vessels near the surface. The extreme inner layer of the synovial tissue forms folds or villi that protrude into the articular spaces (Fig. 4-20). The articular spaces contain a small amount of viscous fluid. The viscous synovial fluid of the joint has been classified as one of the mucopolysaccharides called hyaluronic acid. The high polymerization of the hyaluronic acid is responsible for its jellylike consistency. Moses[6] states,

> There are several theories about the composition and origin of the synovial fluid or synovia. We appear to have microscopic evidence that there are direct connections between blood vessels and fluid. In fact we believe that we have located a vascular system that is primarily created for that very purpose. We are also able to demonstrate cells that appear to be secreting, and we are also able to demonstrate the degeneration of cells en masse into the synovia. Thus, in one series of sections all theories may be confirmed, making possible the theory that the synovial fluid is the result of the contributions of several mechanisms, each for a specific purpose and dictated by function. In fact, we should like to project the thought that function is the causative agent that influences both the chemistry and cel-

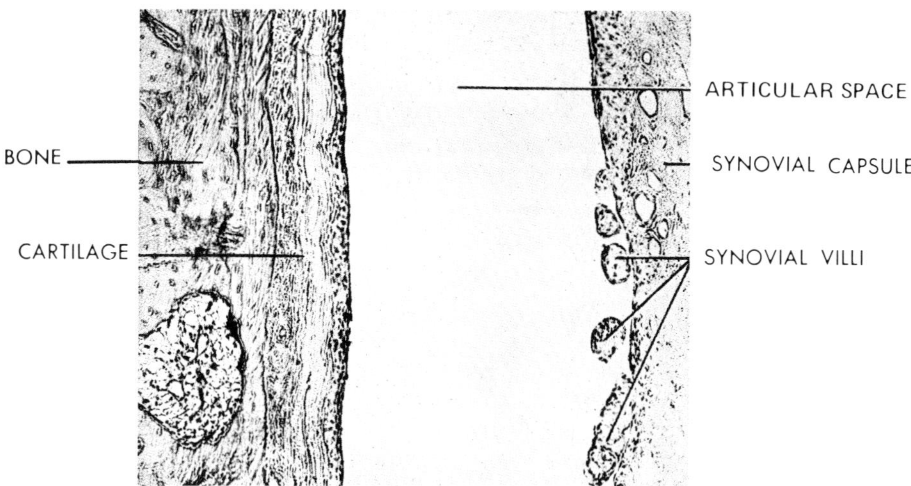

FIG. 4-20. Villi of the synovial capsule of temporomandibular joint. (Orban, B.: Oral Histology and Embryology. ed. 3. St. Louis, C. V. Mosby, 1953)

lular structures of the temporomandibular joint.

The capsule and the structures of the temporomandibular joint are innervated by branches of the auriculotemporal nerve, filaments from the masseteric nerve and the sensory branch of the seventh nerve.[4,11] The nerves are not in a vulnerable position for compression by the heads of the condyles during function. However, the sensory branches of the nerves that innervate the joint are sources of reflex neuralgias. By the process of referred pain, pain may be felt in the head, the neck and other areas of the body. In this area are also found the chorda tympani nerve, branches of the superficial temporal artery, vein and nerve and the anterior tympanic artery, vein and nerve. Trauma can also affect these structures to cause reflex pain in other areas.

The blood supply to the temporomandibular joint is from the superficial temporal branch of the external carotid artery. Branches extend to the medial and lateral walls of the articular disc, but the disc itself is avascular, as is the cartilaginous covering of the bony surfaces of the joint.

REFERENCES

1. Bodecker, C. F.: Histology to operative dentistry and periodontia. J. D. Educ., *4:*171, 1939.
2. Coolidge, E. D., and Hine, M. K.: Periodontia. Philadelphia, Lea & Febiger, 1954.
3. Gettinger, R.: Relationship of orthodontics to oral pathology. Am. J. Ortho. Oral Surg., *24:*1124, 1938.
4. Kronfeld, R., and Boyle, P. E.: Histopathology of the Teeth and Their Surrounding Structures. ed. 3. Philadelphia, Lea & Febiger, 1949.
5. MacKenzie, W. C.: The Action of Muscles. p. 5. New York, Hoeber, 1939.
6. Moses, C.: Studies on the synovial fluid and the synovial membrane of the temporomandibular joint. D. Items Int., *71:*783, 1949.
7. Neumann, H. H., and DiSalvo, N. A.: Does functional effort affect caries activity? J. Dent. Child., *22:*151, 1955.
8. ———: Amazon expedition hunts clues to dental caries. Oral Hyg., *46:*839, 1956.
9. Orban, B.: Biologic principles in correction of occlusal disharmonies. J. Pros. Dent., *6:*637, 1956.
10. ———: Oral Histology and Embryology. St. Louis, C. V. Mosby, 1944.
11. ———: Tissue changes in traumatic occlusion. JADA *15:*2090, 1928.

12. Seipel, R. M.: Trajectories of the jaws, Acta Odont. Scandinav., *8:*81, 1948.
13. Shapiro, H.: Applied Anatomy of the Head and Neck. ed. 2, p. 82. Philadelphia, J. B. Lippincott, 1947.
14. Sicher, H., and Tandler, J.: Anatomie für zahnarzte (Anatomy for dentists). Vienna & Berlin, Julius Springer Verlag, 1928.
15. Sorrin, S.: Interrelationship of occlusion and periodontal structures, J. Dent. Med., *11:*158, 1956.
16. Stedman, T. L.: Stedman's Medical Dictionary. Baltimore, Williams & Wilkins, 1936.
17. Thielemann, K.: Aufgaben und Mittel der orthopadischen Paradentosebehandlung (Orthopedic periodontal treatment). Dtsch. Zahn-Mund-Kieferh., *6:*734, 1939.

Additional Basic References

Arnim, S. S.: The connective tissue fibers of the marginal gingiva., JADA, *47:*271, 1953.

Cheraskin, E., Ringsdorf, W. M., Jr., and Clark, J. W.: Diet and Disease. Emmaus (Pa.), Rodale Books, 1968.

Clark, J. W., Cheraskin, E., and Ringsdorf, W. M., Jr.: Diet and the Periodontal Patient. Springfield (Ill.), Charles C Thomas, 1970.

Sicher, H., and Bhaskar, S. N. (eds.): Orban's Oral Histology and Embryology. ed. 7. St. Louis, C. V. Mosby, 1972.

5 *Physiology of the Stomatognathic System*

In referring to the masticatory organ, its component structures and all of the tissues related to it, the term *stomatognathic system* is used, because this designation includes a number of systematically related organs and tissues that function as a whole. The components of this system are the bones of the skull, the mandible, the hyoid, the clavicle and the sternum; the muscles and the ligaments; the dentoalveolar and the temporomandibular joints; the vascular, the lymphatic and the nerve supply systems; the soft tissues of the head; the teeth. An organ such as the heart or the liver can be dissected anatomically, but a system such as the stomatognathic must be studied as an integrated, physiological, functioning whole. It is important to consider the specific functions that tie this system together rather than the isolated and individual tissues which compose it. Such a comprehensive and functional concept of the entire system will focus attention on the relationship of the teeth to all of the other tissues of the system and will help in understanding both normal and pathological processes.

The stomatognathic system functions almost continuously not only in mastication and deglutition but also in respiration and speech. It also directs the intricate postural relationships of the head, the tongue and the hyoid bone as well as the movements of the mandible. When all parts of the system are in proper functional relationship, each component as well as the system as a whole operates with maximal efficiency and with minimal expenditure of energy. Proper relationship of the mandible and its associated neuromuscular system will cause the minimal degree of neuromuscular tension on muscles, nerves and blood supply during function. Physiological function is essential if the health of the stomatognathic system is to be established and maintained.

Although the teeth are the actual tools of mastication, and although most dental treatment is directed at the teeth, it must be borne in mind constantly that it is the entire stomatognathic system that governs the movement of the mandible and the teeth. Impaired physiological function results in breakdown not only of an individual tissue but also of the interdependent structures involved. Changes in structure and function of any single part of the stomatognathic system will cause corresponding changes in structure and function of other parts, thus setting up something analogous to a chain reaction. Although the operative procedures involved in occlusal equilibration are performed primarily on the teeth, a consideration of the interrelationships of various parts of the stomatognathic system will help the practitioner to plan, create and maintain a physiologic occlusion.

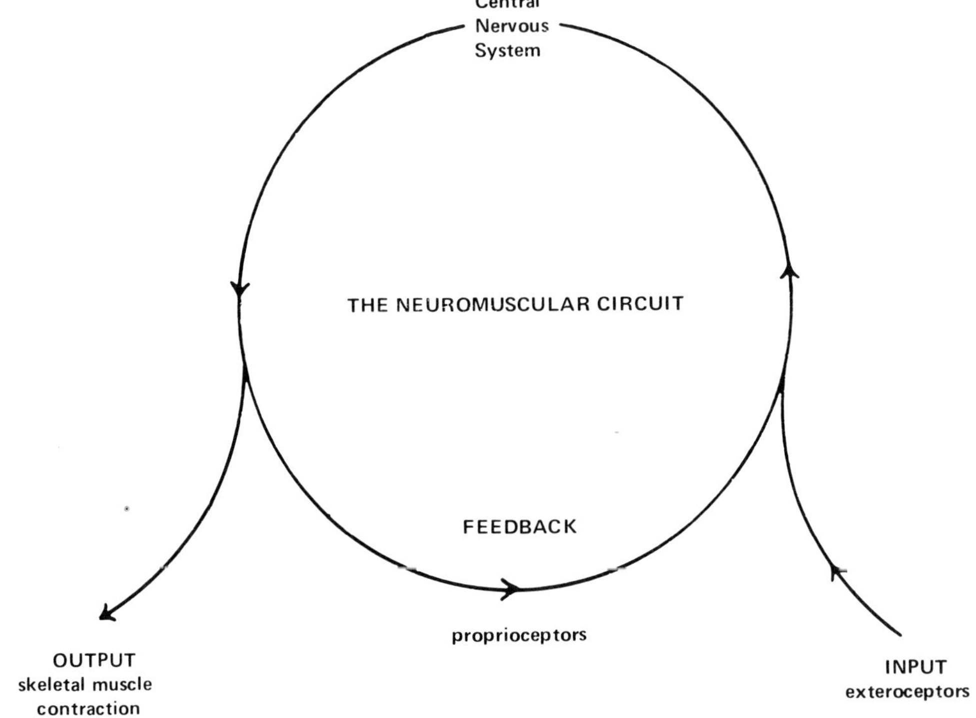

FIG. 5-1. The neuromuscular circuit.

NERVOUS SYSTEM

The three basic functions of the nervous system are perception, integration and reaction. Integration of sensory stimuli takes place in the central nervous system where the appropriate reaction to a given stimulus is determined. Central impulses then stimulate the appropriate motor nerves which, in turn, instigate and regulate the correct muscle reactions.

Figure 5-1 shows the neuromuscular circuit which if blocked creates muscle spasm. A proprioceptor creates feedback which sends messages to the central nervous system. This is the basis of neuromuscular spasm.

Receptors

The sensory aspect of perception is carried on by exteroceptors and interoceptors. A receptor is a specially designed nerve ending responsive to a distinct stimulus or change in environment. The different types of receptors indicate that specific receptors receive specific stimuli. The general relationship of the teeth and the periodontium to receptors is illustrated in Figure 5-2. The receptors that respond to changes in the external environment (pain, touch, pressure and temperature) are called exteroceptors. The receptors that respond to changes in the internal environment (found in periodontal ligaments, tendons, muscles, viscera, etc.) are called interoceptors.

It is interesting to note that the proprioceptors situated in the periodontal membrane (periodontal ligament) and in the muscles of mastication are so exquisitely sensitive that differences in thickness of paper in the order of fractions of a millimeter placed between the teeth may be discerned. Such minute differences cannot be discriminated by the tactile sense.[26]

The proprioceptor is a receptor which responds to change in movement and position and is stimulated by action within the body itself. Proprioceptors are classified alone or as interoceptors. It is the proprioceptors within the periodontal ligaments, the temporomandibular joints, the muscles of the mastication and their tendons that integrate the neuromuscular control of the mandible. The muscle spindles that are sensitive to stretch are proprioceptors.

The free nerve endings perceive pain stimuli and are widely distributed. Pain receptors issue warnings and initiate defense reactions. Merkel's discs and Meissner's corpuscles perceive touch, and the Golgi-Mazzoni end organs differentiate pressure. The pacinian corpuscles are stimulated by deep pressure. Ruffini's corpuscles perceive warmth, and Krause's end bulbs perceive cold. In the physiological state each receptor is specific in its perception. Trauma may affect proprioceptors. One of the functions of the receptor is to be responsive to a specific change and to institute the impulse that is carried by the neuron. All receptors have a critical threshold, and if the intensity of stimulation falls below this threshold, reception and reaction do not occur. This critical threshold varies among individuals and is not constant even in the same individual. If the stimulus changes faster than a determined rate, excitation occurs. For example, a cup of hot coffee may be difficult to drink, but ingestion of liquids of increasing temperatures enables one to tolerate a higher temperature than was possible in the first case. This is the phenomenon of adaptation. In other words, the person adapts to a continued stimulus, and this adaptation raises the critical threshold. This is why continued pressure can cause disease, damage and destruction to the periodontium before the individual becomes aware of it. Pain adapts poorly and therefore acts as a warning signal over a long period of time against the occurrence of pathological conditions.

The periodontal space contains 90 per cent of the nerves of proprioception in the mouth and is responsible for mandibular position. In the fabrication of dentures, this proprioception is lost and mandibular proprioception is mediated solely by the nerves in the temporomandibular joint. It was thought (Fig. 5-3) that the nerves of proprioception were sparse in the temporomandibular joint, but the work of Birgit Theilander proved otherwise.

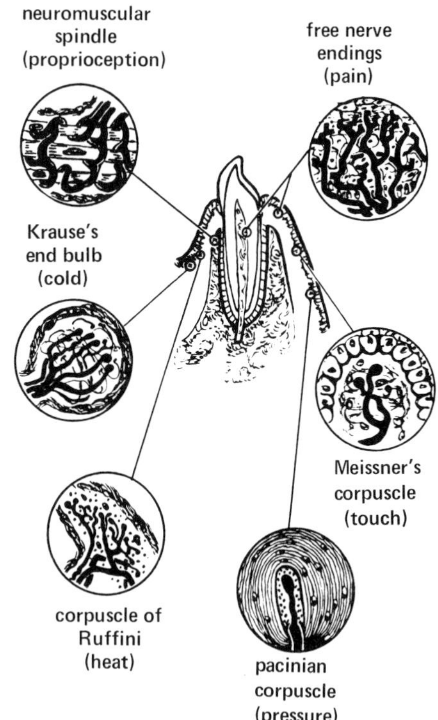

FIG. 5-2. Nerve receptors associated with the oral tissues. (Langley, L. L., and Cheraskin, E.: The Physiological Foundation of Dental Practice. ed. 2. St. Louis, C. V. Mosby, 1956)

Stretch, Extensor, or Antigravity Reflex

The neural mechanism from perception to involuntary response may be called a reflex, which involves a receptor, an afferent limb, a synapse, an efferent limb and an effector. The possible integration of stimuli at the spinal cord level

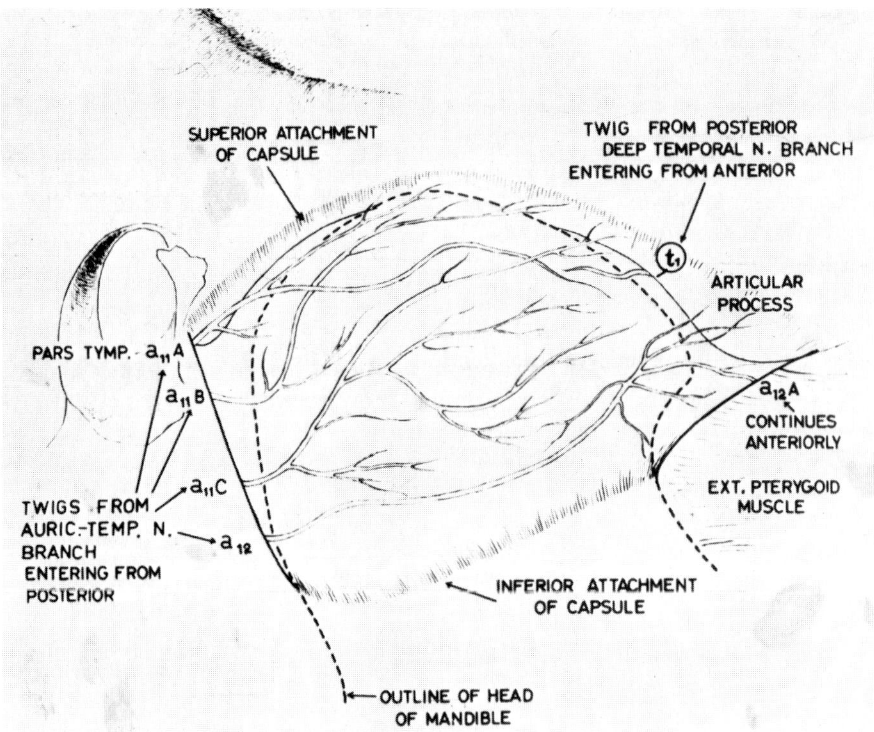

FIG. 5-3. Nerve distribution in the lateral part of the capsule.

is illustrated in Figure 5-4. The purpose of the stretch, extensor or antigravity reflex is to oppose gravity. It is initiated by the stretching of an antigravity muscle fiber, such as that found in temporal, masseter or internal pterygoid muscles.

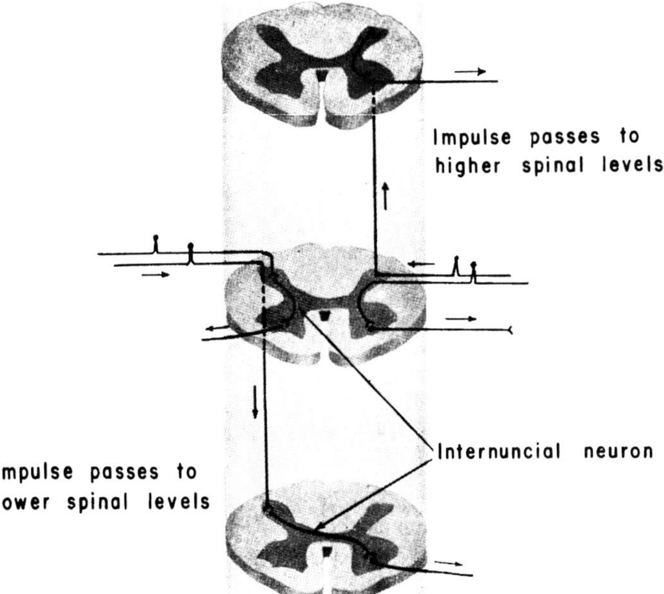

FIG. 5-4. Simple spinal reflex connections; impulses may leave at the same level or at levels above or below the level of entry. (Langley, L. L., and Cheraskin, E.: The Physiological Foundation of Dental Practice. ed. 2. St. Louis, C. V. Mosby, 1956)

The same fibers that were stretched are caused to contract. The antigravity muscles tend to be stretched by the force of gravity, but muscle spindles continually fire impulses that keep the mandible in position. The jaw-jerk stretch reflex (Fig. 5-5), is a specific reflex and is produced by a stretching of the masseter muscle fibers. This sudden stretch of the masseter fibers excites the muscle spindle proprioceptors and, by way of the reflex pathway through the brain stem, the motor nerve causes these same masseter muscle fibers to contract.

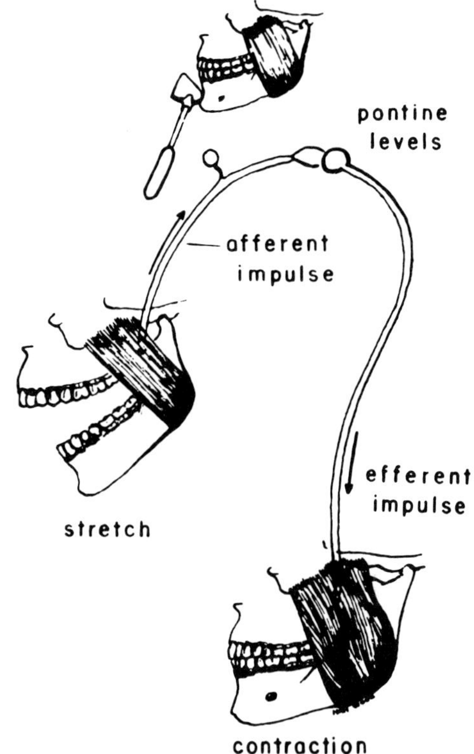

FIG. 5-5. The jaw jerk. Tapping of the chin causes stretch of the masseter, evoking reflex contraction of the same fibers. (Langley, L. L., and Cheraskin, E.: The Physiological Foundation of Dental Practice. ed. 2. St. Louis, C. V. Mosby, 1956)

Flexor Reflex

The function of the flexor reflex is nociceptive or protective. Pain is the primary activator for reflex opening. The flexor reflex is more intricate than the stretch reflex. The stretch reflex activates single muscle fibers, whereas the flexor reflex activates separate muscle bundles and involves internuncial neurons. Abrupt contact of a tooth with a hard object during mastication may cause pain, but it will also cause the muscles that act as the depressors of the mandible to contract and withdraw the tooth from contact with the hard object. Although the stimulus traveled by way of one afferent tract, the movement of the mandible involved the excitation of many efferent neurons. Because the stretch (extensor) reflex works reciprocally with the flexor reflex, the interaction of the two must be syn-

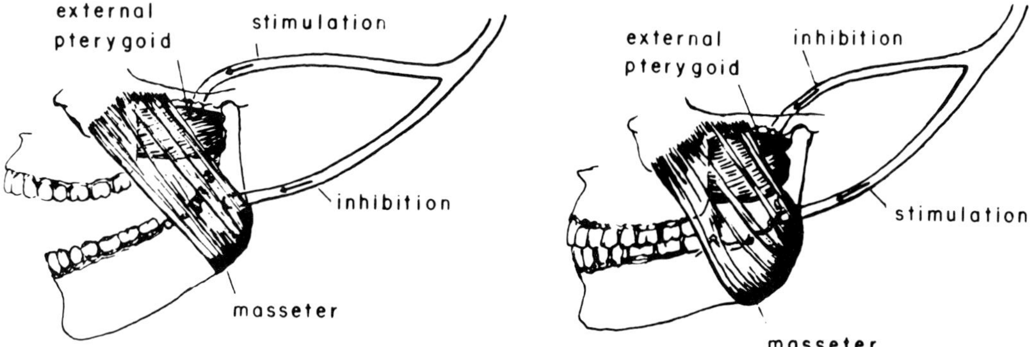

FIG. 5-6. A demonstration of reciprocal innervation. (Langley, L. L., and Cheraskin, E.: The Physiological Foundation of Dental Practice. ed. 2. St. Louis, C. V. Mosby, 1956)

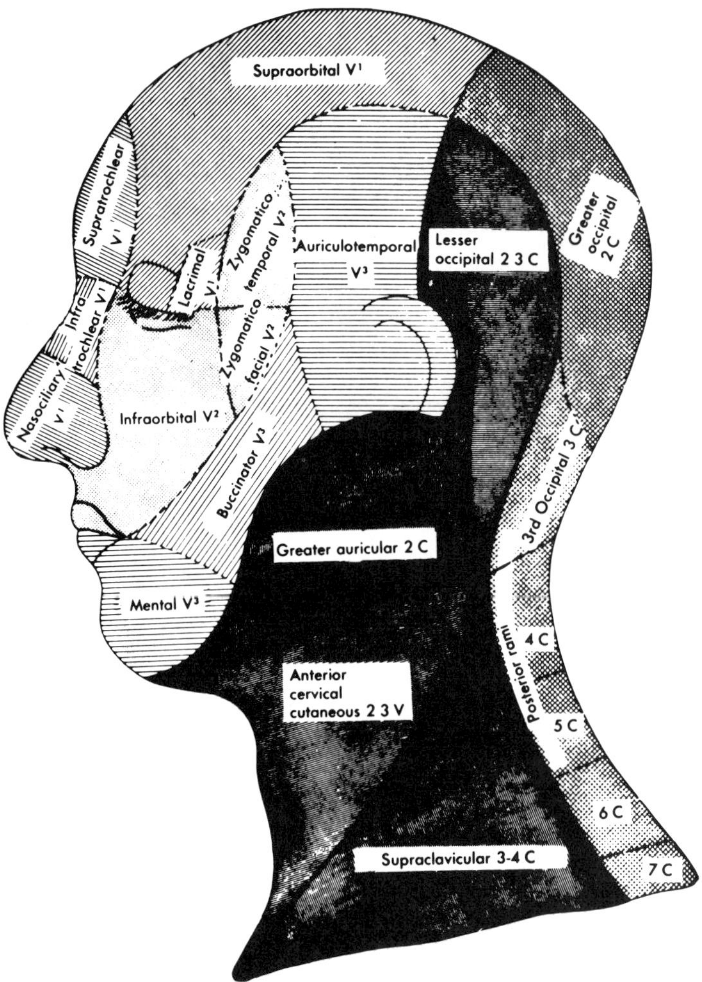

FIG. 5-7. Superficial sensory nerves of head and neck regions. (After Brand, T. W., and Monheim, L. M.: Local Anesthesia and Pain Control in Dental Practice. ed. 4. St. Louis, C. V. Mosby, 1969)

chronized properly. Figure 5-6 illustrates this reciprocal innervation.

The failure of reciprocal action plays an important role in the anterior dislocation of the jaw. It should be recalled that when the mouth is opened (the mandible depressed), the condyle is brought anterior to the glenoid fossa. When the mouth is closed (the mandible elevated), the condyle returns into the glenoid fossa. If, when the elevators of the jaw contract, the M. pterygoideus externus does not relax, then the condyle becomes fixed in front of the articular eminence and the jaw is said to be anteriorly dislocated. The same thing may happen during yawning, the extraction of a tooth, or impression taking.[27]

Learned Reflex

In habitual or reflex actions such as chewing or swallowing, when definite reflex patterns have been formed, integration is unconscious. If no reflex patterns have been formed, the individual is aware of the reaction to stimuli. The latter situation is exemplified by the conscious avoidance of an interfering occlusal contact. However, if the occlusal interference is not corrected, a reflex pattern of avoidance is established and finally takes place habitually. Thus, by repetition, a learned reflex becomes an unconscious reflex.

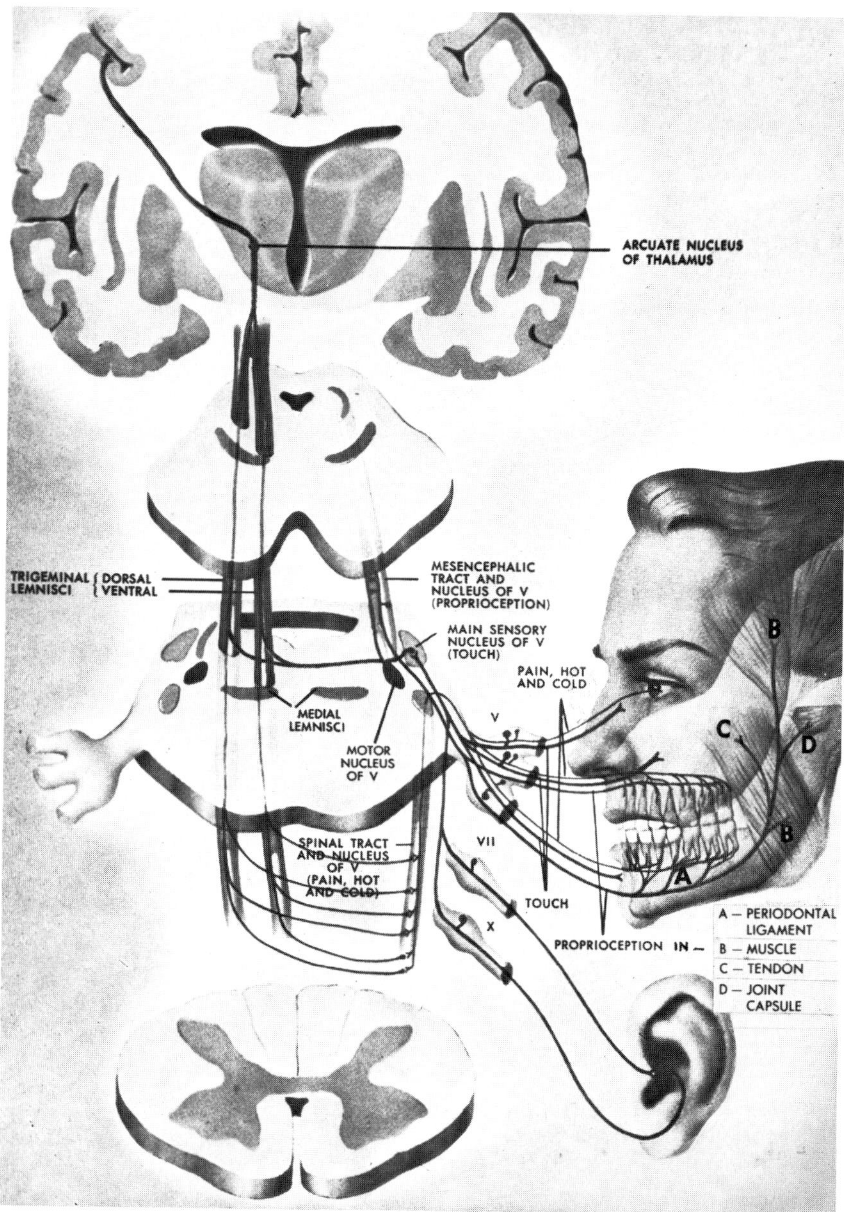

FIG. 5-8. The somesthetic system; head; trigeminal nerve. (After Netter, F.: Ciba Clinical Symposia, Ciba Pharmaceutical Products, Inc., Summit, N. J., 1953)

Innervation of the Head and Neck

The somatosensory innervation of the head and neck is provided by four cranial and three spinal nerves. The cranial nerves (Fig. 5-7) are the 5th (trigeminal), 7th (facial), 9th (glossopharyngeal) and 10th (vagus); the spinal nerves are the 2nd, 3rd and 4th.*

The cutaneous innervation of the face and the scalp is mainly supplied by the trigeminal nerve. It also provides motor

* Mahan, P.: Personal communication, 1973.

innervation to the muscles of mastication. The greater part of the nerve is sensory and gives rise to three divisions: ophthalmic, maxillary and mandibular. The course of the motor part of the trigeminal nerve is associated with the mandibular division. Abrupt contact with a hard object during mastication creates pain which is alleviated by the flexor reflex when the mouth is opened. Although the flexor reflex occurred unconsciously, pain is consciously felt by the person. The impulse is transmitted to the higher levels of the nervous system, and practically at the same time the motor impulse is transmitted to the muscles. An occlusal interference will cause a similar reaction of the neuromuscular system. The interfering contact of the opposing teeth will cause unconscious opening of the mouth and conscious pain. Then the proprioceptors of the periodontal ligament will direct positioning of the mandible to avoid recurrence of the occlusal trauma.

As the mandible is positioned again and again to avoid the interfering occlusal contact, a reflex is created which becomes habitual and is the basis for the habitual convenience mandibular postural relationship.

The sensory proprioceptive fibers lie in the mesencephalon (Fig. 5-8), and are known as the mesencephalic root of the trigeminal nerve. In tracing afferent stimuli, proprioceptors course to the chief sensory nucleus, then by secondary afferents to the posteromedial nucleus of the thalamus and then by way of tertiary afferents to the sensory cortex, but some leave the chief nucleus to pass to the cerebellum.[29] In Figure 5-8 some of the proprioceptors are located in A, B, C and D. The motor nucleus of the trigeminal nerve is at the pontine level (Fig. 5-9).

The auriculotemporal, masseteric and posterior deep temporal branches of the trigeminal nerve innervate the temporomandibular joint, as well as the skin over the joint and the muscles associated with it. As a result of this relationship, dysfunction of the temporomandibular joint frequently causes pain in the muscles of mastication.*

The facial nerve provides the innervation for deep sensation of the face and supplies the motor innervation of the facial muscles, with the exception of the masticatory muscles, the mylohyoid and the digastric. The glossopharyngeal nerve mediates sensation for the base of the tongue (posterior third) and the pharynx, and also provides the motor innervation of the pharynx. The vagus nerve supplies the sensory innervation of the posterior external auditory meatus, the skin behind the ear, and also the pharynx and larynx. It provides the motor innervation of the soft palate, pharynx, esophagus and larynx.[1] The 2nd, 3rd and 4th cervical nerves provide the somatosensory innervation of the posterior half of the head and neck.

In Figure 5-10, as elaborated by Goodfriend, normal dentition and neuromuscular relationships are seen on the right side and missing posterior teeth on the lower left side. Because of the lack of posterior support on the left side, the masseter and the temporalis pull the mandible up into the sore or traumatized joints and cause a myriad of symptoms in the vestibular, auditory, and facial nerves and most important, in the semicircular canals and vestibules.

Referred Pain

The stimulation of a sensory fiber, at any point along its course, will project the sensation to the sensory cortex. From past experience the cortex knows which receptor has been stimulated and pain is believed to arise from this nerve ending. This mechanism is the basis of phantom pain. Another type of referred pain occurs

* Mahan, P.: Personal communication, 1973.

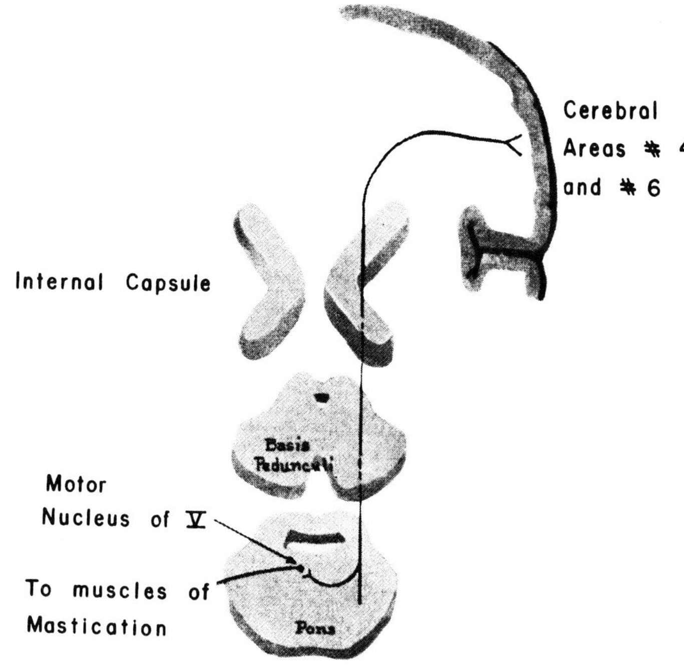

FIG. 5-9. The upper motor component of the trigeminal nerve. (Redrawn from Netter, F.: Ciba Clinical Symposia, Ciba Pharmaceutical Products, Inc. *In* Langley, L. L., and Cheraskin, E.: The Physiological Foundation of Dental Practice. ed. 2. St. Louis, C. V. Mosby, 1956)

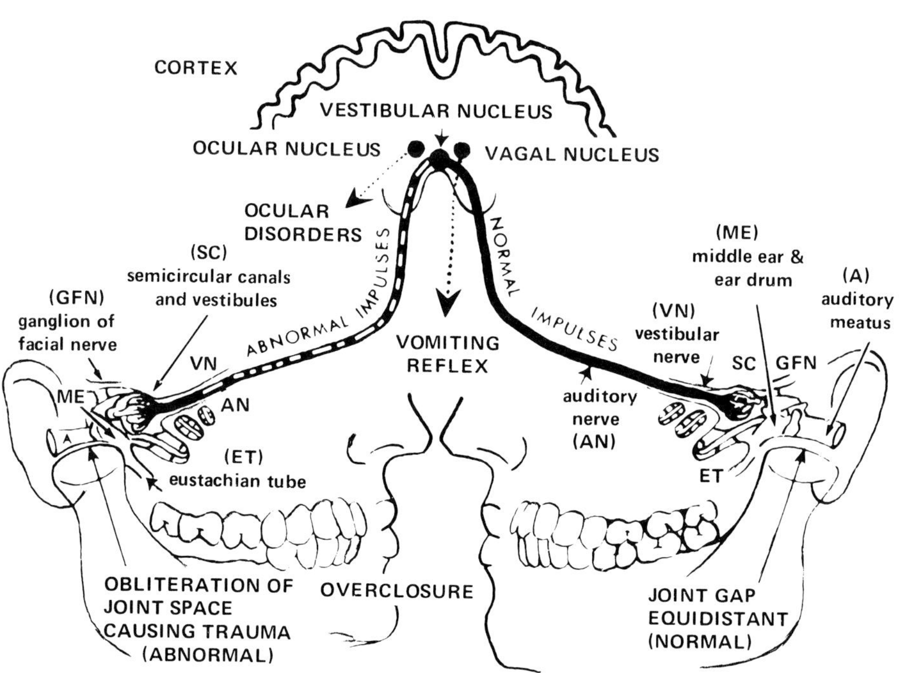

FIG. 5-10. Normal and pathological functions in right and left temporomandibular joints.

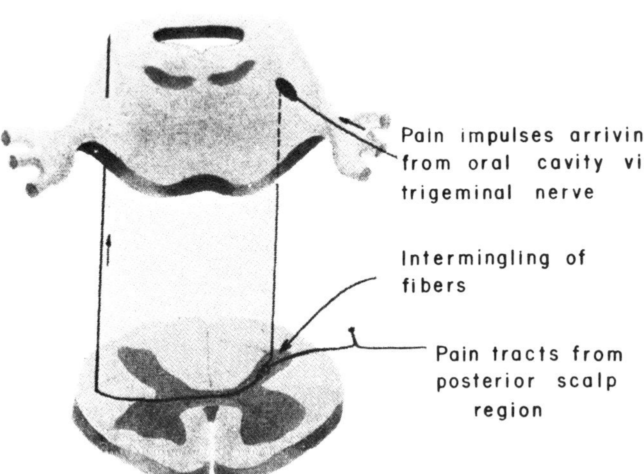

FIG. 5-11. The explanation for referred pain according to the convergence-projection theory. (Redrawn from Netter, F.: Ciba Clinical Symposia, Ciba Pharmaceutical Products, Inc. *In* Langley, L. L., and Cheraskin, E.: The Physiological Foundation of Dental Practice. ed. 2. St. Louis, C. V. Mosby, 1956)

when the pain receptors of the teeth have been stimulated by occlusal trauma and the pain is perceived in the nuchal area of the scalp and the back of the neck. This is due to the close anatomic relationship, at the dorsal horn, of the spinal fifth tract and the afferent fibers of the 2nd and the 3rd cervical nerves innervating the nuchal area. Both afferents ascend by way of the same secondary path, the spinothalamic tract. Thus the cortex mistakenly identifies the *pain stimulus* from the teeth as *pain* in the nuchal area. This anatomical intermingling (Figs. 5-8 and 5-11) explains this phenomenon. Other similar anatomical relationships exist which help explain referred pains in the head, the neck, the shoulder and the arms.

Of the two theories of referred pain, the facilitation theory and the convergence-projection theory, the latter seems to be more tenable.

Threshold of Pain

"The stimulus which possesses just sufficient strength, and no more, to set up an impulse is said to have an intensity of threshold value."[2] It has been found that the threshold value may be decreased as much as 35 per cent in the zone of noxious stimulation which results in hyperalgesia[18] of the area so stimulated. The observations of Robertson et al.[46] on the lowering of the pain threshold of teeth following noxious stimulation are similar to the observations of Lewis and Hess[46] and of Schumacher[46] on the lowering of pain threshold on the skin.

It has also been demonstrated that an agent was present in the blister fluid of skin injured by heat which was capable of lowering the pain threshold in a healthy site in which the fluid was injected.[46]

Thus, common non-noxious stimuli such as cold or hot can induce pain in a traumatized or diseased tooth. The characteristically throbbing tooth pain can be the result of such ordinarily non-noxious stimuli as cardiac systole, dilation of blood vessels and edema.

Therefore, it can be stated that ordinarily inadequate stimuli become noxious stimuli in a tooth with a lowered pain threshold. The result will be pain and minor tissue changes such as edema and vasodilation; these conditions are capable

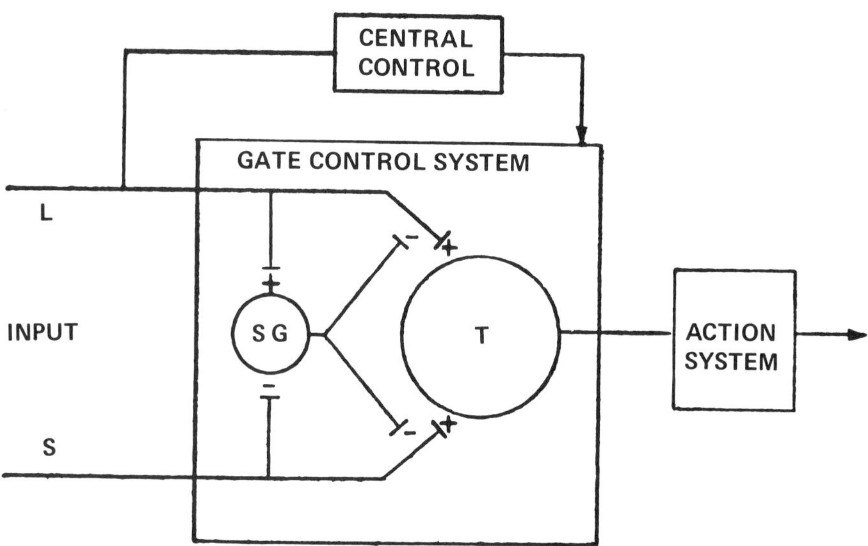

FIG. 5-12. Diagram of the gate control theory of pain mechanisms: L, the large-diameter fibers; S, the small-diameter fibers. The fibers project to the substantia gelatinosa (SG) and first central transmission (T) cells. The inhibitory effect exerted by SG on the afferent fiber terminals is increased by activity in L fibers and decreased by activity in S fibers. The central control trigger is represented by a line running from the large-fiber system to the central control mechanisms; these mechanisms, in turn, project back to the gate control system. The T cells project to the entry cells of the action system. +, Excitation; −, inhibition.

of producing impulses which cause central spread of excitatory effects. The ultimate result is head pain far removed from the point of stimulation.[58]

Gate Control Theory

A relatively recent theory of pain perception is the gate control theory, a description of which follows.*

There are two types of sensory neurons activated by noxious stimuli. Small diameter fibers are slow conducting, usually unmyelinated, and have a relatively high threshold for activation. Large diameter fibers are rapid conducting, myelinated, and have a low threshold for activation.[1] The two different kinds of fibers synapse in the spinal cord both with a substantia gelatinosa (SG) cell, and with a first central transmission (T) cell. Large fibers activate the SG and the T cells; small fibers inhibit SG cells but activate T cells (Fig. 5-12).

The T cell is responsible for the transmission of impulses from both large and small fibers, and the SG cell presynaptically inhibits transmission of these impulses. Thus, an impulse from a large fiber is initially transmitted but lessens in intensity because of simultaneous activation of the SG cell. On the other hand, stimulation of small fibers opens the gate for the transmission of pain-producing impulses by inhibiting the SG cell. In general, whenever a condition inactivates large fibers in excess of small fibers, noxious stimuli will cause the transmission of impulses with resultant pain perception.

Head Pain of Dental Origin

The head pain of dental origin is referred pain. If a maxillary tooth is excessively stimulated electrically, the result

* Mahan, P.: Personal communication, 1973.

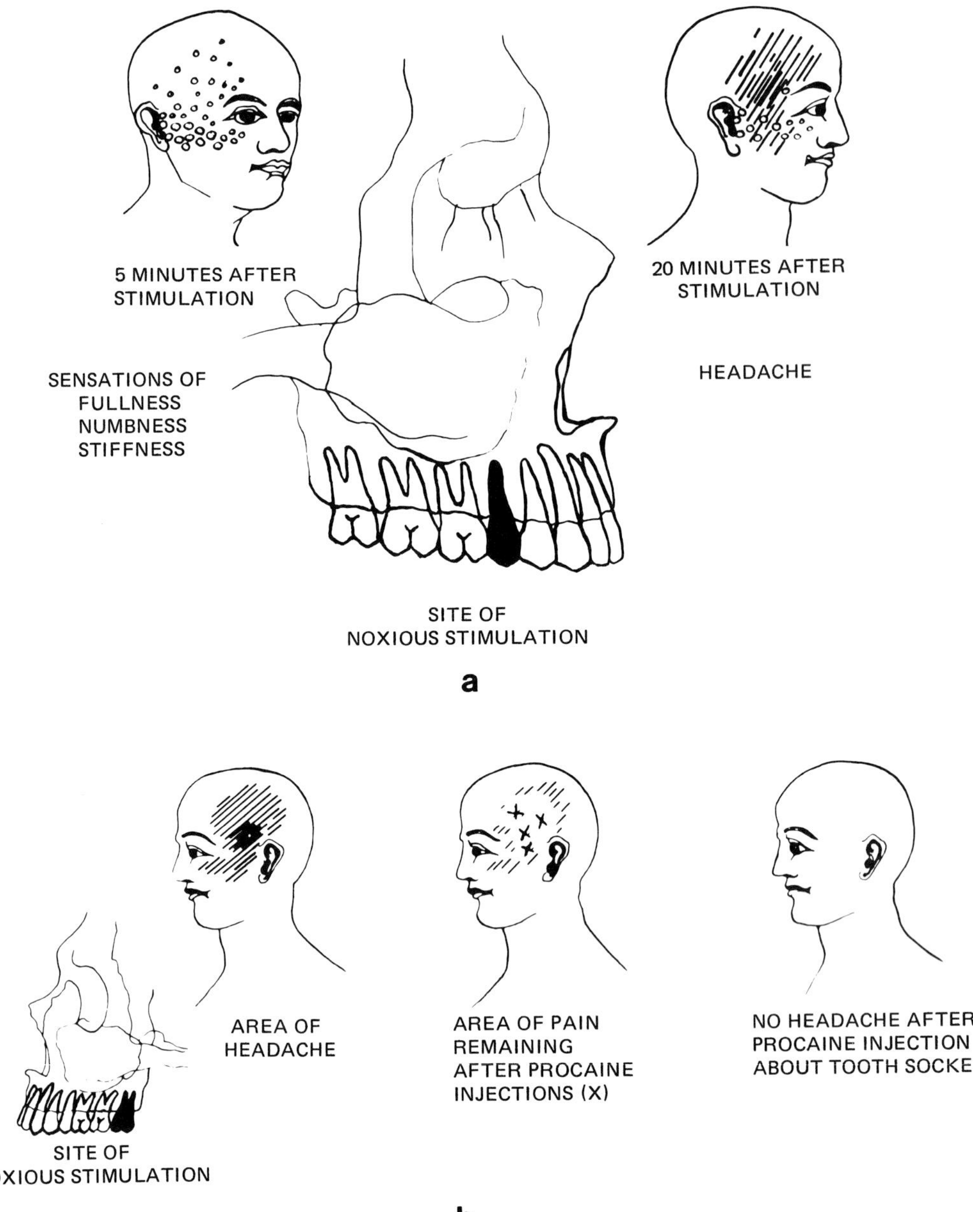

FIG. 5-13. Distribution of sensations of fullness, numbness and stiffness and distribution of headache following noxious stimulation of a tooth on the right side of the upper jaw (*a*). Area of headache following noxious stimulation of a tooth and the effect of injections of procaine into the painful area, as compared with the effect of injection of procaine into the site of noxious impulses (*b*). (Wolff, H. G.: Headache and Other Head Pain. New York, Oxford, 1963)

will be an aching tooth, and the pain will pulse throughout the area supplied by the maxillary division of the trigeminal nerve. It will also radiate to the regions supplied by the ophthalmic and mandibular branches. At the end of electrical stimulation of the tooth, the toothache will disappear, but a pain will persist in

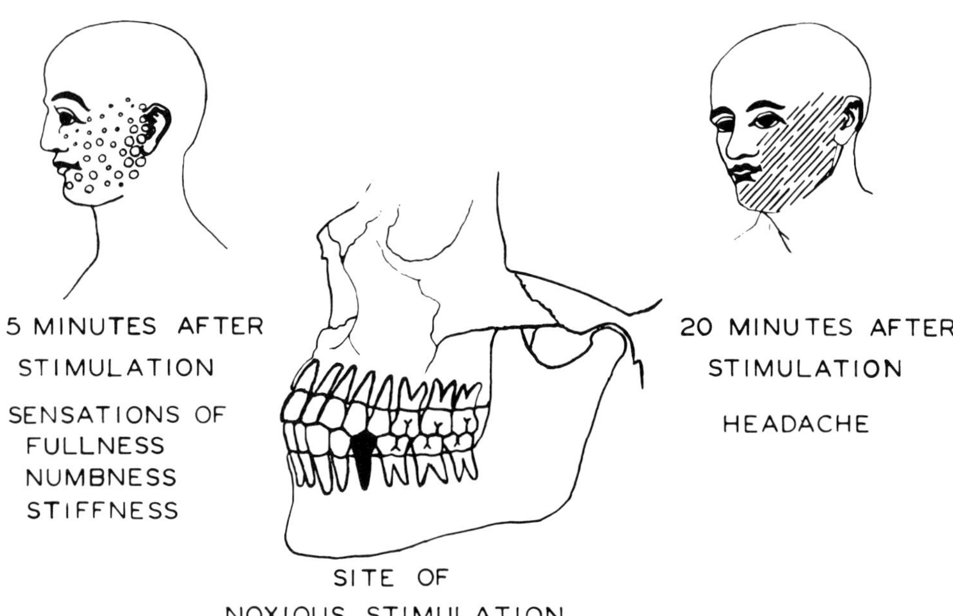

FIG. 5-14. Distribution of sensations of fullness, numbness and stiffness and of headache following noxious stimulation of a tooth in the left side of the lower jaw. (After Wolff, H. G.: Headache and Other Head Pain. New York, Oxford, 1963)

the zygomatic and the temporal areas. The infiltration of anesthetic in the zygomatic and the temporal areas will abate the head pain, but anesthetic infiltration about the tooth will abolish the head pain. This phenomenon is illustrated in Figure 5-13. Similarly, stimulation to a mandibular tooth (Fig. 5-14), will produce a similar phenomenon of referred pain. The areas of the referred pain can be traced through the mandibular division to areas innervated by all three divisions. Continued noxious impulses from the teeth can produce persistent contraction or muscle spasms and pain of the musculature of the head, the face and the neck. Continued noxious stimulation produces effects that are distinctly different from the effects produced by brief stimulation.

A 38-year-old nurse had an excruciating toothache and headache for 2 weeks. The headache extended from the midline of the chin along the lower jaw to the top of the right ear and into the ear, into the upper jaw, into the neck below the jaw and across the back of the head. All the lower teeth on the right side ached and were tender on slight pressure. There was intense pain at the angle of the jaw, and the jaw could be opened no more than .05 cm. because of the contraction and extreme tenderness of the masseter muscle. A monocaine block of the mandibular nerve instantly eliminated all the pain in the face. The teeth remained tender to pressure for 3 to 4 minutes, until analgesia of the entire lower right side of the jaw was complete. The mouth could be opened with but slight discomfort. There remained tenderness and pain in the right side of the neck and both superficial and deep tenderness and headache over both sides of the back of the head and neck. This is illustrated in Figure 5-15.

These observations demonstrate further that the pain resulting from central spread of excitation over all sensory portions of the involved segments is immediately abolished when the primary source of noxious impulses is blocked. In addition, however, these observations show that sustained contractions of the muscles of the head and neck secondary to noxious impulses arising in any part of the head become in themselves a basis of complaint and headache. These persist for some

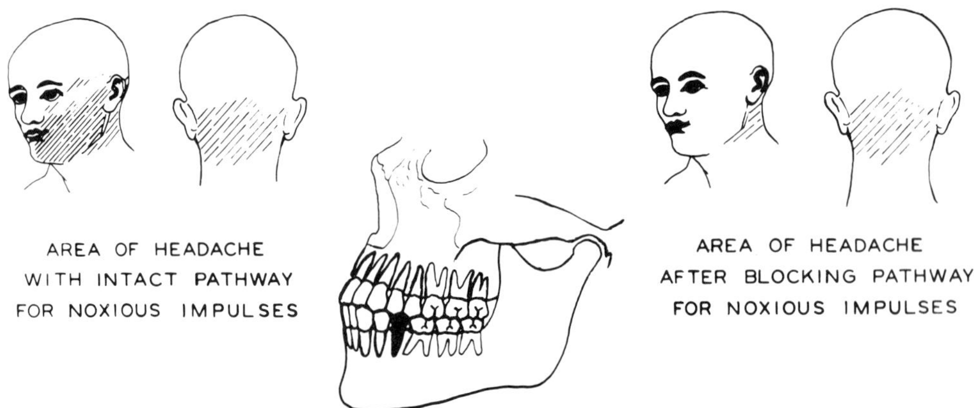

FIG. 5-15. Area of distribution of headache accompanying prolonged noxious stimulation in the lower jaw, showing headache primarily due to the central spread of the effects of noxious impulses arising in the diseased tooth and headache secondarily arising from contraction of muscles in the head and the neck. The former was abolished by blocking the pathway for noxious impulses, whereas the latter persisted for several hours. (After Wolff, H. G.: Headache and Other Head Pain. New York, Oxford, 1963)

time after elimination of the primary source of noxious impulses. Such a residual muscle pain is similar to that which occurs after the vascular components of migraine headache have been eliminated by ergotamine tartrate. In the case of the teeth, this pain from sustained muscular contraction is notably in the masseter and temporalis muscles, in addition to the muscles of the occiput and neck. Occasionally, therefore, pain from such sustained muscular contraction may be a dominant feature of the discomfort from noxious impulses arising in the teeth.[59]

Cerebellum

The cerebellum is the center of integration and coordination. It modifies muscular activity in relation to sensory data. Proprioceptive impulses that traverse the dorsal and the ventral spinocerebellar tracts and the chief sensory nucleus of the trigeminal nerve reach the cerebellum, and it is these sensory data that are used to modify muscular activity. These proprioceptive impulses through the chief sensory nucleus of the trigeminal nerve make the individual aware of varying tension on temporomandibular joints, ligaments and musculature of the stomatognathic system.

In the cerebellum, proprioceptive impulses from all parts of the body are integrated and sent to the appropriate cerebral motor cortex area. The motor cortex fires the cerebellum, which in turn modifies muscular response.

It is the stimulation of the proprioceptors in the periodontal ligament and their direct connection with the cerebellum that probably initiate habitual and other mandibular occlusal positions.

In order to understand the great significance of proprioceptive guidance, one has to study the normal automatic closing movement of the average individual with a full and normal dentition. If one opens the jaws wide and then snaps the jaws shut, the closing muscles pull the jaws unerringly and unhesitatingly into the position of full occlusion. In a mouth with a normal or even with an average dentition, there is no meeting of cusps on inclined planes, no gliding along these surfaces, no "premature" or "initial" contact but an instantaneous and correct intercuspation, vertical and horizontal overlap. In this position, the condyles, in the overwhelming majority of individuals, are slightly in front of their "most retruded" position; in other words, the capsule is not in a state of unique tension but is in all its parts more or less relaxed. This in turn must be interpreted as ruling out proprioceptors of the capsule as directing the automatic closing of the jaws. The only precise guiding signals are the proprioceptive stimuli originating in the periodontal ligaments. If the upper and lower teeth are brought into full contact, the sum total of periodontal stress and, therefore, the sum of all periodontal proprioceptive stimuli, is wholly unique and of an unsurpassed exactness and accuracy. . . . Since these stimuli are set off only at the moment of closure, how can they *lead* the movement into closure exactly in the median occlusal position?

We have to remember that a directed movement, such as that described, is not unique in our body. Neurologists, testing proprioceptive nerves and neural pathways, have long since used a simple movement among their battery of tests. The patient, with his eyes closed or bandaged, is asked to touch the tip of his nose with the tip of his forefinger. If there is no nervous disease, he will be able to do so without any difficulty—but still with some slight variations that may amount to two or three mm. to one side or the other. Here again, proprioceptive signals play the role of leading the movements of shoulder, elbow, wrist, and finger into a certain efficient, though not precise, position. These stimuli, forming in their totality a recognizable and retainable pattern, arise, of course, in all participating muscles and joints. This pattern must be retained in the "memory banks" of our brain, in all probability in what neuroanatomists know to exist as closed neuronal circuits. Evidently, as proved by the experiment, this proprioceptive memory is efficient enough, but not in any way as accurate and precise as that leading the muscle action in mandibular closure. The precision of this movement depends on the precision of periodontal load, by far surpassing that of muscle tension or stimuli in a capsule that is not in an extreme (and therefore unique) position. The "memory" of the periodontal stimulation in full occlusal position leads, therefore, during automatic closure of the jaws, by a feedback to the acting muscles.

One more fact, however, has to be taken into consideration. The "engram," that is the neuronal representation of the proprioceptive memory, cannot be rigid and perpetual. The eruptive movements of the teeth, their attrition followed by mesial drift, and other changes of their position make it unquestionably necessary that this "engram" changes almost continually. Such an engram has to be "reinforced" or reestablished ever so often if it is to function as part of a memory bank. In the case of closing the jaws, this reinforcement takes place every time we close automatically into the full occlusal position, for instance during swallowing.

However, the necessary adaptability of the closing movement has, as a consequence, a rather fast fading out of the existing engram, so that it may be changed into the new pattern that is as exact as the old one.

Thus we arrive at the inevitable conclusion that an edentulous patient is an individual whose mandibular musculature has lost its *precise* guiding signals, especially in the closing movements of the jaws. It is this loss of the periodontal proprioceptors that causes the wavering, uncertain pattern of the "bite" of edentulous patients.[48]

It should be noted that, normally, 90 per cent of the proprioception for jaw closing arises from the proprioceptors of the periodontal ligaments; the remaining 10 per cent is from the temporomandibular joint. When all of the teeth are lost, the periodontal space disappears, and with it 90 per cent of the proprioceptive guiding signals necessary for accurate jaw closing. Thus, when a patient has lost all his teeth and is being fitted for dentures, he has only 10 per cent of the normal degree of proprioception; this is why obtaining an accurate fit is such an extremely difficult problem.

Muscular movement is highly complex and usually involves the use of four types of muscles: prime movers, which move the part of the body; antagonists, which oppose the prime movers; synergists, which aid the prime movers; and fixation muscles, which control the joints to effect appropriate movement of the part.

For example, in order to close the mouth, the M. masseter acts as a prime mover. This muscle is aided by the action of the M. temporalis and M. pterygoideus internus. These latter muscles are considered to be synergists. All of these muscles are opposed by the action of the M. pterygoideus externus and M. mylohyoideus, for example, which are antagonists and serve as a brake, limiting and smoothing the action of the prime movers. The M. temporalis, by its ability to retrude the jaw, acts as a fixation muscle and limits the action of the temporomandibular joint.[28]

The cerebellum coordinates the complex interaction of the four groupings of muscles but does not inaugurate their motor activity.

There are several important things to note with respect to the relationship between the nervous system and the oral cavity:

1. Exteroceptors initiate chewing by touch and taste.
2. Pain receptors serve as a warning mechanism.
3. The proprioceptive mechanism is responsible for awareness of motion and position.
4. The proprioceptive mechanism is responsible for the control of the position of the mandible.
5. Integration in the central nervous system regulates muscle reaction and can be either conscious or unconscious.

MUSCLES

The muscles of the stomatognathic system are masseter, temporal, internal pterygoid, external pterygoid, mylohyoid, geniohyoid, digastric, infrahyoid, sternothyroid, sternocleidomastoid, sternohyoid, thyrohyoid and the muscles of facial expression. From the point of view of function, the muscles in and about the oral cavity may be divided into three groups: mastication, deglutition and facial expression. A muscle may act in more than one group; muscles do not act singly but in groups. The problems of neuromuscular physiology and their pathological possibilities are distinctly related to daily practice.

The muscle fiber is the basic unit of muscles. A motor unit is made up of a muscle fiber and its innervating motor neuron. A single neuron may innervate many fibers, but the more specialized the muscular activity, the less fibers per neuron. This allows small groups of fibers to act without involvement of adjoining muscle bundles. The muscular activity in the head and the neck is highly specialized, as illustrated by the complex and infinitely fine movements of the tongue.

Work is produced by muscle action only when one end is held stabilized or fixed while the muscle contracts. This is isotonic contraction which occurs when a muscle shortens and the tension is maintained. Stimulation of the masseter when the mouth is open will cause the mouth to close; this is isotonic contraction. Isotonic contraction occurs in all movements of the mandible.

However, the greatest pressures are developed when a muscle contracts isometrically—that is, when both ends of the muscle are stationary, as when the teeth are together and there is contraction of the muscles. This produces muscle strain and the greatest degree of force on the periodontium. The neuromuscular physiology of the stomatognathic musculature plays an important part in the understanding of the clenching habits, muscle spasms or hypertonicity, and dysfunction of the whole system.

Because muscle fibers obey the all-or-none law, the stimulation of only one fiber will cause it to contract completely or not at all. By recruitment, added units of graded stimuli of higher threshold produce gradation in contractile forces. In the phenomenon of summation we see that muscle can be stimulated again, during the contraction phase before it can relax, and thus produce continuous contraction or tetany. On the other hand, the state of contracture of a muscle can exist because of fatigue, a state of muscle shortening or partial contracture without conventional neural stimuli.

Muscle tonus is a state of partial contraction or resistance to passive tension or stretch, brought about by a continuous flow of impulses to the muscles. Muscle tonus keeps the mandible from sagging by keeping the antigravity muscles in a state of partial contracture. These originate in the muscles themselves. The so-called "rest position" of the mandible is not one of absolute rest, since the muscles of the antigravity group which maintain the jaw in this position must be in a state of slight contraction maintained by the tonus mechanism. This phenomenon has been demonstrated by Moyers[34] in his electromyographic experiments. If muscular resistance is encountered in trying to open the mouth of a patient, and if the resistance is involuntary on the part of the patient, this state of resistance is called hypertonus. Hypotonus exists when the patient's mouth hangs open and there is a lack of resistance to tension. Tonus depends upon neural integration. Hypertonus, due to the overactivity of the innervating nerves, produces a state of spasticity. Hypertrophy is the increase in the bulk of the individual muscle fiber but not of the number of fibers. Hypertrophy is the result of intensified functional activity. Disuse of muscle fibers results in their diminution in size; this result is called atrophy.

The activators of the cycle which results in muscle action are the sensory receptors in the body.

A specialized sensory end organ, the spindle, found in the muscles and the proprioceptors in the periodontal ligaments, acts to relate the position or the posture of related structures to their environment (i.e., tooth relation to alveolus by way of the periodontal ligament; mandibular relation to the skull by way of the muscles). The proprioceptors in the periodontal ligament are thus actively integrated with the muscles of mastication.

The Masseter Muscle

The masseter muscle is rectangular and stretches from the zygomatic arch to the angle of the mandibular ramus (Fig. 5-16). The superficial portion attaches to the lower border of the zygomatic bone, and its fibers extend down and back to their insertion on the angle of the ramus. The upper third of its outer surface is covered by tendinous fibers, but the muscle itself is formed by an intricate arrangement of tendinous and fleshy bundles. The net effect of this construction is to make the muscle an extremely powerful one. The deep portion of the masseter is fused anteriorly to the superficial portion but is separable from it posteriorly. Its fibers attach to the entire length of the zygomatic arch (unlike the superficial portion, which does not attach to the temporal part of the arch at all), and it inserts into the base of the coronoid process and the upper part of the ramus. The masseter is innervated by the masseteric nerve, which enters the muscle through the semilunar notch of the mandible. The blood supply is the masseteric artery, a branch of the internal maxillary artery. The masseter functions as an elevator of the jaw, and its deep portion acts as a retractor as well.[48]

The Temporal Muscle

The temporal muscle is a fan-shaped muscle originating on the lateral surface of the skull and inserting on the coronoid process and along the ramus (Fig. 5-16). The anterior fibers of the muscle are vertical, the middle are oblique, and the posterior are almost horizontal. Its terminal tendon is attached to the apex of the coronoid process. Other fibers attach to the lateral surface of the coronoid process and still others to the posterior end of the alveolar process. The most superficial fibers of the temporal muscle are fused with the deep portion of the masseter. The muscle itself is constructed similarly to the masseter, insofar as it has the same alternation of fleshy and tendinous parts. It is innervated by the three temporal nerves of the third division of the trigeminal nerve, and its blood supply is from

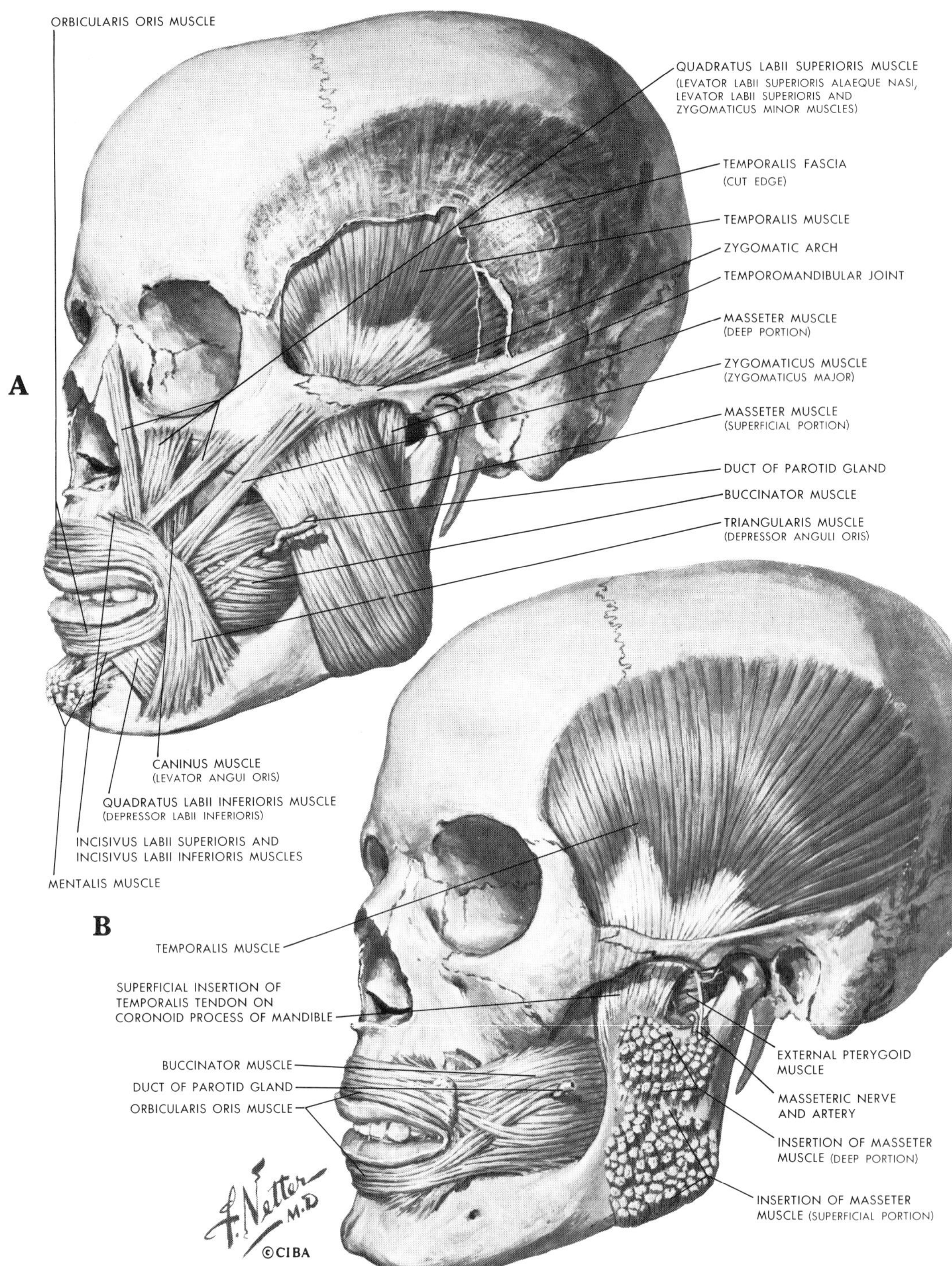

FIG. 5-16. Drawing of the masseter and temporal muscles, viewed from the left side. (*A*) the masseter is intact; (*B*) it has been out away, showing the insertion of its deep and superficial fibers, as well as the insertion of the tendon of the temporal muscle. (© Copyright 1959 CIBA Pharmaceutical Company, Division of CIBA-GEIGY Corporation. Reproduced, with permission, from THE CIBA COLLECTION OF MEDICAL ILLUSTRATIONS by Frank H. Netter, M.D. All rights reserved.)

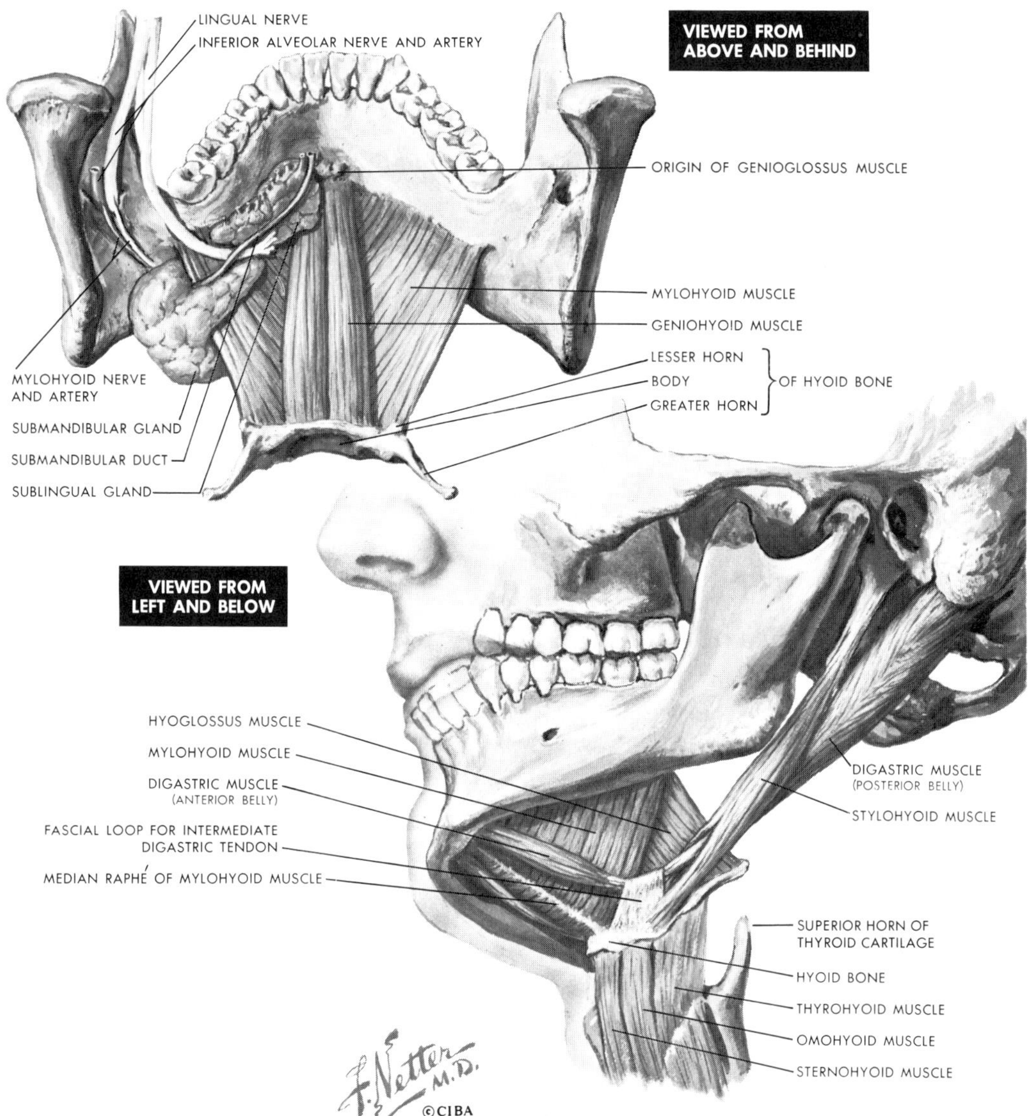

FIG. 5-17. The suprahyoid muscles: (*Top*) view from above and behind; (*bottom*) view from the left and below. (© Copyright 1959 CIBA Pharmaceutical Company, Division of CIBA-GEIGY Corporation. Reproduced, with permission, from THE CIBA COLLECTION OF MEDICAL ILLUSTRATIONS by Frank H. Netter, M.D. All rights reserved.)

the middle and deep temporal arteries. The temporal muscle functions primarily as an elevator of the lower jaw, although its horizontal posterior fibers may also serve as retractors.[48]

The Suprahyoid Muscles

The suprahyoid muscles are the stylohyoid, mylohyoid, digastric and geniohyoid (Fig. 5-17). The most important of these in terms of mandibular movements are the digastric and the geniohyoid.

The digastric muscle consists of an anterior and a posterior belly connected by a strong round tendon. The posterior belly, which is considerably longer than the anterior one, attaches to the mastoid process, and the anterior belly attaches to

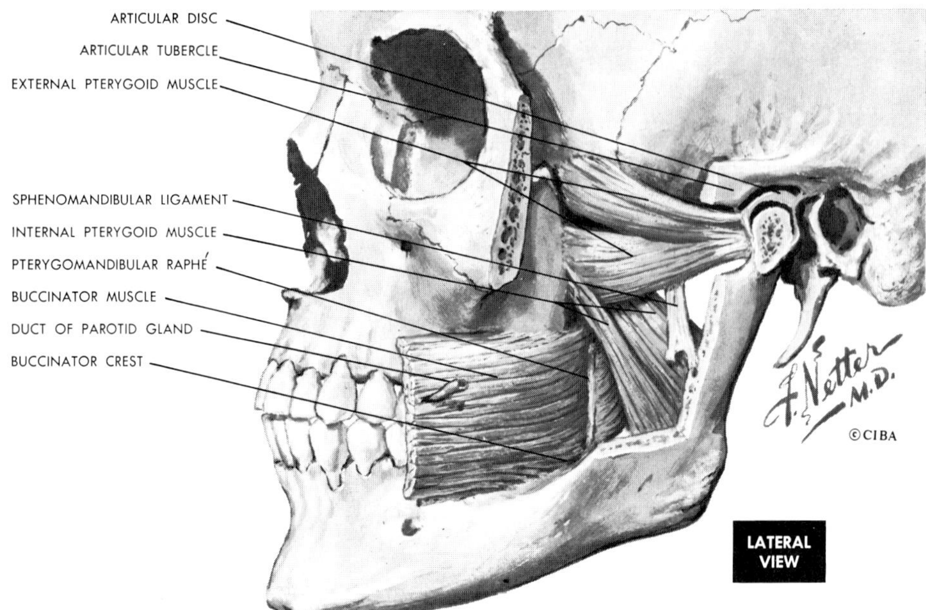

FIG. 5-18. Lateral view of the medial and lateral pterygoid muscles. (© Copyright 1959 CIBA Pharmaceutical Company, Division of CIBA-GEIGY Corporation. Reproduced, with permission, from THE CIBA COLLECTION OF MEDICAL ILLUSTRATIONS by Frank H. Netter, M.D. All rights reserved.)

the digastric fossa near the middle of the front of the mandible. The intermediate tendon attaches to the hyoid bone by means of fibers of the deep cervical fascia, which forms a loop around the tendon. The innervation of the posterior belly is from a branch of the facial nerve; that of the anterior belly is from a branch of the mylohyoid nerve. The function of the digastric muscle is to pull the mandible back and down.

The geniohyoid muscle attaches from the midline to the mental spines of the mandible and inserts on the upper half of the hyoid bone. The muscle is wider posteriorly than anteriorly, and like the digastric, acts to pull the mandible back and down.[48]

The Medial Pterygoid Muscle

The medial pterygoid muscle is essentially the counterpart of the masseter. It is located on the medial side of the ramus, and like the masseter is a rectangular muscle, although it is less powerful (Fig. 5-18). It arises from the medial surface of the lateral pterygoid plate and runs down and back to its insertion on the medial surface of the mandibular angle. Like the masseter, its construction is characterized by an alternation of fleshy and tendinous parts. It is innervated by the medial pterygoid nerve, which branches off the third division of the trigeminal nerve, and it is supplied by a branch of the internal maxillary artery. Its primary function is to elevate the mandible.[48]

The Lateral Pterygoid Muscle

The lateral pterygoid arises with two heads; the inferior attaches to the outer surface of the pterygoid plate, and the smaller superior head attaches to the infratemporal crest of the greater wing of the sphenoid bone. The two heads form a tendon of insertion in front of the temporomandibular joint (Fig. 5-19). In his recent work on the anatomy of the lateral pterygoid muscles, Porter chose the superior approach to the dissection of the

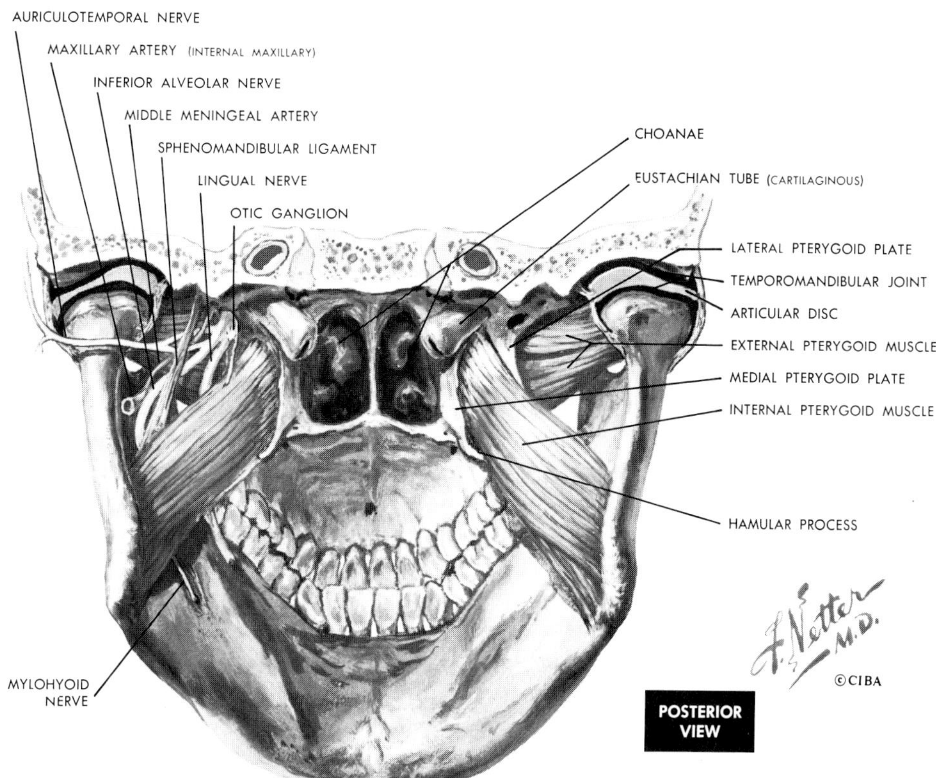

FIG. 5-19. This is a posterior view of the left temporomandibular joint illustrating the external pterygoid muscle. (© Copyright 1959 CIBA Pharmaceutical Company, Division of CIBA-GEIGY Corporation. Reproduced, with permission, from THE CIBA COLLECTION OF MEDICAL ILLUSTRATIONS by Frank H. Netter, M.D. All rights reserved.)

muscle as that which would result in the least distortion.[42]

Figure 5-19 is a posteroinferior view showing the external pterygoid muscles at a 45° angle from the origin to the insertion. Usually lateral views of the sections of the temporomandibular joint are seen and one does not think of the condyle as looking like a fist. We must realize that the mandible is a single bone with two complex joints at the ends of the bone. Porter's investigations show that most of the fibers of the superior head insert into the anterior portion of the meniscus and that some attach to the anterior medial and medial portions, extending to the posterior end of the meniscus. The fibers of the inferior head attach to the pterygoid fovea on the neck of the condyle, with some fibers attaching as well to the medial portion of the condyle.

The lateral pterygoid is innervated by a branch of the masseteric nerve, and the blood supply is from a branch of the internal maxillary artery. Its primary function is as a protractor of the jaw. Function on only one side results in a shift of the mandible toward the nonfunctioning side (Bennett movement). The medial attachment of the lateral pterygoid to the condyle and the meniscus is significant in stabilizing the temporomandibular joint during bilateral protrusion and retrusion of the mandible. This muscle is particularly important in cases of temporomandibular joint dysfunction (for a full discussion, see Chap. 8).

BONES

The forces produced by a functioning stomatognathic system are transmitted to a complex of bones—skull, mandible, hyoid, clavicle and sternum. Bone is one of the most plastic of all tissues, readily adjusting its structure and form to adapt to external forces. The forces involved in occlusion, mastication, deglutition, speech, respiration and facial expression influence the architecture of bone as to type, amount and distribution.

The hyoid bone is important in deglutition and in all movements of the mandible. During deglutition the mouth is closed, and the mylohyoid, the geniohyoid and the digastric muscles raise the hyoid bone which, in turn, elevates the larynx and the lower part of the pharynx. When the hyoid bone is stabilized by the infrahyoid muscles, the contractions of the mylohyoid, the geniohyoid and the digastric muscles pull the mandible downward.

PERIODONTAL LIGAMENT

Essentially, the periodontal "membrane" functions as a ligament. As in all ligaments, the fibers are arranged in accordance with the functional demands upon them. In the case of the periodontal ligament, the functional demands upon the teeth affect the arrangement of the fibers. The basic functions of the periodontal ligament are to cushion the transmission of occlusal forces to the bone, to act as shock absorbers, to maintain the teeth in their normal functional positions and, through the proprioceptive mechanism, to alert the individual to abnormal occlusal relationships. The physiology of the dentoalveolar joint, so closely associated with the periodontal ligament, has been discussed in Chapter 4.

VASCULAR SYSTEM

The basic function of the vascular supply of the stomatognathic system is to provide the metabolites and to remove the waste products of metabolism. Because of the high level of metabolism of the stomatognathic system, nature has supplied it with a rich vascular complex with many anastomoses between individual vessels. The vascular system is also important as a protective mechanism. It contains both cells and plasma elements that are needed to resist, combat and repair the ravages of inflammatory reactions, bacterial invasions and traumatic insults. A detailed description of the vascular supply to the stomatognathic system may be found in any standard text on anatomy.

GROWTH AND METABOLISM

Inherent growth force must be differentiated from growth resulting from functional stimulation. The former is growth that occurs because of the genetic configuration and without any known functional stimulation. It is the force that causes tooth buds to develop into teeth.

Metabolism is of prime importance in the establishment of the occlusion. Bone development and composition, tooth formation and muscle tone all depend upon proper metabolism. Any metabolic disturbance may upset the normal rhythm of growth with direct and deleterious consequences to the occlusion. As a specific example, calcium deficiency not only causes rickets but also affects the growth of the jaws, interferes with tooth calcification, delays eruption and induces muscle hypertonicity.

Muscle action is a primary functional stimulus for the development of the maxilla and the mandible. Proper growth and development of these bones are essential if the size and the shape of the dental arches are to be normal and if there is to be correct alignment and adequate space for the teeth. The lips, the cheeks and the tongue act directly in forming and maintaining the occlusion. Especially during the act of swallowing, the lips and the cheeks press on the labial and the buccal surfaces of the teeth in reaction to the expanding force of the tongue.

Normal and harmoniously functioning temporomandibular joints are important prerequisites for a correct occlusal relationship of the teeth. Should the movements of one condyle be limited in a young growing person, the shape of the fossa and the articular eminence will be altered because of decreased function during an active period of growth. This unilateral mastication, in turn, changes the axial inclinations of the teeth.

Every time a human being swallows, atmospheric pressure acts as an important force. In the final stage of deglutition, a partial vacuum is created in the oral cavity, and the atmospheric pressure in the nasal cavity forces the bony palate to descend. This is especially evident during the stages of active growth when the palatal bones are thin and react readily to pressure. This downward growth of the palate helps to expand the upper arch.

The development of the *anteroposterior curve of Spee* and the *transverse curve of Wilson* results from muscle action and degree of slope of the articular eminence. The transverse curve is caused by lateral mandibular movements. The curve of Spee extends from the incisal edges of the lower incisors backward to the buccal cusps of the bicuspids and the molars. This curve should not be confused with the compensating curve which describes an arrangement of a series of artificial teeth in a curve so designed that certain mechanical advantages may be gained when they are used in chewing.

HORIZONTAL AND VERTICAL OVERBITES

The horizontal overbite or overjet is the distance in the horizontal plane between the lingual surfaces of the upper teeth and the labial surfaces of the lower teeth, H.O. (Fig. 5-20). An edge-to-edge bite displays a zero horizontal overbite.

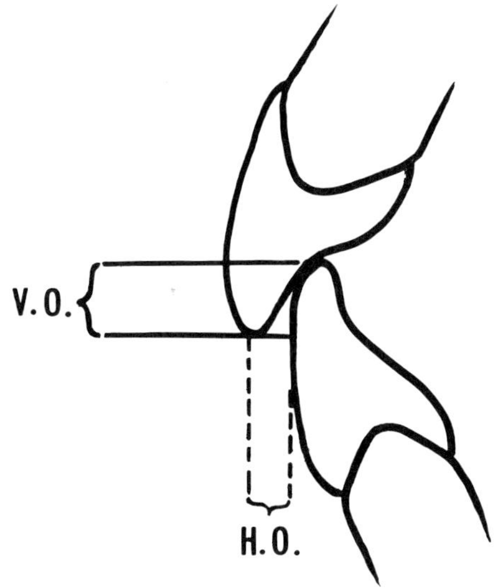

FIG. 5-20. The horizontal and the vertical overbites.

The vertical overbite is the vertical distance between the incisal edges of the upper and the lower incisors when they overlap, V.O. (Fig. 5-20). An edge-to-edge bite exhibits a zero vertical overbite. In occlusions which "grind themselves in," such as occur among tobacco chewers, there is a tendency to create a zero vertical overbite. Frequently, the vertical overbite is so great that lateral mandibular movements are impossible. In such cases, the upper cuspids are usually responsible, although the upper laterals and centrals may also be guilty.

When a patient exhibits a deep vertical overbite, it does not necessarily follow that the vertical dimension is closed. The deep vertical overbite may be normal for that individual because of his genetic pattern. In making an accurate diagnosis it is important to recognize a deep normal overbite. If such a condition exists, the operator must not attempt to restore a vertical dimension which has never been lost. The criteria are the rest position of the mandible, the interocclusal distance, and the shape of the glenoid fossa.

For the teeth to occlude properly, the arch forms of the mandible and the maxilla must be congruent. Should the arch forms be in conflict, the teeth will be unable to meet in their correct inclined plane relationship.

DETERMINANTS OF MANDIBULAR MOVEMENT

The heredity of the individual determines the relative size of the jaws, the occlusal anatomy of the teeth and the anatomy of the temporomandibular joint. Forces that undertake to establish and maintain a physiologic occlusion must act within the limits established by heredity. Different schools of thought place greater or lesser emphasis on the action of the neuromuscular system, the inclined planes of the teeth and the anatomy of the temporomandibular joints as the basic factors that determine the occlusion. However, careful consideration will indicate that each of these factors has an important role in the formation and the maintenance of the occlusion. Mandibular movements are a result of neuromuscular action, but the various paths that the mandible traverses are dictated by the anteroposterior and the mesiodistal slopes of the mandibular fossae.

As the teeth erupt, their positions are determined by the inclined plane relationships, the muscles of the tongue, the lips, and the cheeks and the arcs traversed by the mandible, as dictated by the slopes of the joints in all functional masticatory movements. The curve of Spee and the transverse curve result because of both the anteroposterior and the mesiodistal slopes of the articular eminences and because of the action of the muscles which forces the inclined planes of the teeth to assume positions that attempt to prevent interference in the different mandibular movements. The lips and the cheeks act as counterbalances to the expanding force of the tongue, and this interaction helps to keep the erupting teeth in correct position while the alveolar process is growing and providing firmer anchorage.

TEETH

The teeth are not mere tools—they bear a definite physiological relationship to every component of the stomatognathic system and to the system as a whole. If the dentist is to treat the entire system successfully, he must understand the ties that bind or relate the individual parts of the stomatognathic system to each other and to the entire system. The teeth are the most important parts of this system because without them or their substitutes, physiological function of the stomatognathic system is impossible. They are the structures toward which the function of all other parts of the system is directed. Specifically, the occlusal surfaces of the teeth are the connecting links between the various parts of the stomatognathic system. When they are in harmony with each other and with all the other parts of the system, normal function takes place, stimuli are correctly transmitted from the periodontal ligament to the neuromuscular system, and normal muscular movements result. However, if there are interfering occlusal contacts, this orderly and integrated system is disrupted, and abnormal jaw movements, disease, degeneration and destruction inevitably result. The final result of this degenerative process is that the teeth can no longer perform their normal functions in mastication and deglutition.

The end result of dentistry should be the establishment of a physiologic occlusion wherein every tooth is of proper form and in proper function. However, to establish a normal occlusion the dentist must have a definite goal and concept in mind. A physiologic occlusion is one which is initiated by a correct centric-relation occlusion and produces maximal tooth contact in all ranges of occlusal articulation.

The terms "occlusion" and "articulation" mean different things to different people, and it is important to define them carefully. *Occlusion* refers to the closed position. It connotes a static state and therefore should always be considered as referring to a static closed position. *Articulation,* on the other hand, connotes movement and therefore should always be used to refer to the dynamic relationship of the teeth during mandibular movements. It is important also to emphasize the concept that *centric-relation occlusion exists when there is maximal intercuspation of the maxillary and the mandibular teeth in harmony with centric relation.*

TOOTH ANATOMY AND FUNCTION

To render the function of mastication most efficient, nature has provided man with teeth of various anatomic forms. In an omnivorous diet, neither cuspless teeth nor teeth with cusps so long that they interlock and prevent lateral movements will function effectively. Cusps, fossae, sulci, marginal ridges and inclined planes are so designed that they permit a complex rotary motion of mastication with maximal tooth contact in all ranges of occlusal articulation. A theoretically ideal anatomy of the teeth would provide that the cusps, the fossae, the sulci, the marginal ridges and the inclined planes of the teeth of one arch will interdigitate correctly and precisely with the teeth in the opposite arch. However, since nature constantly deviates from perfection of form and size in all other parts of the body, it is not surprising to find similar deviations from the ideal in the anatomy of the teeth. These variations may interfere with centric-relation occlusion.

Proximal contacts between the teeth act as stabilizers. They are responsible for continuity of arch form and for the prevention of individual tooth movement. When teeth make contact during function, there is always some slight movement, but the continual contacts act as buffers and hold the teeth in their proper positions. By doing this they help to maintain the correctly established physiologic occlusion.

The axial inclinations of the teeth are determined by the inclined plane relationship and the anterior component of force. The former determines the buccal inclination of the upper teeth and the lingual inclination of the lower teeth. The anterior component of force is responsible for the mesial inclination of the posterior teeth and the labial inclination of the anterior teeth.

Missing teeth disturb the occlusion by permitting the teeth of the same jaw to migrate and by allowing the teeth of the opposite jaw to elongate because of diminished resistance. This affects the whole pattern of occlusion by altering the inclined plane and other relationships. Unless missing teeth are replaced immediately, the occlusion cannot maintain itself in proper physiological condition.

WEAR AND OCCLUSAL TOPOGRAPHY

In his investigations of the jaws of pre-Norman-Conquest Britons, Keith[23] observed an end-to-end occlusion in the incisor region. This was the result of attrition caused by a gritty diet. In 1929, Williams[55] reported some interesting facts in his studies of Eskimos, whose diets consisted mainly of dried foods and who used their teeth to soften skins. As a result of such vigorous usage, the Eskimos' teeth were badly worn. However, they seemed to be immune to caries and to periodontitis simplex. Even though there was great wear, the teeth of the Eskimos, Williams found, were functionally efficient because of the worn enamel edges, the cupped-out portion of the dentin and the powerful musculature. He also deter-

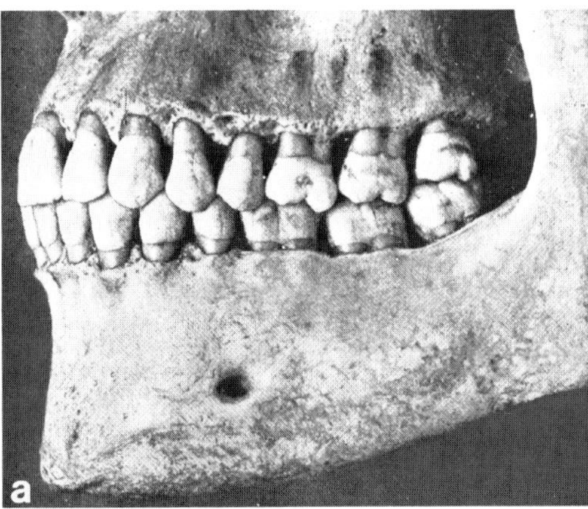

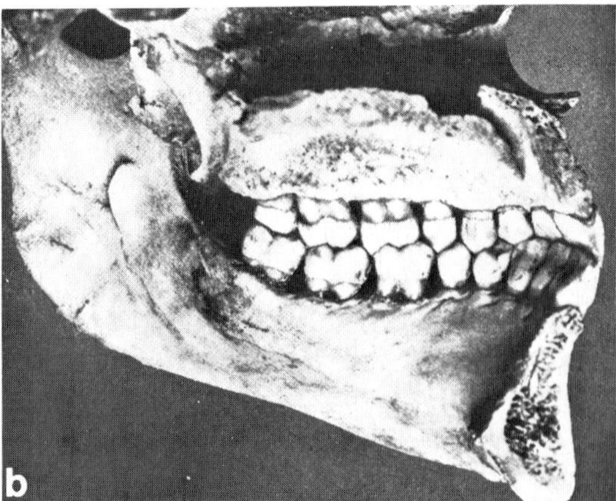

FIG. 5-21. Lateral (*a*) and lingual (*b*) views of the teeth in occlusion. (Turner, C.: American Textbook of Prosthetic Dentistry. Philadelphia, Lea & Febiger, 1932)

mined that up to the age of 68, the Eskimos have an average of 29.5 teeth present. The Eskimo occlusion tends to be functional, and there is elimination of the vertical overbite and development of an end-to-end occlusion. Eighty-seven per cent of the Eskimos studied by Williams had a zero vertical overbite. Williams' findings may be summarized as follows: distribution of the occlusal load to all the teeth; conversion of oblique to axial loading; shortening of the extraalveolar lever arm; appearance of functionally efficient inverted cusps with sharp edges of enamel as the tooth wears; postponement of closed-bite effects until the fourth degree of wear despite the large amount of wear.

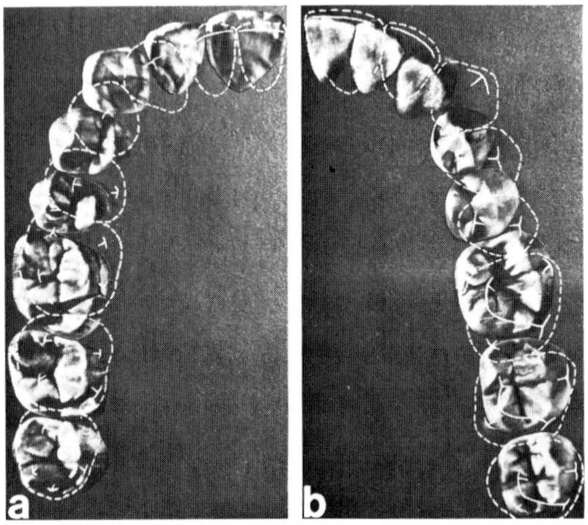

FIG. 5-22. Centric-relation occlusion: the superimposition of the teeth of the opposite arch. Outline of lower teeth superimposed on upper teeth (*a*). Outline of upper teeth superimposed on lower teeth (*b*). (Friel, E. S.: The relation of function to the size and form of the jaws. Proc. Roy. Soc. Med., *22*:53, 1921)

Many investigators[2] contend that natural wear is the proper adjustment of the occlusion. However, they do not consider the fact that a modern diet consists, for the most part, of cut and cooked foods and requires very little masticatory effort.

The equilibration of the occlusion will assist nature in her program of coordination of the cusps to produce an equal distribution of forces to as many teeth as possible as well as to produce the other side effects that take place in natural wearing of the teeth. Attrition is a compensatory mechanism in nature's plan to provide the proper physiological tolerances for the various parts of the functioning organ.

TOOTH POSITION, OCCLUSION AND ARTICULATION

The concept of centric-relation occlusion is inextricably associated with arch form, and this intimate relationship must

FIG. 5-23. Centric-relation occlusion. Numbered cusps fit into numbered fossae; lettered cusps fit into lettered fossae.

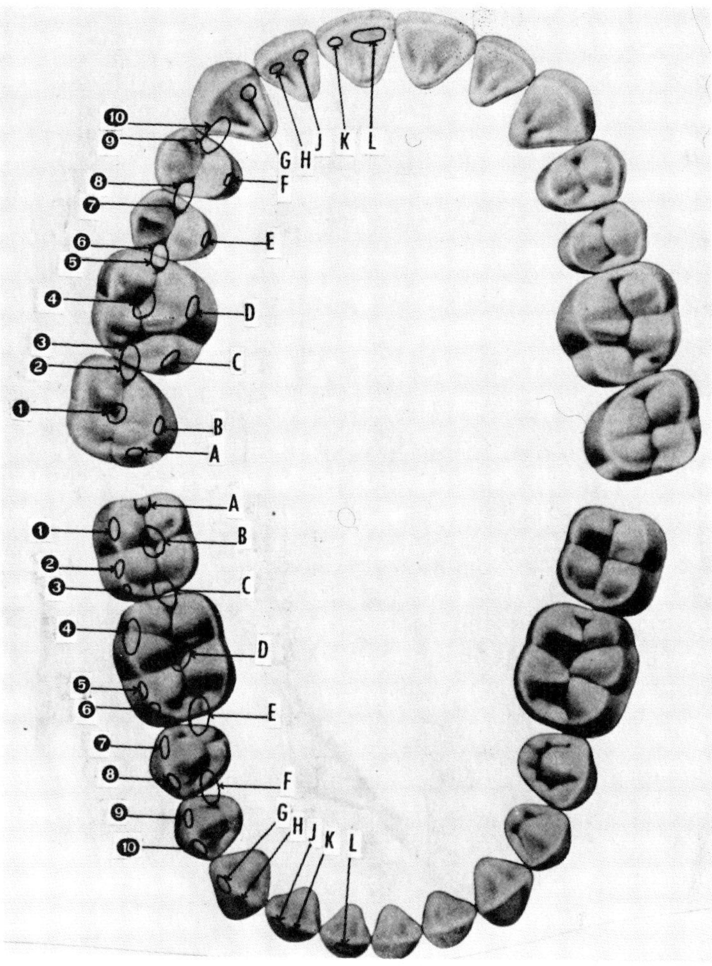

be borne in mind constantly. The tooth-to-tooth relationships are largely determined by the form of each arch and by the relationship between the form of one arch and that of the opposing one. The correctness or the defectiveness of the arch form and the tooth-to-tooth relationship becomes evident in an examination of the occlusal contact relationships. If the arch form and the tooth-to-tooth relationships are normal, the occlusal contact surfaces usually will be normal.

A thorough knowledge of the contacts in centric-relation occlusion is a prerequisite for proper procedure in occlusal equilibration. Understanding of what constitutes the normal will make recognition of deviations readily evident to the practitioner who is examining a patient's mouth prior to embarking upon occlusal equilibration.

Figure 5-21 illustrates the occlusion of the teeth from a lateral and lingual view. Figure 5-22*a* demonstrates the contact of the teeth in centric-relation occlusion; the dotted outlines of the mandibular teeth are superimposed on the maxillary teeth. Figure 5-22*b* demonstrates the contact of the teeth in centric-relation occlusion; the dotted outlines of the maxillary teeth are superimposed on the mandibular teeth. Figure 5-23 demonstrates the contacting surfaces of the teeth in centric-relation occlusion: cusp 1 fits into

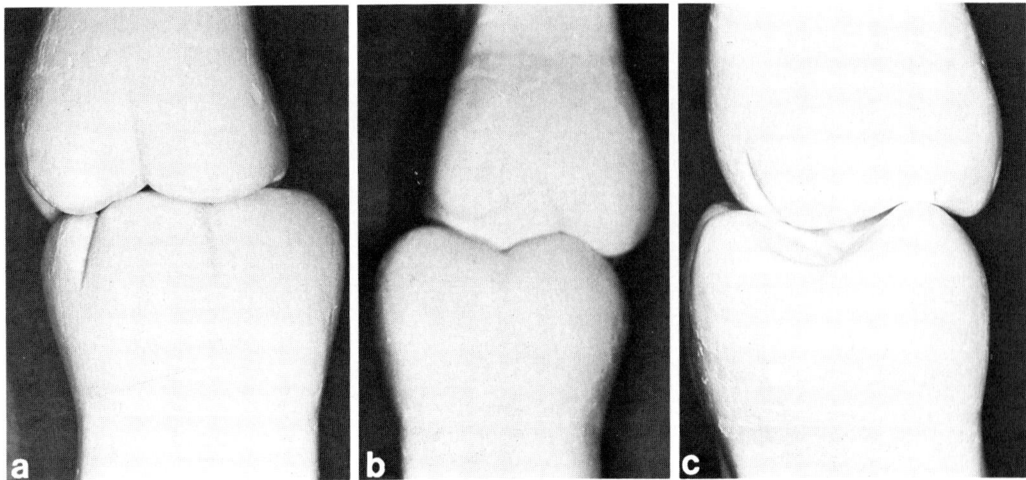

FIG. 5-24. Views of molars in centric-relation occlusion: buccal (*a*), lingual (*b*), and distal (*c*).

fossa 1; cusp 2 fits into fossa 2; and so on.

A pair of first molars illustrates the various centric and eccentric positions of the teeth. Figure 5-24 demonstrates the buccal, lingual and distal views of the maxillary and the mandibular first molars in centric-relation occlusion.

As the mandibular teeth move through the functioning range of articulation, the concept of masticatory movement must be borne in mind. The mandible moves downward and laterally until the buccal cusps of the mandibular molars are under the buccal cusps of the maxillary molars. The mandible then moves upward, and the buccal cusps of the lower molars move against the lingual inclines of the buccal cusps of the upper molars. Simul-

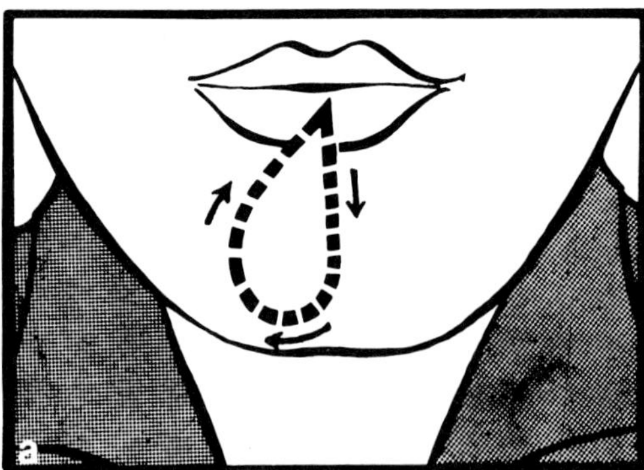

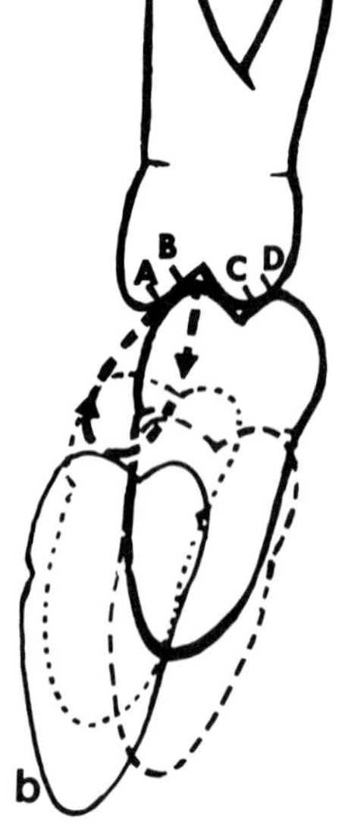

FIG. 5-25. The right functioning envelope of motion described by the mandible (*a*) and the mandibular molar (*b*).

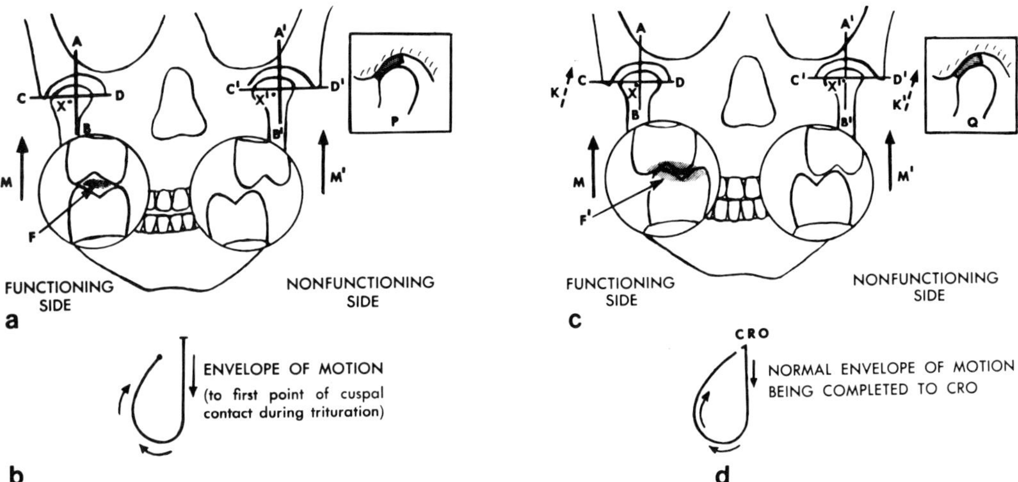

FIG. 5-26. Diagram of the mechanics that are set in motion on the functioning and the nonfunctioning sides during the envelope of motion phase of mastication.

taneously, the buccal planes of the lingual cusps of the lower molars move against the lingual cusps of the upper molars. The normal envelope of motion for the right lateral mandibular movement is illustrated in Figure 5-25*a*. The tooth-to-tooth relationships are based upon this envelope of motion. Figure 5-25*b* demonstrates the cycle of movements of the mandibular molar which is describing the envelope of motion. The glide planes AB and CD of the upper molar should be in harmony with the temporomandibular joint movement.

Figure 5-26 demonstrates the mechanics of ideal mandibular movement during the right functioning range and the left nonfunctioning range of articulation. The forces in the masticating cycle are exerted mainly on the functioning side from functioning position toward centric relation. The following conditions are present in (*a*): In trying to triturate the food, F, the elevator muscles M and M′ pull upward with equal force until the food, F, is reached and begun to be incised by the cusps. The dots X and X′ are equidistant from the original

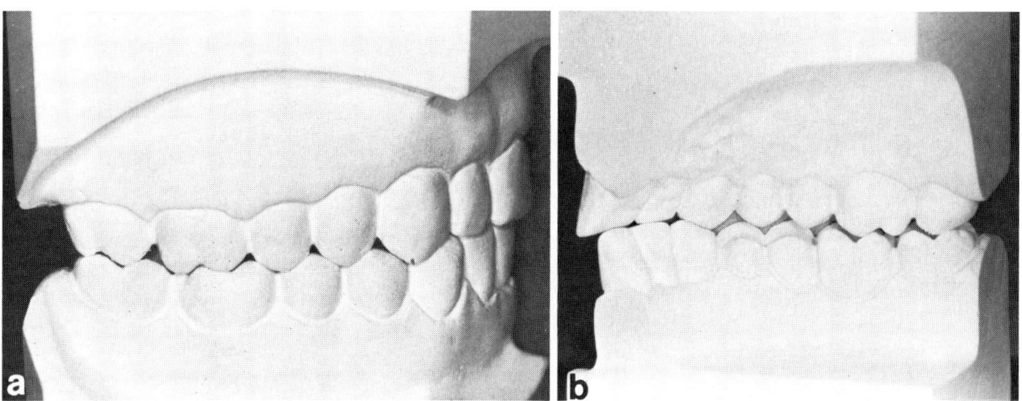

FIG. 5-27. Maxillary and mandibular teeth in the functioning position: buccal view (*a*), lingual view (*b*).

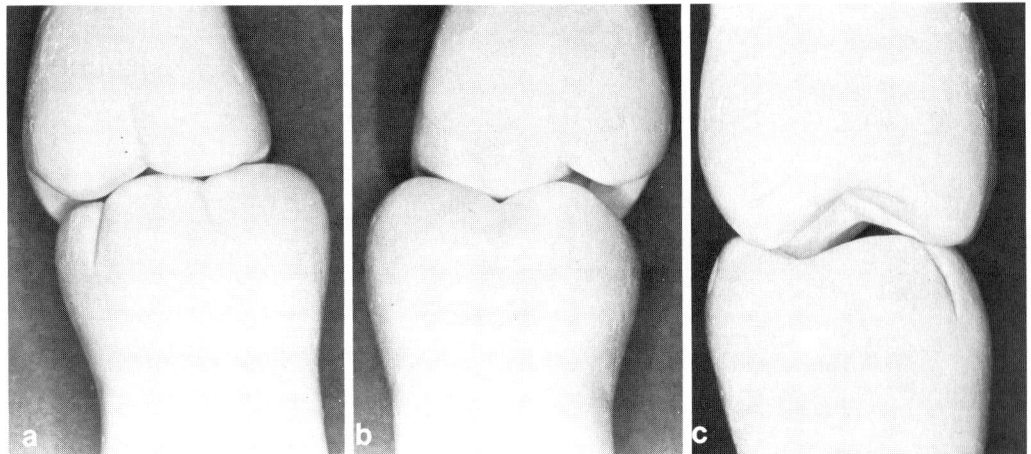

FIG. 5-28. Views of an opposing pair of right first molars at the beginning of the functioning range: buccal (*a*), lingual (*b*), and distal (*c*).

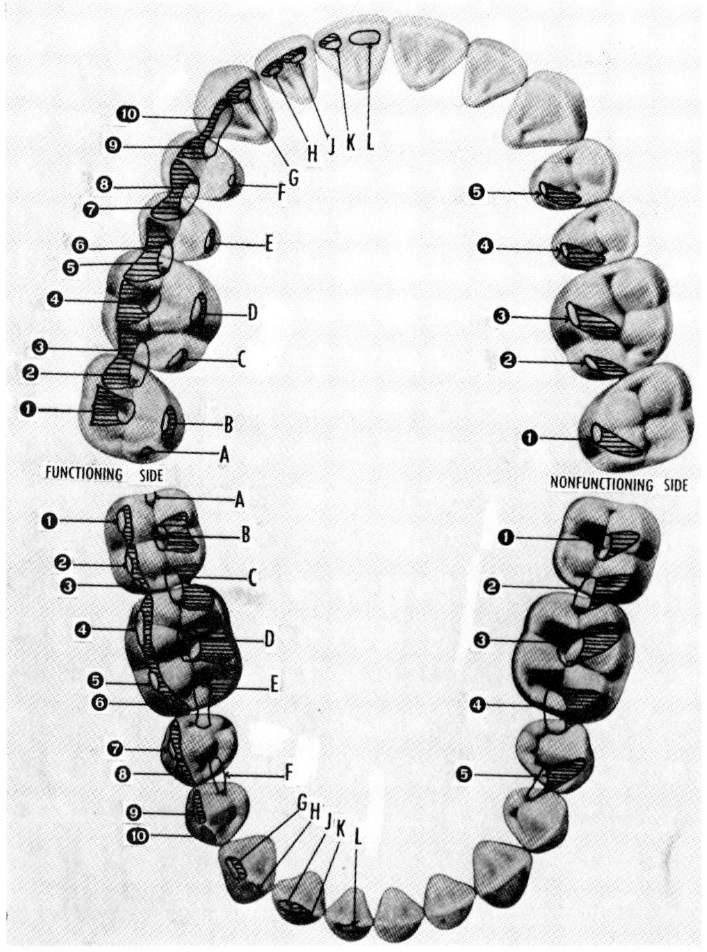

FIG. 5-29. Functioning range of articulation: The lower buccal cusps (numbers) move across shaded areas of the upper buccal cusps (corresponding numbers). Similarly, the shaded areas of the lower lingual cusps (letters) move across the upper lingual cusps (corresponding letters). Nonfunctioning range of articulation: The shaded areas of the lower buccal cusps (numbers), move across the upper lingual cusps and shaded areas (numbers).

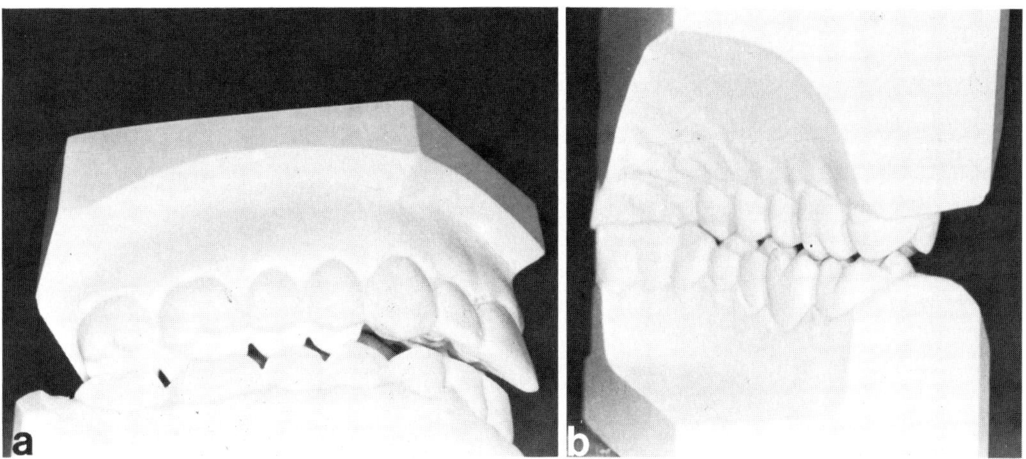

FIG. 5-30. Right nonfunctioning position of occlusal articulation, buccal (*a*) and distolingual (*b*) views.

CRO (centric-relation occlusion) centers ABCD and A′B′C′D′.

In Figure 5-26 the mandible has moved through the envelope of motion and has reached the first point of cuspal contact. In P, the profile view of the left temporomandibular joint, close contact exists between the condyle and the meniscus as the condyle travels posteriorly into the glenoid fossa. In (*c*), the ideal mandibular movement is further illustrated with the following conditions. The muscles, M and M′, continue to exert equal force, and the mandible moves in the direction of K and K′. The food, F, is further triturated by the cuspal contacts on the functioning side. The dots, X and X′, continue to be equidistant from the original CRO centers ABCD and A′B′C′D′. In Q, the profile view of the temporomandibular joint, close contact continues to exist between the condyle and the meniscus as the condyle travels posteriorly and laterally into the glenoid cavity. On the functioning side, the condyle is beginning to traverse the Bennett movement. In (*d*) the normal envelope of motion is almost complete to CRO. In this idealized manner the mandible moves through the envelope of motion with synergistic function of all the parts of the stomatognathic system.

Figure 5-27 demonstrates the appearance of the maxillary and the mandibular teeth in the functioning position of occlusal articulation from the buccal view and the lingual view of the right side. Figure 5-28 demonstrates the maxillary and the mandibular first molars at the first point of contact before the cusps slide on the planes of the teeth during the functioning range of occlusal articulation (buccal, lingual and distal views).

Figure 5-29 demonstrates the contacting tooth surfaces in the functioning range of occlusal articulation. Lower cusp 1 contacts and moves across the shaded area from upper fossa 1; upper cusp A contacts and moves across the shaded area from lower fossa A. This number-to-number and letter-to-letter relationship of the cusps and the fossae continues throughout the arches. The outlined unshaded areas maintain centric-relation occlusion. The mandibular movements in mastication are more complex and varied than the diagrams indicate, but the purpose of the drawings is to simplify the occlusal-contact relations to facilitate understanding.

The mandible may be pictured as a U-shaped bone as one observes the movement of the mandible downward and laterally on the functioning side and then

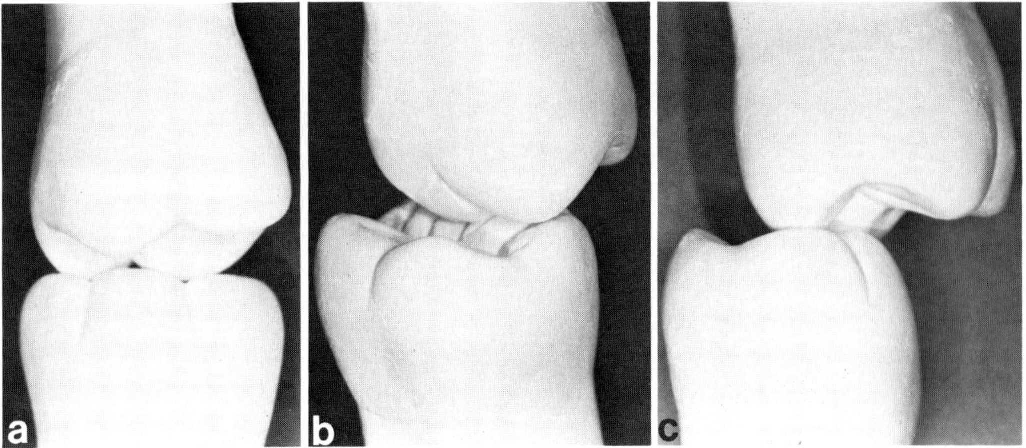

FIG. 5-31. Views of an opposing pair of right first molars at the beginning of the nonfunctioning range of articulation: buccal (*a*), distolingual (*b*), and distal (*c*).

upward as the initial tooth contacts are made. On the nonfunctioning side, the cusps of the teeth, in an empty mandibular movement, make contact. In most mouths with natural dentition, nonfunctioning occlusal contacts are not usually present.

Figure 5-30 demonstrates the appearance of the maxillary and the mandibular teeth in the right nonfunctioning position of occlusal articulation, buccal and distolingual views, on the right side. Figure 5-31 demonstrates the maxillary and the mandibular first molars at the first point of contact before the cusp slides on the planes of the teeth during the right nonfunctioning range of articulation (buccal, distolingual and distal views). Figure 5-29 demonstrates the normal contacting surfaces in the left nonfunctioning range of occlusal articulation. Cusp 1 contacts fossa 1 and moves across the shaded area; cusp 2 contacts fossa 2; and so on.

Cuspal interferences on the nonfunctioning side keep the functioning side open. This results in torque on the teeth and the mandible.

The occlusal surfaces of the contacting teeth in the protrusive ranges of articulation are the distal planes of the cusps of the maxillary teeth and the mesial planes of the cusps of the mandibular teeth of the posterior dentition (Fig. 5-32).

In the anterior region, the contacts on the lingual of the maxillary teeth are located from the point of incisal contact in protrusive position and then gingivally to the point of centric-relation occlusion.

Figure 5-33 demonstrates the appearance of the maxillary and the mandibular teeth in protrusive position (buccal and lingual views).

The protrusive positional relationship of the teeth is a momentarily static one which exists at the instant of complete incision of food by the anterior teeth. As these teeth incise food, they meet almost in end-to-end relationship. In most patients with natural dentition, the incisal contact of the anterior teeth is the only one present in the protrusive positional relationship.

PHYSIOLOGY OF MASTICATION

The act of mastication is a complicated pattern of oral function involving the coordination of all parts of the stomatognathic system. Although the teeth are anatomically designed to act as instruments which incise, crush and triturate food, they can act efficiently only when nerves, muscles, temporomandibular joints, tongue, lips, cheeks and supporting structures are functioning properly. Mastication prepares the food for swallowing, increases surface area of the food so that the digestive juices may operate effectively, liberates the taste stimulants to increase the flow of digestive juices and protects the digestive tract from hard, sharp or harmful material by pulverizing the food and by giving the tactile sensation of the teeth, the tongue, the lips and the cheeks an opportunity to reject injurious substances.

The act of mastication may be divided into three phases: incision, crushing and trituration or mastication proper. During incision the lower jaw is depressed and moves forward. Then, with the food between the teeth, the lower jaw is elevated and slightly retracted so that the incisal edges of the upper and the lower teeth fall opposite each other. This is the so-called protrusive position. The incising movement continues with the incisal edges of the lower teeth passing over the lingual surfaces of the upper anterior teeth until the position of centric-relation occlusion is reached. Incision in lateral positions occurs in a similar manner. The functioning-side condyle goes downward, forward and laterally into the lateral protrusive position. On the functioning side, the buccal planes of the lower buccal cusps contact the lingual planes of the upper buccal cusps. The functioning-side condyle then retraces its path to centric-relation occlusion and repeats the cycle several times. Because of

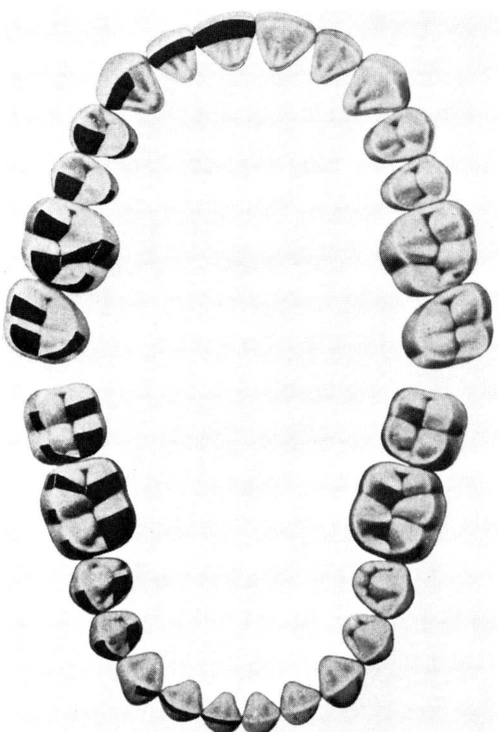

FIG. 5-32. Protrusive range of articulation. The contact surfaces, as the lower teeth move across the upper teeth, are marked in black.

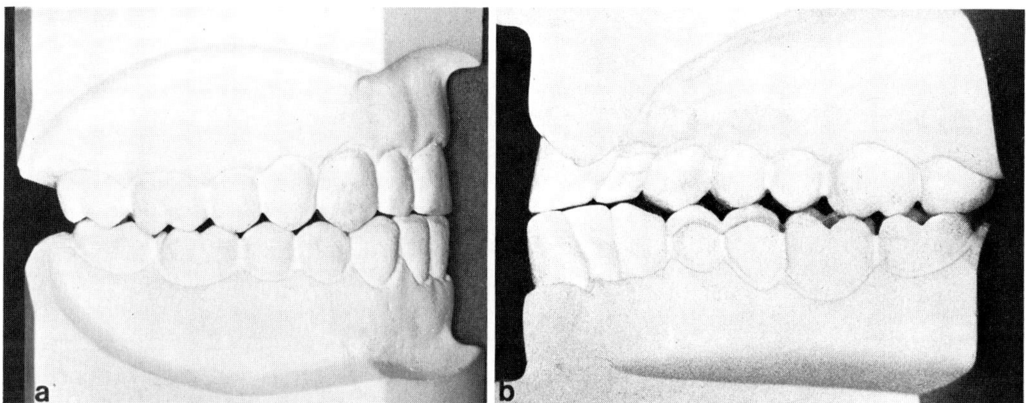

FIG. 5-33. Views of the protrusive position: buccal (*a*) and lingual (*b*).

the shape of the mandible, accompanying movements are made by the condyle on the nonfunctioning side.

When food of satisfactory size has been incised, the action of the tongue and the cheeks places it on the occlusal surfaces of the posterior teeth for the next two phases of mastication: crushing and trituration. Direct crushing is accomplished by a hingelike opening and closing movement of the mandible. In a bracing action, the condyle is set well into the fossa before the teeth make contact. This action is repeated a few times.

Trituration or mastication proper is accomplished by dropping the mandible in a hingelike motion and shifting to a left or right functioning position. On the functioning side, the buccal cusps of the mandibular teeth lie below the buccal cusps of the maxillary teeth. The envelope of motion is completed as the mandible returns to the position of centric-relation occulusion. The moving point-to-point and plane-to-plane contacts of the opposing teeth triturate the food during the latter part of the cycle. The tongue then positions the bolus of food between the teeth of the opposite side, and the trituration movement begins again. These complex masticatory movements are repeated until the food is sufficiently comminuted to enable deglutition to take place. In normal mastication, in which there are no interfering occlusal contacts, the mandible moves back into centric relation with the condyle head on the functioning side set well into the fossa to brace against the pull of the muscles as they force cuspal penetration into the bolus. This bracing action enables the teeth to contend with vertical force only. However, when there is an interfering occlusal contact, the mandible is forced to move into a convenience relationship to provide cuspal contact between the maxillary and the mandibular teeth. This movement pulls the head of the condyle away from its centric-relation position in the fossa, thus negating the bracing action. Consequently, the periodontium is subjected not only to the normal vertical force but also to the much more destructive lateral forces.

PHYSIOLOGY OF DEGLUTITION

The act of deglutition, which carries the triturated food from the mouth to the stomach, may be divided into three stages. In the first stage, which is entirely voluntary, the teeth are in contact, and the tongue is pressing against the lingual surfaces of the teeth and the hard palate, thus preventing food from escaping. The pressure of the tongue against the palate forces the food back toward the posterior wall of the pharynx. The second stage involves the passage of the food through the pharynx to the esophagus and is an involuntary reflex action. When the bolus passes the isthmus of the fauces, it contacts certain sensory areas which initiate a series of coordinated muscular contractions of the tongue, the pharynx and the larynx and a momentary suspension of respiration. The base of the tongue rises and moves backward driving the bolus of food down the pharynx. The third stage is the passage of the food through the esophagus to the stomach.

The importance of swallowing in relation to centric-relation occlusion lies in the fact that the teeth make contact every time the act of swallowing takes place. It is generally assumed that the teeth make contact only during the act of mastication, or less than a total of an hour a day. The fact is that the teeth make contact during every act of swallowing, or about 1,500 times daily. This contact during swallowing attempts to take place in centric relation, but it occurs in the convenience relationship that exists in the patient's mouth. The presence of interfering occlusal contacts in centric relation means that the teeth and their supporting structures are subjected to constant microtraumata. To prevent or minimize damage to the teeth and their supporting structures, the protective proprioceptive mechanism attempts to establish convenience mandibular-maxillary relationships by shifting the mandible. This protective reaction becomes habitual, and abnormal masticatory and swallowing patterns develop. When the mandible does succeed in closing in centric relation, the interfering teeth are traumatized. Because the teeth do make contact so many times a day, it is of the utmost importance that occlusal equilibration be performed so that the teeth occlude in centric relation. This will ensure even distribution of forces to all the teeth, both in mastication and during deglutition.

Many people are so-called forceful swallowers whose teeth are brought into contact with excessive force every time they swallow. This habit may depress the teeth and produce tooth movement with general sequelae of periodontal degeneration as a direct result.

SYNERGY OF MASTICATORY COMPONENTS

The movement of the mandible plays an important role in speech, mastication and deglutition. This section is concerned primarily with mastication. The mandible is connected to the skull by a complex joint arrangement, muscles, ligaments and other soft tissues. The neuromuscular pattern of the movements of the mandible is important. The primary function of the mandible is mastication. All muscle forces involved in mastication are expended through the teeth to the mandible and the maxilla. The mandible may be compared to a handle, to which the actual instruments of mastication, the teeth, are attached.

The masticatory organ is composed of a synergism of the temporomandibular joint, the neuromusculature and the occlusal relationship of the teeth as it is maintained by the periodontium. If one of the components of this closely related system is altered, effects are produced upon all the other components. The relationships of the main parts of this system may be conceived of as a constant and lifelong battle for survival between the temporomandibular joint, the periodontium and the teeth, with the neuromuscular system providing the force. In patients who have weak or hypermobile joints, breakdown results in temporomandibular joint syndrome. However, if the temporomandibular joint is strong enough to resist breakdown, the periodontium supporting the teeth will give way. Proof of the fact that the temporomandibular joint is stronger than the periodontium lies in the truth that, at the age of 80, all human beings still possess their temporomandibular joints, but few of them have good teeth supported by a strong periodontium.

TEMPOROMANDIBULAR JOINT

The anatomical structure of the temporomandibular joint (a ginglymoarthrodial or gliding-hinge joint) makes it possible for the mandible to assume many positions. This joint is one of the compensatory mechanisms common to the stomatognathic system. Involved and integrated in mandibular movement are the shape of the mandibular fossae, the degree of tension on the associated ligaments, the meniscus, the neuromuscular system and the guiding inclines of the teeth. Every complex system must have parts that give and compensate for wear, change in structure, poor relationships in other parts of the system, etc. It is of both theoretical and practical value to visualize this joint as an organ of integrated activity.

The Articulating Bodies

The mandibular condyle is the articulating surface of the mandible. It is about

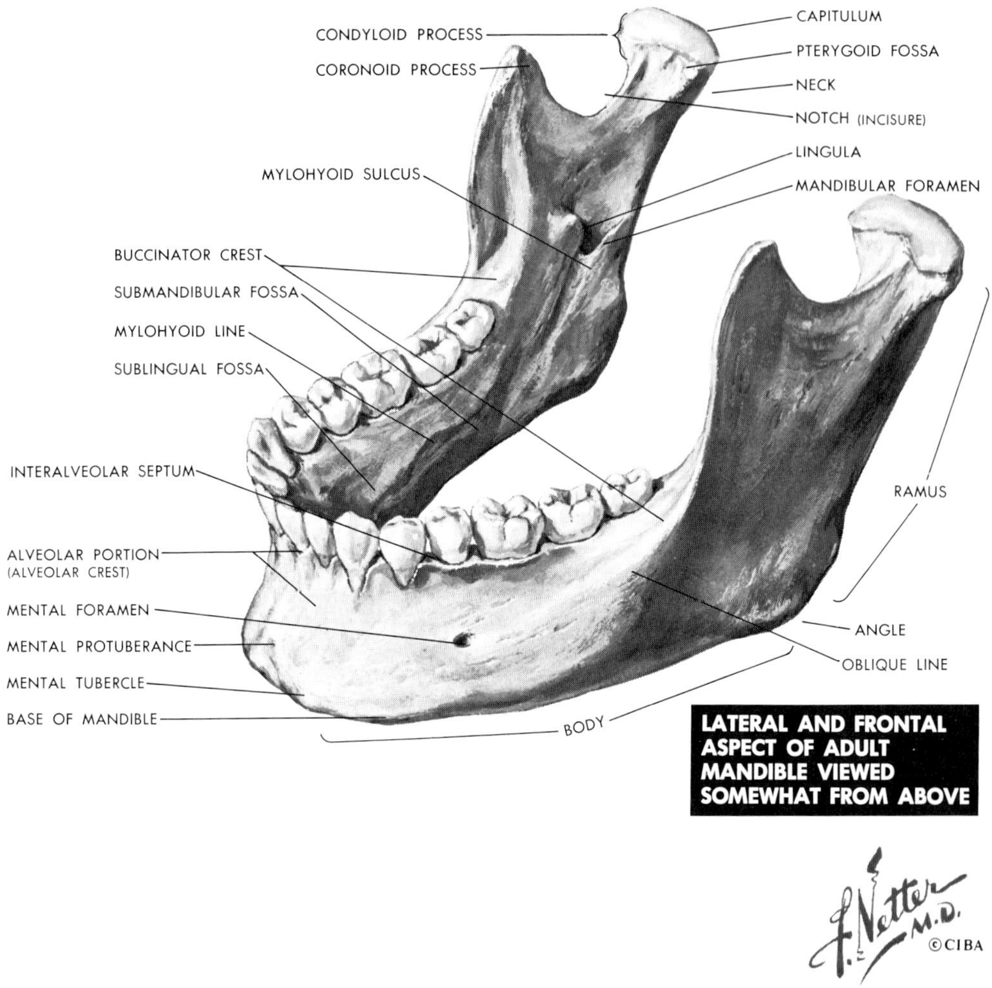

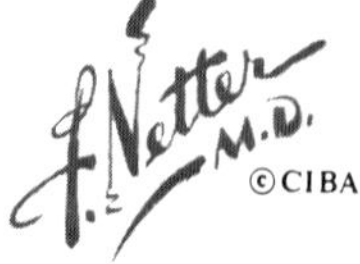

FIG. 5-34. Drawing of the mandible. (© Copyright 1959 CIBA Pharmaceutical Company, Division of CIBA-GEIGY Corporation. Reproduced, with permission, from THE CIBA COLLECTION OF MEDICAL ILLUSTRATIONS by Frank H. Netter, M.D. All rights reserved.)

15 to 20 mm. long, the long axis being at right angles to the ramus, and 8 to 10 mm. thick (Fig. 5-34). It is very convex in an anteroposterior direction, but only slightly so mediolaterally. Although laterally the condyle stands out only slightly from the ramus, it does extend considerably beyond the inner surface of the ramus.[48]

The articulating surface of the temporal bone is made up of the articular or glenoid fossa and the articular eminence. The glenoid fossa is just in front of the tympanic opening, with the elevated, cone-shaped postglenoid process between (see Fig. 5-35). It should be noted that the roof of the glenoid fossa is quite thin; in fact, a light held inside the cranium will shine through it. Clearly it is not meant to bear stress. Instead the stress-bearing elements of the articulation are the articular eminence and the meniscus. The articulating surfaces of the joint are covered by fibrocartilage, which is adapted to bearing pressure, rather than by hyaline cartilage, which is common in

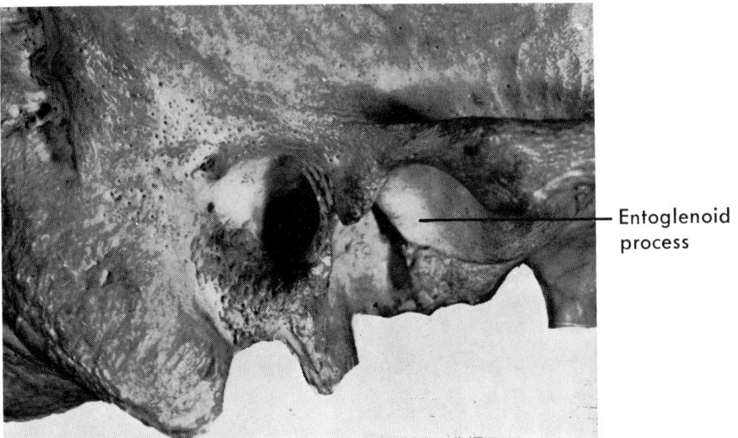

FIG. 5-35. The temporal bone, showing a well-developed postglenoid process. (Sicher, H., and DuBrul, E. L.: Oral Anatomy. ed. 5. St. Louis, C. V. Mosby, 1975)

other joints. The eminence is quite convex anteroposteriorly, with a radius of curvature of 5 to 15 mm., and slightly concave mediolaterally. Its anterior slope is slight compared to the posterior slope—a feature that prevents anterior dislocation of the jaw during wide opening, when the condyles may move beyond the height of the articular eminence. On its medial side, the glenoid fossa is bounded by a bony lip that leans against the angular spine of the sphenoid bone; this structure prevents a medial dislocation of the condyles.[48]

Ligaments of the Temporomandibular Joint

There are four ligaments associated with the temporomandibular joint. The *capsular* ligament is attached to the temporal bone and surrounds the temporomandibular articulation and the condyle. Its primary function is to hold the two bones together and thus to form a joint. The *temporomandibular or external lateral* ligament runs from the outer temporal part of the zygomatic arch and the articular tubercle to insert on the lateral and posterior margins of the neck of the condyle. This is the main suspensory ligament of the mandible during moderate opening movements and it strengthens the lateral aspect of the capsule. The *sphenomandibular* ligament runs from the spine of the sphenoid bone to the lingula. It is also a suspensory ligament of the mandible and functions when the latter opens wider. When this occurs, the temporomandibular ligament relaxes, and the sphenomandibular ligament becomes taut in the manner of a guy rope. The *stylomandibular* ligament runs from the styloid process of the temporal bone and inserts on the posterior border of the mandible. It acts as a brake for the mandible, preventing excessive anterior drift of the mandible during extreme opening. These ligaments are illustrated in Figure 5-36. In experimental recordings, even though the muscles have been fatigued, the recordings of the hinge-axis are always the same. Therefore, it follows that the ligaments play a definite part, although *only* a part, in the synergy of neuromuscular posture and motion.

The Meniscus and Joint Capsule

Between the temporal and mandibular elements of the joint is the interarticular disc, or meniscus. Surrounding and sup-

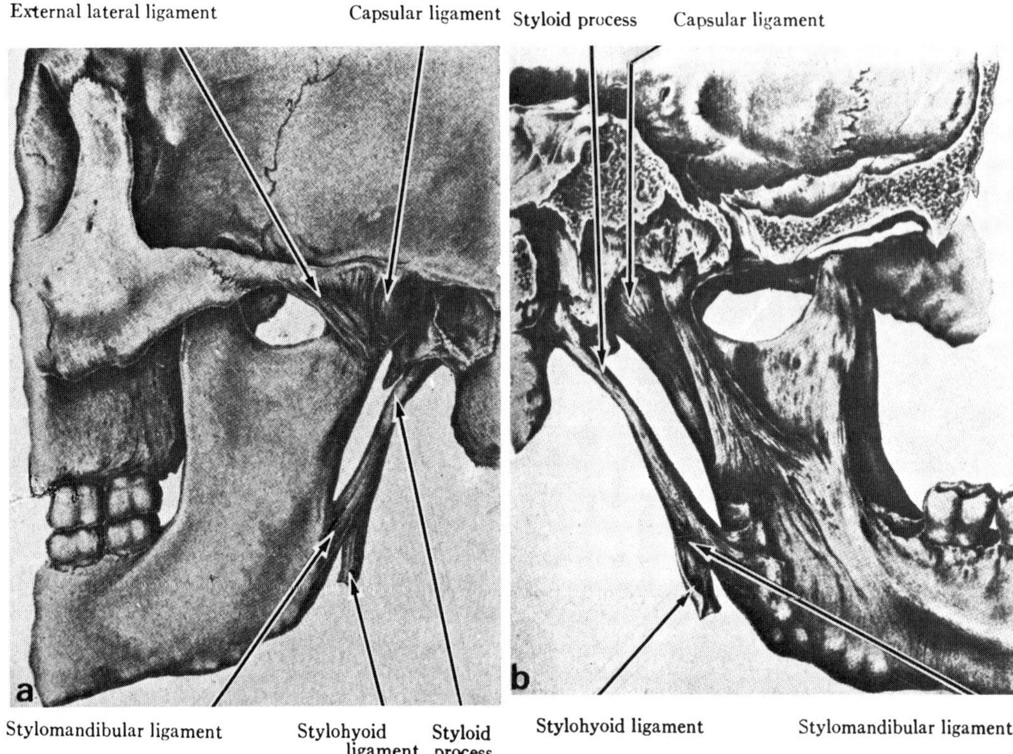

FIG. 5-36. The four ligaments associated with the mandibular joint: external view (*a*) and internal view (*b*). (Deaver, J.: Surgical Anatomy of the Head and Neck. Philadelphia, Blakiston, 1904)

porting the articulating elements of the temporomandibular joint is the joint capsule. The synovial membrane lines all structures of the joint not subject to pressure and is characterized by a rich supply of blood vessels.

Rees[44] made a comprehensive study of the temporomandibular joint, involving its structure and function. Though the work was done on fresh cadavers, portions of the paper are quoted because it answered with clarity the problem of what takes place in the joint in vivo during function.

Gross Anatomy of the Meniscus

Its inferior surface is everywhere concave and is oval in shape like the condyle with which it is in contact, with its long axis placed transversely. The superior surface is convex posteriorly but anteriorly it is saddle-shaped, being slightly convex from side to side and slightly convex from before backward. From

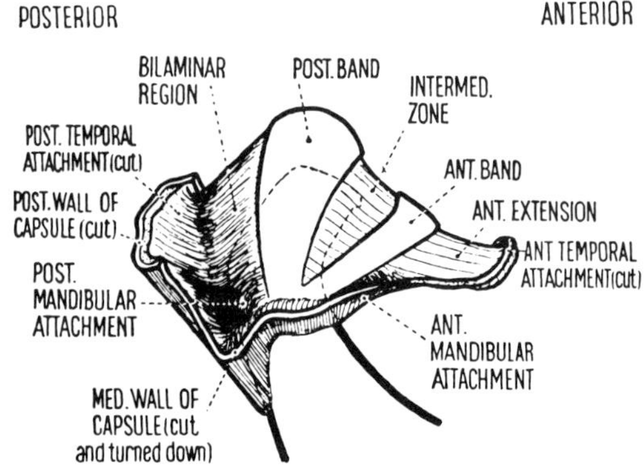

FIG. 5-37. The parts of the meniscus in relation to the condyle. (Rees, L. A.: The structure and function of the temporomandibular joint. Br. Dent. J., *96:*125, 1954)

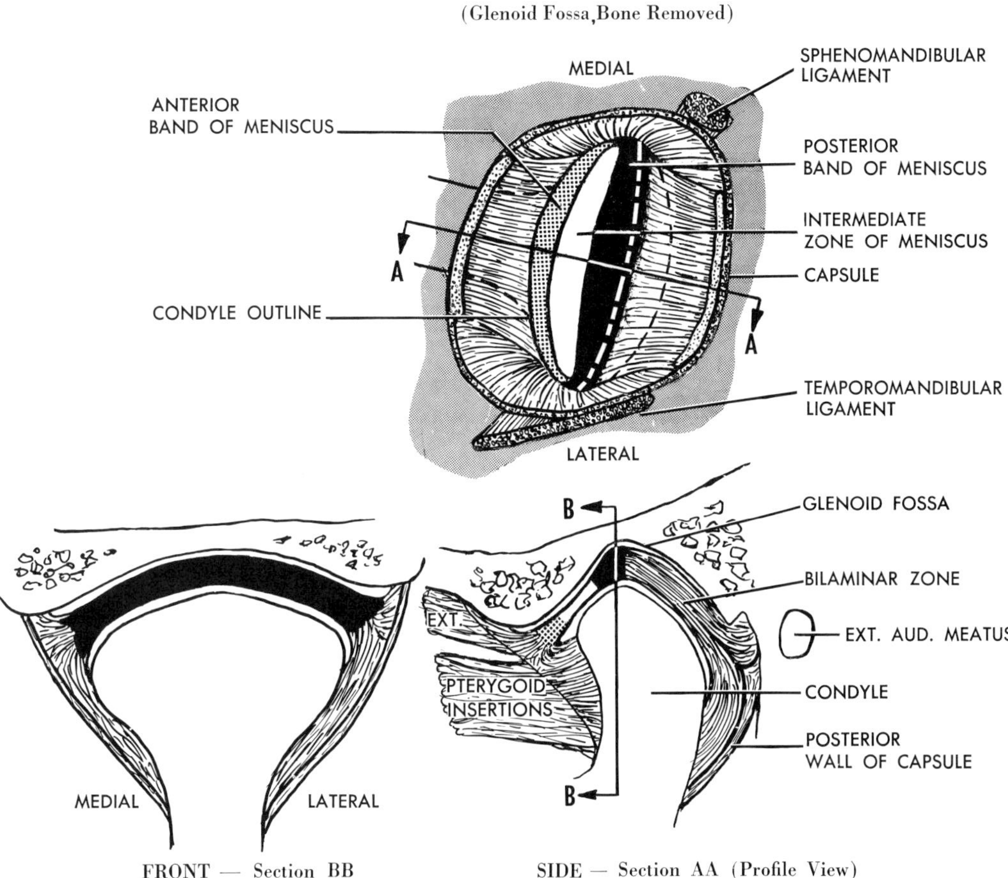

FIG. 5-38. The basic structures of the left temporomandibular joint, showing top, front and profile views oriented to each other at sections AA and BB. (After Rees)

above, the disc appears pear-shaped with the apex anteriorly. Its general form, when the jaws are opposed, is that of a schoolboy's peaked cap covering the condyle and extending forward in front of the condyle in relation to the articular eminence of the temporal bone.

The disc is not equally thick throughout but exhibits four clearly defined transverse ellipsoidal zones (Fig. 5-37) which may be termed the anterior band, the intermediate band, the posterior band, the bilaminar zone. These zones are much wider in the transverse direction than in the anteroposterior owing to the narrowness of the disc on its medial and lateral sides where it is attached to the mandible.

The anterior band is moderately thick but relatively narrow from before backward. The intermediate band is much thinner than the others, and is also narrow. The posterior band is much the thickest of the three and is also the widest from before backward. The bilaminar zone consists of an upper stratum which is attached to the posterior wall of the glenoid fossa and the squamotympanic suture, and a lower stratum which is attached to the back of the mandibular condyle.

Attachments of the Meniscus

Medially and laterally the meniscus blends with the capsule, and both are attached together to the medial and lateral poles of the condyle. Anteriorly the disc is attached above to the anterior margin of the articular emi-

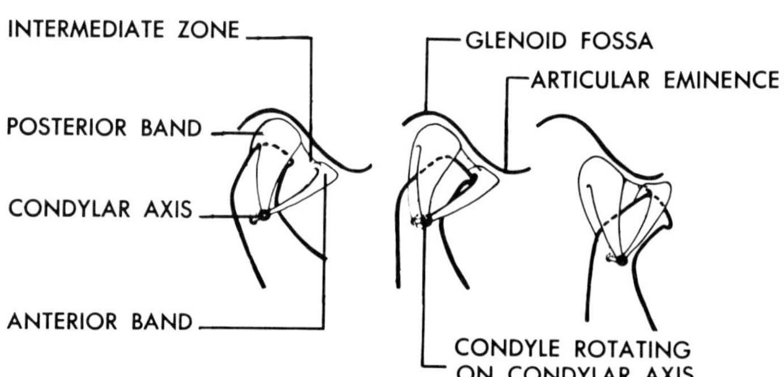

FIG. 5-39. The forward movement of the condyle in relation to anterior, intermediate and posterior transverse bands of the meniscus. (Rees, L. A.: The structure and function of the mandibular joint. Br. Dent. J., *96:*125, 1954)

nence and below to the front of the articular margin of the condyle. Posteriorly the attachments of the disc by way of the bilaminar zone have already been described.

In addition to the bony attachments mentioned the disc is also attached to neighboring muscles, namely, the external pterygoid, masseter and temporalis. In the case of the external pterygoid, tendinous fibers merge with the disc to form a true insertion. The connections with the masseter and temporalis muscles are less strong, consisting of fibrous bands at right angles to the direction of the muscle fibers which are continued from the perimysium and epimysium into the anterolateral portion of the disc.

Anatomy of the Capsule and the Temporomandibular Ligament

Posteriorly the capsule is inseparably blended with the posterior surfaces of both upper and lower strata of the bilaminar zone of the disc. The capsule fibers are distinguishable only because they run directly from temporal bone to mandible (Fig. 5-38, profile view).

Medially the capsule is loose and weak and is separated from the disc by a deep synovial extension of the upper compartment except below where the capsule and disc are jointly attached to the medial pole of the condyle as seen in the top view.

Anteriorly the capsule is absent, the upper and lower attachments of the disc alone delimiting the synovial cavities. It is here that the external pterygoid attachment to the disc is found (Fig. 5-38, profile view).

The lateral wall of the capsule is loose and thin behind, but nevertheless it is stronger than the medial wall. More anteriorly it is strongly reinforced by the temporomandibular ligament as seen in the top view. This is a flat sheet of dense collagenous tissue without elastic fibers which is so inseparably blended with the capsule as to be regarded as a thickened part of it. It passes downward and backward from the root of the zygoma to the neck of the condyle below the lateral pole.

Anatomy of the Mandibular Condyle

The shape of the articular surface varies somewhat from individual to individual but in general it is shaped like a gabled roof in that it presents a transverse ridge at its summit and anterior and posterior surfaces sloping inferiorly from it. The anterior sloping surface is approximately 5 mm. in width, the posterior 12 mm. The lateral and medial poles of the condyle, just below the articular surface, are usually marked by distinct bony tubercles for the attachment of the capsule and meniscus.

Movements Between the Condyle and the Meniscus

In the retrusive position [centric-relation occlusion position] (Fig. 5-39), the posterior thick band of the meniscus lies just in front of the transverse condylar ridge. As the condyle is moved forward its ridge passes 5 or 6 mm. across the posterior thick band on to the intermediate thin zone of the meniscus. When the jaw is forced forward as far as it will go, the ridge crosses the anterior band and comes to rest just in front of it. From the extreme retrusive position to the extreme protrusive one the

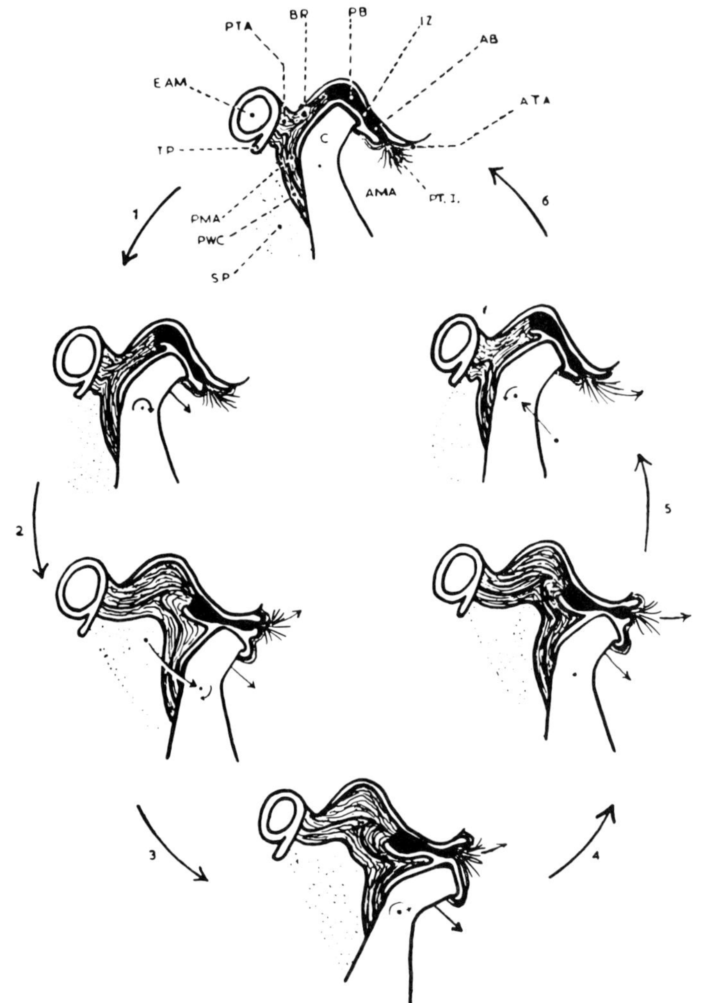

FIG. 5-40. Phases of condylar movement.
AB—anterior band
AMA—anterior mandibular attachment
ATA—anterior temporal attachment
BR—bilaminar region
EAM—external auditory meatus
IZ—intermediate zone
PB—posterior band
PMA—posterior mandibular attachment
PTA—posterior temporal attachment
PT.I—lateral pterygoid insertion
PWC—posterior wall of capsule
SP—soft tissue pad
TP—tympanic plate
(Rees, L. A.: The structure and function of the mandibular joint. Br. Dent. J., *96:*132, 1954)

excursion of the condylar ridge relative to the meniscus is not more than 8 mm.

Movements Between the Meniscus and the Temporal Bone

Since the total forward excursion of the condylar ridge relative to the temporal bone is at least 15 mm., and since it has been found that the maximal movement of the ridge relative to the meniscus is 8 mm., we should expect that the meniscus should move forward on the temporal bone at least 7 mm., between the most retrusive and the most protrusive positions of the mandible. This was confirmed by actual observations.

It is evident that the movement of the condyle and meniscus forward out of the glenoid fossa necessitates something else moving in to take their place. In dissected joints the back of the meniscus curls downward away from the temporal bone leaving an air space when the condyle is moved forward. In unopened joints and in the living subject of course the meniscus must remain in contact with the temporal bone, since no air can enter the joint. The appearance of a depression on the surface of the face behind the condyle when the jaw is opened in the living subject supports the view that soft tissues at the back of the joint move into the vacated glenoid cavity, and this is confirmed in specimens frozen in the protrusive position before sectioning, when the glenoid fossa is occupied by the bilaminar zone of the disc. This relatively thick but loose structure has evidently been wedged forward into the space vacated by the condyle (Fig. 5-40, movement 2).

Correlation of Structure and Function

The forward movement of the meniscus when the mouth is opened is evidently due to the pull of the lateral pterygoid muscle and the attachment of the meniscus to the condyle on either side. These attachments, however, are near the condylar axis so that the condyle is able to rotate relative to the disc and a different part of the disc is in contact with a given region of the condyle for each position of the mandible—first the posterior band, then the thin intermediate band and, finally, the anterior band coming into contact with the ridge of the condyle as the latter moves forward. In other words the excursion of the condyle is greater than the excursion of the disc as they both move forward owing to relative movements between the condyle and disc.

The significance of the varying thickness of the disc in its different zones is not altogether clear, but it seems likely that it subserves two purposes: (1) the interposition of a thin zone between two thicker zones should make the disc more flexible and enable it the better to alter its shape from concave below to convex above as it slides forward from the articular fossa on to the articular eminence; (2) the condyle, being separated in its retrusive position [centric-relation position] from the temporal bone by the thickest part of the disc, and by the thinnest part of the disc when it moves on to the articular eminence, is not constrained to follow the sinuous contours of the temporal surface but can move in a straightforward arc of a circle with its center near the lingula.

It has been contended that forward movements of the disc cannot occur because of its attachment posteriorly to the temporal bone. This attachment, however, has been shown to consist of loose fibroelastic tissue stretchable to the extent of 7 to 10 mm. in the dissected specimen, which is enough to allow for the amount of forward movement of the disc required in moving from the most retrusive to the most protrusive position, so that the abovementioned contention is invalid. The structure of this bilaminar portion of the disc, moreover, is ideally suited to its role in filling the vacated glenoid fossa in the protrusive position. The great vascularity of the bilaminar portion also makes one suspect that its volume may possibly increase by venous engorgement when it is occupying the glenoid fossa.

The return of the disc when the condyle moves backward seems to be brought about by its attachments to the condyle particularly the nonelastic lower stratum of the bilaminar zone. This is perhaps aided by the elastic recoil of the upper lamina of the bilaminar zone. No special muscular mechanism seems to be involved in the return of the disc as it is in the forward movement.

The attachment of the disc to the perimysium and epimysium of the temporalis and masseter muscles may or may not be of functional significance. It might be, however, that these attachments counteract the tendency of the external pterygoid to pull the disc medially as well as forward.

The general weakness of the capsule and its absence anteriorly are such as to absolve it from any duties in restraining the free movements of the condyle and disc. The strong temporomandibular ligament, however, is fairly taut in all positions of the joint and no doubt serves to keep condyle, disc and temporal bone firmly opposed. Limitation of forward movement, however, seems to result from the restraint offered by the posterior fibers of this ligament and of backward movement by the anterior fibers, while limitation of lateral movement results from the tension of the ipsilateral ligament and of medial movements by the contralateral ligament.

Summary of Movements Taking Place at the Mandibular Joints

The movements taking place at the mandibular joints can, for purposes of analysis, be divided into six phases (Fig. 5-40). These are:

1. *Occlusal Phase.* The jaws are closed so that the teeth meet and interlock in the occlusal position. The posterior band of the meniscus occupies the deepest part of the glenoid fossa, while the condylar ridge lies just behind its inferior surface (Fig. 5-39). The bilaminar region and its temporal attachment are relaxed, but the mandibular polar attachments of the meniscus are taut. Hence, in further movement in a backward direction

(which can occur to a small extent in the most retrusive position) the condyle will draw the meniscus back with it. Retrusion is finally limited by the temporomandibular ligaments and by the tension of the meniscus from its anterior attachments.

2. *Retruded [Centric Relation] Opening Phase.* The condyles commence to rotate around the bicondylar axis while this axis remains more or less stationary. The condylar ridge slides forward 5 to 6 mm., on to the intermediate zone of the meniscus. Meanwhile the upper surface of the meniscus slides forward on the temporal bone, and this phase is continued smoothly into the next.

3. *Protrusive Opening Phase.* The bicondylar axis moves in a downward and forward direction as the condyles continue to rotate around this axis. Simultaneously, the condylar ridge moves further forward on the lower surface of the intermediate zone. The latter remains interposed between the anterior slope of the condylar articular surface and the articular eminence during this moverment; the bilaminar region and its temporal attachment stretch some 6 to 9 mm. to allow for this movement. The posterior mandibular attachment of the meniscus is relaxed so that it can be folded on the back of the lower surface of the meniscus by soft tissues which are sucked in from behind and from the sides of the joint.

4. *Extreme Protrusive Opening Phase.* During the previous phase the back of the meniscus has been stretched nearly to its limit. The bicondylar axis continues to move downward and forward and the condylar poles move further forward relative to the posterior transverse band. Meanwhile the condyle is still rotating upon the bicondylar axis, and, near the full extent of opening, the condylar ridge slips forward (with a jump in some people which may produce a "clicking" sound) over the anterior transverse band. This occurs when the meniscus has been drawn forward to the full extent permitted by its temporal attachment behind. The extent of forward movement of the condyle is limited by its attachment to the temporal bone by means of the polar attachments of the meniscus at the sides and the posterior temporal attachments of the meniscus behind, and also by the temporomandibular ligaments. When the mouth is open to its full extent the amount of soft tissue sucked in from posterolateral aspects of the joint is at its maximum.

5. *Closing Phase.* The condyles rotate backward on the bicondylar axis as the latter moves in a backward and upward direction. The condylar ridge returns to the intermediate zone, the external pterygoid acting to hold the meniscus forward while it does so. The rest of the movement in this phase is the reverse of that occurring in the protrusive opening phase: the intermediate thin band remains interposed between the anterior slope of the condylar articular surface and the slope of the articular eminence, the relation of these structures being maintained by the external pterygoid muscle (and perhaps the masseter too) acting on the condyle and meniscus. The degree of backward slide of the meniscus on the eminence is 6 to 9 mm. This phase continues smoothly into the next.

6. *Retrusive Closing Phase [Centric-Relation Occlusion].* The bicondylar axis has returned almost to its retrusive position but the condyles continue to rotate backward around it. The posterior thick band has almost reached the deepest part of the glenoid fossa. In the backward rotation the condylar ridge slips behind the posterior thick band, the external pterygoid muscle holding the front of the meniscus forward to enable it to do so. This automatically draws tight the previously slack mandibular attachment of the bilaminar region; the meniscus is thereafter drawn back with the neck of the condyle to the occlusal position, and beyond this to the most retrusive position.

In phases 5 and 6, the soft tissue previously sucked in is forced or allowed to return to the posterolateral aspects of the joint.

The principal conclusions from this work were that the attachments and structure of the meniscus are such as to allow a considerable range of movement relative to the temporal bone, and that such movement does occur; that the meniscus is not homogeneous in structure and that different parts of the meniscus are interposed between condyle and temporal bone in different positions of the mandible.[44]

HINGE-AXIS

In its initial opening and final closing movements, the mandible acts as a hinged joint. McCollum[30] referred to the axis of rotation of the mandible as the

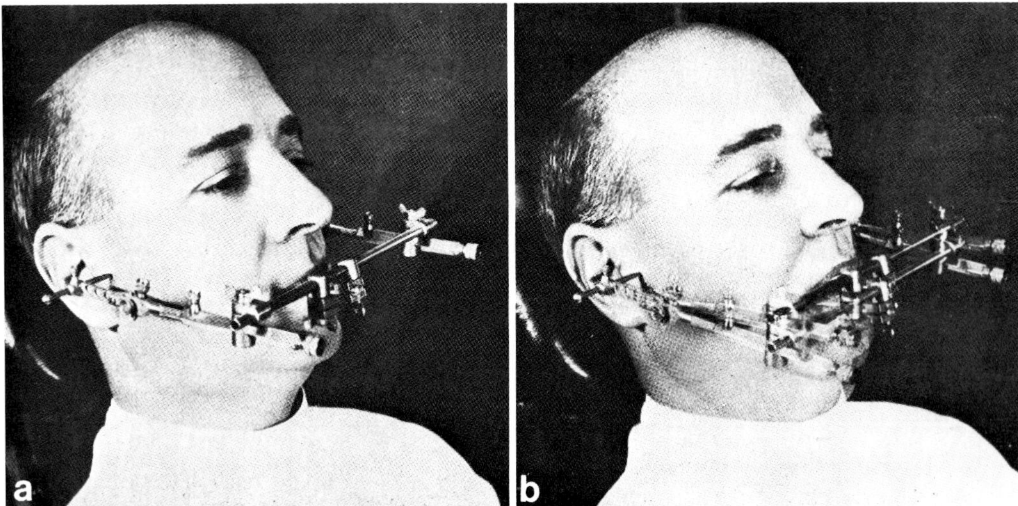

FIG. 5-41. The three-piece adjustable face-bow attached to the stem of the mandibular clutch (*a*). When the caliper pin is in correct position, "letting the mouth drop open" does not displace the point: it only rotates (photograph is a double exposure) (*b*). (McCollum, B. B., and Stuart, C. E.: A Research Report. p. 44. South Pasadena, Calif., Scientific Press, 1955)

"hinge-axis." Both right and left condylar heads of the mandible have their own distinct axes of rotation, as a wheel has a rotational axis which controls the arc within which the wheel rotates.

Another illustration of this idea may be found in the hinge of a door. While the hinge slides on its own pin, the axis of the arc that the door actually describes is an imaginary one buried in the center of the pin.

The determination and the proof of the hinge-axis is accomplished by the following procedure. An aluminum clutch is cemented to the mandibular teeth, and a stud is fixed to attach the clutch to the face-bow bar (Fig. 5-41*a*). To each end of the bar are attached the arms which carry the pins to the area of the tragus of the ear (*b*). While the patient opens and closes his mouth repeatedly, the caliper pin will describe an arc. Steadily but slowly, the caliper pin is adjusted until it rotates but does not describe an arc. When the axis of rotation has been reached, it will rotate around a fixed point, thus demonstrating a hinge-axis. Because they assumed that the head of the condyle pivots on the fossa, many investigators confused this pivotal action with the rotational axis in the head of the condyle. Confusion is caused by the lack of understanding of the fact that an axis of rotation lies within the head of the condyle and may be determined.

The importance of the hinge-axis can be demonstrated by the following line of reasoning. The upper stone cast is attached to the face-bow for mounting on the articulator. One point of orientation between the face-bow, the patient and the articulator is the hinge-axis. The importance of the proper use of the face-bow is demonstrated as follows. The face-bow orients the maxilla to the hinge-axis movement of the mandible with relation to the skull. If correctly transferred to the articulator, this axis becomes the axis of the articulator. If casts are mounted on an articulator without the use of a face-bow, they may be positioned incorrectly anteroposteriorly, superoinferiorly, or to the left or the right, or there may be a combination of these errors.

Because no basic terminology has been universally adopted, each investigator in the field of occlusion has had to establish his own. The identical movement or relationship has been called different things by different authors, and the inevitable result is confusion. To understand the abstract problems that must be solved in any discussion of occlusion, it is important to establish clear concepts. No investigator has actually seen condylar movement in the living human being. Information about reactions within the joint are conjectural and are based largely upon fluoroscopy, roentgenography and various types of graphological instruments. It is the interpretations of the readings from these machines that cause the confusion both in terminology and in the practical articulator concepts which have been based upon them.

CENTRIC RELATION

All mandibular movements must be thought of as skull-to-mandible relationships. Although these positions may also be considered as the mandible-to-maxilla, condyle-to-fossa and various other relationships, it is only by stressing the concept of mandibular position as a skull-to-mandible or a bone-to-bone relationship that there can be any basis for explaining mandibular movements. The skull, the mandible, the temporomandibular joint, muscles, nerves and occlusal surfaces of the teeth are all integrated in mandibular movements, and this integration and coordination serve as the basis for mandibular movement. It is the neuromuscular system that integrates and coordinates mandibular movement.

There seems to be no *single* anatomical reason for the centric relationship of the mandible. The joint capsule and the ligaments are loose; the muscles are in various states of tonus; and there seems to be no fulcrum posterior or superior to the head of the condyle. Nevertheless, the interaction of the neuromuscular mechanism, the temporomandibular joint, the teeth and the ligaments creates a basically accurate and constantly reproducible posture and pattern of movement. The muscles protect the temporomandibular ligaments from strain by their very rapid protective reflex actions.

However, a purely muscular reflex of the proprioceptor mechanism is not enough to explain the accurate readings yielded by a hinge-axis recording.

The National Society of Denture Prosthetists[45] defined centric relation as follows: "The mandible is in centric relation when the heads of the condyles are in their most retruded positions from which the jaw can make free lateral movements." This definition is based on Gysi's arrow-point tracings.

One group of investigators has maintained that the intercuspal position and the arrow-point tracing must be identical. Others believe that the correct mandibular position is about 1 mm. anterior to the arrow-point tracing. The latter group considers the apex of the arrow-point as a "retruded" or "strained" relation. A third group contends that the mandible may be moved actively or passively posterior to the arrow-point and into a "strained" relation.

The various interpretations of the apex of the gothic arch or arrow-point tracings have given rise to the following set of confusing terms: centric occlusion,[15,41] centric position,[51] centric relation,[17,36,50] dorsal position,[54] gothic arch centric relation,[6] habitual rest occlusion,[14] retruded centric relation,[22] retruded rest position,[49] terminal occlusion,[10] terminal occlusal position,[24] true centric relation,[13,20,31,50] unstrained centric relation,[16,] centric or physiological rest position,[19] centric relation, true centric position,[9] eccentric jaw relationship,[32] eccentric intercuspation,[33] functional centric position,[25] functional centric relation,[5,16] normal centric relation,[5] rest or centric relation, true relaxed

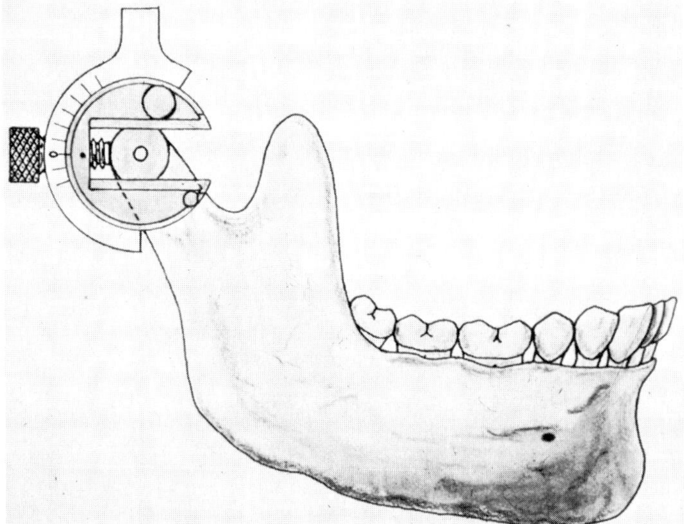

FIG. 5-42. Many dentists believe that the mandible is a Hanau articulator. (After Wilson)

centric relation,[53] true centric position,[12] true mandibular centric position,[52] true relaxed centric occlusion,[27] true rest centric position, working or rest centric position.[8]

Many dentists think of the temporomandibular joint as being purely mechanical (Fig. 5-42).

There has been a multiplicity of additional definitions and descriptive terms, but in effect the term "centric relation" has been bestowed upon the apex of the gothic-arch tracing, positions anterior to the apex and various other positions. Applying the same term to different points inevitably caused confusion.

Centric-Relation Definition

Centric relation is a skull-to-mandible relationship. The mandible is in centric relation when the heads of the condyles exhibit pure rotary motion around the hinge-axis while the mandible traverses an

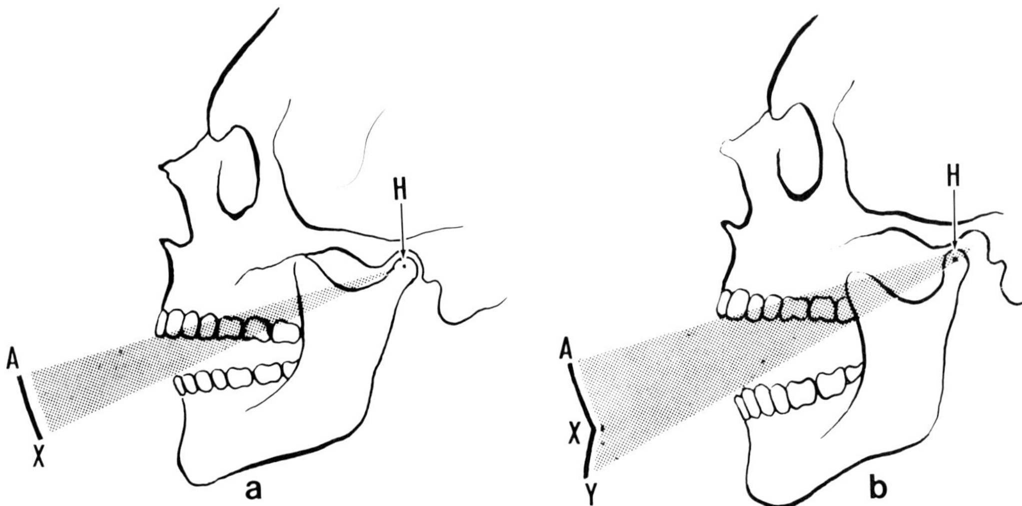

FIG. 5-43. The relationship between the rotary and the translatory condylar movements. The rotary movement (*a*) describes arc AX; the translatory movement (*b*) describes XY.

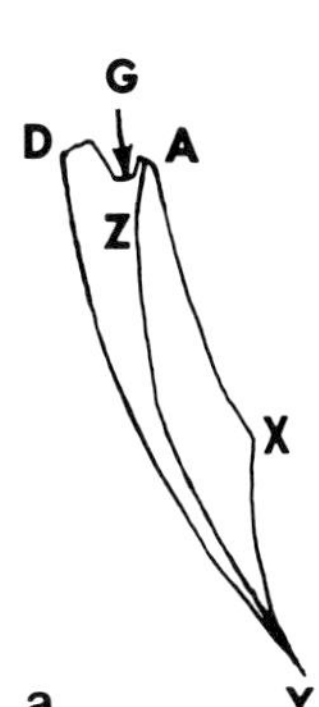

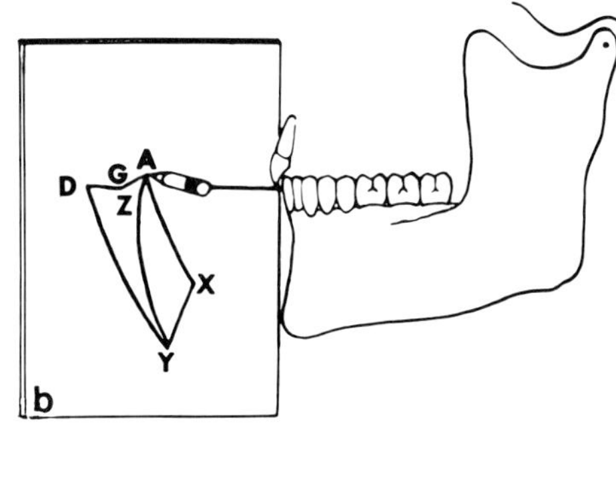

FIG. 5-44. The schematic inscription of median plane tracing (*a*). In the patient's tracing (*b*), D represents the extreme protrusive border position; A, centric-relation occlusion; G, the protrusive position; AX, the centric-relation arc; XY, the translatory arc; AZY, the line of habitual opening and closing during mandibular movements. (After Posselt, Hayek *et al.*)

arc, before translatory movement of the head of the condyle occurs. This is illustrated in Figure 5-43. The hinge-axis is the fixed point, H, while the mandible rotates and describes arc AX, the centric-relation arc. After point X is reached, the mandible exhibits translatory movement XY with an added bit of rotary motion, and the hinge-axis moves with the head of the condyle.

The arc through which the mandible moves from A to X (Fig. 5-43) is the centric-relation arc. The intercuspal distance of this arc will average from 0 mm. (centric-relation occlusion) to 26 mm. with a large amount of variation among individuals. The important point is that the hinge-axis exhibits only rotary movement and does not show translatory movement when the arc is inscribed.

Definitions of centric relation have always stressed the most retruded, unstrained position of the mandible from which lateral movements are possible. Basically, these considerations are not the guiding principles of centric relation. Rather, it is the traverse of the mandible through the centric-relation arc that is the basic consideration.

Moyers[34] has demonstrated electromyographically that the action potential of the musculature in the centric-relation arc closure is equal on both sides. This is evidence of the coordinated relationship between the neuromuscular system and the operations of the temporomandibular joint and the posture of the mandible.

Centric-Relation Occlusion—Definition

When the terminal closure of the mandible on the centric-relation arc exhibits intercuspation of the teeth, centric-relation occlusion occurs.

MANDIBULAR REST POSITION

The rest position is a variable postural relationship that depends upon the tonus of the muscles attached to the mandible. Mandibular rest position is an equilibrium between the tonus of the gravity or jaw-opening muscles and the antigravity or jaw-closing muscles. This posture will vary, depending upon the position of the head at different times. Other factors which influence muscle tonus and, consequently, the rest position are function, sleep, pathological conditions and normal aging processes. Because of variations in muscle tonus, rest position is not constant. The registration of a habitual rest position is fraught with uncertainty. It is impossible to record rest position as accurately as the centric-relation arc can be recorded. Posselt[43] has shown that the rest position does not lie on the centric-relation arc. He says:

The rest position shows in the majority of cases a comparatively great displacement of the mandible as a whole when it moves from the intercuspal position [centric-relation occlusion] to the rest position and conversely.

The rest position will usually be found 2 to 4 mm. from A on the line AZY (Fig. 5-44).

Research in the field of electromyography[33] demonstrates that the minimum of action potential in a muscle is recorded during the rest position.

There is no occlusal contact between the maxillary and the mandibular teeth in rest position. Usually, an interocclusal distance ranging from 2 to 4 mm. can be measured between the maxillary and the mandibular anterior teeth. This is called the free-way space and varies among individuals.

If the vertical dimension is abnormally increased—so-called "bite raising"—thus eliminating the free-way space, the teeth will be in constant contact. This eliminates the rest position and creates continuous tension on the muscles of mastication, and stress on the teeth and the supporting structures.

The importance of the rest position lies in the fact that it permits the tissues of the stomatognathic system to rest and thus to repair themselves. It has been shown that even slight pressure, if it is constant, will cause pathological tissue changes. Intermittent pressure, on the other hand, provides a period of rest during which self-repair can take place.

Centric-relation occlusion is the terminal point on the centric-relation arc, A in Figure 5-43. It is at this point that the maxillary and the mandibular teeth make maximal intercuspal contact. The practical significance of centric-relation occlusion as a basic factor in the health of the stomatognathic system is that it is the goal of occlusal equilibration to provide intercuspal contact of the maxillary and the mandibular teeth in harmony with centric relation.

ECCENTRIC MANDIBULAR MOVEMENT REGISTRATIONS

The eccentric mandibular movements have been recorded by means of tracers, photographic registrations and roentgenograms. Many investigators[9,15,25] made valuable contributions to this field. Since registrations obtained by means of the gothic-arch tracer are the most practicable from the point of view of the practicing dentist, they must be considered in great detail. The many available types of gothic-arch tracers are all built upon the basic principle of a fixed plate that receives the tracing on one arch and a pin, that is fixed to the other arch, that does the actual tracing (Fig. 5-45*a*). As the mandible moves to the extreme positions in the horizontal plane, or border movements, the tracing starts with a gothic arch and takes on the shape of a rhomboidal pattern. Border movements of the mandible are the farthest limits of the eccentric mandibular positions and are determined by the temporomandibular joints and the soft tissues. The limits or borders vary with different degrees of jaw opening. The angle BAC formed on the tracing table that is attached to the mandible represents the posterolateral border paths, BA and CA, in lateral movements from the posterior border position, A. This is the gothic arch. A is the posterior border position, and D is the anterior border position, thus making AD the protrusive path. Note that when making a gothic-arch tracing, it is the plate attached to the mandible that moves, while the pin attached to the maxillary arch scribes the tracing but remains stationary. For this reason, the tracings are in inverted relationship to their respective anatomic movements. In the figure, AC is the result of the left lateral border movement from centric relation, and AB is the result of the right lateral border movement from centric relation.

As the patient inscribes the gothic-arch tracing, BAC (Fig. 5-45*b*), the patient is

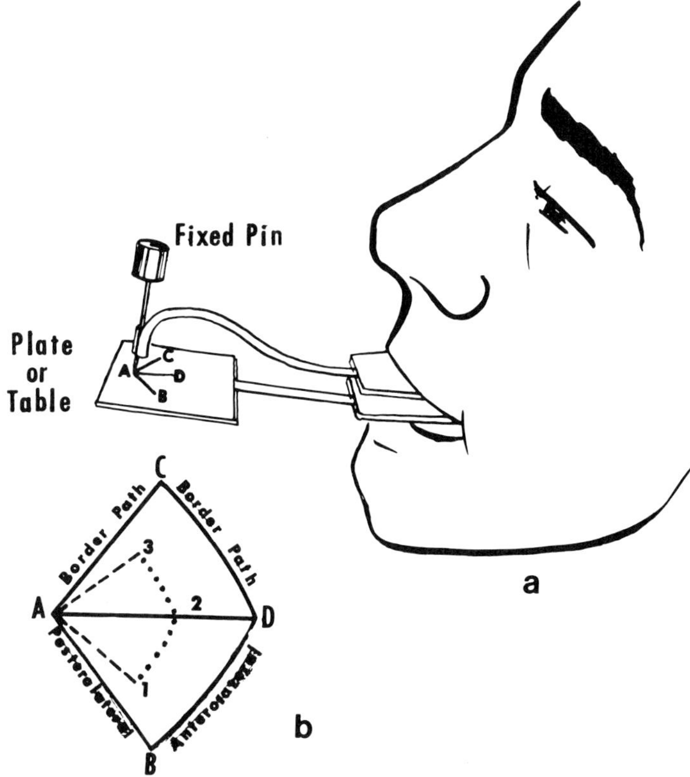

FIG. 5-45. The inscription of a gothic-arch tracing on the tracing plate by the fixed pin (*a*). A completed tracing (*b*) of all the extreme lateral border positions ABCD. The average functioning area of the patient is within the area A1, 2, 3.

instructed to assume point B and to protrude his mandible anteriorly toward the protrusive position. This action will create the marking BD. Then the patient should move similarly on the opposite side, whereupon he will trace line CA. As the mandible assumes the anterolateral border positions, the rhomboidal pattern, ABCD, is traced. Although the shape has been called rhomboidal for the sake of clarity, the figure is not an actual geometric rhombus.

In the same individual, the shape of the border movements is essentially the same at different degrees of jaw opening, even though the sizes of the area may vary. However, there is no relationship among different individuals either in size or shape of the border movement areas at the same degree of jaw opening. The lateral angles, DBA and DCA, are acute, whereas the anterior angle, BDC, and the posterior angle, BAC, are obtuse. The posterolateral border movement paths, AB and AC, seem to follow a straight course. The anterolateral border movement paths, DB and DC, seem to be slightly curved. This is probably owing to the inclination of the walls of the glenoid fossa. However, the individual functions within a small area. In Figure 5-45*b* enclosed in the border movement diagram, ABCD, is the functional diagram A 1, 2, 3. Every patient records a distinctive functional diagram. Pure protrusive incision takes place along the path A2. Mastication takes place somewhere in the path A1 or A3, depending on which side functions. The length of these paths is approximately 2 mm.

To record a tracing in the sagittal plane, a profile tracing is made with the scribing point attached to the mandible and the tracing plate parallel with the sagittal plane (Fig. 5-44*a*). To explain this tracing, consider a representation of

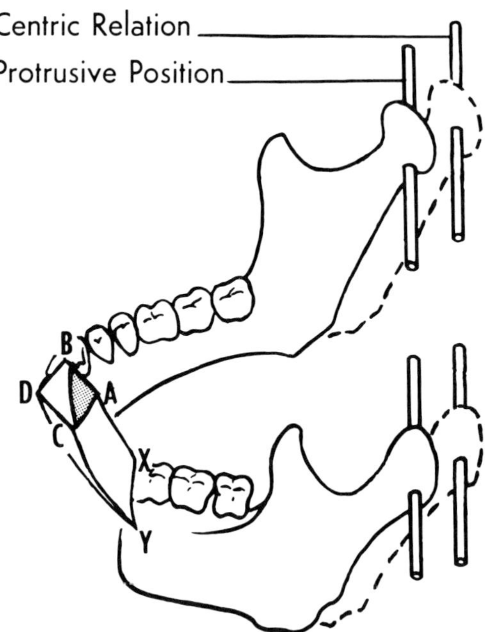

FIG. 5-46. A composite three-dimensional representation of the horizontal and median plane recordings as traced by the mandible. This is a summation of Figures 5-43, 5-44, and 5-45. As illustrated, each condyle has its own axis. (After Fisher)

an actual tracing (*b*). Recording of the anterior border path in the median plane from the protrusive position, D, with a minimum of jaw opening to the maximum open position, Y, gives curve DY. When the mandible opens from the posterior border position, A, it first inscribes arc AX. This is the centric-relation arc. At point X, the mandible begins to move forward in translation as it rotates and continues to open until it arrives at point Y. The mandible is protruded and retruded along the protrusive glide path, AD. The shape of the path AD in the average patient is determined by the lingual inclines of the upper anterior teeth until it reaches point G.

Then the continued protrusion of the mandible subsequently makes the path GD, which is caused by other cuspal and planar contacts. The habitual movements in the median plane lie between the anterior and the posterior border movements and are indicated by line Z. The rest position is found along the line Z. Figure 5-46 demonstrates both the composite-horizontal and the median-plane recording as traced by the mandible.

Certain conclusions may be drawn from the research that has been undertaken in mandibular movements and from the techniques that have been devised to record them.[13] Border movements are rarely if ever used. Habitual movements take place within the border movements. The rest position is a variable habitual position in the sagittal plane and represents a bodily shift of the mandible. Mandibular border movements can be reproduced accurately in the same individual, but because of their instability, habitual movements cannot be reproduced accurately.

The degree of convexity of the articular eminence and the degree of concavity of the mandibular fossa affect all mandibular movements.

In many people who are double-jointed, the temporomandibular joint is also hypermobile. Usually, the extent of mandibular opening ranges from 33 to 45 mm., but normal recordings of 60 mm. have been made. The shape of the head of the condyle varies among individuals and influences mandibular movement by its relationship to the shape of the fossa. There is a close functional relationship between left and right temporomandibular joints. Movement in one is definitely influenced by movement in the other.

MANDIBULAR OPENING AND CLOSING MOVEMENTS

All mandibular movements result from neuromuscular action. Since there is such a wide range of mandibular movements, it must be realized that the muscles act in various synergistic-antagonistic patterns with each other at different times.

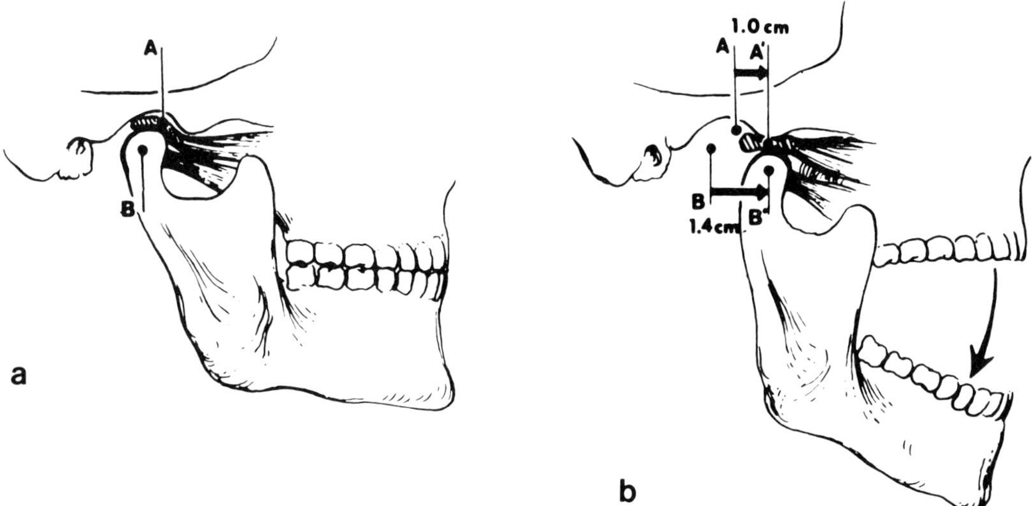

FIG. 5-47. In the closed position of the right temporomandibular joint (*a*), the center of the disc is at A and the center of the condyle at B. Note that the upper fibers of the lateral pterygoid attach to the disc and the lower fibers attach to the neck of the condyle. In opening, while the disc moves a distance of 1.0 cm, the condyle must move 1.4 cm (*b*).

The forward movement of the mandible results primarily from the contraction of the external pterygoid muscles which pull the condyles forward. To prevent the mandible from falling, the elevating muscles exhibit a slight degree of contraction. The depressors of the mandible relax. When the mandible is retracted, the deep portion of the masseter muscles and the posterior fibers of the temporal muscles contract strongly. At the same time, the geniohyoid and the digastric muscles (depressors) and the elevators synergistically balance each other to maintain the mandible in the horizontal plane.

Opening movements of the mandible are caused by the synergistic action of the external pterygoid muscles and the depressors of the mandible. Although the external pterygoid pulls the condyle and the disc forward, the geniohyoid, the mylohyoid and the digastric muscles pull the mandible downward and backward. This blending of muscle action makes possible the rotary and translatory movements of mandibular opening.

Mandibular closure may be divided into two phases. At first there is an interaction between the retracting portions of the masseter and the temporal muscles and the retracting portions of the depressors. During this action the mandible glides backward with little upward motion. The second phase begins with the contraction of the masseter, the internal pterygoid and the temporal muscles and ends when there is occlusal intercuspation of the teeth. Without this delicate neuromuscular balance there would be a possibility of temporomandibular joint dislocation. At the end of the opening movement, the head of the condyle is at the center of the articular eminence and, in some cases, a little anterior to it. If the powerful elevators of the mandible were to function before retraction occurs, the condyle would slip forward to the front of the articular eminence, thus producing a dislocation of the head of the condyle. Sagittal opening and closing movements exhibit a straight line when viewed frontally because of the harmonious coordinated action of the neuromuscular system of both sides, especially the external pterygoid muscles.

Figure 5-47 diagrams the relationship of disc and condyle in the normal case (*a*) when the mouth is closed and (*b*) when it is open. The structure of the joint is such that during opening the disc is moved forward through a distance of 1 cm. from point A to A′, while at the same time, in order to maintain a harmonious relationship with the disc, the condyle must move through a distance of 1.4 cm. from point B to B′. Clearly, the two bodies of the lateral pterygoid act as two coordinating muscles. The result is that on each side, two different muscles must move at two different rates of speed coordinately for the joint to function normally and for a person to be able to open his mouth in a straight line.

Because the lateral pterygoid has two distinct points of insertion (Figs. 5-18 and 5-19)—the anterior and medial borders of the meniscus (*a*) and the neck of the condyle (*b*)—it acts essentially as two coordinating muscles, one of which moves the meniscus and the other the condyle.

LATERAL AND BENNETT MOVEMENTS OF THE MANDIBLE

In the lateral movements of the mandible, asymmetrical muscular patterns develop on each half. On the nonfunctioning side, the external pterygoid muscle contracts, and simultaneously the elevators of the same side contract slightly to prevent the jaw from dropping. On the other side, the contralateral retracting parts of the elevators hold the condyle in a relatively fixed position to prevent much anterior movement.

However, the condyle does rotate and glide medially, and this is the basis of the Bennett movement, which takes place across the glenoid fossa mediolaterally during lateral excursions. The importance of this phenomenon is its relationship to the occlusal surfaces of the teeth. The Bennett movement is the power movement and takes place on the functioning side with the head of the condyle set well into the fossa under tremendous muscle pressure. Although masticatory movements are highly complex, they become automatic in each individual as a result of the integration of the proprioceptive mechanism and muscular action. There is variation among individuals, depending upon neuromuscular reflex formation, but each person's masticatory movements are characterized by a high degree of stability. However, stability does not mean that there can be no change. The proprioceptive mechanism has a protective function. Interfering occlusal contacts act as stimuli to the proprioceptors in the periodontal ligament. The established neuromuscular pattern is then changed to prevent the reception of these stimuli. In this way, a new pattern which avoids the interfering occlusal contacts is established. However, this new pattern affects the position of the head of the condyle in its relation to the mandibular fossa in the various mandibular movements. Anatomical positioning is altered, and the head of the condyle may be constantly delivering a series of microtraumata to susceptible tissues with resultant temporomandibular joint and reflex disturbances.

SUMMARY

The ideal occlusion is one that provides for the maximum number of tooth contacts in centric-relation occlusion and in all the eccentric ranges of articulation. To approach this ideal, cusp heights, inclined planes, curve of Spee, curve of Wilson, neuromuscular action and movements within the temporomandibular joint must all be harmonious. The teeth themselves are very important to the freedom and the harmony of mandibular movement.

In the following situations, one or

more teeth are out of harmony with the muscle action, the temporomandibular joint and the rest of the dentition, and thus can interfere with mandibular movement. Any disturbance of occlusal level, axial inclination and tooth position limits mandibular movement. Elongated upper cuspids prevent freedom in lateral movements. Inclined planes that are out of harmony and other anatomical anomalies prevent the maximum number of tooth contacts in all mandibular movements. Deep fossae and long cusps tend to lock the dentition in centric relation. Teeth that have extruded into spaces in the opposite jaw as a result of tooth loss interfere with mandibular movements. Any type of restoration involving the occlusal surfaces that is placed in an unequilibrated mouth usually accentuates and exacerbates the disharmony. Restorations that are not anatomically harmonious with the other teeth and with the rest of the stomatognathic system prevent proper mandibular movements. Interfering occlusal contacts on the nonfunctioning or the functioning sides prevent the maximum number of tooth contacts in eccentric mandibular movements. The conditions mentioned above usually cause interfering occlusal contacts of the teeth in centric and eccentric mandibular movements and prevent proper mandibular movement.

Variations in relative jaw sizes will cause abnormal tooth relationships with consequent disharmony of mandibular movements. Deep overbites usually result in a vertical masticatory stroke.

The concept of the mandible as a lever developed from the traditional comparison of the crushing movement of the mandible with the action of a nutcracker. Different authorities have considered the mandible as a first, second or third class lever, or a combination of classes. It is important to remember that the fibrocartilaginous coverings of the head of the condyle, the fossa, the bone forming the condyle and the articular eminences are designed to bear pressure. This design is manifested histologically. The muscles of mastication provide the power, and the actual work is performed by the teeth which crush and triturate the food. Nevertheless, because of the intricacies of condylar movements, it is inaccurate to compare the actions of the mandible with those of a simple mechanical lever.[7]

REFERENCES

1. Bell, W. E.: Synopsis: Oral and Facial Pain and the Temporomandibular Joint. pp. 7, 15, 16. Dallas, E. Bell, 1967.
2. Best, C. H., and Taylor, N. B.: The Physiological Basis of Medical Practice. p. 904. Baltimore, Williams & Wilkins, 1950.
3. Beyeler, K.: Leitfaden fuer das beschleifen der zaehne bei paradentose (Manual for grinding of the teeth in cases of periodontal disease). Bern, 1944.
4. ———: Ueber paradentose und artikulationsstoerungen (Paradentosis and disturbances of articulation). Paradontologie. *2:*130, 1948.
5. Boos, H.: Centric and functional bite relations. JADA, *30:*262, 1943.
6. Brenner, G. P.: Functional occlusion for artificial dentures. JADA, *30:*1030, 1943.
7. Brown, A. H.: Movements of the mandible not provided for in present-day articulators. JADA, *17:*982, 1930.
8. Central Nebraska Study Club: Complete denture service with balanced functional occlusion using the patient as his own articulator. JADA, *30:*375, 1943.
9. Denen, H. E.: Movements and positional relations of the mandible. JADA, *25:*548, 1938.
10. Eltner, E.: Die anatomische articulator Eltner in der praxis (The anatomic articulator Eltner in practice). Schweiz. Vierteljhrschr. Zahnh., *22:*7, 1912.
11. Fischer, R.: Die oeffnungsbewegungen des unterkiefers und ihre Wiedergabe am artikulator (The opening movements of the mandible). Schweiz. Monatsschr. Zahn., *45:*867, 1935.
12. Gillis, R. R.: Establishing vertical di-

mension in full denture construction. JADA, *28:*430, 1941.
13. Granger, E. R.: Biologic factors in partial denture design. J. 2nd Dist. D. Soc., *31:*5, 1945.
14. Gysi, A.: Kieferbewegung und zahnformen (Mandibular movement and forms of teeth). Vienna, Schiff, Handbuch der Zahnheilkunde, 1929.
15. ———: Practical application of research results in denture construction (mandibular movement). JADA, *16:*199, 1929.
16. Hall, R. E.: Full denture construction. JADA, *16:*1157, 1929.
17. Hanau, R. L.: Articulation defined, analyzed and formulated. JADA, *13:*1694, 1926.
18. Hardy, J. D., Goodell, H., and Wolff, H. G.: Studies on pain: observations on the hyperalgesia associated with referred pain. Am. J. Physiol., *133:*316, 1941.
19. Harris, E.: Centric relation of the mandible. JADA, *37:*565, 1948.
20. Hight, F. M.: Graphic reproduction of mandibular movements in full denture construction. JADA, *17:*1489, 1930.
21. ———: Intra-oral method of establishing maxillomandibular relation. JADA, *19:*1019, 1932.
22. ———: Registration and recording of maxillomandibular relations. JADA, *21:*1660, 1934.
23. Keith, (Sir) A.: Concerning certain structural changes which are taking place in our jaws and teeth. Br. D. J., *45:*1243, 1924.
24. Koehler, L.: Statik und mechanik (Statics and mechanics). Dtsch. Monatsschr. Zahnh., *39:*705, 1921.
25. Kurth, L. E.: Occlusion in dentistry. JADA, *25:*1067, 1938.
26. Langley, L. L., and Cheraskin, E.: The Physiological Foundation of Dental Practice. pp. 28, 76. St. Louis, C. V. Mosby, 1956.
27. Ibid: p. 106.
28. Ibid: p. 115.
29. Lindblom, G.: Om balanserad artikulation samt dess betydelse for den marginala paradentitens behandling. Svensk Tandlak. Tidskr., *25:*353, 1932.
30. McCollum, B. B., and Stuart, C. E.: A research report, fundamentals involved in prescribing restorative remedies. D. Items Int., *61:*522, 641, 724, 852, 942, 1939.
31. McLean, D. W.: Diagnosis and correction of occlusal deformities prior to restorative procedures. JADA, *26:*928, 1939.
32. ———: The physiology of mastication. JADA, *27:*226, 1940.
33. ———: Pathologic occlusion: a major clinical problem. JADA, *31:*1586, 1944.
34. Moyers, R. E.: Temporomandibular muscle contraction patterns in Angle Cl. II, Div. 1 malocclusions, an electromyographic analysis. Am. J. Ortho., *35:*837, 1949.
35. ———: An electromyographic analysis of certain muscles involved in temporomandibular movement. Am. J. Ortho., *36:*481, 1950.
36. National Society of Denture Prosthetists, Report. JADA, *17:*1122, 1930.
37. Parma, C.: Research on prehistoric jaws, Paradontologie, *2:*123, 1948.
38. ———: Die kompensationskurve von Spee (Spee's compensation curve). Dtsch. Zahn-, Mund- Kieferh., *17:*350 (Nos. 9 & 10), 1953.
39. ———: Zur funktionsmechanik in der paradontologie (Mechanical function in periodontia). Oesterr. Ztschr. Stomatol., *51:*294 (No. 6), 1954.
40. ———: Die zahnwanderung (Movement of the teeth). Oesterr. Ztschr. Stomatol., *51:*474 (No. 9), 1954.
41. Phillips, G. P.: Diagnostic value of a practical study of the temporomandibular joint. D. Cosmos., *67:*1184, 1925.
42. Porter, M. R.: The attachment of the lateral pterygoid muscle to the meniscus. J. Pros. Dent., *24:*555, 1970.
43. Posselt, U.: Studies in the mobility of the human mandible. Acta Odont. Scand., *10* (Suppl. 10):3, 1952.
44. Rees, L. A.: Structure and function of the temporomandibular joint. Br. D. J., *96:*125, 1954.
45. Report, National Society of Denture Prosthetists. JADA, *17:*1122, 1930.
46. Robertson, S., Goodell, H., and Wolff, H. G.: Headache, the teeth as a source of headache and other pain. Arch. Neurol. Psychiatr., *57:*277, 1947.
47. Robinson, M.: Temporomandibular joint: theory of reflex controlled nonlever

action of the mandible. JADA, *33:*1260, 1946.
48. Sicher, H.: Oral Anatomy. ed. 2. St. Louis, C. V. Mosby, 1952.
49. Sears, V. H.: Problems of occlusion in partial denture construction. JADA, *17:*434, 1930.
50. Simpson, H.: Registration of centric relation in complete denture prosthesis. JADA, *26:*1682, 1939.
51. Stuart, C. E.: Articulation of human teeth. D. Items Int., *61:*1029, 1939.
52. Thompson, J. R.: The rest position of the mandible and its application to analysis and correction of malocclusion, Angle Ortho., *19:*163, 1949.
53. Thompson, J. R., and Craddock, F. W.: Functional analysis of occlusion. JADA, *39:*404, 1949.
54. Wild, W.: Unterkieferbewegungen und kaubewegungen (Mandibular and masticatory movements). Rev. Mens. Suisse Odont., *56:*897, 1946.
55. Williams, C. H. M.: Correction of abnormalities of occlusion. JADA, *44:*749, 1952.
56. ———: Present status of knowledge concerning the etiology of periodontal disease. Oral Surg., *2:*729, 1949.
57. ———: Normal physiology of the periodontium as it is affected by occlusal function. J. Periodont., *25:*22, 1954.
58. Wolff, H. G.: Some observations on pain, The Harvey Lectures, *39:*39, 1943, 1944.
59. ———: Headache and Other Head Pain. p. 440. New York, Oxford, 1948.

Additional Basic References

Ackermann, F.: Le Mecanisme des Machoires (The mechanism of the jaws). Paris, Masson, 1953.

Afonsky, D.: The trigeminal nerve. Oral Surg., *5:*913, 1952.

Anderson, D. J.: Measurement of stress in mastication. J. D. Res., *35:*664, 1956.

Arstad, T.: The Capsular Ligaments of the Temporomandibular Joint and Retrusion Facets of the Dentition in Relationship to Mandibular Movements. Oslo, Akademisk, 1954.

Brandnup-Wagnsen, T.: Present conceptions of the movements and functional positions of the human lower jaw. J. Pros. Dent., *2:*780, 1952.

Carlsoo, S.: Nervous coordination and mechanical function of the mandibular elevators. Stockholm, Acta. Odont. Scand., 1952.

Chick, A. O.: The relation between mandibular movements and the occlusal form of teeth in man. Br. D. J., *92:*29, 1952.

Corbin, K. B., and Harrison, F.: Function of the mesencephalic root of the fifth cranial nerve. J. Neurophysiol., *3:*423, 1940.

D'Amico, A.: The canine teeth-normal functional relation of the natural teeth of man. J. South. Calif. D. A., *26:* 1958.

Gibilisco, J. A., Shira, R. B., Shore, N. A., and Travell, J. G.: Panel on a Medical/Dental View of Temporomandibular Joint Dysfunction and Muscle Spasm. ADA 115th Annual Session, 1974.

Granger, E. R.: The establishment of occlusion: the articulator and the patient. D. Clin. North Am., Nov., p. 536, 1960.

Hildebrand, G. Y.: Studies in the Masticatory Movements of the Human Lower Jaw. Berlin, de Grauzter, 1931.

Hiltebrandt, C.: Die unterkieferbewegungen und ihre bezeihungen zum kiefergelenk (The movements of the mandible and their relation to the temporomandibular joint). *Z.* R., *47:*941, 1938.

Hjortsjo, C. H.: Studies on the Mechanics of the Temporomandibular Joint. Lunds Univ. Arsskrieft, C. W. K. Gleerup, 1955.

Huffman, R., Regenos, J., and Taylor, R.: Principles of Occlusion. Columbus, H. R. Press, 1969.

Kaplan, R. L.: Concepts of occlusion. D. Clin. North Am., p. 587, Nov., 1963.

Landa, J. S.: Integration of structure and function of the temporomandibular joint. New York J. Dent., *24:*290, 1954.

Long, J. H.: Location of the terminal hinge axis by intraoral means. J. Pros. Dent., *23:*11–24, 1970.

Lytle, R. B.: Vertical relation of occlusion by the patients' neuromuscular perception. J. Pros. Dent., *14:*12, 1964.

McCollum, B. B.: The mandibular hinge axis and a method of locating it. J. Pros. Dent., *10:*428, 1960.

Mahan, P. E.: Research in physiology of significance to dentistry. JADA, *72:*1448, 1966.

Mann, A. W., and Pankey, L. D.: Oral rehabilitation utilizing the Pankey-Mann instrument and functional bite technique. D. Clin. North Am., 215, 1959.

———: Oral rehabilitation, J. Pros. Dent., *10:*135, 1960.

———: The P. M. philosophy of occlusal rehabilitation. D. Clin. North Am., 621, 1963.

Melzack, R., and Wall, P. D.: Pain mechanism: A new theory. Science, *150:*3699, 1965.

Nagle, R. J.: Temporomandibular function. J. Pros. Dent., *6:*350, 1956.

O'Leary, T. J., Shanley, D. B., and Drake, R. B.: Tooth mobility in cuspid protected and group-function occlusion. J. Pros. Dent., *27:*21, 1972.

Pankey, L. D.: Seminar manual. Pankey Institute for Advanced Dental Education, Miami.

Perry, H. T.: Muscular changes associated with temporomandibular joint dysfunction. JADA, *54:*644, 1957.

Posselt, U.: Range of movement of the mandible. JADA, *56:*10, 1958.

Pound, E.: The mandibular movements of speech and their seven related values. J. South. Calif. D. A., *34:*435, 1966.

Pruden, W. H., II: Occlusion related to fixed partial denture prosthesis. D. Clin. North Am., p. 121, Mar., 1962.

Ramfjord, S. P., and Ash, M. M.: Occlusion. ed. 2. Philadelphia, W. B. Saunders Company, 1971.

Sarnat, B. (ed.): The Temporomandibular joint. ed. 2. Springfield, (Ill.), Charles C Thomas, 1964.

Schuyler, C. H.: Factors in occlusion applicable to restorative dentistry. J. Pros. Dent., *3:*722, 1953.

———: An evaluation of incisal guidance and its influence in restorative dentistry. J. Pros. Dent., *9:*374, 1959.

Sicher, H.: Functional anatomy of the temporomandibular joint. *In* Sarnat, B. (ed.): The Temporomandibular Joint. ed. 2, pp. 28–58. Springfield, (Ill.), Charles C Thomas, 1964.

Silverman, M. M.: The speaking method in measuring vertical dimension. J. Pros. Dent., *3:*193, 1953.

Walsh, J. P.: Neurophysiological aspects of mastication. Dental J. Australia, *23:*49, 1951.

Wolff, H. G.: Headache and Other Head Pain, New York, Oxford University Press, 1963.

6 Examination for Temporomandibular Joint Dysfunction

HEAD PAIN AND THE TEMPOROMANDIBULAR JOINT

Most people expect a thorough examination when they visit a physician, especially for the first time, but very few have been educated to understand the necessity for similar thoroughness when they visit a dentist.[14] The emergency patient who is in pain expects and should receive immediate treatment, but for all others a thorough examination should be performed before any treatment is undertaken. Because it is impossible to separate temporomandibular joint dysfunction from every other aspect of dentistry, this examination should be sufficiently detailed to cover every aspect of the patient's stomatognathic system.

Examination. It is most important that the examination of the patient be thorough. Caries can becloud the patient's pain pattern, and the occlusion of the teeth may do likewise.

The Diagnosis. The diagnosis should be the assessment of all clinical signs and symptoms.

Prevention. There is no question that we agree on caries prevention (fluorides, home care, etc.), nor is there any question about the necessity for the prevention of periodontal disease. By the same token, occlusion-related pathology prevention should be equally stressed. Therefore, it follows that along with caries and periodontal treatments, preventive occlusal treatments are indicated.

The dental practitioner should be alerted to the widespread existence of this syndrome and of the diagnostic criteria that will aid him in the recognition of this clinical entity. He should have a system of recording the symptoms and of checking the progress of the condition.

Examination of New Patient

In the course of the preliminary examination of a new patient, it is important that a few pertinent questions be asked such as:

1. Do you have pain in the region of the temporomandibular joint and the ear?
2. Do you have difficulty in opening or closing your mouth?
3. Does opening or closing your mouth produce any facial pain?
4. Do you have headaches?
5. Do you have clicking in the temporomandibular joint?

If the dentist elicits positive answers to these questions, a comprehensive temporomandibular joint examination is indicated.

Although some practitioners may prefer not to use a printed form in taking the personal history, the outlines suggested below should be used as a guide. Some dentists may want to use an actual printed form so that it may be enclosed in the patient's folder along with all other records of the case.

Form I is a detailed questionnaire for head pain and temporomandibular joint examination. The rationale for the questions therein may be found in other publications by the author. Form II is a pictorial representation of

Form I
PERSONAL HISTORY

Date__________ No.______

Mr.____
Name Mrs.____ ____
Miss____ Last Name First Name Middle Initial

Residence____ Tel. ________
No. Street City Zone State Area Code:

Occupation_______________________ Firm's Name__________________
If housewife, write housewife Leave blank, if housewife

Firm's Address ____________________________________ Tel.________
No. Street City Zone State

Date of Birth__________ Marital Status__________ Ages of Children__________

Spouse's Name____
Last Name First Name Middle Initial

Spouse's Occupation____________________ Firm's Name__________________

Firm's Address____________________________________ Tel. ________
No. Street City Zone State

Who referred you to us? ______________________________________

Address____ Tel.________

Name of your regular physician__________________________________

Address____ Tel.________

Name of your regular dentist____________________________________

Address____ Tel.________

On the lines below, please list any physicians; dentists; neurologists; ear, nose, throat specialists; orthopaedists; chiropractors; psychiatrists; or clinical teams. Also, please list their specialties and briefly describe their diagnosis and treatment.

Dr.______________________ MD DDS Specialty____________________

Address____ Tel.________
Area Code:

Diagnosis and Treatment_______________________________________

____

____

Dr.__________________________ MD DDS Specialty__________________________

Address____ Tel.__________ Area Code:

Diagnosis and Treatment____

____

____

Dr.__________________________ MD DDS Specialty__________________________

Address____ Tel.__________ Area Code:

Diagnosis and Treatment____

____

____

Dr.__________________________ MD DDS Specialty__________________________

Address____ Tel.__________ Area Code:

Diagnosis and Treatment____

____

____

Dr.__________________________ MD DDS Specialty__________________________

Address____ Tel.__________ Area Code:

Diagnosis and Treatment____

____

____

Dr.__________________________ MD DDS Specialty__________________________

Address____ Tel.__________ Area Code:

Diagnosis and Treatment____

____

MEDICAL HISTORY

Please answer as many of these general health questions as possible with *YES* or *NO*. However, write freely on the discussion questions.

A. Have you had: Arthritis?_____ Osteoarthritis?_____ Rheumatoid arthritis?_____

Sinus infection?_____ Ear infection?_____ Swollen glands?_____

Blood vessel disease?_____

B. Do you have frequent headaches?_____ What area of the head?_____ How long do they last?__________ Migraine?_____

C. Have you ever had a severe blow to the head?_____

What part of the head?__________ Date __________

D. Have you ever suffered nutritional deficiencies?_____ Colitis?_____

E. Ulcers?_____

F. Do you regularly take any medication?_____ Which?____________________

Are you allergic to any medication?_______ Which?____________________

G. If you have any current nondental physical problems, please describe them:_____

____

H. Do you have any emotional problems regarding your teeth? Please describe them:

____

I. Please indicate anything else about yourself which you suspect may be related to your condition____

PAIN SYMPTOMS

1. Is there pain in the right joint?______________ Left joint?______________
2. When did the symptoms start in the right joint?__________ Left joint?__________
3. Indicate kinds of pain: Sharp____ Dull____ Aching____ Deep____ Superficial____
4. Is the pain constant?________________ Intermittent?________________
5. How often do you have pain?________________________________
6. Does pain start abruptly?________________ Gradually?________________
7. Does pain disappear abruptly?______________ Gradually?______________
8. What time of day or night is pain most severe?______________________
9. What is the longest period you have gone without pain?________________
10. Does rest increase pain?________________ Decrease pain?______________
11. What medication, if any, do you take to relieve pain?__________________

12. Please describe any method of positioning the jaw that you have found for relieving pain________________

13. Do any of the following normal daily activities cause pain? (Answer either *YES* or *NO*.) If yes, where do you feel pain?

    Yawning________ Chewing________ Swallowing________ Speaking________

    Singing________ Shouting________ Brushing teeth________ Turning head________

    Brushing or combing hair______ Hunching shoulders______ Moving the neck______

    trunk________ shoulders________ arms________

14. Do your teeth hurt? Upper right________ Lower right________ Upper left________

    Lower left________

15. Did the symptoms start after any of the following conditions:

    Severe emotional upset____________ Excessively large bite or yawn ____________

    Blow on jaw______________ Irregular or raised dental filling______________

    Excessive opening of mouth during dental extraction________________

    Dental treatment utilizing a head cap________________

    Traction for cervical arthritis________________

ORAL SYMPTOMS OTHER THAN PAIN (Answer the following questions either *YES* or *NO*.)

16. Do you feel that your "bite" is closed?________________

17. Are your jaws clenched when you awaken from sleep?________________

    Do you grind your teeth when asleep?______________ Awake?______________

    Do you clench or grind your teeth when Driving?________ Gardening?________

    Golfing?________ Bowling?________ In moments of concentration?________

18. Are your jaw muslces ever tired?______________ When?______________

19. How do you chew your food? Comfortably?____________ Angrily?____________

    To get it down as quickly as possible?________________

20. Do you ever notice excessive warmth in your jaw muscles?________ When?________

21. Have you ever noticed salivary changes?______ Increase?______ Decrease?______

22. Do you have a salty taste in your mouth?__________ A coppery taste?__________

    A sour or lemony taste?________________

23. Do you ever feel pressure or tenderness about the right eye?______ Left eye?______

24. Do tears form in your eyes for no apparent reason?________________

25. Does your face swell?____________ What part?____________ When?____________

26. Do you ever get dizzy?____________________ How often?____________________

27. Do you ever feel faint?____

28. In which ear (R or L) do you ever notice: Ringing? (R)______ (L)______ Popping noises? (R)_____ (L)_____ Stuffiness? (R)______ (L)_____ Pain? (R)_____ (L)_____ Itchy feeling? (R)______ (L)______ A hearing change? (R)______ (L)______

29. Do you have a tic or nervous twitch about the face?__________________________

    Where?______________________________ When?______________________________

30. Is there a family history of temporomandibular joint dysfunction?____________

31. Have you been treated by an orthodontist?____________ Periodontist?____________

Finally, by referring back to the names of doctors in Section I, please answer:

32. Did any of their treatments make you feel better? If so, which helped the most? In what manner?____

    ____

    ____

33. Did any of the treatments make you feel worse? Which ones? In what manner?

    ____

    ____

    ____

the distribution of pain areas. Form III is a follow-up symptom chart.

Form I consists of a folded sheet of paper, divided into four pages, each page measuring 8½ by 11 inches. It is divided into three parts: Personal History, Medical History and Clinical Examination. The patient fills out the first two parts. For the clinical examination, long experience has shown that the use of a simple code (√ for positive, X for negative findings) enables the dentist to dictate his findings to his assistant, leaving him free to concentrate on the examination procedure. Only rarely will written information have to be filled in. The purpose of this head pain and temporomandibular joint examination is to correlate pertinent signs and symptoms in order to differentiate between temporomandibular joint arthrosis and other diseases with similar symptoms.

Name________________________ Date________________________
Code: √ Positive; X Negative

CLINICAL EXAMINATION

A. Course and Distribution of Pain on Palpation: (R) (L)

1. Frontal .... __ __
2. Temporal .... __ __
3. Vertex.................................... __ __
4. Occipital................................ __ __
5. Parietal.................................. __ __
6. Supraorbital .... __ __
7. Infraorbital............................ __ __
8. Zygomatic .... __ __
9. Nasal .... __ __
10. Angle of mandible................ __ __
11. Mental .... __ __
12. Preauricular .... __ __
13. Auricular............................... __ __
14. Postauricular.......................... __ __
15. Inferior maxillary nodes .... __ __
16. Submandibular nodes .... __ __
17. Deep cervical nodes .... __ __
18. Throat constricture .... __ __
19. Tongue tip (burning) .... __ __
20. Palatal region......................... __ __
21. Cervical region .... __ __
22. Shoulder................................ __ __
23. Arm .... __ __
24. Does raising arm cause pain? __ __
25. Fingers.................................. __ __
26. Furrowing brow area............. __ __
27. Ear lobes:
    Tenderness .... __ __
    Swelling............................... __ __

B. Muscle Examination (Tenderness and Pain on Palpation):

1. Temporal:
   Anterior fibers........................ __ __
   Middle fibers.......................... __ __
   Posterior fibers....................... __ __
   Body .... __ __
2. Masseter:
   Origin.................................... __ __
   Anterior body......................... __ __
   Posterior body........................ __ __
   Insertion................................ __ __
3. Internal Pterygoid:
   Insertion................................ __ __
4. External Pterygoid:
   Insertion................................ __ __
5. Infratemporal Fossa:
   Tenderness .... __ __
   Swelling................................. __ __
6. Sternocleidomastoid:
   Origin.................................... __ __
   Body .... __ __
   Insertion................................ __ __
7. Sternocleidomastoid reflects pain in:
   Heart__Chest __ __
8. Trapezius:
   Origin.................................... __ __
   Body .... __ __
   Insertion................................ __ __
9. Hypertrophy of any muscle
   ____
10. Other muscle involvement
    ____

C. Ear Examination:

1. Anterior wall tenderness........ __ __
2. Excessive wax........................ __ __

D. TMJ Symptoms Other Than Pain:

1. Noises (audible):
   Crepitation............................. __ __
   Click....................................... __ __
2. Clicking:
   a. Sagittal opening click
      Immediate .... __ __
      Intermediate...................... __ __
      Full opening .... __ __
   b. Sagittal closing click
      Immediate .... __ __
      Intermediate...................... __ __
      Terminal closure.............. __ __
   c. Clicking in eccentric ranges

Right functioning range ... __ __
Left functioning range...... __ __

3. Noises (stethoscopic):
   a. Crepitation opening .... __ __
   b. Crepitation closing........... __ __
   c. Crepitation in eccentric ranges ....
      Right functioning range ... __ __
      Left functioning range...... __ __
   d. Rubbing .... __ __
4. Fremitus................................. __ __
5. Abnormal condyle movement revealed by palpation............. __ __
6. Hypermobility of condyle....... __ __
7. Hypomobility of condyle........ __ __
8. Subluxation of condyle.......... __ __
9. Dislocation of condyle........... __ __
10. Swelling of TMJ area .... __ __
11. Are you double-jointed?......... __ __

E. Mandibular Movements (Empty) Causing Pain—Area Involved (note which):

1. Centric Relation:
   a. Opening ____________
   b. Closing ____________
2. Rt. Functioning Range ____________
3. Lt. Nonfunctioning Range ____________
4. Lt. Functioning Range ____________
5. Rt. Nonfunctioning Range ____________
6. Protrusive Range ____________

F. Interfering Occlusal Contacts:

1. Centric Relation____________
2. Rt. Functioning Range ____________
3. Lt. Nonfunctioning Range ____________
4. Lt. Functioning Range ____________
5. Rt. Nonfunctioning Range ____________
6. Protrusive Range ____________

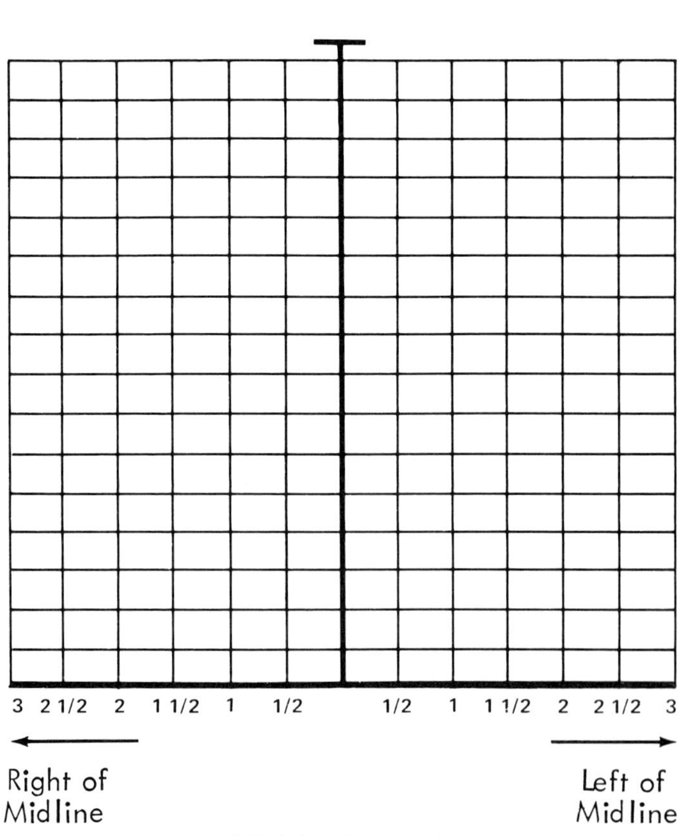

G. Sagittal Pattern of Mandibular Movement Deviation from Straight Vertical Opening-and-Closing Movements as Seen by Examiner:

*H. Widest Interincisal Opening*______mm.

Overbite______mm.

Total opening______mm.

I. Classification of Pathological Mandibular Relationships:

1. Protrusive______________________
2. Retrusive ______________________
3. Increased vertical______________________
4. Medial mandibular shifts due to bite relationships ______________________
5. Reduced vertical______________________

J. Temporomandibular Joint Roentgenographic Findings—comparing the right and left joint:

1. Lateral view, closed position—oblique lateral-transcranial projection
   a. Glenoid fossa: contour __________

      density______________________
   b. Articular eminence: contour _____

      density______________________
   c. Joint gap: anterior __________

      superior______________________

      posterior ______________________
   d. Condyle head: contour __________

      density______________________
2. Lateral view, open position—oblique-lateral-transcranial projection
   a. Angle of inclination of the posterior wall of the articular eminence

      ____
   b. Relation of center of the condyle head to the center of the articular eminence ______________________
   c. Distance traversed by the condyle head ______________________
3. Midorbitomeatal baseline—corner-of-the-mouth projection
   a. Mediolateral position of the condyle head with relation to the fossa

      ____
   b. Contour and density of the posterior wall of the articular eminence

      ____
   c. Gap between the posterior wall of the articular eminence and the condyle head______________________
   d. Contour and density of the condyle head______________________

K. Summary of TMJ X-Ray Findings:

Closed position left______________________

____

Closed position right______________________

____

Open position left______________________

____

Open position right______________________

____

*L. Summary of General Examination:*__

____

____

*M. Clinical Analysis:*______________________

____

____

*N. Diagnosis:*______________________

____

____

*O. Plan of Treatment:*______________________

____

____

Form II

Name ____________

Date ____________

DISTRIBUTION OF PAIN AREAS

A

B

Form II is a visual representation of the areas of pain distribution. There are two types of pain or tenderness experienced by the patient or elicited by palpation: superficial or deep. To distinguish between them, use a red pencil for marking the areas of superficial pain or tenderness and a blue pencil for indicating the areas of deep pain. The horizontal lines can be used for explanatory notes. The figures (*A*) and (*B*) portray a cutaway of the right and left

Form III

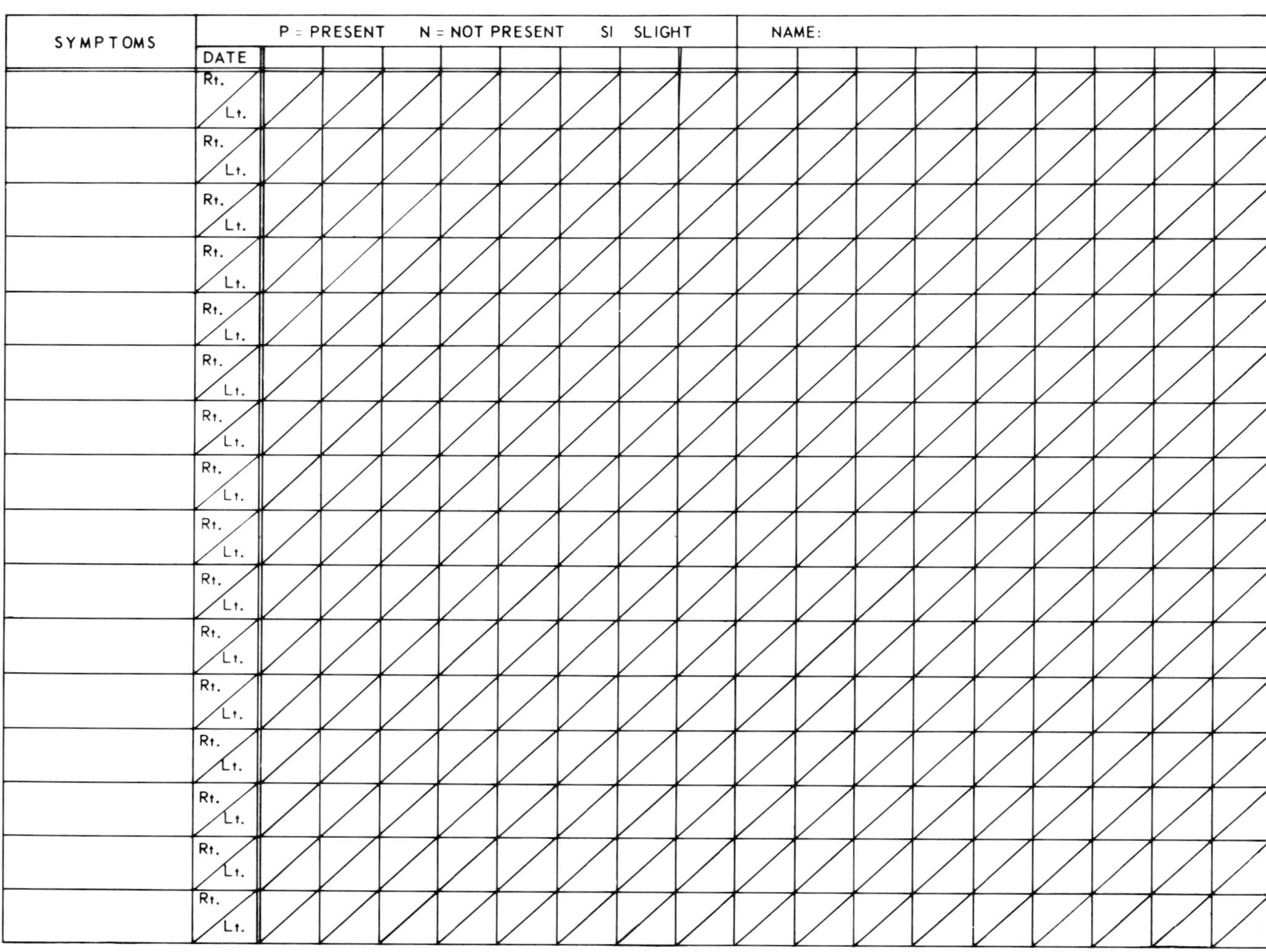
SYMPTOMS

P = PRESENT N = NOT PRESENT Sl SLIGHT

NAME:

DATE

Rt. Lt.

Rt. Lt.

Rt. Lt.

Rt. Lt.

Rt. Lt.

Rt. Lt.

Rt. Lt.

Rt. Lt.

Rt. Lt.

Rt. Lt.

Rt. Lt.

Rt. Lt.

Rt. Lt.

Rt. Lt.

Rt. Lt.

Rt. Lt.

sides of the face, respectively, for the purpose of demonstrating the right and left external and internal pterygoid muscles.

After all the information has been filled out on the examination sheet (Form I) and on the chart (Form II), and the patient has left the office, list these symptoms in the appropriate column in Form III. Using the code printed at the top of Form III, note the status of each symptom. Since Form III is printed on both sides of a single sheet of paper, it is possible to list 32 symptoms, and to trace their progress for 18 visits. There is a box at the top of each column to insert the date of the visit. In those unusual instances in which the patient has more than 32 symptoms, the simultaneous use of two sheets will regularize what might otherwise become a chaotic procedure. The positive symptoms are highlighted and a plan of treatment can then be formulated quickly. Form III has proved a tremendous timesaver, because the symptoms do not have to be relisted at each visit and a symbol can be used to indicate the status of the particular symptom. Its use prevents the possibility of failing to check on any symptom. In addition, the patient's progress can be evaluated at a glance.

In most instances of temporomandibular joint dysfunction, the symptomatology is so extensive and varied that no patient can be relied on to remember with any degree of accuracy all of his symptoms. Once the patient begins to feel better and his symptoms abate, he has a tendency to forget the original severity of his pain and the extent of his other symptoms. By noting the status of the pain areas and other symptoms at each visit, a visual pattern becomes evident. These charts are of inestimable value to the dentist, since they can be used to demonstrate graphically to the patient the range and course of symptoms and the eventual result of treatment. The systematic use of Form III will provide an accurate method of checking on every symptom, as well as a means of ascertaining at a glance the progress made by each patient.

DISCUSSION OF THE HEAD PAIN AND TEMPOROMANDIBULAR JOINT EXAMINATION

Complications in temporomandibular joint dysfunction treatment can be avoided by a thorough head pain and temporomandibular joint examination. The difficulties that may occur during and after temporomandibular joint treatment can be avoided if complete and accurate medical and dental histories are taken beforehand. While the compiling of complete medical and dental histories should be a well-established procedure in every phase of dental practice, it is especially important when temporomandibular joint dysfunction treatment is to be undertaken. A series of routine questions is asked of the patient with an aim to uncovering pertinent data in his history. For example, in contacting former dentists and physicians, it may be discovered that the patient has certain drug allergies, neuroses, an inability to tolerate appliances, etc. Such a history may give information which would contraindicate certain types of treatment or might indicate precautionary measures which must be taken before, during or after treatment.[3] The questions based on the symptomatology of systemic conditions which are important for their effect and interrelationship with temporomandibular joint dysfunction are discussed under "Differential Diagnosis" in Chapter 9. The affirmative answer to some of these questions may be insignificant to the patient; however, careful evaluation and further questioning will determine the significance of an answer.

The medical history is not intended as a substitute for a medical examination by a physician. It is a check on the patient's medical background for the purpose of protecting him during the course of dental treatment.

The analysis of the findings of pain is of major importance. The time interval between the onset of first symptoms, their distribution, duration, frequency and type serve basically to determine whether we are dealing with any of the major or minor neuralgias. The area of onset, the distribution and the course of the pain symptoms are particularly significant. The common symptoms of temporomandibular joint arthrosis, such as cervical, nuchal, vertex and temporal pain, etc., seem to be unrelated and usually are reported to the physician rather than to the dentist. The correlation of these symptoms with pathological function creates a basis for the diagnosis of joint dysfunction. Form II is used to chart the distribution of superficial and deep pain areas and other pertinent data. The relation of pain to function, the triggering device and the analysis of painful mandibular movement provide information regarding pathological muscle function, muscle spasm and disturbances in joint function. Vertigo is a common symptom of many diseases as well as a common diagnostic symptom of temporomandibular dysfunction. Oral symptoms of pathologic occlusion may be clenching of the teeth and jaws during sleep or waking hours, salivary changes and muscle fatigue.[9]

Temporomandibular joint sounds may either be audible or inaudible to the examiner. The inaudible type requires stethoscopic examination, although the sounds are always audible to the patient. These sounds consist of clicking, rubbing and crepitation. Many patients believe that these noises are normal. A tape recorder microphone may be placed next to the temporomandibular joint in order to record the various types of clicking before treatment and to verify the absence of it after treatment. Subluxation, dislocation and swelling may often be symptoms of joint dysfunction.

The ear is often affected by disturbances of the temporomandibular joint. Tinnitus, popping noises, stuffiness, change in hearing ability, tenderness, swelling of the ear lobe, and excessive wax formation due to disturbance of the wax-forming organ are common symptoms. The importance of the muscle examination as a diagnostic procedure is its correlative feature with the other symptoms of temporomandibular joint arthrosis. The areas of painful muscles are plotted on Form II.

The interfering occlusal contact is the key to the diagnosis of pathologic occlusion. Its detection in all the ranges of articulation cannot be overemphasized.

The dentist, undertaking restorative procedures on a patient whose temporomandibular joint difficulty is unrecognized, is unknowingly dealing with a "bomb" which may be triggered to explode at any time during or after treatment. He will have problems in adapting the restorations to the existing pathologic occlusion. It should be emphasized that such restorations have been adapted to a habitual pathologic-occlusion relation. The restoration will function in this pathological relation; however, if the restored tooth is examined as an entity, it will be found that the tooth has not been restored to normal form and function.

Patients with temporomandibular joint dysfunction usually have a wide range of symptoms which must be charted systematically. It is of utmost importance, therefore, to employ a system of record-keeping that is comprehensive, accurate, and timesaving. The use of such a system is necessary to make a precise diagnosis, formulate a plan of treatment, and record and evaluate the treatment performed. Unless the practitioner uses a foolproof method of recording and checking the progress of every one of the patient's symptoms, comprehensive care is impossible.

The summary of the medical and the dental histories and the clinical examination will make evident the pertinent facts that are necessary for evaluation and further exploration. The correlation of the medical and the dental histories, the clinical examination of the stomatognathic system, the roentgenographic summaries and the clinical analysis will become a reasonable pursuit and lead to clarity of thought and a logical rationale for diagnosis and treatment not possible previously.[10]

CLINICAL ANALYSIS

A concept of dentistry that goes beyond the local treatment of individual teeth and groups of teeth to an understanding of the mouth as a masticatory organ and the restoration of that organ to optimal health and function must be based not only upon careful history and examination, such as have been described earlier, but also upon systematic clinical analysis. Only when these three steps have been taken can diagnosis be accurate, plan of treatment logically constructed and ultimate prognosis favorable. Although there is no doubt that functional occlusion can exist over a wide range of conditions, it is also true that many apparently normal occlusions are revealed to be actually pathological when they are subjected to careful and critical clinical analysis. Too frequently, an erroneous diagnosis of normalcy is made as a result of a static view of the mouth and the teeth as they present themselves at examination. However, if the entire masticatory organ is considered dynamically, if the process whereby it has reached its present state is revealed and understood, an orderly course of degeneration is frequently brought to light, and clues may be found to aid in preventing further deterioration.

Deviations from normal, no matter how slight, should be detected and recorded. Such deviations may be the beginnings of serious collapse of the dentition. Any deviation from the normal should be evaluated critically in the light of its potential to damage the organ of mastication. The medical history, the dental history and examination and the clinical analysis will reveal such deviations.

The emphasis here is on predictive dentistry. A thorough examination reveals a "predictive profile." The slightest deviations may predict serious problems. Such predictions pave the way for preventive dentistry. The dentist evaluates deviations and formulates a plan of treatment to correct them.

The clinical analysis is one of the relationships of the approximating teeth to each other and to their antagonists, of the teeth to the investing bone and the soft tissues, and of the mandible to the maxilla and the skull. Through casts and roentgenograms, all deviations from normal, as well as the effects of such deviations upon the masticatory organ as a whole, are noted and correlated. When the clinical analysis has been completed and recorded, it will be a detailed blueprint of the stomatognathic system. This blueprint will trace the history of the case from its present condition backward to its origins and will enable the dentist to plan efficiently and effectively for restoration to optimum health and function. In addition, the completed and recorded clinical analysis serves as an excellent aid in the important process of educating the patient.

To assure accuracy and standardized procedure, the clinical analysis should be based on the outline of the examination, and the findings of the analysis should be recorded.

Since the type of examination and history suggested by the outline is unusual in its thoroughness and in its attention to the general condition of the patient as well as to the details of his tooth and mouth structure, it might be well to discuss the purposes served by such a detailed procedure as well as the importance of such thoroughness.

As the dentist takes the patient's medical history, he has an opportunity to lead the patient toward an understanding of the interrelationships of the teeth and the mouth with the other organs of the body and with general health.[6]

The taking of a detailed history and the subsequent clinical examination at the chair serve a dual purpose. First, they enable the dentist to ascertain, note and evaluate all pertinent facts in the case. Second, they provide an additional opportunity to explain to the patient the relationships between his teeth and mouth and his general well-being, what the dentist plans to do and why certain things should be done. The clinical examination must be an organized, habitual, routine and standardized procedure. It must not neglect or fail to consider even the slightest deviation from normal. To minimize the possibilities of future error and to provide a record for planning treatment and for future surveillance, all findings should be committed to writing on a chart, such as Form III.[2,12]

Although the rationale for most of the procedures outlined above is familiar to all dentists, as are the techniques involved in carrying them out, it might be well to discuss some of them in greater detail, especially as they bear upon the problems involved in stomatognathic dysfunction.

Discussion of Analysis of Articulated Casts

The casts are used to note past effects on the masticatory organ and to plan future adjustments and reconstructions.[4] For a proper analysis of occlusal dysfunction, two types of examinations of the casts must be made. First, there is a static analysis consisting of an examination of the casts at rest. Second, there is a dynamic analysis or the examination of the casts in action on an articulator. Lindblom[7] calls the latter the functional analysis. The primary purpose of the dynamic or functional analysis is to reveal interferences in articulation which cannot be observed directly in the mouth. The articulated casts are also useful because they enable the dentist to examine the pattern of wear caused by the skid into habitual convenience relationship.

It is extremely difficult to observe articulation and centric-relation closure directly in the mouth. Casts mounted upon suitable instruments not only make observation easier but also enable the dentist to make his studies at his convenience and thus to assure thoroughness. The articulator is a machine that *approximates* the relationship between the upper and the lower casts to the relationship between the maxillary and the mandibular teeth in the patient's mouth. Since most articulators are built to average measurements, they can yield only approximations rather than precise relationships for an individual patient.

To achieve the greatest possible degree of accuracy in the articulated mounting, it is necessary to consider three planes of reference: vertical, horizontal and anteroposterior. These three planes are established through the use of the face-bow. The centric-relation bite establishes the upper cast into the bite fork, and the bite fork carried by the face-bow itself establishes vertical, horizontal and anteroposterior relationships of the teeth to the hinge-axis of the articulator. The marker on the face-bow is used to establish the Frankfort plane, the Camper plane, the axis-orbital plane, or any other horizontal plane that is constant. The McCollum, Guichet, and Stuart face-bows (and articulators) make possible a more accurate location of the hinge-axis.[5] For those dentists who do not want to go through the procedure of a hinge-axis articulator mounting, a Galletti articulator may be used. However, the Pankey-Mann method of articulation is the safest and most practical that can be used by the general practitioner in complete mouth rehabilitation. Whichever method is used, its principles should be understood and techniques and procedures involved in its operation standardized and mastered. The lower cast is oriented to the upper by means of a centric-relation wax bite. The technique for obtaining this bite is explained in Chapter 13. The necessity for using the centric-relation wax bite in mounting the upper and the lower casts on the articulator will be discussed in a later section. Suffice it to say at this time that a mounting approximating the relationships between the upper and the lower teeth and between the teeth and the relevant parts of the skull is necessary in each case if an accurate clinical analysis and diagnosis and a logically constructed plan of treatment are to be achieved.

It is important for the dentist to explain to the patient that the health and the function of his mouth depend not only on the number of teeth that are present but also on which teeth are present. One patient, for example, may be missing all six lower molars, while another may have six teeth missing in a more random pattern throughout his mouth. The relative masticatory efficiency of these patients is entirely different. A masticatory efficiency of 100 per cent would require that each group of teeth function at full capacity—all incisors cutting, all cuspids tearing, all bicuspids crushing, all molars triturating. In the case of the patient who has lost all six molars, the triturating efficiency is zero because the upper molars are unopposed, and trituration cannot take place. In the case of the second patient, only part of the total efficiency for each group of teeth has been lost because only some of the teeth in each group are unopposed and hence, nonfunctional. Therefore, it is evident that although the same number of teeth are missing in both cases, the first case presents a more serious problem.

Only through a careful comparison of each tooth on the patient's cast with its counterpart on a normal cast can changes of position of the teeth be detected. Conditions such as tipping, migration and open interproximal spaces should be noted. As teeth drift or contacts open, many important changes take place in the periodontium. Many conditions can be detected by observing the occlusal level on the articulated casts. Such conditions as the "roller coaster" effect of the occlusal plane and the presence of extruded teeth should be noted carefully. The type of occlusion should also be noted as should teeth or segments of the arch which are end-to-end, in cross-bite or in mixed bite.

The observation of the horizontal and the vertical overbites is necessary in order to plan the reshaping of the teeth in the eccentric ranges of articulation.

In every case, vertical dimension should be determined so that evidences of change may be ascertained. Study of the articulated casts supplemented by study of the roentgenograms of the temporomandibular joint will enable the dentist to differentiate between a vertical overbite which is normal for a particular patient and a decreased vertical dimension. The importance of making this differentiation *before* initiating any treatment cannot be overemphasized. If a normal vertical overbite is "opened," further intrusion of the teeth and other undesirable sequelae may be expected.[7]

Discussion of the Roentgenographic Analysis

The primary purpose of roentgenography of the teeth from a periodontal point of view is the revelation of bone structure. While it is obviously important to secure all the facts that a roentgenogram can reveal about a case, the basic problem is to determine the present height, quantity and quality of the bone structure and to utilize this information in a dynamic analysis of the case under treatment.

Whether or not all the teeth are present, fourteen periapical and four bite-wing exposures of teeth and alveolar bone should be taken routinely in every case. Under special circumstances, additional exposures may be necessary.

It may be possible to look at the standard size dental film casually and cursorily, but the methodical study that is really necessary if roentgenography is to be used to its fullest advantage must be carried out on a projected enlargement. Tiny details and variations from normal, which may escape unnoticed on the small film viewed directly, will appear clearly on the enlargement.

Check the crown-root ratio, that is, the relation of the height of the clinical crown to the length of the root. This ratio and the number of roots present become very important factors to consider if a tooth is to be used as an abutment. After noting whether the roots of a tooth are in line with the masticatory forces on the teeth, a basis for treatment may be designed to restore the dentition or to prevent further movement. The width of the periodontal space should be observed. In many cases the width of the periodontal space is indicative of the occlusal force sustained by the tooth. Note whether the space is of normal or abnormal width around the root and whether the cervical, the middle or the apical areas vary in width.

Next, the lamina dura should be studied carefully. Starting at the distal of the tooth and following the lamina dura all around the root, the height and the quality of the lamina dura should be noted. Since dense bone is laid down next to the periodontal space in response to tensile force, this procedure will enable the dentist to estimate past and existing forces on each tooth. The trabecularization and the density of the alveolar bone, the interseptal bone and the supporting bone must be carefully observed. The quality of the bone is an important criterion for diagnosis.

Roentgenographic examinations always should be concluded with a general summary of the findings. The act of summarizing will lay a firm foundation for diagnosis.

The purpose of temporomandibular joint roentgenograms is to provide the correlative information of the temporomandibular joint and the occlusion. This relationship is elaborated further in the chapters on temporomandibular joint roentgenography and case histories.

DIAGNOSIS

Although the procedures involved in history taking, clinical examination and clinical analysis may seem inordinately time-consuming, they are essential if the highest aims and major objectives of good dentistry are to be accomplished. Each part is important because it helps to furnish the facts that are necessary for diagnosis and planning of treatment. In addition, each part constitutes an important phase in the education of the patient which enables him to appraise his condition intelligently and to cooperate with the dentist in restoring his teeth and mouth to optimal health and function.

It might be well to restate and reconsider the objectives of dentistry at this point so that the necessity for a broader concept of diagnosis as a basis for achieving them may be emphasized and understood. The objectives of dentistry are:

1. To recognize and remove any factors disturbing the physiological function of the masticatory organ
2. To repair and reconstruct the dentition, distributing the forces of occlusion and articulation to as many teeth as possible in harmony with the supporting structures and the temporomandibular joint
3. To plan for the maintenance of normal function

The dental diagnosis is based primarily upon the evaluation of:

1. The static and the dynamic analyses of the masticatory organ
2. The periodontal analysis
3. The status of the dentition. All of the information from the clinical analysis forms the basis of the dental diagnosis. As all the basic facts in the case are revealed, and as all the fundamental elements that lead to the diagnosis are considered, the general diagnosis will seem to emerge almost automatically.

PROGNOSIS

Every case must be planned around the following periods:

1. The treatment period during which an attempt is made to restore the dentition to a physiological state
2. The autoreparative period during which bone and connective tissues, blood vessels, nerves, gingival tissues and teeth undergo physiological repair
3. The maintenance period during which the temporomandibular joint func-

tion is continually checked by means of roentgenography, checking of the occlusion and the articulation, prophylaxis and other procedures. The prognosis depends upon the course of these periods.

PLAN OF TREATMENT

The treatment of temporomandibular joint dysfunction requires an orderly and well-planned procedure.[1] The improper relationships of the teeth, neuromusculature, and temporomandibular joint means that we have to answer the question, "Can we bring this patient to normal function?"

The diagnosis has clarified the cause-and-effect relationships of the problem at hand. The plan of treatment sets up a *modus operandi* for solving these problems.

Every aspect that affects the planning of the treatment must be considered in the light of the following objectives:

1. To establish control over the destructive forces in the mouth that were revealed during the static and the dynamic analyses
2. To establish control over the temporomandibular joint
3. To establish control over the state of the teeth
4. To provide maintenance control over the three problems mentioned above
5. To educate the patient in his cooperative role in achieving the four objectives mentioned above.

If any change in the occlusal level of the teeth is indicated, study can be facilitated by adding wax to the occluding surfaces of the teeth of the mounted casts and carving them to approximate correctness. By this method, interfering tooth surfaces may be trimmed or wax may be added where necessary, and the casts may be studied carefully before any operations are performed on the teeth themselves. Such study will assist in achieving final success by enabling the dentist to see how each tooth must be reshaped, moved orthodontically or otherwise treated. In the unusual case of totally collapsed dentition, the reconstruction of the masticatory organ can be planned and actually executed on the stone cast with restorations in wax before any work at all is done in the patient's mouth. The Pankey-Mann articulator serves very well in this capacity. The additional procedures necessary in such cases are integrated in the plan of treatment. The only difference in procedure is the extension of the treatment period to provide for sufficient time for the patient to wear a Shore Mandibular Autorepositioning Appliance (see Chap. 11) or other appliances so that his comfort on the new occlusal level may be tested.[13]

REFERENCES

1. Bartels, J. C.: Diagnosis and treatment planning. J. Pros. Dent., *7:*657, 1957.
2. Blass, J. L.: Non-technical aids in diagnosis and patient education. New York J. Dent., *17:*241, 1947.
3. Brodie, A. G.: Differential diagnosis of joint conditions in orthodontia. Angle Ortho., *4:*160, 1934.
4. Chestner, P.: A methodical approach to the analysis of study casts. J. Pros. Dent., *4:*622, 1954.
5. Contino, R. M., and Stallard, H.: Instruments essential for obtaining data needed in making a functional diagnosis of the human mouth. J. Pros. Dent., *7:*66, 1957.
6. Friend, D., *et al.:* The Dentist and His Patient. New York, New Organization, 1946.
7. Lindblom, G.: The value of bite analysis in modern dentistry eliminating uncertainty and lack of planning in the treatment of human dentition. Br. D. J., *80:*87, 1950.
8. McCollum, B. B.: Consideration and treatment of the mouth as an organ of digestion. JADA, *16:*1426, 1929.
9. Miller, S. C.: Diagnosis and treatment planning in periodontics. J. D. Med., *9:*109, 1954.

10. Moore, D. S.: The importance of a case history. J. Ontario D. A., *29:*124, 1952.
11. Mossberg, D.: Basic principles versus systems. Am. J. Ortho., *37:*594, 1951.
12. Rochon, R.: Prognosis—the stepchild of oral diagnosis. J. D. Educ., *14:*191, 1950.
13. Seides, H. M.: A diagnostic and technical approach to complete oral rehabilitation. D. Survey, *23:*250, 1947.
14. Thoma, K. H.: Oral Diagnosis and Treatment Planning. Philadelphia, W. B. Saunders, 1937.
15. Ziskin, D. E.: Oral diagnosis as it functions today. JADA, *20:*1703, 1933.

7 Stress

Temporomandibular joint dysfunction, like many other afflictions of modern man, is a syndrome of complex etiology and inevitably there is a strong emotional component. The problem must not be thought of as psychosomatic in origin; rather, it is somatopsychic. It is the pain that causes the neuroses, not the neuroses that cause the pain.

The stress with which the patient lives may either trigger or exacerbate the symptoms. Therefore, it is important that the dentist have an understanding of stress—its causes, some of its effects, successful and unsuccessful mechanisms for coping with it, and the position of temporomandibular joint dysfunction in this overall picture.

Why different people react to stress in completely different ways is a many-sided problem; there are no simple or comprehensive answers to the question. One person will react to a stressful environment by developing hypertension, or ulcers; another will develop temporomandibular joint dysfunction; and an exceptional person, under equal or even greater stress, may remain symptom free. Undoubtedly, there are predisposing physical factors which help to explain the differences; a multitude of psychological causes might also be invoked. But there is no one satisfactory explanation for the disparity. However, most temporomandibular joint dysfunction patients have to some extent developed maladaptive responses to stress, and these responses have played a role in creating the temporomandibular joint problem.

Definition

According to Selye, stress is the "nonspecific response of the body to any demand made upon it."[5] This is a very broad definition: the response is said to be *nonspecific,* that is, there is a general adaptation of the whole body to meet the demand; and further, the response is to *any* demand, not just to a severe or an unpleasant one. It is important to understand this point, for we may be accustomed to thinking of stress as bad. Yet while unreasonable pressure from an overbearing employer or incapacitating, financially draining illness is clearly a stress-producing situation; so also is seeing a good movie, or receiving a coveted promotion, or falling in love. Stress is fundamental to life. It is not an entity to be avoided or conquered; we all are subject to it and live with it our entire lives. Selye has implied that complete freedom from stress would be death.[6] Without stress, life would lack challenge and color. Although too much stress can be incapacitating, too little is not motivating enough.

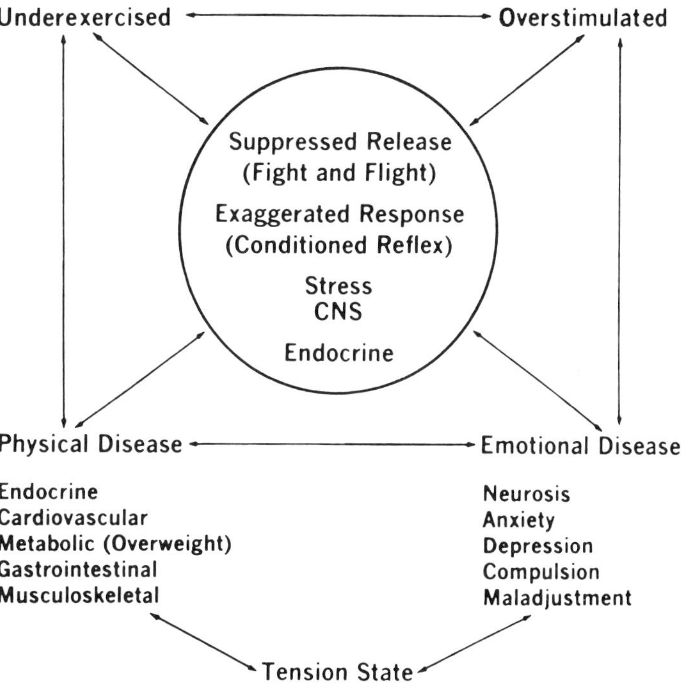

FIG. 7-1. Fight-or-flight response of the mechanical, urbanized individual. (After Krause, H.)

Fight or Flight

The classic model of stress is the familiar fight-or-flight response. A threatening situation is perceived and the entire body is put on the alert (Fig. 7-1). Muscles tense, peripheral circulation increases, digestive processes shut down, and the body is poised, ready to meet the situation head on or to flee from it. In our society, however, the fight-or-flight response is rarely acted out as such, for neither fighting nor fleeing is usually appropriate. As stress-provoking conditions become more complex, so must the response, and problems most often begin with the person's difficulty or inability in finding an appropriate response. Although stress per se is neutral, neither good nor bad, it becomes the concern of the physician or dentist when its effects become harmful, debilitating, or incapacitating. This, no doubt, is why we tend to think of stress only in terms of its negative potential.

General Adaptation Syndrome

Common to all stress is what Selye terms the general adaptation syndrome.[7] First comes alarm. Then comes adaptation, during which bodily and mental resources are mobilized to deal with the situation. However, if the stressful condition persists indefinitely, the final stage of exhaustion begins. One's "adaptation energy," or adaptive capacity, is highly individual. A degree of stress that is highly stimulating to one person may verge on incapacitation for another. All stress is wearing and uses up some of this finite supply of energy. Whether the energy is used recklessly and wastefully ("burning the candle at both ends") or slowly and productively over a long and fulfilling lifetime is a choice left to the individual. One cannot replenish the store of adaptation energy, or determine how large the store is to be, but one may decide how it is to be used.

Yet a major problem in our complex society is that more and more, people feel they do not have a real voice in choosing the life they will lead or in determining how their energies will be used. This is one reason why stress has become an entity of such concern to the healing professions.

> . . . if man loses hope of changing his situation, anticipating more of the miserable sameness day after day, year after year, dispirit can breed specific disease, with symptoms which conventional doctors can chart and follow, but not always understand—and very seldom cure.[2]

Not only has our society produced the compartmentalized man who cannot break out of dispiriting sameness, but it is also characterized by a frighteningly accelerated rate of change—in ideas, technology, social stratification, and standards—of a magnitude never seen before. Implicit in this change are intense demands for adaptation; in other words, intense stress. As Brunwald put it,

> . . . we stand at the threshold of, and have in fact already begun to experience, enormous upheavals in all aspects of our lives—personal and professional. As medical scientists and physicians and dentists we will, in addition to our present objectives, be forced to find ways to strengthen man's ability to adapt to the greater environmental and mental stresses that await him. . . . It is clear that if we are to survive the storm individually and collectively, our adaptive abilities will be strained to the utmost, and we shall be forced to cope successfully with the many new problems posed by "future shock."[4]

Not surprisingly, stress tends to be a bigger problem in urban environments. Cities can provide the excitement and challenge necessary to a productive life, yet they can also easily trap people in narrow, unfulfilling life patterns. The major stressors of the twentieth century—excessive change and overcompartmentalization—are particularly active in cities. Consequently, the city is often the locus of a high percentage of stress-related disease. However, suburban and rural environments are not exempt. Instant communication affects every stratum of society and every type of community, making escape from complex, global problems next to impossible.

Coping

The incidence of stress-related disease has become alarmingly high because of the problems mentioned above. It is not that stress is harmful in itself—as we have seen, it is not, nor is it avoidable. The *degree* of stress plus the availability of options for dealing with it are the crucial factors. It is when the individual is so overwhelmed by events that he can no longer find effective means for adapting, that stress leads to life-threatening disease and dysfunction.

As an example, visualize three dolls—one of glass, one of celluloid plastic, one of steel. If a 25-pound hammer labeled "disease attack" struck the glass doll, the object would shatter. If the hammer struck the celluloid plastic doll, the object would be dented or would break. If the hammer struck the steel doll, the object would produce a musical sound. The disease attack is the same in each case; it is the resistance that is different.

The fact that emerges quite clearly is that the possible results of excessive stress are numerous. Most common are diseases of the heart and blood vessels, the number one killer in America today. Another favorite target is the digestive system. It is also becoming increasingly clear that the body's immunological system may be affected by stress, possibly rendering susceptible individuals prone to infectious diseases, allergies, rheumatoid arthritis, and even cancer.

Effect of Stress on Muscles

Of major interest to the dentist concerned with temporomandibular joint dysfunction is the effect stress has on the muscles. Stress that cannot be effectively dealt with frequently leads to tension. As part of the fight-or-flight response, the muscles of the entire body become tense in anticipation of action. However, when no direct physical response is possible or appropriate, the muscular tension cannot be worked out in action, and this unrelieved tension has the effect of shortening the muscles.

Most individuals who do not earn their living through physical labor are underexercised. Their muscles are in a weakened state from lack of activity and are therefore susceptible to the damaging effects of tension arising from stress. The chronically tense muscle is in a state of perpetual, if unproductive, overuse and will eventually react by going into intensely painful spasm. Further, the muscle that is shortened through tension and lack of activity will begin to lose its elasticity, so that when it must perform, extra contraction must be initiated. Another damaging result of muscular tension is that once tension has resulted in painful, sore muscles, the individual will usually respond by tensing the same muscles again, resulting in further shortening of those muscles.

Stress and Tension in Temporomandibular Joint Dysfunction

In the case of temporomandibular joint dysfunction the predisposing physical cause is pathologic occlusion resulting in malposition of the mandible. The basic problem is that the occlusal disharmony may lead to abnormal muscle activity and tension, which then lead to painful spasm and temporomandibular joint dysfunction. Stress plays a major role in establishing this pattern. According to Bell,

> the role of tension is of great importance. . . . The most important activator of occlusal disharmony is believed to be emotional tension, and it acts in several ways: it increases clenching and bruxism; it increases all muscular activity; it raises muscle tonus, causing increased interarticular pressure which may lead to functional interference; it induces fatigue which may lead to spasm, and it increases the patient's anxiety and alarm, thus setting up a vicious cycle.[1]

Weinberg emphasizes that it is meaningless to attempt to categorize temporomandibular joint dysfunction patients as suffering either from emotional stress or from an occlusal disharmony: the two factors are intimately related and cannot be viewed in isolation.[8] However, temporomandibular joint dysfunction always implies an occlusal problem, and once the dysfunction is established, it becomes a source of stress in itself, and as such becomes self-perpetuating.

Profile of the Temporomandibular Joint Dysfunction Patient

Learning to cope successfully with stress is of utmost importance to the patient with temporomandibular joint dysfunction. The dentist plays a vital role in this process. The complex physical-psychological nature of temporomandibular joint dysfunction is such that therapeutic intervention on the strictly physical level cannot suffice. The dentist must view his patient as a whole person rather than concentrating only on his localized physical difficulty. As part of this process the practitioner should try to learn something of his patient's emotional makeup, his life situation and its stresses, and his inner strengths and weaknesses. The latter is especially significant, for only when the patient's strengths have been disclosed can the dentist help him to exploit these positive qualities successfully and to utilize them in the fight against the debilitating effects of stress.

Until recently, most temporomandibular joint dysfunction patients were female, hypertensive, short, blond, and between 35 and 45 years of age. This typical profile has changed radically. Now patients with temporomandibular joint dysfunction may be as young as 10 years old, and at least 25 per cent of them are male. Why the change? We have suggested that temporomandibular joint dysfunction is commonly an accompaniment or result of stressful circumstances. Formerly, it was middle-aged and older patients who suffered the most from stressful emotional and life-adjustment problems. Yet of late society has placed ever more pressure for achievement on its younger members. All the way down through the elementary schools, the demands for scholastic achievement and rapid advancement are growing. In addition, adolescence is inevitably a time of great stress, as the individual must cope with changing body image, temperament and identity, as well as with peer pressure and parental expectations. It is hardly surprising that this intense pressure should be reflected in a rising incidence of temporomandibular joint dysfunction in young people, and the dentist must therefore be aware of any manifestations of this syndrome in younger as well as middle-aged patients.

It is the responsibility of the dentist to help the patient perceive his problems in a more realistic light: only then can the patient begin to learn more effective means of dealing with stress. The approach used in each case will be highly individual, for no two patients are alike. In every case, however, it should be borne in mind that competent coping can never take place in an atmosphere of ignorance.

People with temporomandibular joint problems frequently delay seeking treatment, and this behavior may be seen as one manifestation of their difficulty in coping with stress. One reason for delay is the hope that the problem will simply disappear by itself; another is the mistaken impression that clicking or painful joints are quite normal. A large number of patients live with the dread that their symptoms are the result of incurable cancer or a brain tumor; this fear is so great that they simply cannot confront the problem and deal with it in a constructive fashion. Therefore, the dentist must use his consultation room as a "listening room." The patient should be encouraged to ventilate his fears and anxieties. For his part, the dentist, having done a thorough examination and made a sound diagnosis, must be able and willing to answer the patient's questions, to maintain a reassuring attitude toward him, and to instill in him a sense of hope.

The Dentist's Responsibility

It is important that the dentist explain to the patient and discuss the totality of his temporomandibular joint problem, for the patient is in no position to cooperate in his treatment if he is left in the dark about his difficulty. It is also important that members of the patient's family understand the problem; the dentist should explain the origin and character of the problem and the course of treatment. It is extremely supportive to the patient to have those close to him directly involved in his therapy.

Because temporomandibular joint dysfunctions run the gamut from the almost purely physical to the almost purely emotional, the dentist must develop a keen sensitivity toward his patients. Only then can he locate in each case the point along this physical-psychological spectrum at which the problem lies. By explaining the situation to his patient, the dentist can enlist him as a partner in his treatment. When the patient understands the emotional component of his temporomandibular joint dysfunction, both he and the dentist will be able to deal with the problem more effectively.

As Reiner* states in her illuminating

* Assistant Professor, Educational Foundations, Hunter College of C.U.N.Y.

article on "Psychological Aspects of Dentist-Patient Relationships,"

in the last decade an awareness of the psychological aspects of interpersonal relationships has assumed increasing importance in the conduct of dental and medical practices. The result has been greater success in both treatment and attitudes toward dental care. However, the obvious failure of preventive dental health programs to significantly change the dental habits of Americans indicates a need for dental educators to give more serious consideration to the inclusion of psychological approaches to human interaction in the professional curriculum. Clinical procedures which utilize many of the significant aspects of the patient's reactions to dental care would modify the generally negative approach to treatment. A unique aspect of dentistry is that in most instances the patient associates the dentist with producing pain. In contrast to this is the physician who is usually perceived as relieving pain. Generally, the determining factor for seeking dental care is not preventive measures but rather the final stages of dental problems closely related to pain.

The dentist, in his professional relationship with his patients is dealing primarily with stress and anxiety; first, the anxiety of the patient and himself which operate independently of each other; second, the anxiety which occurs as a result of their interactions with each other. Stress or anxiety can be psychologically understood as a specific emotion or state of tension or arousal that stirs an organism to observable action or to internal change. Stressful conditions include a situation involving conflict, frustration, ambivalence, and guilt. Stress is coped with in a unique fashion, each individual having developed his own life's pattern of emotional response. In the face of severe stress, physiological changes may occur to further complicate the situation.

The young child acquires his deepest gratifications through his mouth and oral activity. At the same time he develops anxiety related to his oral cavity because of inevitable adult interference with oral pleasure-seeking needs. Dental treatment incorporates infantile guilt and anxiety associated with his mouth. It is symbolic, for the adult, of his early life situation with feelings of helplessness and dependency upon an individual in a superior role. Regression, or childlike adaptive behavior, occurs because of the similarity of dependency upon the dentist to early dependency on individuals in authority, namely, parents.

Throughout our development, various organs or parts of our bodies assume an increased importance. There develops an hierarchy of physical organs wherein teeth generally are assigned an important position. Unconsciously teeth are symbolic of aggressive weapons, strength, health, decay and sexuality. They appear with frequency in our dream life as an indication of our unconscious thoughts.

Research indicates that anxiety is the strongest factor in dental absenteeism and neglect of teeth. The patient's anxiety is a dread of a danger which is out of proportion to the real situation, and dread of an unknown danger as well. Frequently his own masochistic and self-destructive needs form an intervening barrier against maintaining his dental health and cosmetic appeal at their optimum. The patient requires an indication that he is in the hands of a professional worker who understands and respects his fears, thereby providing him with an element of safety necessary for trust.

In order to overcome much of a patient's resistance to treatment and to understand the patient's problems, communication with the dentist is a vital factor. The dentist's own anxiety in which he can be immersed, intervenes. It is the rare dental practitioner who does not experience serious anxiety from time to time regarding his own ability. To counteract this emotion, unconsciously he denies it and represses it. Overtly he manifests a confidence and egocentricity that does not leave room for reconsideration of a difficult case or consultation with a colleague. In addition, the dentist has feelings of guilt because he is perceived by his patients in the generally uncomplimentary image of causing pain as well as anger.

The average dental practitioner often feels that the treatment of temporomandibular joint dysfunction is beyond his capabilities. With this in mind, he often overlooks the problem, or if cognizant of it and not knowing what to do, plays down the symptoms of temporomandibular joint dysfunction, meanwhile hoping that the pain will go away. It will not. What the practitioner does not realize is that the treatment of temporomandibular joint dysfunction *is* within his capabilities but that he must have a logical plan of procedure.

Reiner continues:

In interpersonal relationships with his patients, the dentist faces several sources of anxiety. First, he must decide the professional image he wants to project and second, to what extent it must modify his responses to his patients and to others in his personal and social milieu. The security felt by making a "friend" of each patient whose loyalty hopefully cannot be questioned is counteracted by the possible loss of a "friend" should there ensue a dental parting of the ways.

The dentist's psychological need for approval and recognition cannot always be satisfied appropriately. The patient is not always in a position to judge the quality of the dental work and frequently complains and is hostile. The dentist finds himself in the difficult position of being alone in judging his work. He has to supply his own ego rewards.

The dentist experiences additional anxiety in regard to establishing his own criteria of success. These may be in conflict with those of his professional milieu, or may set him on the frustrating, never-ending pursuit of the most lucrative practice, or the most highly respected reputation. No matter what is his decision, its fulfillment is dependent upon his patients who remain indifferent to his emotional needs.

The tension, hostility, and ambivalence which occur as a result of the dentist's emotional problems reduce his effectiveness with patients. He experiences a diminution of the psychic energy which is needed to cope with daily pressures. The dentist must understand and deal effectively with his own anxieties in order to be able to direct his attention to fulfilling his patient's needs, which in clinical situations are dominant. . . .

The dental practitioners seek procedures to improve the confidence, rapport, motivation, and comfort of their patients. Several well-conducted research studies have been reported that provide some insight into the needs and concerns of the patient. . . . A review of several studies reveals that patients indicated that their choice of dentists was affected by specific factors in the following rank order of importance:

1. Personality of the dentist
2. Reputation of the dentist
3. Quality of workmanship
4. Convenience (e.g., location, schedule of appointments)
5. Fee of the dentist

It is interesting to note that in a large sampling of individuals in varied income brackets, the fee of the dentist was of least importance in selecting a dentist. This substantiates other observations that dental neglect is as prevalent in upper income groups as in lower groups. Obviously it is not lack of money that prevents proper dental care, although this is frequently the rationalization proffered.

Patients have indicated their preferences regarding the length of time for treatment in the dental chair. There is a significant preference for the half-hour appointment over a one-hour appointment. Long hours in the dental chair should occur only by mutual agreement. Psychologically it must be recognized that anxiety increases with time and is complicated by feelings of captivity and loss of control.

When evaluating the dentist's personality, patients indicated that the most desired characteristic is that he be sympathetic. This seems to be even more important to women than to men. The dentist is perceived by the patient as an authority figure with power over his captive and with formidable instruments to assist him. He is perceived, as well, as a threat to body integrity, and hence there is a strong desire for an assurance of safety.

Patients rejected the talkative dentist. Quiet accompanying the dental experience was preferred by many except for the very fearful patient. He preferred music which has become a usual office background over the talkative dentist. Music acts as a buffer to the painful experience, whereas the dentist's voice draws patients into the situation where he experiences discomfort.

It is not possible to treat solely a specific area of the body. It is necessary to know the total individual in order to relate to him effectively. Each patient has his unique physical and behavioral response to severe anxiety and he gives consistent clues which should not be ignored.

The following psychologically sound practices should be helpful to the practitioner:

1. Explain each procedure before its application, thereby providing the patient with some safeguards against anxiety.

2. Encourage mutual participation with the dentist, conveying your awareness and respect for the patient's feelings.

3. Become sensitive to the patient's behavior and attempt to respond appropriately.

4. Know the patient as a person as thoroughly as you know his mouth.

Dentist-patient relationships are potential conflicts, because each participant is confronted with emotionally charged drives. The patient may be fearful of pain, anxious about the results of treatment, resentful of the authority-figure dentist, and concerned over the expenses involved. The dentist may find emotional stress in not being able to please his patient, not having his treatment fully appreciated for its worth, and in having to cope with the patient's outward expressions of dissatisfaction.

Relationships between dentists and their patients have been known to improve when communication between them becomes frank and friendly. The practitioner can motivate and instill confidence in his patient when he understands that dentistry is concerned not only with the oral cavity but also with the total person. Dentist-patient relationships depend on mutual trust and understanding.[3]

REFERENCES

1. Bell, W.: Recent concepts in the management of temporomandibular joint dysfunction. Oral Surg. *28:*596, 1970.
2. McQuade, W., and Aikman, A.: Stress. pp. 13–14. New York, E. P. Dutton, 1974.
3. Reiner, M.: Psychological aspects of dentist-patient relationships. J. Oral Med., *27:*79, 1972.
4. Roche Laboratories: Coping with Stress. 1975.
5. Selye, H.: Stress Without Distress. p. 27. Philadelphia, J. B. Lippincott, 1974.
6. Ibid: p. 32.
7. Ibid: pp. 38–40.
8. Weinberg, L. A.: Temporomandibular dysfunction profile: a patient-oriented approach. J. Pros. Dent., *32:*312, 1974.

8 *Temporomandibular Joint Dysfunction and Pathologic Occlusion*

Since the components of the stomatognathic system are closely interrelated, pathological conditions in one part always affect other parts to a greater or a lesser degree. Abnormal or pathologic occlusion results in abnormal function of all the other parts of the stomatognathic system and especially of the temporomandibular joint. A change in the position of the teeth usually results in a change in the position of the mandible and of both condyles. If the condyle in one joint moves in one direction, the other condyle must make a corresponding and compensatory movement because the mandible is a single U-shaped bone. If these shifts are caused by abnormal or pathologic occlusion, minute or gross pathological effects on the structures of the temporomandibular joint must take place, and these will be accompanied by various symptoms. It is the direction and the frequency of stress that are most important. The fundamental research of Bernard[2] and Cannon[3] into the complex interrelationships between structure and function showed that whenever there is interference with normal function, there is disease.

An examination of the temporomandibular joint usually reveals that the shape

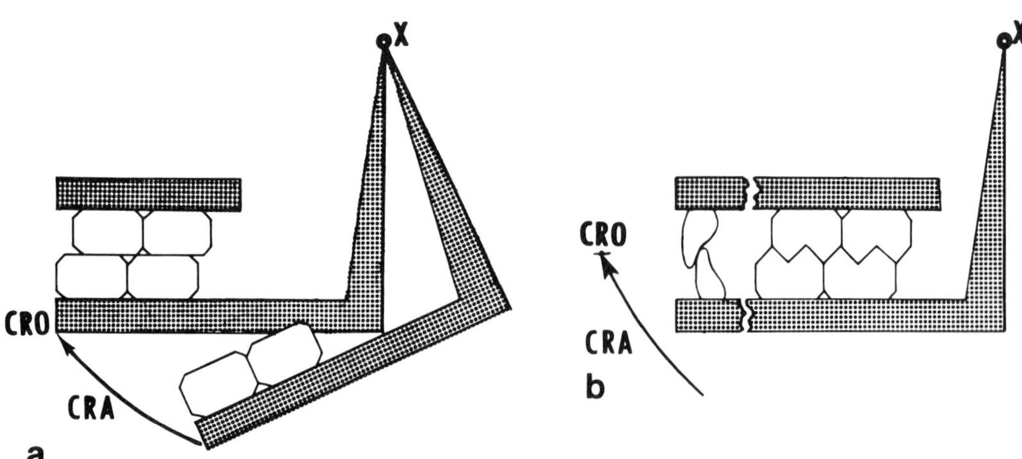

FIG. 8-1. A diagram (*a*) of the centric-relation arc, CRA, closure on the hinge-axis, X, into centric-relation occlusion, CRO. A diagram (*b*) of centric-relation occlusion, CRO. The mandible closes in centric-relation arc, and the cusps rest in their opposing fossae. This is in harmony with the hinge-axis at X.

of the condyle and the glenoid fossa vary according to the occlusion and the articulation of the teeth. This fact helps to explain mandibular movements. In the temporomandibular joint, as in all other joints, structure influences function, and the structure is the means or the tool whereby functional operations take place.

Since it is an accepted principle of physiology that structure is modified by function, it should be realized that abnormal function will cause modifications and alterations in the structure of the temporomandibular joint. In a deep vertical overbite it is usual to find a deep mandibular fossa and steep inclines on the cusps of the teeth. On the other hand, in a zero vertical overbite, it is usual to find a shallow fossa and flattened cuspal inclinations. Wild and Bay[10] show that the temporomandibular joint in general and the condyle in particular undergo gradual changes to compensate for wear and loss of teeth. In cases of temporomandibular joint dysfunction and pathologic occlusion, in which the teeth, the periodontium and the alveolar bone are strong, the temporomandibular joint will succumb to the abnormal stresses and show gross symptoms. If all the factors in the masticatory organ are equally strong, minute changes will take place in all of them until such time as the resistance of the body is low; then accelerated degeneration of the weakest parts will take place.

PRINCIPLES OF CENTRIC-RELATION OCCLUSION

It is important to consider the basic principles of centric-relation occlusion. Centric-relation occlusion exists when the teeth occlude in harmony with centric relation. The basic factors that determine centric-relation occlusion are the teeth, the periodontium, the neuromuscular system, the bones and the temporomandibular joint. The hinge-axis of the condyles is the center of the centric-relation arc. Before translation occurs, rotary movements are made about this hinge-axis. It is this rotary motion about this single axis that is sought, whether or not teeth are present. In Figure 8-1*a*, in which all of the cusps have been removed for the purpose of demonstrating what would happen in full closure under such circumstances, the mandible closes in a hinge movement. Note the representation of the condylar hinge-axis at X, and the centric-relation arc, CRA. When teeth are present, cuspal interdigitation must harmonize with the centric-relation arc. In centric-relation occlusion, the mandible closes in a centric-relation arc and the cusps rest in their opposing fossae. This action is demonstrated in (*b*). Note the hinge-axis at X and the upper and lower incisor relationship at the completion of the centric-relation arc into centric-relation occlusion, CRO.

As a patient opens from and closes to centric-relation occlusion, he moves through the centric-relation arc (Fig. 8-2). For future discussion, it is important to understand this figure fully. Figure 8-2*a* depicts centric-relation occlusion, CRO. The teeth have passed through the centric-relation arc and are now in terminal closure. The dot, X, in the center of the condyle, represents the hinge-axis. The point at which lines AB and CD cross represents the hinge-axis of the centric-relation arc. In centric-relation occlusion, the dot on the condyle and the cross-point of AB and CD are always identical. The normal joint gap is depicted at F. Note the equal spacing of the joint gap between the fossa and the condyle.

Figure 8-2*b* illustrates all the mandibular occlusal contacting surfaces in centric-relation occlusion and the normal condyle-fossa relationships. Figure 8-2*c* demonstrates the frontal view of the mandibular movement in the sagittal plane.

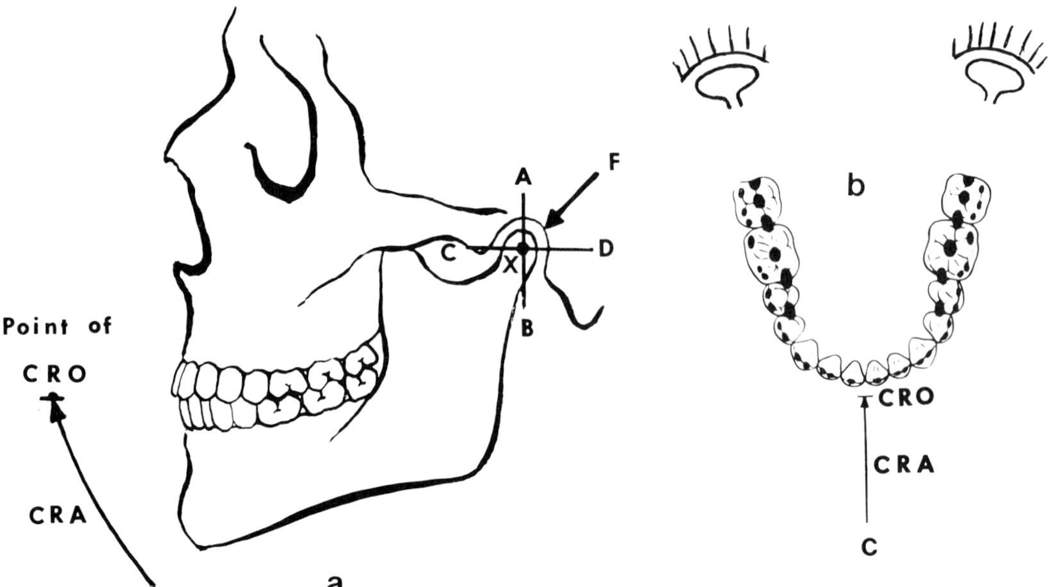

FIG. 8-2. Profile view (*a*) of the arc of closure, CRA, to the terminal position, CRO, in harmony with the hinge-axis, X, of the temporomandibular joint; mandibular centric-relation occlusion contacting surfaces (*b*); frontal view of the centric-relation arc in the sagittal plane (*c*).

The mandible passes through the centric-relation arc, CRA, to terminal closure or centric-relation occlusion, CRO. Compare this diagram with the profile view of the centric-relation arc in Figure 8-2*a*.

ETIOLOGY OF CENTRIC-RELATION AND ECCENTRIC-RANGE INTERFERING OCCLUSAL CONTACTS

Since the interfering occlusal contact is the primary cause of pathologic occlusion and temporomandibular joint dysfunction, its etiology should be discussed before going on to a consideration of the classes of pathologic occlusion. This will clearly point the way to an understanding of pathologic occlusion and temporomandibular joint dysfunction.

There are two categories under which the etiology of interfering occlusal contacts may fall. One is the direct cause, which consists of abnormalities of tooth and arch form; the second is the indirect cause, consisting of abnormalities of other tissues which, in turn, affect the teeth and the arch form.

Direct Causes of Interfering Occlusal Contacts

Every individual has a pattern of growth that is predetermined by his genetic constitution. Because of the multiplicity of possible genetic combinations, the sizes of the maxillary and the mandibular arches may not be harmonious. In such cases, although the teeth may be quite normal, the disparity in arch size may not permit them to occlude in normal relationship. Hereditary factors may also cause variations in the size and the anatomy of the teeth. Though slight in themselves, these variations may not permit the development of a normal occlusal relationship.

Excessive occlusal wear of a full or nearly full dentition, or the loss of posterior support will cause a closed-bite type of pathologic occlusion. Unreplaced lost teeth may permit extrusions of opposing teeth and rotations and migration of adjacent teeth. These conditions will result in abnormal occlusal relationships. Extensive caries and loss of tooth structure produce results similar to those attributable to actual tooth loss. Restorations which are in supra-occlusion and are anatomically inharmonious are detrimental to the stomatognathic system because they become iatrogenic interfering occlusal contacts.

Occlusal rehabilitation, improperly performed, may result in increased vertical dimension with resultant pathologic occlusion and condylar displacement. Orthopaedic procedures that attempt to "reposition the mandible" usually result in pathologic occlusion and temporomandibular symptoms. Supernumerary teeth, over-retention and premature loss of deciduous teeth and improper eruption of the permanent teeth are direct causes of interfering occlusal contacts by altering tooth position and arch form.

Another direct cause of interfering occlusal contacts is the eruption of a third molar which causes buckling of the anterior teeth and disturbance of the arch form. In dealing with direct causes, the treatment is focused on those teeth that are the direct causes of the interfering contacts.

Indirect Causes of Interfering Occlusal Contacts

In this category, abnormal tissues move the teeth, create an interfering occlusal contact and thus create pathologic occlusion. Periodontal and periapical pathological conditions may cause tooth movement with resultant pathological tooth relationships. Among these pathological conditions are abnormal wandering of the teeth, destruction of alveolar bone, pressure of inflammatory granulation tissue in the periodontal pockets,[6] etc.

Various habits which cause tooth movement, such as pipe smoking, tooth clenching and lip biting, as well as occupational habits, may also result in pathologic occlusal relationships. Various types of cysts and tumors, usually benign, can cause malposition of the teeth by exerting pressure on the roots. Though occurring infrequently, enlarged tuberosities may interfere with centric-relation closure by contacting the retromolar area of the mandible before the teeth occlude. Therefore, the patient must move into a habitual convenience relationship in order to occlude his teeth.

External trauma and diseases of the tissues of the stomatognathic system during the developmental and the adult stages of the individual may each have effects in producing a pathologic occlusion. Congenital malformation, diseases and fractures of the temporomandibular joint will result in pathologic occlusion. Reduced, unreduced and improperly reduced fractures of the mandible and the maxilla will change occlusal relationships which in turn create pathologic occlusion. Condylectomy, mandibular resection, and similar osseous surgery of the jaws will also result in occlusal changes. Paralysis of motor nerves of the stomatognathic system and injuries to or diseases of the muscles of the stomatognathic system cause lack of muscular coordination and unphysiological action during function. Endocrine disease may cause variations in structures of the stomatognathic system, resulting in pathologic occlusion. Restorations that are placed in infraocclusion may allow the opposing tooth to elongate and create an interfering occlusal contact during the excursive movements.

In those orthodontic cases which evidence tooth movement, pain, etc., after completion of the case, the reason can generally be ascribed to an interfering contact in centric-relation closure or any of the functional mandibular movements.

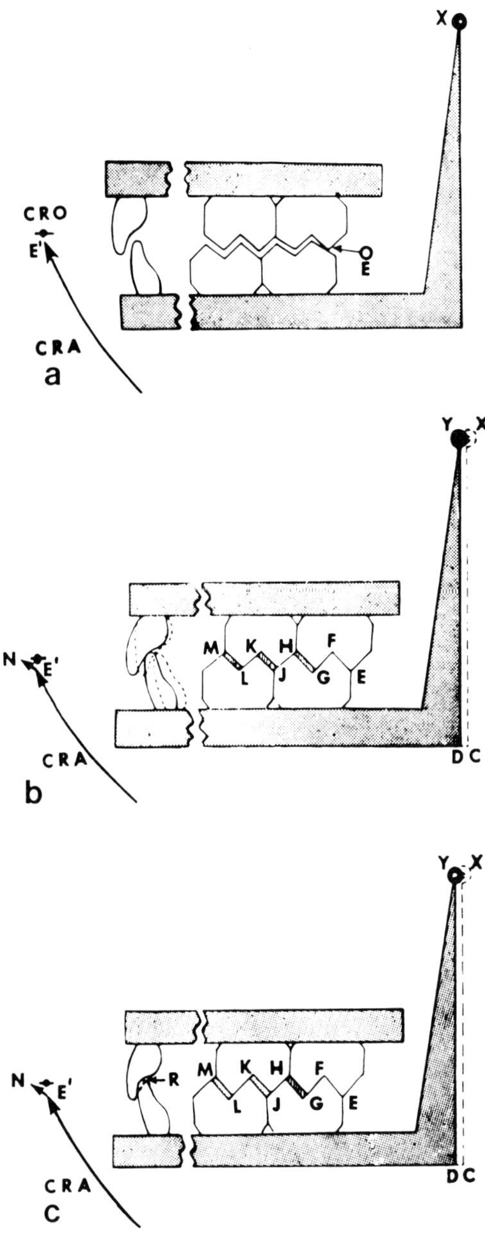

FIG. 8-3. The representation of an interfering occlusal contact at E in centric relation (*a*). CRA, as indicated by the large arrow, is the centric-relation arc. E′ indicates the interfering occlusal contact. CRO, as indicated by —●—, is centric-relation occlusion. The representation of habitual convenience relationship caused by interfering occlusal contact at E, resulting in a protrusive shift of the mandible from E′ to N and a forced movement of the incisors (*b*). The representation of habitual convenience relationship (*c*) in the presence of resistant bone results in the gouging out of the teeth at R. Note shift in direction of the arrow as the mandible strikes the interfering contact and shifts into habitual convenience relationship, E′N.

Thompson[9] discussed this matter at length in "Function—the Neglected Phase of Orthodontics."

In cases involving indirect causes, treatment is focused first upon these indirect causes, as necessary in each case; then occlusal equilibration is performed on the dentition as a whole.

THE CENTRIC-RELATION INTERFERING OCCLUSAL CONTACT

A centric-relation interfering occlusal contact exists when the mandible closes on the centric-relation arc and part of one tooth comes into contact with part of another tooth in the opposing arch before the closing movement has been completed in the terminal position.

Figure 8-3*a* illustrates a point of interfering contact in centric relation. At this stage of closure, the full mandibular force is exerted against the mesial plane of the distal cusp of the upper second molar and against the distal plane of the distal cusp of the lower molar at E. Note that X is the center of rotation or hinge-axis, and also note the centric-relation arc to the point of contact, E′.

Figure 8-3*b* illustrates the habitual convenience-relationship occlusion. As the cusp slides or skids on the inclined plane of the interfering contact, E, the mandible moves into a convenience relationship. The teeth occlude, but the mandible has been pushed anteriorly from point X, the hinge-axis, to point Y, the new location of the axis of the condyle. Dotted line XC represents the normal location of the posterior border of the mandible, whereas line YD represents the

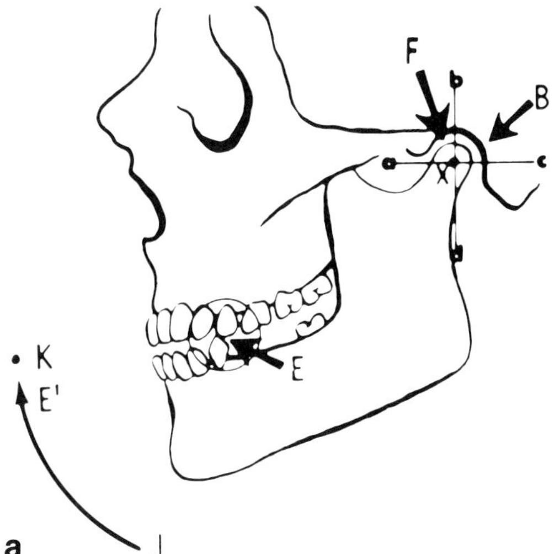

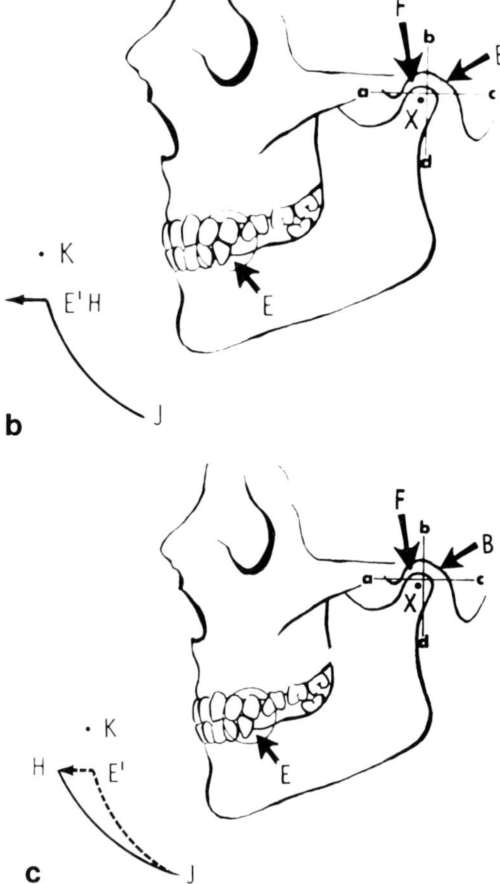

FIG. 8-4. Patient is closed into centric relation. Note that the interfering occlusal contact at E is keeping the lower teeth from intercuspation. The space at F is normal centric relation (*a*). Closing from centric-relation arc into pathologic occlusion, JE′H (*b*). Mandibular function is determined by the engram. The patient learns to function in a pathological protrusive relationship, HE′ (*c*).

new location of the border. The solid line, EF, illustrates the plane to which the interfering occlusal contact adjusts itself, and the width of the cross-hatched lines, GH, JK and LM represents the distance forward that the condyle has been displaced. The upper anterior teeth supported by weak alveolar bone have been pushed forward from their positions indicated by the dotted lines. Note that closure has not been completed on the centric-relation arc; it has shifted protrusively as shown by arrow E′N.

Figure 8-3*c* shows the mandible again in habitual convenience-relationship occlusion, but this time the encasing bone around the anterior teeth is strong, and the teeth are gouged out at R. Note that the condyle is pulled forward to Y, as in (*b*).

According to Angle[1] there are 138 contacting surfaces in centric-relation occlusion. Therefore, if an interfering occlusal contact is present, all the cuspal contacts of the teeth are thrown into incorrect relationship, the centric-relation arc is changed, the condylar positions are changed, and the neuromuscular system is thrown out of balance.

In understanding occlusal trauma and temporomandibular joint dysfunction, it is important to stress the fact that it is not the cusps of the teeth that are improperly constructed, but that it is the angulation of the cusps that is incorrect. The primary disturbance lies in the improper angulation, which becomes the guiding incline that deflects the mandible into an abnormal position. This results in a secondary disturbance of the temporomandib-

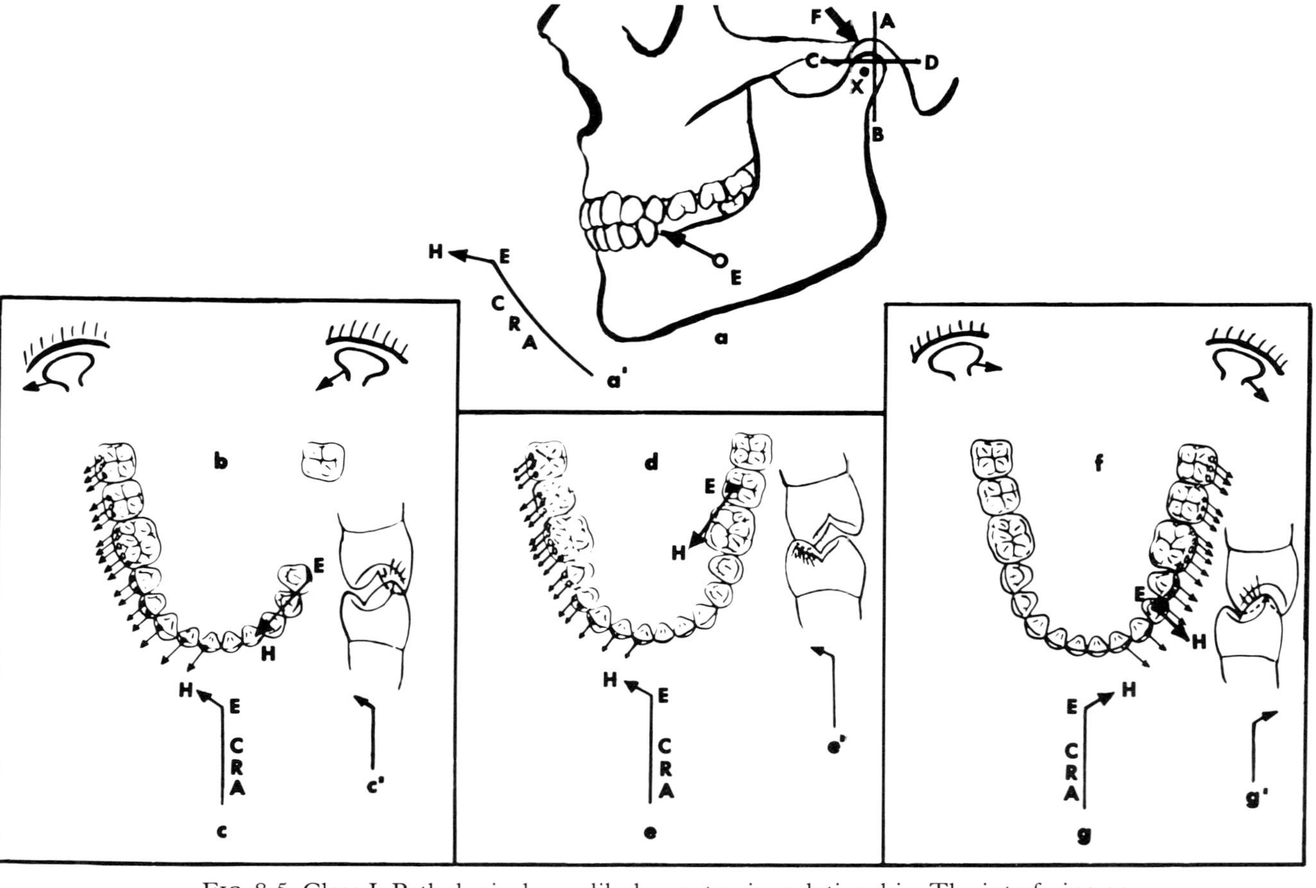

FIG. 8-5. Class I. Pathological mandibular protrusive relationship. The interfering occlusal contact (*a*), IOC at E caused a general anterior displacement of the mandible (*b–g*). The planes of the cusps that make up the interfering occlusal contact determine whether the mandible shifts medially or laterally from the point of interference. The occlusal and frontal diagrams (*b–e*, *f* and *g*) show the various contacting combinations that cause medial and lateral protrusive mandibular displacement.

ular joint structures, the suspensory ligaments and the neuromusculature of the stomatognathic system. Occasionally, the symptoms of the secondary disturbance become so severe that the primary disturbance is overlooked. The practitioner then tends to treat the severe symptoms rather than the primary cause, which is the interfering occlusal contact.

Centric relation up to the first point of contact, as it travels the path JE′H is seen in Figure 8-4. As the mandible in (*b*) passes through the centric-relation arc (CRA) toward terminal closure (K), the interfering occlusal contact at E takes place, preventing the mandible from going to K. This is a centric-relation registration (JE′H). When the mandible is deflected into the habitual convenience relationship at H, the mandible follows the path E′H. In Figure 8-4*c*, when there is an occlusal interference as in E, the patient learns a habitual convenience relationship and function—not from J to E′, but functions along the arc JH. This is the patient's engram.

The previous illustrations have demonstrated the basic concept of the centric-relation arc and cuspal interference with centric-relation occlusion. A proper understanding of the interference in centric relation makes it possible to form a basis for the interpretation and the understanding of pathological mandibular positions caused by centric-relation interfering occlusal contacts.

CLASSIFICATION OF PATHOLOGICAL MANDIBULAR RELATIONSHIPS

It is possible to classify pathological mandibular positions caused by centric-relation interfering occlusal contacts by establishing a set of standards. There are five classes of pathological mandibular positions or habitual convenience relationships caused by interfering occlusal contacts in centric relation. These classifications are based upon the investigations of H. G. Morris.[8]

Class I. Pathological Mandibular Protrusive Relationship

In the pathological mandibular protrusive relationship caused by an interfering occlusal contact in centric relation, the most common finding is a unilateral interfering occlusal contact. More infrequently, a bilateral interfering occlusal contact is found. Figure 8-5 illustrates pathologic mandibular protrusive occlusion. At E, there is an interfering occlusal contact between the mesiolingual plane of the buccal cusp of the upper second bicuspid and the distobuccal plane of the buccal cusp of the lower second bicuspid. As the mandible passes through the centric-relation arc, CRA, toward terminal closure, the interfering occlusal contact, E, takes place. The mandible is then deflected into the habitual convenience relationship, H, moving through the protrusive medial path, EH. This is shown on the profile diagram (*a*′), the occlusal diagram (*b*), and in the frontal view of mandibular movement (*c*). The dot, X in (*a*), has now been forced to move from the hinge-axis position, ABCD. The left condyle is now positioned anteroinferiorly and medially. The joint gap, F, demonstrates these changes. In the occlusal diagram (*b*), the shift of the mandible is protrusive and medial in the direction of the arrows. The small arrows indicate the areas of contact that the buccal cusps of the lower teeth may make with the buccal cusps of the upper teeth because of this medial shift. The large arrow starts at the interfering contact, E. The insert (*c*′) portrays the medial view of the interfering contact between the mesiolingual plane of the buccal cusp of the upper second bicuspid and the distobuccal plane of the buccal cusp of the lower second bicuspid.

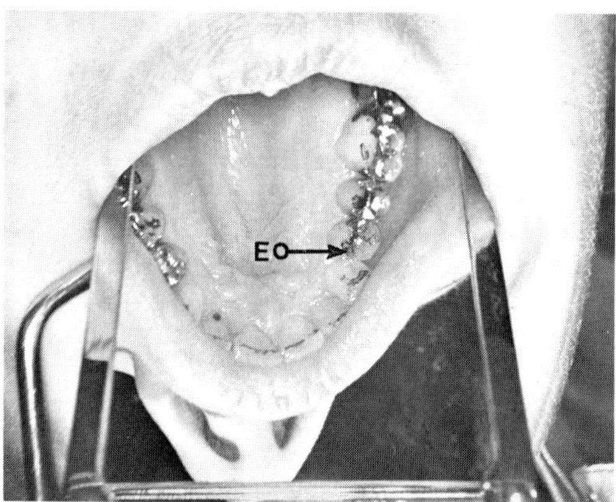

FIG. 8-6. The commonly occurring interfering occlusal contact on the mesiobuccal plane of the lingual cusp of the upper first bicuspid at E.

The small arrow under the insert illustrates the path of movement of the lower bicuspid. This is the same interfering contact that is illustrated in (*a*).

In the occlusal diagram (*b*), the shift of the mandible diagonally in the direction of the arrows results in trauma to the upper and lower teeth of the side opposite the interfering contact; this may cause a labial movement of the upper anterior teeth with many periodontal signs and pain symptoms. *This is called the diagonal manifestation of symptoms, since the original cause is an interfering occlusal contact diagonally opposite the site of the symptoms.*

When an interfering occlusal contact exists between the mesiolingual plane of an upper lingual cusp and the distobuccal plane of a lower lingual cusp, the mandibular shift is also in the protrusive medial direction as in (*d*). A mandibular shift of 1 to 3 mm. is not at all uncommon. In (*d*) and (*e*), the interfering occlusal contact is made by the mesiolingual plane of the mesiolingual cusp of the upper second molar and the distobuccal plane of the mesiolingual cusp of the lower second molar. The insert (*e'*) illustrates the mandibular shift which takes place as the tooth strikes the interfering contact and travels to the habitual convenience relationship. The small arrow under the insert illustrates the path of movement of the lower molar. This type is the most common Class I pathological mandibular protrusive medial relationship. This pathological movement is also exhibited by both condyles in the temporomandibular joints. In (*b*), as one condyle moves anteriorly and medially, the other condyle may move posterolaterally, laterally, or anterolaterally. This condition accounts for mesial alveolar process pathosis adjacent to the lower molars and bicuspids. These are the most numerous interfering occlusal contacts.

In about 15 per cent of cases treated, the initial interfering occlusal contact occurs as the mesiobuccal plane of the lingual cusp of the upper first bicuspid (E in Fig. 8-5*f*) contacts the distal plane of the buccal cusp of the lower first bicuspid, causing a protrusive lateral shift of the mandible. This is also illustrated in (*g*), the frontal view, and (*g'*), the insert. In the case of the protrusive lateral shift of the mandible, both the direction of the lower arch's movement and the pain symptoms are on the *same* side as the interfering occlusal contact. In most cases the pain is in the tooth that is in interfering contact.

There are several reasons for the existence of this particular interfering contact. The lower first bicuspid may be irregular in shape and it may be in either buccal or lingual version. Another possibility is that the lingual cusp of the lower first bicuspid may not be high enough to articulate properly with the upper first bicuspid. Therefore, the upper tooth may elongate because of the lack of proper occlusal anatomy of the lower first bicuspid. Another reason may be that the upper first bicuspid may erupt considerably earlier than the lower first bicuspid and thus be in an elongated position. An actual case is illustrated in Figure 8-6.

In summary, the following conditions

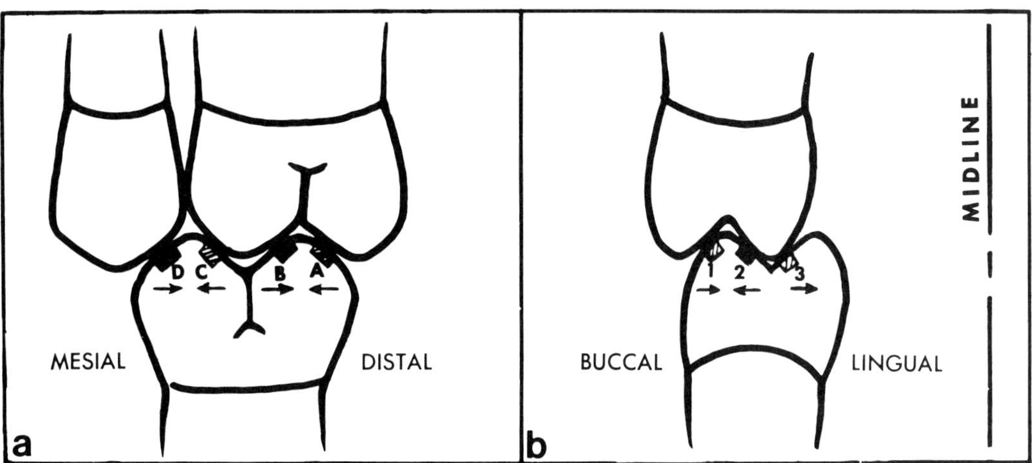

FIG. 8-7. In (*a*) the lower molar distal plane interfering contacts, A and C, will produce protrusive shifts of the mandible in the direction of the arrows underneath A and C. Mesial plane interfering contacts, B and D, will produce retrusive shifts of the mandible. The lower molar buccal plane interfering contacts, 1 and 3, produce medial shifts of the mandible in the direction of the arrows underneath 1 and 3, while the lingual plane contact 2 will produce a lateral shift of the mandible (*b*).

exist in the various Class I pathological mandibular movements. The planes of the lower teeth that make the interfering occlusal contact control the movement or the shift of the mandible from the point of interfering contact. There are three possible mandibular shifts: protrusive, medial and lateral. The mandibular shift is usually a combination of these movements.

In normal and nearly normal occlusions, the following situations are found. When an interfering occlusal contact exists between the mesiolingual plane of the upper buccal cusp and the distobuccal plane of the lower buccal cusp, the result is a protrusive medial shift of the mandible. When an interfering occlusal contact exists between the mesiolingual plane of the upper lingual cusp and the distobuccal plane of the lower lingual cusp, the result is similar to that described in the first case, namely, a protrusive medial shift of the mandible. When an interfering occlusal contact exists between the mesiobuccal plane of the upper lingual cusp and the distolingual plane of the lower buccal cusp, the result is a protrusive lateral shift of the mandible.

If the interfering occlusal contact exists on the distal planes of cusps of lower teeth, as A and C in Figure 8-7*a*, the mandible will shift in a protrusive direction. If the interfering occlusal contact exists on the mesial planes of cusps of the lower teeth, as B and D, the mandible will shift in a retrusive direction. If the interfering occlusal contact exists on the buccal planes of cusps of lower teeth, as 1 and 3 in (*b*), the mandible will shift medially from the point of interference toward the midline. If the interfering occlusal contact exists on the lingual planes of cusps of lower teeth, as in 2 of the same figure, the mandible will shift laterally from the point of interference away from the midline. Mandibular movements are combinations of (*a*) and (*b*). If the side of the mandible with the interfering occlusal contact moves medially, the opposite side moves laterally, and vice versa.

Figure 8-8*a* illustrates a case of protrusive lateral shift of the mandible; (*b*) illustrates the centric-relation interfering

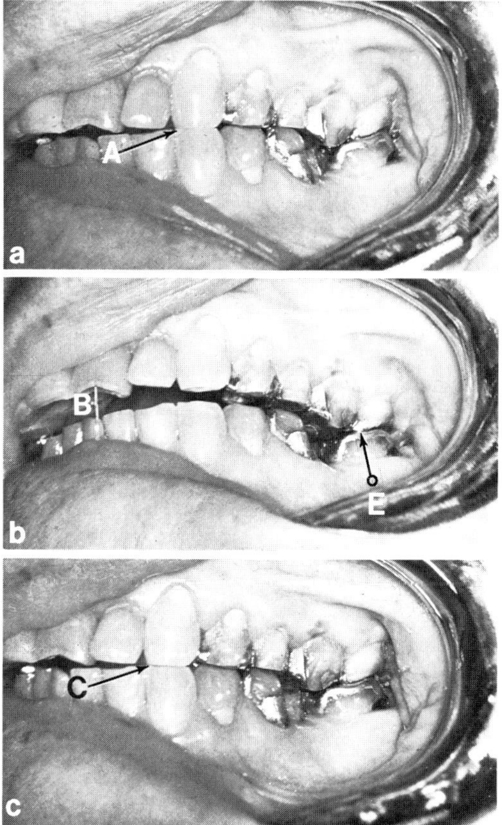

FIG. 8-8. Protrusive lateral shift of the mandible. Convenience relationship with the lateral shift (*a*); the centric-relation interfering contact on the second molars (*b*); the equilibrated case in centric-relation occlusion (*c*).

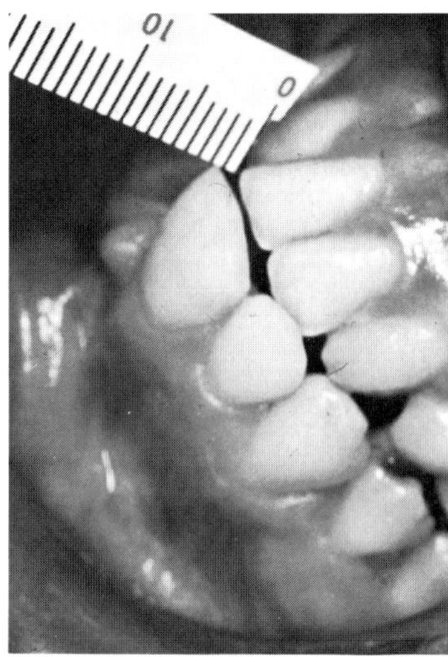

FIG. 8-9. Pathologic occlusal registration.

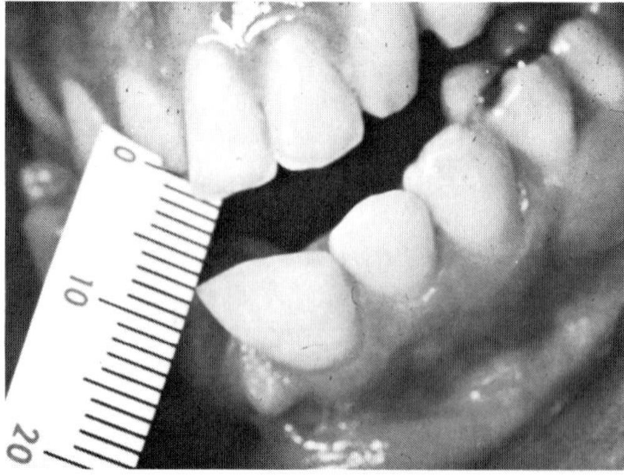

FIG. 8-10. Interfering occlusal contact in central relation.

contact on the second molars; (*c*) illustrates the centric-relation occlusion after equilibration. In (*a*) the cuspids are in an edge-to-edge relationship at A. In (*b*) it is well to observe both the space between the incisal surfaces of the upper and the lower anterior teeth at B and the flat incisal wear. In (*c*) the lower cuspid at C is lingual to its position in (*a*). This is evidence that the mandible is now posterior and medial to its position in (*a*).

As illustrated in Figure 8-9, the pathological occlusal registration is shown by the 1-mm. distance between the incisal of the lower central to the incisal of the upper central.

Upon training the patient to give a

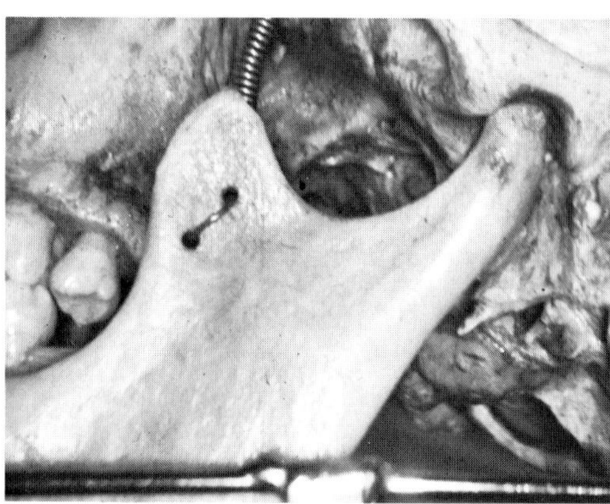

FIG. 8-11. Pathological position of condyle as caused by an interfering occlusal contact.

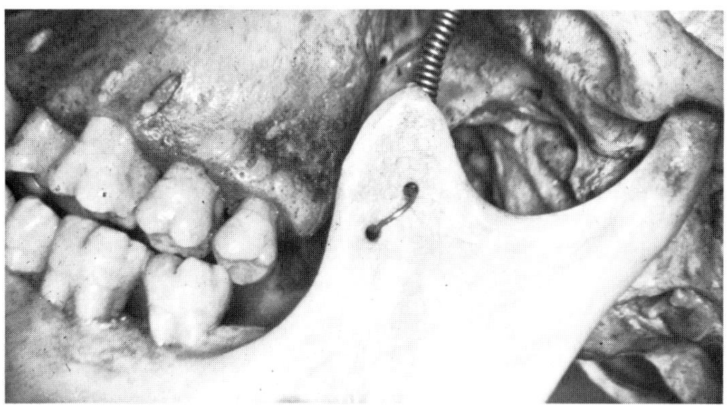

FIG. 8-12. The position of the condyle with equidistant joint gap.

centric-relation registration, an interfering occlusal contact is demonstrated in the posterior region which causes the interincisal distance to be 7 mm. (Fig. 8-10). This means that the condyle, as well as the lateral pterygoid muscle, is retruded 6 mm., and this was probably causing spasm and pain.

In Figure 8-11, the mandible has gone into a habitual convenience protrusive bite because of the way the upper left third molar strikes the lower left second molar. This can be seen by the position of the condyle resting on the posterior wall of the articular eminence and the absence of a uniform joint gap.

In Figure 8-12 the upper left third molar is seen striking the distal of the lower left second molar. The mandible has closed in a centric-relation arc and the joint gap is equidistant. This supports the theory that normal condyle placement within the fossa should result in an equidistant joint gap.

Figure 8-13 illustrates A. J. Drew's[4] presentation of a case of a medial mandib-

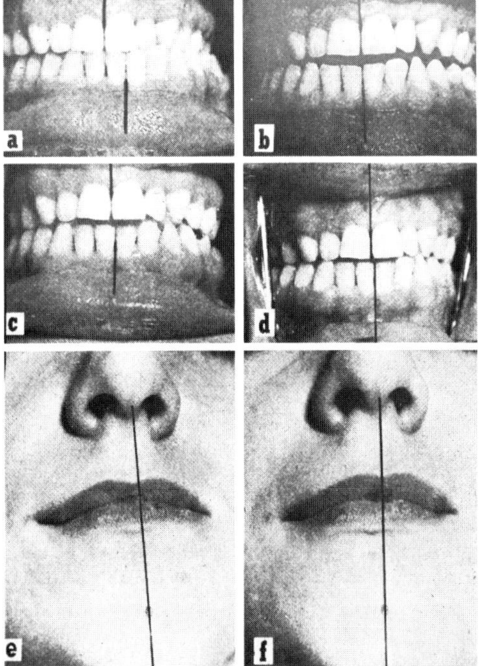

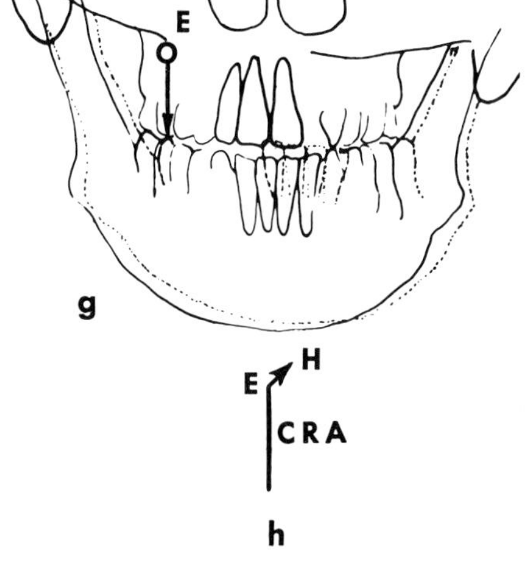

FIG. 8-13. A case of medial mandibular displacement corrected by occlusal equilibration. (Drew, A. J.: Unusual lateral displacement corrected by grinding. D. Survey, *25*:1624, 1949)

ular displacement corrected by equilibration. This case illustrates to what extreme an occlusal interference can displace the mandible. In (*a*) observe the convenience relationship of the teeth which created the cross-bite on the left side. In (*b*) the mandible is at the point of interfering contact on the centric-relation arc. The contact is between the buccal plane of the mesiobuccal cusp of the lower right molar and the lingual plane of the buccal cusp of the upper first molar. It should be noted that there is no cross-bite on the centric-relation arc. The beginning of the medial shift of the mandible as the lower buccal cusp glides on the upper buccal cusp is illustrated in (*c*), with (*a*) demonstrating completion of the mandibular shift. The chin displacement in (*e*) should be noted. The results of occlusal equilibration are illustrated in (*d*), with concomitant chin repositioning illustrated in (*f*). In the cephalometric tracings illustrated in (*g*), the solid line mandible demonstrates the position of the mandible in (*b*) with the interfering contact at E. The superimposed dotted line tracing illustrates the medial shift of the mandible as seen in (*a*). In the mandibular closure diagram (*h*), the centric-relation arc is normal until it strikes the interfering occlusal contact at E, then it traverses the path, EH. At first glance this would seem to be a case of cross-bite relationship, but thorough clinical examination demonstrated that the apparent cross-bite relationship was actually caused by an interfering occlusal contact. This is similar to the false Class III orthodontic classification. The small mandibular shift that occurs from the point of the interfering occlusal contact to the convenience relationship is illustrated by the arrow in the small insert of Figure 8-5, at *b*, *d*, and *f*. This demonstrates mandibular movement at the area of the point of contact. When viewed frontally (*c*, *e*, and *g*), the movement is magnified because of its greater distance from the pivot, which is the condyle.

Class II. Pathological Mandibular Retrusive Relationship

In the pathological mandibular retrusive relationship caused by an interfering occlusal contact in centric relation, the usual finding is a unilateral interfering occlusal contact. Figure 8-14 shows this pathological retrusive relationship.

As the mandible traverses the centric-relation arc, it is stopped by the interfering occlusal contact at E. The mandible then closes into the habitual convenience relationship, H, moving through the retrusive path, EH. The dot, X, has now been forced to move from the position ABCD. The condyle is now positioned posteroinferiorly. This posteroinferior relationship is caused by the rocking action of the mandible on E, the fulcrum, as the patient tries to bring his teeth together. This results in a narrower joint gap, F, posteriorly and a wider gap superiorly and anteriorly. When the mesial plane or the marginal ridge of the cusps of the lower third molar makes an interfering contact with the distal marginal ridge of the cusps of the upper second molar, the mandible is guided distally, and there is an attendant movement of the condyles in the mandibular fossae. In the earlier stages of this condition, there is a proprioceptive sense of discomfort about which the patient is vague and which he finds difficult to describe. Aside from the occlusal disharmony, other symptoms may be tenderness of the joint, a tearing and crackling sound and a clicking noise. Other types of interfering occlusal contacts than those caused by unopposed erupting teeth may also result in this mandibular retrusive relationship.

Class III. Increased Vertical Relationship

This interfering occlusal contact relationship is almost invariably caused by the insertion of a restoration in supraocclusion. In Figure 8-15, as the patient closes in the centric-relation arc, CRA, the

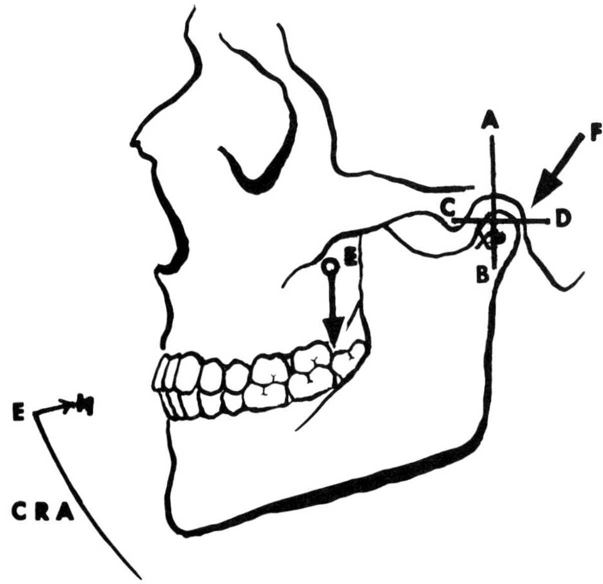

FIG. 8-14. Class II. Pathological mandibular retrusive relationship caused by the interfering contact at E, the condyle center indicated by the dot, X, has shifted posteroinferiorly from original position at intersection of lines ABCD. Mandibular closure is along the centric-relation arc, CRA, and after striking the interfering occlusal contact, E, the mandible shifts in the direction of the arrow, EH.

interfering occlusal contact, E, acts as a fulcrum on which the mandible rocks in a teeter-totter manner as the muscles attempt to bring the mandible into centric-relation occlusion. Because of the interfering occlusal contact at E, the mandible closes into the habitual convenience relationship, H, slightly anterior to the CRO position. The dot, X, has now been forced to move from the centric-relation axis position, ABCD. The condyle is positioned inferiorly, thus increasing the width of the joint gap, F. An alternate closing of the joint gap, F, occurs when

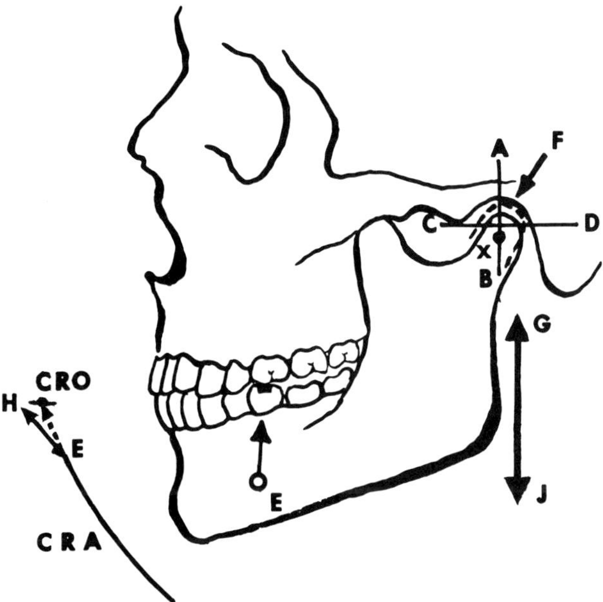

FIG. 8-15. Class III. Increased vertical relationship caused by interfering contact, E, on the restoration, resulting in a teeter-totter action of the mandible.

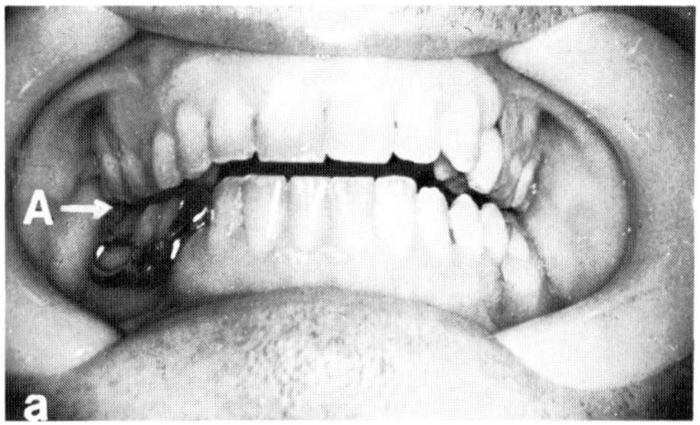

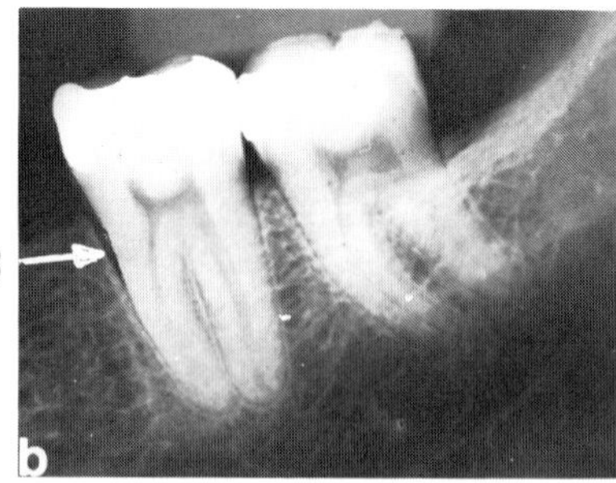

FIG. 8-16. A Class III increased vertical relationship caused by a molar occlusal rest of a partial denture at A. The patient is in centric relation on the interfering contact, which, in turn, is producing the space between the anterior teeth. At B, the roentgenogram of the clasped molar demonstrates, in turn, the wide periodontal space and heavy lamina dura at the mesial of the second molar.

there is a teeter-totter action as first the teeth anterior to E are in closure and then the teeth posterior to E are in closure. The arrows HE and GJ show movement in both directions. Morris[8] claims that this rocking action of the mandible causes temporomandibular joint derangement by stretching or causing tension on the suspensory ligaments and the internal pterygoid and masseter muscles (the mandibular sling) at the angle of the mandible. Figure 8-16 illustrates a lower partial denture exhibiting a centric-relation interfering occlusal contact produced by the occlusal rest. This interference results in an open bite in centric relation. To bring both arches into apposition, the mandible must rock on the high point.

Another category of open-bite cases consists of a natural dentition with bilateral occlusal contact only at the second and the third molars. This is a damaging situation because fewer teeth share the masticatory load, and mastication itself is impaired. This condition creates a teeter-totter mandibular action with subsequent joint involvement, as though high restorations were placed on the occluding posterior teeth. If the freeway space is normal, the occlusion of the remaining teeth can be built up. An alternative procedure may be the actual closing of the bite of the contacting molars in centric relation until the bicuspids are brought into contact. Figure 8-17*a* shows the case as it presented itself with bilateral oc-

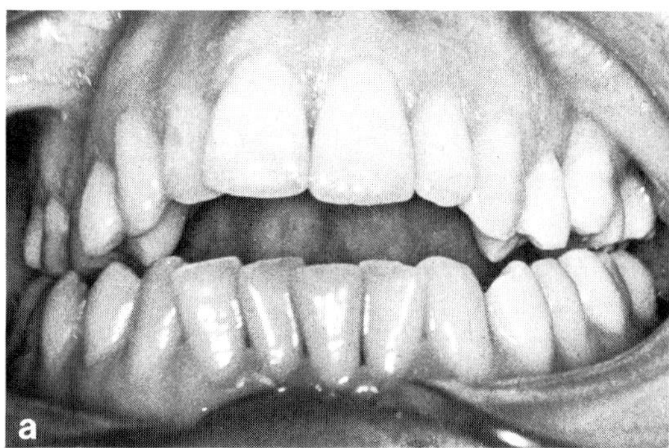

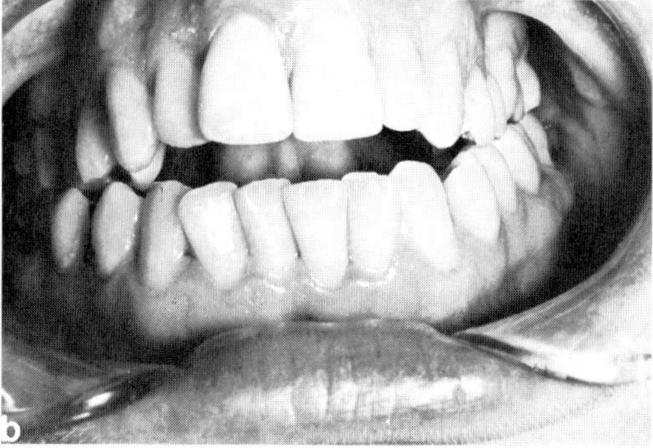

FIG. 8-17. An open-bite case with occlusal contact only in the second and the third molar region (*a*). The same case after occlusal equilibration; now first and second bicuspids contact as well (*b*).

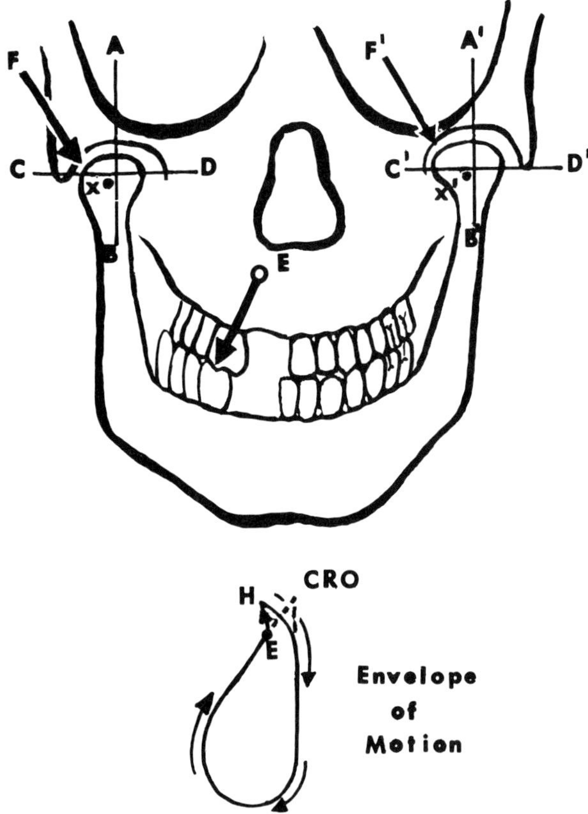

FIG. 8-18. Class IV. Pathological lateral shift of the mandible due to a cross-bite relationship and the effects produced within the temporomandibular joints and the envelope of motion.

clusal contacts on the second and third molars only. In (*b*) contact up to and including the first bicuspids was obtained. This is done by careful, judicious, selective reshaping of the occlusal surfaces. These cases require a great deal of preliminary study before treatment is inaugurated. It is sometimes necessary to bring single teeth into occlusal contact by using occlusal restorations.

In their dentofacial study of 500 students between the ages of 16 and 32, Huber and Reynolds[7] found that 0.2 per cent have occlusal contact only as far forward as the bicuspid region. The study of 1,036 cases by Hellman[5] roughly confirms this percentage.

Another type of pathologic occlusion due to increased vertical dimension is the creation of a new level of occlusion by bridgework or partial or full dentures which partially or totally obliterate the freeway space. Even though the completed case may be in centric-relation occlusion, the absence of a freeway space which provides the physiological rest position will create abnormal muscle tension which will, in turn, result in muscle spasm.

Class IV. Pathological Medial or Lateral Protrusive Shifts of the Mandible Due to Cross-Bite Relationships

In the pathological medial and lateral protrusive shifts of the mandible due to a cross-bite interfering occlusal contact in centric relation, it is usually found that as the patient completes the cycle of closure, the mandible is shifted to the right or to the left. This lateral shift is illustrated in Figure 8-18. This type of interfering occlusal contact is usually found in cross-bite cases involving one or more pairs of teeth in the cuspid, the bicuspid or the molar regions. As the mandible closes in centric relation, the buccal plane of the buccal cusp of the upper tooth strikes the lingual plane of the buccal cusp of the lower tooth. This interfering occlusal contact guides the mandible laterally and protrusively as it continues the cycle of closure. This creates a vise for the mandible and initiates a tremendous struggle between the teeth and the musculature. The dotted lines at the peak of the envelope of motion, CRO, represent the beginning of the mandibular movement from centric-relation occlusion and its normal return. Normally, the path continues through E to CRO. H represents the habitual convenience relationship. The interfering occlusal contact is represented by E, and the lateral path by EH. Because of the interfering occlusal contact at E, the mandible has shifted laterally. The dots, X and X′, have been forced to move from the normal condyle centers, ABCD and A′B′C′D′. The condyle at ABCD is positioned laterally and inferiorly, and the joint gap, F, is narrower laterally but is wider superiorly and medially. The condyle at A′B′C′D′ is positioned medially and inferiorly, and the joint gap, F, is narrow medially but wider superiorly and laterally.

Figure 8-18 illustrates a lateral shift of the mandible due to the interfering contacts described. A medial shift of the mandible is produced when the lingual plane of the upper buccal cusp strikes the buccal plane of the lower lingual cusp. This mandibular shift will generally be accompanied by a slight mandibular protrusion. The bodily shift of the mandible can be observed as a deviation of the midline of the face as the patient closes into a habitual convenience relationship. It has been demonstrated on skulls that in such cases the medial portion of the condyle and the lateral wall of the fossa may be damaged.[10]

Class V. Reduced Vertical Relationship

The pathological reduced vertical relationship may be caused by a loss of posterior teeth, excessive wear of the occlusal surfaces of a full dentition or partial eruption of the permanent dentition. The pathological reduced vertical relationship due to loss of posterior supporting teeth may be bilateral or unilateral. Figure 8-19 illustrates bilateral loss of supporting posterior teeth. The mandible traversed the centric-relation arc, CRA; reached centric-relation occlusion, CRO; and because the posterior teeth were missing, the mandible was as a result guided up and backward to point H by the muscles and the lingual inclined planes of the upper anterior teeth. An accompanying movement takes place in the temporomandibular joint. The dot, X, is displaced superiorly and posteriorly to the axis representation, ABCD.

Figure 8-20 illustrates unilateral loss of supporting posterior teeth. The result is unilateral function. Unilateral mastication may cause a posteromedial shift of the condyle of the unsupported side due to the lack of resistance to muscle pull by any teeth. This results in temporomandibular joint symptoms in the unsupported side. It is also possible that symptoms may appear in the temporomandibular region on the unilateral chewing side if there is an interfering occlusal contact and if it is such that it forces the condyle on the functioning side into an abnormal position. Wild and Bay[10] have shown that under such conditions all the components of the temporomandibular joint on the nonfunctioning side and the entire skull will be affected.

In cases of unilateral mastication in which teeth are present only on the functioning side, it is usual to find condylar changes in the opposite temporomandibular joint. This may be explained by conceiving of the mandible as a lever with the teeth acting as the fulcrum. The

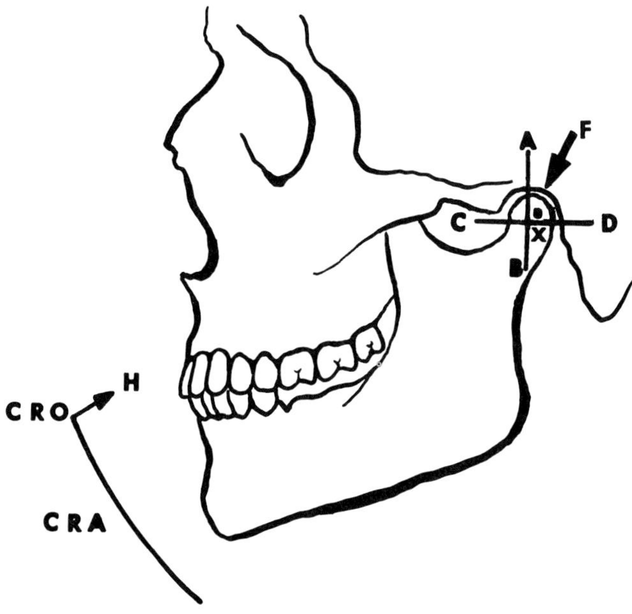

FIG. 8-19. Class V. Reduced vertical relationship caused by the loss of posterior teeth which in turn causes the mandible to be displaced posterosuperiorly in closure.

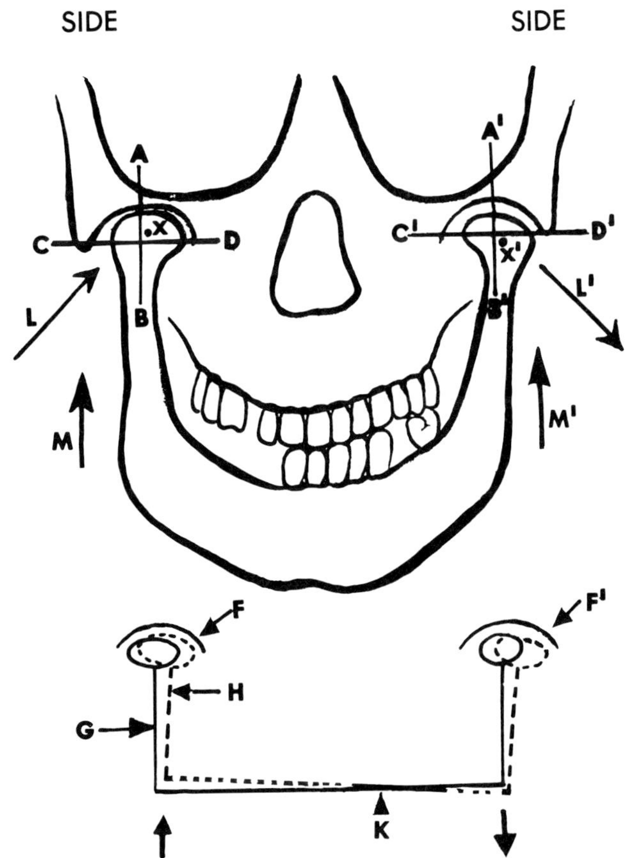

FIG. 8-20. Unilateral loss of posterior teeth, with resultant consequences.

effects are produced in the temporomandibular joint, but chiefly on the side where there are no teeth. This situation is illustrated in Figure 8-20 where the following conditions exist. The teeth on the functioning side act as the fulcrum, K. The muscles, M, on the nonfunctioning side do not have tooth stops, and as a result of muscular contraction intrude the condyle into the fossa. The muscle, M′, on the functioning side undergoes isometric contraction; the teeth act as fulcrums; and, due to lever action, a stretching of the muscles on the functioning side takes place. The dot, X, on the nonfunctioning side has moved superiorly and medially from ABCD to close joint gap F. The dot, X′, on the functioning side has moved inferiorly and laterally from A′B′C′D′. The joint gap, F′, is widened medially and superiorly. The arrows, L and L′, demonstrate the direction of movement of the condyles. The mandible has assumed the strained position, H, in contrast with the normal position, G. The excessive masticatory forces produced by such conditions will cause tooth movement and gradual disintegration of the entire masticatory organ. Morris[8] describes this condition as follows:

If the anterior articular eminence of the temporal fossa were nonexistent, the temporal fossa would be a flat plane parallel to the occlusal plane, and if the anterior teeth articulated in an end-to-end relationship, the hinge-axis could move up, and up only, closing the vertical dimension within the limits of the compressibility or depressibility of the articular capsule. The anterior articular eminence is, however, an inclined plane and the lingual surfaces (guiding planes) of the maxillary incisors are inclined planes and in unison they direct the head of the condyle superiorly and posteriorly. The distance of the movement is controlled by the longest of these two planes, the rapidity or speed of movement controlled by the plane of greatest inclination, and the force controlled by the elevator muscles.

The articular capsule is in part protected from pathological movement by the superior fibers of the external pterygoid, but the sharp anterior border of the condyle, which has moved up and back, comes in apposition to the articular disc and the articular disc is caught between this margin and the articular eminence during mandibular function.

Sicher reports a flattening of the condyle and articular eminence resulting in resorption and reactive proliferation of the bone, degeneration of parts of the capsule and degeneration of the fibers covering the condyle and tubercle. He terms this condition traumatic osteoarthritis deformans. Burket in discussing traumatic disease of the temporomandibular joint (excluding fractures) speaks of acute traumatic temporomandibular arthritis. We may accept either of these terminologies for the advanced stages of the condition. In the primary phases it is simple inflammation, subsequent degeneration, and proliferation over a continued period of time and may result in true osteoarthritis. Sicher also states that in approximately 20 per cent of all skulls there is a flaw of development resulting in a foramen in the tympanic plate. As Class V thrust of the condyle is directed in this general direction, it is reasonable to assume that should there be an inflammation in this region, not only are the tympanic plate, the foramen, and the soft tissue of the foramen involved in this zone of inflammation, but also the acoustic meatus may be included.

Often parotid tissue invades the lateral limits of the area distal to the condyle. Should the invasion be sufficiently deep or the limits of the temporomandibular inflammation be sufficiently extensive, parotid tissue can be involved. Burket mentions joint involvement secondary to suppurative parotitis. We should give more consideration to pyogenic infection of the parotid gland secondary to inflammation of traumatic temporomandibular joint origin.

The auriculotemporal nerve passes posteriorly and down on the inner surface of the external pterygoid muscle after leaving the foramen ovale and then crosses the posterior border of the neck of the condyle. The posterior border of the neck of the condyle is not necessarily within a zone of inflammation, but the neck can be within such a zone, as it associates with the external pterygoid. The auriculotemporal nerve, a specialized nerve receiving and conducting pain, should receive consideration in temporomandibular pathology as a source of clinical evidence of pain.

The chorda tympani, containing taste fibers for the anterior region of the tongue and secretory fibers for the oral glands, anterior, lingual, submaxillary, sublingual, etc., passes in a deep narrow groove (petrotympanic fissure) behind the articular capsule and is separated from the capsule by the bony border of the fossa. It is also within the zone of Class V induced inflammation. The stimulation can produce changes in salivation and excessive sensitivity of the tongue as well as burning and acid taste which are frequently given by patients as their chief complaint.

We do not pretend that all pathology of the temporomandibular area is trauma-induced, or that if and when trauma is a factor, Class V malposition interpretation will answer all questions relative to Costen's syndrome and other vague complaints and symptoms. For example, a furuncle situated on the anterior wall of the external auditory canal can produce symptoms similar to those experienced in temporomandibular disease. The enlargement of the small lymph node just anterior to the temporomandibular joint can be associated with any inflammation in that general area. We should consider that many symptoms are the result of traumatic-induced inflammation and not of the force itself.

Burket in discussing the temporomandibular syndrome, states, "When the symptoms are present they do not arise until 5 to 8 years after the mutilation of the occlusion." If we associate this observation with the incidence of periodontal bone degeneration in young patients, as recorded in the Gibson chart, we will be more alert in both interpretation and diagnosis and be more inclined to practice preventive occlusal adjustment with prevention of inflammation as the goal. If we accept the work of Valy Menkin, we cannot consider the inflammatory phase of temporomandibular disease as strictly a local condition.

The periodontal results of Class V centric are known to be an overburdening of the remaining teeth (an insufficient number of teeth for equitable distribution of forces). The primary traumatism of anterior teeth is quite similar to secondary traumatism of Class I malcentric, and necessarily the pathologic evidence is not dissimilar.

Sensitivity of the necks of anterior teeth, especially anterior maxillary teeth, is often one of the primary symptoms. This can be attributed to trauma-induced hyperemia of the pulp, the inflamed nerve being more receptive to stimuli than a physiologically normal tooth. The observation has been made that not only does the rectification of trauma aid in the reduction of sensitivity but also that the necks of the teeth are less susceptible to caries after correction.

The closed or deep bite is characterized by an increase in the freeway space and a decrease in the vertical dimension when the teeth are in terminal closure. The most common cause of the closed bite is loss of posterior teeth as discussed. The second cause of a closed bite or reduced vertical relationship is excessive wear of the occlusal surfaces of the natural dentition. Excessive wear decreases the height of the crowns of the teeth and results in reduced vertical relationship with possible concomitant sequelae of the temporomandibular joints. The third cause of a closed bite is that the permanent teeth do not always erupt to the proper height. Premature loss and abnormal wear of deciduous teeth may decrease the vertical dimension of the deciduous dentition. Since the permanent first molars erupt to the height partly determined by the deciduous dentition, they will not attain their correct height in such cases. The height of the remaining permanent teeth will, in turn, be determined by the height of the first permanent molars. A closed bite alters the occlusal relationship of the teeth and the interrelationships of all component parts of the stomatognathic system.

All cases of Costen's temporomandibular joint syndrome fall into the first cause of Class V cases since they are caused by loss of posterior tooth support. It should be noted, however, that in Classes I to IV, the patient may exhibit

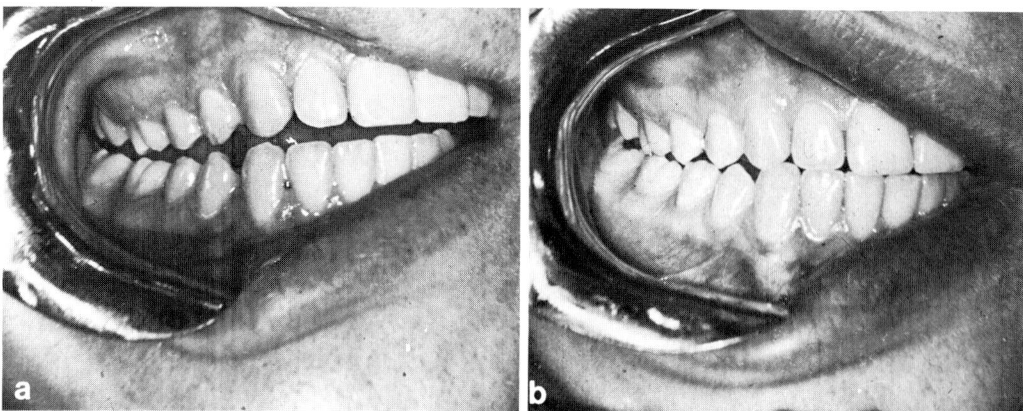

FIG. 8-21. Lack of contact on the functioning side due to nonfunctioning-side interfering contact (*a*). Contact on the functioning side after occlusal equilibration (*b*).

temporomandibular joint symptoms even though there is posterior tooth support. It is this observation that should make the dentist careful not to label all temporomandibular joint symptoms as Costen's syndrome.

INTERFERING OCCLUSAL CONTACTS OF THE FUNCTIONING AND THE PROTRUSIVE RANGES

In pathologic occlusion, it may be inferred that the condyle is not properly placed within the temporomandibular joint. Therefore, it follows that the lateral and protrusive excursions will not follow a definite pattern. Centric-relation occlusion is the foundation or baseline from which all eccentric movements are made. An incorrect, pathologic or convenience-relationship occlusion will cause all lateral and protrusive movements to be basically incorrect. This disorganization is followed by the establishment of a degenerative pattern of lateral and protrusive interfering occlusal contacts. It is impossible to classify the numerous types of possible variations in pathological lateral and protrusive occlusal articulation, but the application of the principles of normal articulation plus occlusal equilibration can be of great aid in the correction of each case.

One of the greatest problems in the functioning range of articulation is the so-called locked bite. If, in the functioning range of articulation, only the cuspids make contact while the posterior teeth are not in functional contact, all the lateral force is taken up by the cuspids. The patient tries to avoid these pathological lateral excursions by masticating with a short choppy stroke. A rocking and jarring effect on the bicuspids is produced, and eventually these teeth are loosened. A hammering effect is produced both upon the occlusion and on the temporomandibular joints. This produces torque on both temporomandibular joints during function. It is possible to draw an analogy between lateral movements and the effect that a matchstick placed under one rocker of a rocking chair will have both upon the motion of the chair and upon the person sitting in it. Every time the rocker hits the matchstick, the entire chair will be jarred, and the shock will be transmitted to the person. A similar effect is produced upon the teeth and the temporomandibular joints when there are interfering occlusal contacts in the lateral ranges of articulation. As the constant jarring will ultimately damage the rocking chair, so will the constant trauma caused by the interfering occlusal contact eventually harm the dentition and the joints.

PLUNGER CUSPS

A very common complaint is interproximal food impaction during mastication. Frequently, this is caused by what is erroneously called a "plunger cusp." Careful analysis and examination of the "plunger cusp" will show that actually it is an interfering occlusal contact that wedges apart two adjoining teeth in the opposing arch during closure. The reshaping of the offending cusp or of the marginal ridges that create the interfering contact will correct this condition. Indiscriminate and routine removal of so-called "plunger cusps" during "preliminary grinding" will result in loss of effective occlusal contacts when and where they are needed. It is an interfering occlusal contact in centric relation that causes the interproximal separation of the opposing teeth, and it should be treated as such.

INTERFERING OCCLUSAL CONTACTS OF THE NONFUNCTIONING RANGES

Interfering occlusal contacts on the nonfunctioning side of the natural dentition constitute a very serious problem. Changes in the occlusal pattern and articulation are the results of nonfunctioning-side interfering contacts. The lingual planes of the buccal cusps of the lower molars or bicuspids and the buccal planes of the lingual cusps of the upper molars and bicuspids on the nonfunctioning side may prevent contact of the teeth on the functioning side. The patient cannot chew on the functioning side without damaging the temporomandibular joint on the nonfunctioning side.

Figure 8-21*a* illustrates a patient who lacks contact on the right side in the functioning range of articulation. The lack of contact is caused by an interfering occlusal contact on the left or nonfunctioning side. The patient cannot masticate properly on the right side because of the lack of occlusal contact. He must force his teeth together to improve his mastication, and this produces trauma in the temporomandibular joint on the nonfunctioning side. Therefore, the patient resorts to unilateral mastication on the left side. This results in degeneration of the stomatognathic system because of the masticatory imbalance. The same patient is seen in (*b*) after the removal of the interfering contacts on the nonfunctioning side.

Figure 5-26, which illustrates normal functioning and nonfunctioning-side movements, should be reviewed. Figure 8-22 demonstrates the mechanisms of the problem of a nonfunctioning-side interference. The forces in the masticating cycle are exerted on the functioning side of the arch from the lateral range toward centric-relation occlusion. The following conditions are present in (*a*). In trying to triturate the food, F, the elevator muscles, M and M′, pull upward with equal force on both sides until point E is reached. The dots, X and X′, are now equidistant from the original CRO centers, ABCD and A′B′C′D′. The interfering occlusal contact, E, on the nonfunctioning side thus prevents the teeth on the functioning side from making contact. In (*b*), the envelope of motion, the mandible has reached point E, the interfering occlusal contact. In P, the profile view of the left temporomandibular joint, close contact exists between the condyle and the meniscus.

In order to triturate food, the teeth on the functioning side of the arch must be brought into apposition. In Figure 8-22*c*, this is further illustrated with the following conditions. The functioning side con-

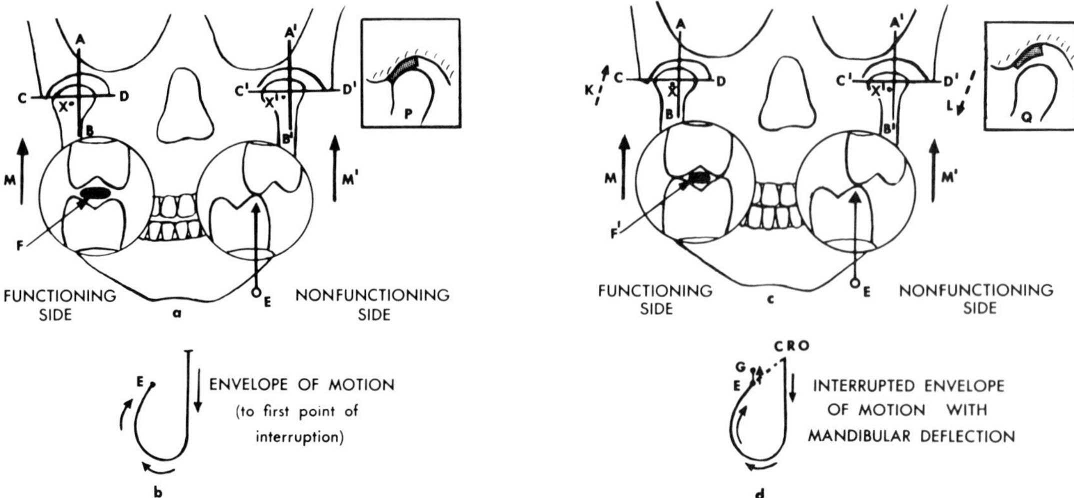

FIG. 8-22. A diagram of the mechanics that are set in motion by an interfering occlusal contact on the nonfunctioning side.

tact has been achieved, but E, the interfering contact, has become a fulcrum. The muscles, M and M′, cannot continue to exert equal force. Muscle pull, M, brings the teeth together on the functioning side in an attempt to set the condyle well into the fossa for the power movement. Muscle pull, M′, is in isometric contraction against the contact, E. Because of the fulcrum effect produced by E during functioning-side closure, there is a downward pull or stretching of the muscle, M′, thus increasing the pull on these muscles during their isometric contraction. On the nonfunctioning side of the arch, the condyle must travel quite a distance posteriorly and laterally to get the mandible back into centric-relation occlusion. Actually, therefore, the condyle on the nonfunctioning side is in free movement during the traverse, and the interfering occlusal contact, E, becomes a fulcrum and forms a lever of the first class. The dot, X, on the functioning side has moved superiorly but is lateral and inferior to the original center, ABCD. The arrow, K, on the functioning side demonstrates the direction of movement of the condyle. The dot, X′, on the nonfunctioning side has moved inferiorly and slightly medially from the original center, A′B′C′D′. The arrow, L, on the nonfunctioning side, demonstrates the direction of the movement of the condyle.

In Figure 8-22*d*, the envelope of motion, it should be noted that the movement from E to G is straight up instead of following the dotted line to CRO. In Q, the profile view of the left temporomandibular joint, the condyle has been detached from the meniscus. The patient will not use the right side as the functioning side because of the discomfort caused by the interfering contacts on the nonfunctioning side. Disuse atrophy is the fate of the periodontium on the right side if this situation continues. Other effects of an interfering occlusal contact on the nonfunctioning side depend upon the outcome of the battle between the periodontium and the temporomandibular joint. In this type of interfering occlusal contact, much lateral force is produced upon the buccal cusps of the mandibular teeth and the lingual cusps of the lateral teeth. Symptoms of pain, mobility and periodontal disturbances are the usual sequelae in the areas of the involved maxillary and mandibular teeth.

HYPERMOBILE TEMPOROMANDIBULAR JOINT

A hypermobile temporomandibular joint is one that allows excessive opening movements with a distinct tendency toward dislocation and subluxation. This is traumatic to the soft tissues of the joint. Patients who exhibit a hypermobile joint are predisposed to temporomandibular joint pain caused by occlusal trauma. Occlusal equilibration will alleviate the pain and, when used in conjunction with drug therapy, should produce excellent results. A patient with a hypermobile temporomandibular joint is instructed never to open his mouth wider than the thickness of his thumb. Within 6 months to 2 years the ligaments tighten and the patient can no longer open his mouth to its former excessive extent. It is interesting to note that many people with hypermobile temporomandibular joints also exhibit the phenomenon of double-jointedness in other areas.

REFERENCES

1. Angle, E. H.: Classification of malocclusion. D. Cosmos., *41:*248, 1899.
2. Bernard, C.: De la physiologie générale, Paris, Hachette, 1872.
3. Cannon, W. B.: The Mechanical Factors of Digestion. p. 8. New York, Longmans, 1911.
4. Drew, A. J.: Unusual lateral displacement corrected by grinding. D. Survey, *25:*1624, 1949.
5. Hellman, M.: Variations and anatomy of jaw bones, JADA, *14:*418, 1927.
6. Hirschfeld, I.: Mechanics of mastication in relation to the health of the periodontium, J. Periodont., *4:*35, 1933.
7. Huber, R. E., and Reynolds, J. W.: A dento-facial study of male students at the University of Michigan in the physical hardening program, Am. J. Ortho., *32:*1, 1946.
8. Morris, H. G.: Pathological temporomaxillary mandibular relation, J. Periodont., *22:*216, 1951.
9. Thompson, J. R.: Function—the neglected phase of orthodontics, Angle Ortho. *26:*129, 1956.
10. Wild, H., and Bay, R.: Lever action of the mandible. JADA, *35:*596, 1947.

Additional Basic References

Beyron, H. L.: Occlusal changes in adult dentition. JADA, *48:*674, 1954.

Blatt, I.: The parotid-masseter hypertrophy-traumatic occlusion syndrome. Laryngoscope, *79:*624, 1969.

Chaput, A.: Occlusion traumatique, Actualities Odonto-Stomatologique, 1956.

Gerry, R. G.: The effects of trauma and hypermobility on the temporomandibular joint. Oral Surg., *7:*876, 1954.

Ingle, J. D.: Determination of occlusal discrepancies. JADA, *54:*6, 1957.

Lucia, V. O.: The gnathological concept of articulation. D. Clin. North Am., pp. 183–197, Mar., 1962.

McLean, D. W.: Occlusal orthopedics. D. Cosmos, *74:*313, 1932.

———: Diagnosis and correction of pathologic occlusion. JADA, *29:*1202, 1942.

Nagle, R. J.: Temporomandibular function, J. Pros. Dent., *6:*350, 1956.

Neff, C. W., and Kydd, W. L.: Open-bite: physiology and occlusion. Angle Ortho., *36:*351, 1966.

Nove, A. A.: Cervico-facial orthopaedia, Dent. Record, *66:*25, 49, 86, 109, 1946.

Pokorny, D. K., and Blake, F. P.: Principles of Occlusion, a Teaching Manual. University of Detroit, Detroit, 1968.

Schuyler, C. H.: Fundamental principles in correction of occlusal disharmony, natural and artificial, JADA *22:*1193, 1935.

———: Correction of occlusal disharmony of the natural dentition. New York State J. Dent., *13:*445, 1947.

———: Factors contributing to traumatic occlusion. J. Pros. Dent., *11:*708, 1961.

Schwarz, L.: Disorders of the Temporomandibular Joint. Philadelphia, W. B. Saunders, 1959.

Schwarz, L., and Chayes, C. M.: Facial Pain and Mandibular Dysfunction. Philadelphia, W. B. Saunders, 1968.

Straussberg, G.: Key to treatment in closed bite cases. D. Survey, *17:*27, 1951.

Subtelny, J. D., and Sakuda, M.: Open-bite: diagnosis and treatment. Am. J. Ortho., *50:*337, 1964.

Sved, A.: Growth of the jaws and the etiology of malocclusion. Int. J. Ortho. Oral Surg. *21:*799, 1935.

Weinberger, A.: Attrition of teeth. Oral Surg., *8:*1048, 1955.

Westbrook, J. C.: A pattern of centric occlusion, J. Periodont., *20:*22, 1949.

Zola, A.: Morphologic limiting factors in the temporomandibular joint. J. Pros. Dent., *13:*732, 1963.

9 Temporomandibular Joint Dysfunction

In the application of physiology to dentistry, the significance of minute degenerative changes of the tissues of the masticatory organ has received insufficient emphasis. The fact of this degeneration will be demonstrated in this chapter, and evidence of its existence will manifest itself in results actually demonstrable in the masticatory organ.[105] One of the consequences of the violation or the misapplication of the laws of biomechanics may be the actual degeneration and destruction of tissue. The course of such degeneration and destruction can be traced from minor beginnings to almost total collapse. Frequently, the onset of this process is so minute and seems so trivial that it is difficult to detect and to distinguish from the picture of normalcy. For this reason the entire masticatory organ must be examined thoroughly for the most minor deviations from the normal. A complete understanding of each sign and symptom, interpreted as a result rather than as a cause for degeneration and dysfunction, will aid in diagnosis.

The four compensating parts of the stomatognathic system are the teeth, the periodontium, the temporomandibular joint and the neuromuscular system. When all the parts function in complete harmony, physiological aging of all component parts results. Should any one part function improperly, the normal stresses and strains of function become greater or lesser on the remaining parts. If the periodontium is stronger, strain and torque will be produced on the temporomandibular joint. If the temporomandibular joint is stronger, the effects will be produced upon the teeth and the periodontium. Concomitantly, effects may also be produced in the neuromuscular system.

This chapter will stress the diagnostic symptoms and signs of the teeth, the periodontium, the soft tissues, the temporomandibular joint, the face and the head. Pain as a symptom will be related to its causative agents. Not all of the symptoms to be discussed occur in every patient, because the resistance of each part determines the appearance of the symptoms.

The careful study of every patient's symptoms of pain probably will lead to fewer mistaken diagnoses of pain of psychosomatic origin. Pain is a most important manifestation of pathologic occlusion because it usually indicates that the process of degeneration has been going on for some time. It is a warning signal, and its perception is subjective and intensely individual. The cause of the symptomatology may be different in each patient, but the pain itself is most vivid and real to the patient. It is the problem of the examiner to classify all symptoms according to their proper relationship or pattern.

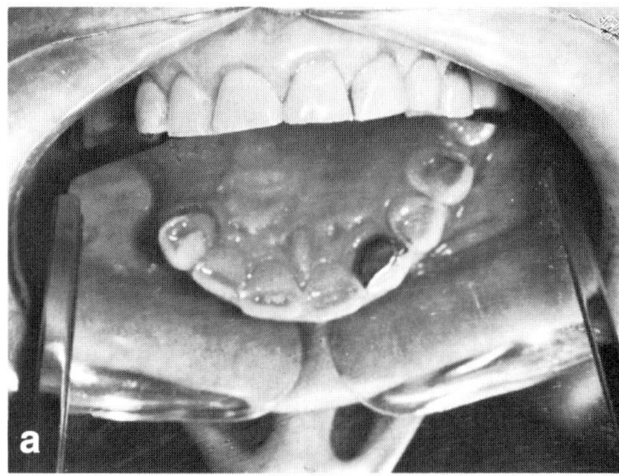

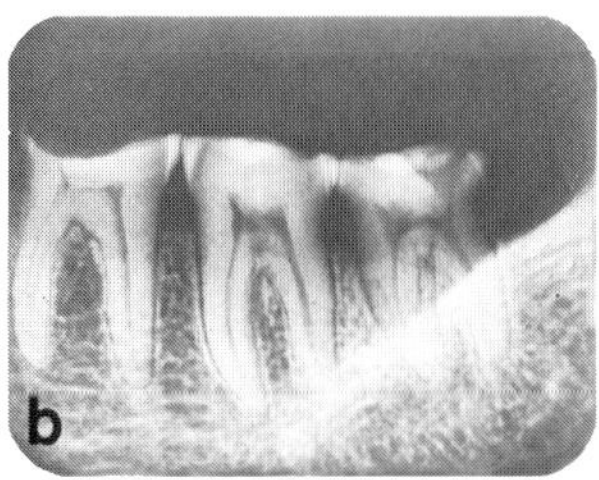

FIG. 9-1. Worn-flat incisal and occlusal surfaces laying bare the dentin (*a*). Roentgenogram portraying exposure of the dentin (*b*). (Pohto, M.: Sekundaaridentiinin. S.H.T. Finisk T.F.H., *49:*143)

There are three categories of head pain which are related to the stomatognathic system:[1]

1. Pain emanating from the tissues of the stomatognathic system
2. Pain referred from the tissues of the stomatognathic system to other areas
3. Pain referred from other areas to the stomatognathic system

The first and the second categories will be discussed in relation to other manifestations of pathologic occlusion. The third category is discussed in the section on differential diagnosis.

MANIFESTATIONS OF PATHOLOGIC OCCLUSION

Manifestations of Occlusal Trauma Produced in Crown, Root and Pulp

The effects of occlusal trauma may be revealed in a study of the occlusal contours or occlusal topography. The following signs indicate occlusal trauma:

1. Cusps that show no wear at all—an indication that other teeth are bearing the burden that should have been borne by the unworn teeth
2. Large facets and flat occlusal areas (Fig. 9-1*a*)—an indication of the presence of overload beyond tolerable physiological limits
3. Jagged, slashed or broken incisors
4. Cusps that are partially or completely sheared off
5. Abraded areas and exposed dentin (Fig. 9-1*b*) (dentin wears more rapidly than the harder enamel)
6. Gingival erosion

Not only the natural dentition but also restorations show signs of occlusal trauma. As manifested on restorations, the signs of occlusal trauma are persistent fracture of an amalgam restoration, which may be caused by occlusal trauma and may be a sign that the restoration is in interfering occlusal contact; and wear facets on gold and silver restorations.

The roots may also show symptoms of occlusal trauma. Root resorption may occur when teeth are subjected to abnormal stress. This condition can be observed in the roentgenogram of the tooth or the group of teeth that is subjected to such stress (Fig. 9-2). Roentgenograms will also reveal localized cementum hypertrophy as an abnormal amount of cementum deposited in the area around the

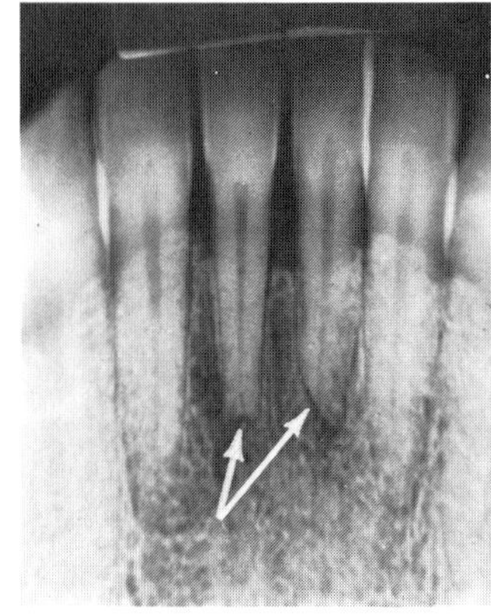

FIG. 9-2. Root resorption due to occlusal trauma.

root of any teeth that have been subjected to great stress. These extensions of cementum provide a larger surface area for the attachment of periodontal fibers, thus making the anchorage firmer (see Fig. 4-17).

Frequently, unexplained fractures of the apical third of the roots of the lower anterior teeth will be revealed in a roentgenogram (see Fig. 4-18); such fractures may be due to occlusal trauma. Occlusal trauma may cause gingival recession with consequent exposure of cementum. This may result in cervical pain. Uneven wear which exposes dentin results in sensitive incisal or occlusal surfaces because the dentin is not adequately protected against extremes of temperature. Frequently, the patient will complain of pain, but examination will reveal neither caries nor exposed dentin or cementum. In such cases, the pain may be the result of trauma caused by an interfering contact in centric relation or in one of the ranges of articulation.

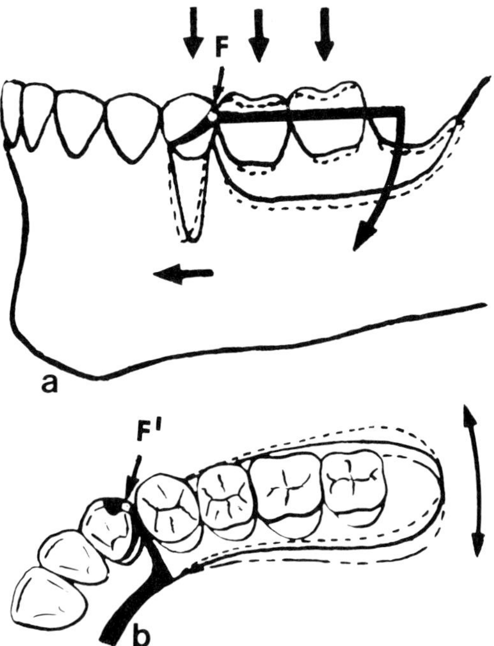

FIG. 9-3. The loads carried by abutments because of the pump-handle action of partial dentures (*a*). The tooth and the partial denture are displaced in the direction of the dotted lines. The fulcrum is at F. The torque produced by the lateral action of the partial denture saddle as the patient functions in the lateral ranges (*b*). The fulcrum is at F′. (After Krough-Poulsen, Loos)

Diagnostic Symptoms of Occlusal Trauma

The following symptoms of occlusal trauma are manifested in the pulp. Often a tooth is observed which is sensitive to thermal changes due to a hyperemic pulp. In such cases, the cause of the difficulty may be occlusal trauma. When the forces are abnormal and the resistance of the pulp tissue is low, pulpitis and eventual pulp death may result. However, when the resistance of the pulp is high, it will react to abnormal stress by laying down secondary dentin to protect itself from the occlusal stresses. Some of the effects of occlusal trauma on the pulp may also be observed roentgenographically. There will be recession of the pulp owing to the laying down of secondary dentin. Occlusal trauma may also result in obliteration of the pulp chamber and canal as well as in the formation of denticles or pulp stones.

The teeth, themselves, may evidence many manifestations of occlusal trauma. Among these may be migration and malposition with a corresponding loss of occlusal contact. Restorations that are in interfering occlusal contact transmit the overload and trauma to the abutment teeth. Partial dentures that are not constructed to function physiologically in centric-relation occlusion and the eccentric ranges of articulation result in a pump-handle action which traumatizes the abutments (Fig. 9-3). In this manner the clasps act as orthodontic appliances which move the abutment teeth and may also cause periodontal symptoms.

Food impaction is another manifestation of occlusal trauma on the teeth. In the case of the interfering occlusal contact that occurs between a cusp that makes contact with opposing marginal ridges and wedges them apart, vertical food impaction usually takes place. A nonfunctioning-side occlusal contact will cause unilateral mastication as a preferred condition of mastication, thus causing hyperfunction on one side and hypofunction on the other.

Manifestations of Occlusal Trauma Produced in the Periodontium

The manifestations of occlusal trauma in the periodontium will be discussed under the following headings: soft-tissue manifestations, periodontal-space manifestations and bone manifestations.

Glickman wrote:

Occlusion and the Periodontium

Since mastication is the major function of the dentition and since the periodontium constitutes the supporting mechanism which enables the teeth to fulfill this function, consideration of the interrelation between the forces of occlusion and the periodontium is basic in periodontology.

In an analysis of the effect of occlusal forces upon the periodontium, the tooth, periodontal membrane, alveolar bone and cementum are best considered as a functional unit. From a morphologic viewpoint, the cementum and bone constitute the support for the principal fibers of the periodontal membrane. The functional balance between the periodontal membrane and the alveolar bone is a particularly sensitive one. These tissues respond more readily to alterations in occlusal force than does the cementum. Although changes do occur in the cementum associated with pronounced alterations in occlusal force, such changes occur secondary to, and to a less severe degree, than the changes seen in the periodontal membrane and alveolar bone. Both the periodontal membrane and alveolar bone are dependent upon the functional stimulation for the preservation of their structure. The removal of functional forces has a deleterious effect upon them. In addition to being united in a close morphologic and functional relationship, the periodontal membrane, alveolar bone and cementum, because of their common mesenchymal origin, are mutually involved in the destructive and reparative phenomena arising from injury.[41]

The Role of Trauma as a Primary or Secondary Factor in the Causation of Periodontal Disease

It is unlikely that a categorical positive or negative answer to the above aspect of trauma from occlusion will evolve from clinical observation alone for the following reasons:

1. It is difficult in routine practice to obtain clinical information under properly controlled conditions. When the operator is confronted with both periodontal disease and occlusal disharmony it is generally not feasible to determine the sequence in which they occurred.
2. Because of the close physiologic relationship which exists between the forces of occlusion and the maintenance of the periodontium, it is extremely hazardous to dogmatically rule out the existence of an unfavorable modification in this relationship despite the absence of gross occlusal disharmonies.
3. The effect of systemic influences upon the periodontal tissues is such that subtle variations in the former may impair the ability of the periodontium to withstand generally acceptable occlusal forces, even in those cases in which no notable systemic disease exists.

An inflexible attitude regarding the problem of whether trauma from occlusion is primary or secondary in the causation of periodontal disease is somewhat untenable in a complex biological system such as that which exists between the individual, the periodontium and occlusal forces.[43]

Soft-Tissue Manifestations

Occlusal trauma may be manifested by a number of signs and symptoms of the soft tissues.

1. Excess stress on the teeth produces inflammatory changes in the soft tissues. These will result in changes in the color of the gingiva. A comparison of the color of the gingiva with the color of the hard palate will help the dentist to detect the inflammation caused by occlusal trauma.

a. Occlusal trauma may cause changes in the tone and the texture of the gingiva.

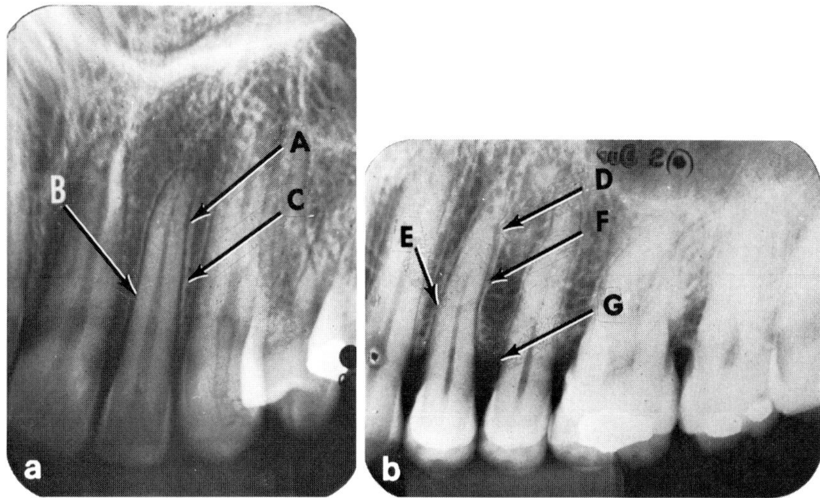

FIG. 9-4. Wide periodontal space at A, an hourglass stricture at B, a heavy lamina dura at C, in a case of high adaptive capacity (*a*). Wide periodontal space at D, an hourglass stricture at E, a heavy lamina dura at F, loss of crestal bone at G, in a case of low adaptive capacity (*b*).

There may be redness and congestion of the marginal gingiva, an absence of stippling, inflammation of the gingiva, edema and glossiness of the tissues, or a combination of these conditions.

b. There may be changes in the structure and position of the gingiva caused by occlusal trauma. The effects of occlusal trauma may be recognized by epithelial nodules, traumatic crescents, gingival festoons, gingival clefts, blunting of the crest of the interproximal papillae, linear depressions, distended veins in the mucosa, hypertrophy of the gingiva, bleeding, recession of the gingiva, or any combination of these conditions.

2. In the presence of occlusal trauma, the papillae and other gingival tissues are usually tender and sore.

a. Occlusal trauma may also bring about changes in the condition and the position of the papillae. These are very sensitive indicators of the health of the gingiva. Occlusal trauma may also be manifested in the gingival sulcus. When a periodontal pocket coexists with occlusal trauma, the trauma will induce further destructive changes in the periodontium. Other manifestations are periodontal abscesses and pus in the crevicular exudate. Miller[77] states that traumatic occlusion may create a situation in which lowered local resistance may result in chronic necrotizing ulcerative gingivitis.

Periodontal-Space Manifestations

Clinically, the periodontal space is examined roentgenographically. Abnormal forces on the teeth produce the following effects on the periodontal space:

1. With high resistive capacity of the tissues (Fig. 9-4*a*) the hourglass shape of the periodontal space at A becomes more pronounced.

2. With low resistive capacity of the tissues (*b*), the bone is resorbed at the crest at F, and the periodontal space is increased at D (see Fig. 4-8).

3. Periodontal abscess may be a manifestation of occlusal trauma.[77]

4. Mobility may be an indication of occlusal trauma and can be detected roentgenographically by greater width of the space mesially, distally and/or api-

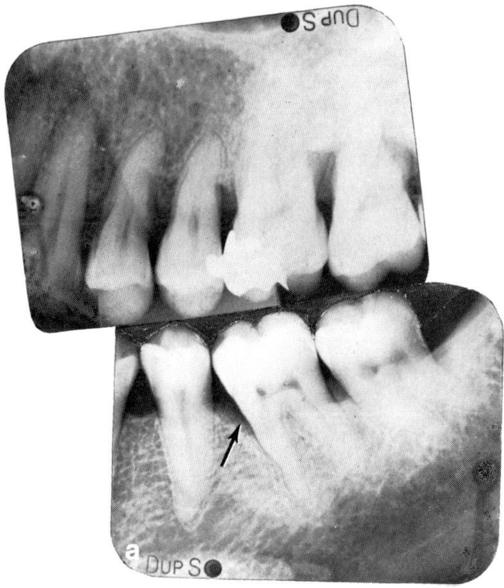

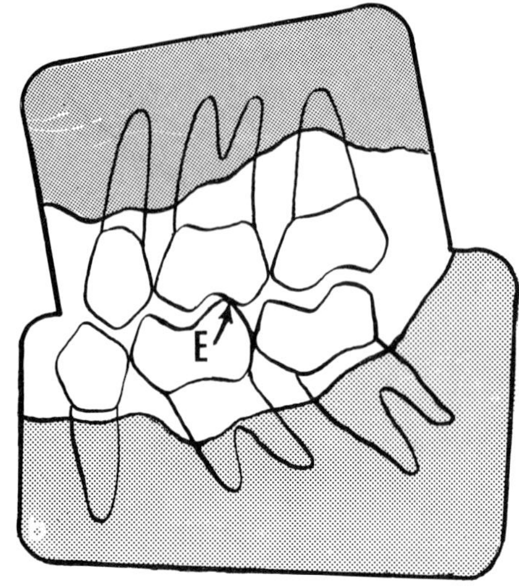

FIG. 9-5. Roentgenogram and diagram showing bone loss produced by an interfering occlusal contact, E, in centric relation. Note the level of bone on the mesial of the lower first molar and the upper first molar. Observe the upward slope of bone toward the distal surface of the lower second bicuspid root. Incipient stages will show the same type of resorption in a milder degree.

cally. The increase in the space width may also be detected by luxation of the tooth buccolingually. Muhlemann[81,82,86,87] and others[57,58,84,88] have demonstrated that tooth mobility is closely interrelated with occlusal function and abnormal stress.

The work of Jozat[62] and others[30,66,85] on the width of the periodontal space and function concludes that:

1. Periodontal width is not definite.
2. The periodontal space is increased with age and function.
3. Through youth and middle age, the periodontal spaces of the mandibular teeth are larger than those of the maxillary teeth; after 60 years of age, the situation is reversed.
4. Tooth function influences periodontal space width. Functioning teeth have a greater periodontal space width (0.359 to 0.307 mm.) than nonfunctioning teeth (0.275 to 0.263 mm).
5. Abutment teeth which support prosthetic appliances usually have the greatest periodontal space width.
6. The masticatory pattern influences the width of the periodontal space. In cases of little or no overbite, the periodontal space is greater than in cases with a large vertical overbite.
7. The smallest periodontal space width measured was 0.055 mm. and the largest was 0.605 mm. All measurements were taken at the middle of the root.

Bone Manifestations

It is the periodontal ligament that transmits forces to the alveolar bone. The roentgenogram makes it possible to view the effects of these forces on the bone. The manifestations of force on the bone can be any of the following: resorption, condensation or a change in the substance of the bone.

Normal forces stimulate the bone and maintain the lamina dura in a physiological condition. An abnormal force, if it is associated with good anabolic processes, will cause the lamina dura to thicken in order to compensate for the occlusal stresses. However, should the catabolic phase of metabolism predominate, an excessive occlusal force will cause the degeneration and eventual destruction of the lamina dura. The supporting bone reacts to abnormal force in a similar manner. With a high resistive capacity, the trabeculae rearrange themselves and increase in size, thus presenting a denser roentgenographic appearance. Abnormal stress associated with a low resistive capacity causes rarefaction of bone, which is also evident in the roentgenogram.

Clinically, some of the characteristic manifestations of occlusal trauma on the alveolar bone are loss of bone on the mesial of the lower molars or bicuspids and on the distal of the upper molars or bicuspids. Figure 9-5 is a roentgenogram showing the effects of a centric-relation interfering contact upon the bone. Note the level of the bone on the mesial of the lower molar and the distal of the upper molar as compared with the level of the bone in the rest of the roentgenogram. Bone loss can occur because of an interfering contact in any of the eccentric ranges of articulation. Figure 9-6 illustrates alveolar bone loss as a response to excessive force in a case of nonfunctioning-side interfering occlusal contact.

Kellner[67] as well as others[45,46] have come to the following conclusions:

1. The state of the lamellar bone that limits the periodontal space is related to the functional demands made upon it.
2. Function influences the retroalveolar spongiosa. Hyperfunction induces heavy trabecularization, and hypofunction results in decrease in the trabecularization of the alveolar bone.

Functional stimulation of bone is physiologically necessary for its maintenance. Occlusal trauma interferes with the normal pattern of mastication and often results in disuse atrophy of portions of alveolar bone which support teeth that are not in function.

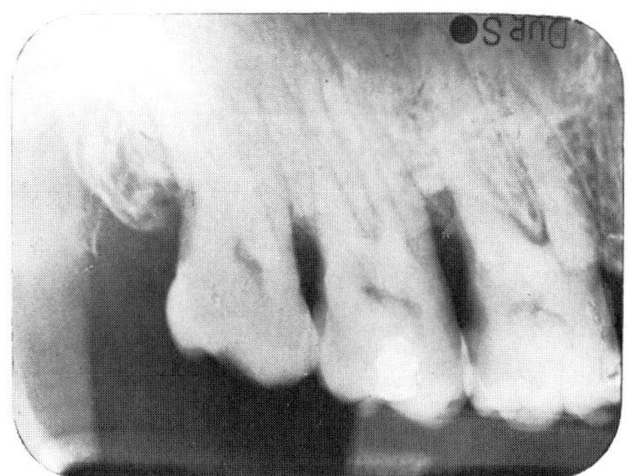

FIG. 9-6. The roentgenogram shows bone loss around an upper left first and second molar due to a nonfunctioning-side interfering contact. The patient in this case complained of looseness of these teeth and of pain in the temporomandibular joint on that side. Removal of the interfering contact in the nonfunctioning range brought about a cessation of these symptoms.

Pain of the bone at the base of a tooth is the result of repeated microtraumata to the tooth which have been transmitted to the bone. This type of pain may be lik-

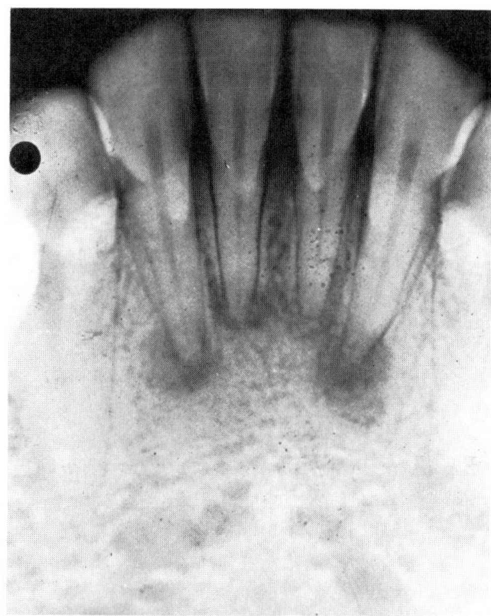

FIG. 9-7. Periapical osteofibrosis caused by occlusal trauma.

ened to a bone bruise; the tooth acts as the traumatizing agent to the periodontal ligament which is unable to prevent transmission of force to the bone.

Figure 9-7 illustrates a case of periapical osteofibrosis caused by occlusal trauma in which the destroyed bone has been replaced by fibrous tissue. The pulp test of the involved teeth proved to be positive. In the next stage of this condition, the fibrous tissue is replaced with cementum, forming cementomas.

Clinical Implications of Occlusal Trauma

Regarding the clinical implications of trauma from occlusion and periodontal disease, Glickman says:[42]

The following facts are pertinent to a basic orientation regarding the significance of trauma in the clinical management of periodontal disease:

1. With the exception of a few isolated conditions, trauma from occlusion is a complicating or predisposing rather than an initiating factor in chronic destructive periodontal disease.
2. The correction of occlusal disharmony in the treatment of periodontal disease is predicated on the assumption that the occlusal forces are injurious to the tissues and that their alleviation will have a beneficial effect.
3. The importance of the correction of occlusal forces in the overall treatment of periodontal disease depends upon the degree to which such forces are contributing to the destruction of the periodontal tissues.
4. When trauma from occlusion produces destructive changes in the periodontium, it constantly stimulates the normal reparative processes of the tissues. The reparative processes remove the degenerated tissue and form new tissues necessary for the reconstruction of the area. It is important to think of injurious forces in terms of both the destructive and reparative changes that they stimulate. The reason a force is traumatic is because the destructive changes it induces exceed the reparative capacity of the tissues. Alleviation of the force enables the reparative changes to predominate, and restoration of the tissue in the area of injury follows.
5. The degree to which the correction of occlusal forces will benefit the periodontium is dependent upon the reparative capacity of the tissues.
6. Local irritants such as calculus, food impaction, and overhanging fillings induce inflammatory changes which impair the reparative capacity of the tissues and therefore diminish the therapeutic effectiveness of the correction of occlusal forces.
7. The existence of systemic disturbances capable of altering the periodontal tissues will also impair their reparative capacity and diminish the therapeutic effectiveness of the correction of occlusal forces.
8. In order to obtain the maximum benefit from the correction of occlusal relationships as part of the overall treatment of periodontal disease, it is imperative to eliminate all other factors capable of impairing the reparative capacity of the tissues.

Held,[56] on the other hand, states:

To sum up, taking into account the clinical observations of parodontolysis (diseases characterized by a progressive atrophy of the parodontium) on the one hand, and the histopathological findings on the other, we can describe the pathogenesis of parodontolysis as follows:

1. Gingivitis simply does not develop into parodontolysis as long as the bone resorption does not occur following a dystrophic factor of endogenous origin.
2. In cases where traumatic occlusion and articulation do not intervene, parodontolysis develops independently of subjacent inflammatory lesion, whatever its origin.
3. When the periodontium is injured by functional disturbances (occlusal trauma) or dystrophic disturbances (periodontosis), the inflammation of the gingiva and periodontium meet and form a true parodontitis (inflammatory form of parodontolysis) with bony tissues taking part in the inflammatory phenomena.
4. The development of a parodontolysis always comprises a dystrophic factor; simple inflammatory lesions of mechanical origin (heavy trauma) or of infectious origin (medicamental or infectious parodontitis) are reversible by eliminating the cause, since bone has the power to regenerate in such cases.

Careful inspection and exploration of the tissues will reveal these signs of oc-

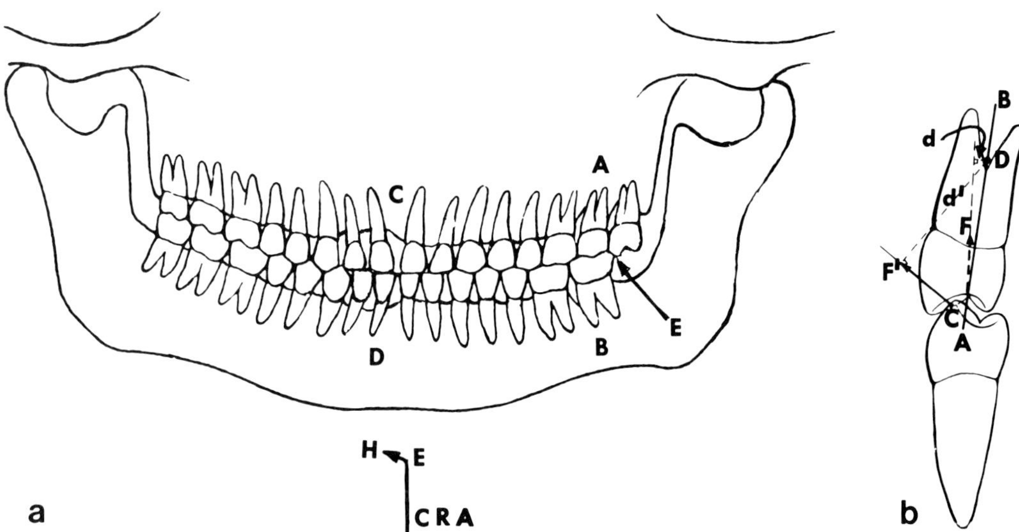

FIG. 9-8. A medial protrusive shift of the mandible caused by the interfering occlusal contact, E, and the resultant manifestations at A, B, C and D (*a*). The frontal diagram, CRA, portrays the direction of mandibular movement during the shift from E to H. The mechanism of the development of excessive movements of tipping (F′ × d′) caused by the convenience relation contacts after an interfering occlusal contact has resulted in a medial or a lateral protrusive mandibular shift (*b*).

clusal trauma before periodontal involvement becomes so extensive that they are masked. It is important to uncover these signs and symptoms as a preventive measure so that corrective therapy may be instituted to ensure against further and more serious degeneration of the soft tissues.

Manifestations of Occlusal Trauma and Pathologic Occlusion in Other Soft Tissues

Occlusal trauma may be manifested by pain and swelling in other soft tissues of the stomatognathic system:

1. Infratemporal fossa—palpation of this structure may reveal swelling, edema and intense tenderness and pain.

2. Salivary glands—the parotid, the submaxillary and the sublingual glands swell, and increased salivation is often a symptom of neural derangement indirectly due to occlusal trauma.

3. Lymph nodes—the superior deep cervical nodes behind the angle of the mandible are often sensitive to palpation in cases of occlusal trauma.

4. Pain and swelling in the soft tissues. The neuromuscular (motor) and the neural (sensory) manifestations of pathologic occlusion are discussed in later sections of this chapter.

Protrusive Medial and Protrusive Lateral Manifestations of a Centric-Relation Interfering Occlusal Contact

In Chapter 8 under Class I, pathologic protrusive medial and lateral shifts of the mandible were analyzed. To help explain the symptomatology of this complicated situation, let us consider again the sequence of events which lead up to a protrusive medial shift of the mandible. This is illustrated in Fig. 8-5*a*, *b*, and *d*. The patient closes in centric relation, strikes the interfering occlusal contact and shifts the mandible medially, directed by the gliding inclines of the teeth in interfering occlusal contact, causing the buccal planes of the buccal cusps of the lower teeth on the opposite side to strike the lingual planes of the buccal cusps of the upper teeth on that side, thus traumatizing the upper and the lower teeth on that side.

The protrusive lateral shift of the mandible is similarly produced by an interfering occlusal contact, except that this contact causes the mandible to shift laterally from the point of contact in a direction away from the midline, traumatizing the teeth on the same side. It is the convenience relationship of the mandible that applies force to the traumatized side in each case. Statistically, it should be noted that the possibilities of a protrusive medial shift of the mandible are twice that of the possibilities of a lateral shift of the mandible (Fig. 8-3*b*). Clinically, however, because of the arrangement and the height of the involved cusps, the percentage of protrusive medial shift occurrences is nearer 85. Therefore, when a patient complains of pain in an apparently normal tooth, the cause of this symptom in about 85 per cent of cases may be an interfering occlusal contact diagonally opposite the affected tooth. In the other 15 per cent of cases, the pain may be on the same side as the interfering contact.

To illustrate, it is quite common to find an interfering occlusal contact between the mesial of an extruded upper third molar and the distal of the lower second molar, as in Figure 9-8*a*. This is due to the nonexistence of a lower third molar. Depending upon the contacting planes of the cusps, the mandible may shift protrusive medially or protrusive laterally, but in either case, in a protrusive movement. In *a* the shift depicted is protrusive medially, and the manifestation is diagonally opposite to the interfering contact, E. The following manifestations present themselves:

1. Labioversion and diastema formation at C
2. Alveoloclasia at AB caused by the interfering-contact trauma and alveoloclasia at CD caused by the trauma due to the convenience-position mandibular shift with resulting mobility
3. Inflammation and recession of the gingiva at A and B
4. Wear on the lingual surfaces of the upper teeth and the labial surfaces of the lower teeth at A and B

The reasoning behind the periodontal disturbances and pain that constitute the protrusive medial manifestation is based upon the following:

1. The medial mandibular movement causes the buccal planes of the lower buccal cusps to strike the lingual planes of the buccal cusps of the upper teeth located diagonally opposite the interfering contact.
2. This contact is usually made by one, two or three pairs of teeth, and only these teeth bear the brunt of the trauma in the convenience relationship.
3. Normally, a pair of teeth will contact cusp-to-fossa, with the force being aligned parallel with the long axis, AB (Fig. 9-8*b*). Thus the perpendicular distance, d, from the line of action of force, F, to the fulcrum, D, is extremely small, and the result is a small moment. This moment is tenable physiologically.
4. Because of the mandibular shift, the upper tooth is struck at C. The direction of the force, F, is at an angle approximately perpendicular to the long axis of the tooth, thereby creating a large moment arm, d′. The result of the large moment arm is a multiplication of the force factors about the fulcrum, D, of the tooth. Because the buccal plate of bone on the upper arch is thin and is not constituted to withstand the forces in that direction, the upper tooth is forced buccally. The resulting trauma causes periodontal disturbances and pain.

The protrusive lateral movement of the mandible, caused by an interfering contact, exhibits similar manifestations of tooth movement, pain and periodontal involvement on the same side as the interfering contact, rather than on the

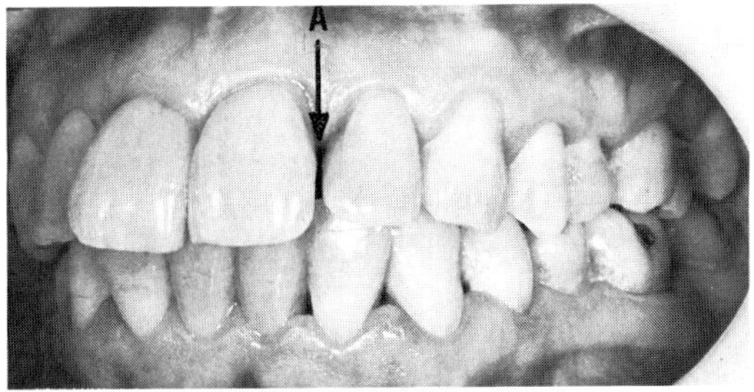

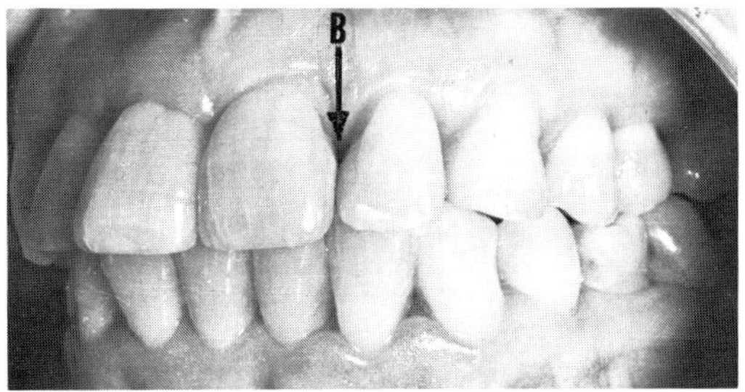

FIG. 9-9. An interfering occlusal contact causing diastema at A shown closed at B after occlusal equilibration was performed.

diagonally opposite side. This type of mandibular movement occurs less frequently than the protrusive medial mandibular and therefore may be overlooked unless the examination is conducted carefully.

Many times an anterior tooth or teeth will wander or elongate for no apparent reason. This phenomenon may be explained by the protrusive medial or lateral shifts of the mandible. A clinical illustration of the diagonal manifestation is seen in Figure 9-9. Note the diastema at A between the upper left central and lateral. Further examination revealed gingival involvement and pain in the area. An interference analysis revealed an interfering occlusal contact between the right upper and lower first molars diagonally opposite. Note the same area at B after occlusal equilibration has removed the interfering contact in the molar region. The diastema and the pain have disappeared, and the gingival condition has improved.

Retrusive Manifestations of a Centric-Relation Interfering Occlusal Contact

In the 1890's Warnekros[127] and Alkory[2] described the diagonal manifestations of interfering contacts. Their conception of the diagonal manifestation consisted in mobility and movement of teeth and gingival symptoms on the side diagonally opposite the centric-relation interfering contact. Thielemann[113] in 1939 elaborated this idea. The diagonal manifestation of Thielemann is illustrated in Figure 9-10. The interference is the lower left molar in black; this situation was created when the upper molar was removed and the lower molar extruded. The effects are retrusion of the mandible owing to the interfering occlusal contact at E; an interference to mandibular movement into the right lateral range of articulation owing to nonfunctioning-side interference at E; and an in-

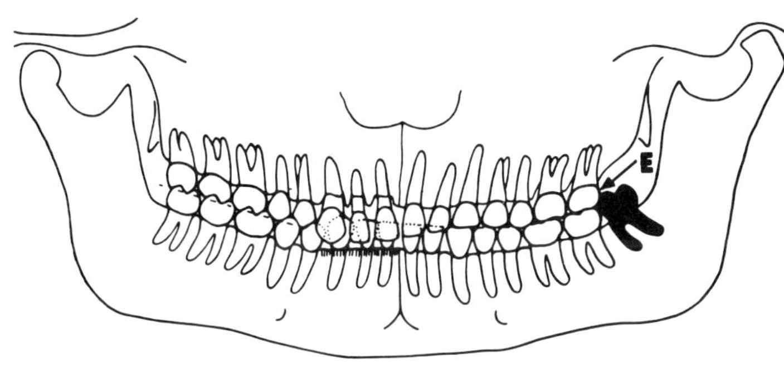

FIG. 9-10. A retrusive shift of the mandible caused by an interfering occlusal contact, E, and the resultant manifestations. (Thielemann, K.: Biomechanik der Paradentose. Munich, Barth, 1956)

terference to mandibular movement in the protrusive range of articulation at E.

Thielemann[113] presented the following symptoms in this type of case, as seen in Figure 9-10.

On the left side:

1. Temporomandibular joint symptoms due to the forced retrusion in the convenience relationship
2. Excessive cuspal wear on the posterior teeth
3. Loss of mesial and palatal bone around the upper molars owing to the fact that they receive the impact of the interfering occlusal contact

On the right side:

1. Unworn cuspal surfaces on the posterior teeth
2. Retrusive convenience relationship created space between the lingual surfaces of the upper anteriors and the labial surfaces of the lower anteriors
3. Elongation of the upper and the lower anteriors because of lack of contact and causing marked increase in vertical overbite
4. Unworn anterior teeth
5. Labioversion of the upper anterior teeth with resultant diastemas
6. Marked periodontal changes of the upper and the lower anterior teeth:
   a. Gingival recession
   b. Alveolar bone resorption
   c. Mobility
   d. Upper anterior hypertrophic changes
   e. Pocket formation, exudate and calculus

It is interesting to note that somewhat similar symptoms (i.e., diastemas, periodontal involvement, etc.) that appear around the anterior teeth may be caused by diametrically opposed mandibular movements—the protrusive medial and the retrusive shift. Compare Figure 9-9 with Figure 9-10.

Habit Manifestations

Pathologic occlusion and interfering occlusal contacts may result in the following habits:

1. Unilateral mastication
2. Perverted swallowing
3. Bruxism
4. Tooth clenching and grinding during waking hours

Unilateral Mastication. This is usually the result of discomfort on one side of the arch during mastication. This discomfort may be caused by restorations placed in supraocclusion and interfering occlusal contacts that cause sensitive teeth.

The results of this discomfort are conscious shifting of all masticatory function to the side of the arch that enables the patient to masticate comfortably. In time, this becomes an unconscious habit.

Perverted Swallowing. This is often the result of mandibular malposition caused by an interfering occlusal contact in centric relation. The patient will have to place the mandible in an abnormal position to swallow. The result is an unbalanced musculature of the swallowing mechanism.

Bruxism. The grinding or the gnashing of teeth during sleep is called bruxism or Karolyi's phenomenon, la bruxomania, stridor dentium and occlusal neurosis. Boyens[23] includes under bruxism, clenching, audible gnashing, cusp doodling and contacts made in abnormal mandibular excursions. Tishler's[117] occlusal neurosis referred to the grinding, the pounding and the clenching of the teeth when the mouth is empty. This nocturnal activity has a similar etiology to daytime clenching and grinding and follows the same course. These mandibular movements are the result of the patient's unconscious search for centric-relation occlusion and the elimination of any interference toward the attainment of this position. One patient described this as comparable to turning and twisting in a search for a comfortable spot on a lumpy mattress. If the emotional background of the patient is not such as to predispose him to bruxism, an interfering contact will not initiate the habit. However, if there is an emotional predisposition to the habit, the interfering occlusal contact will become

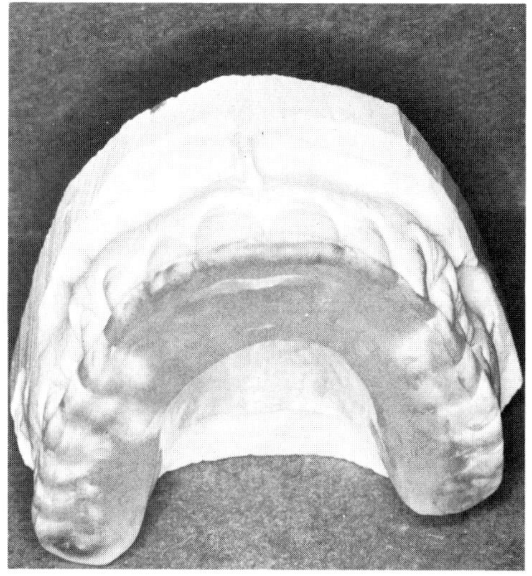
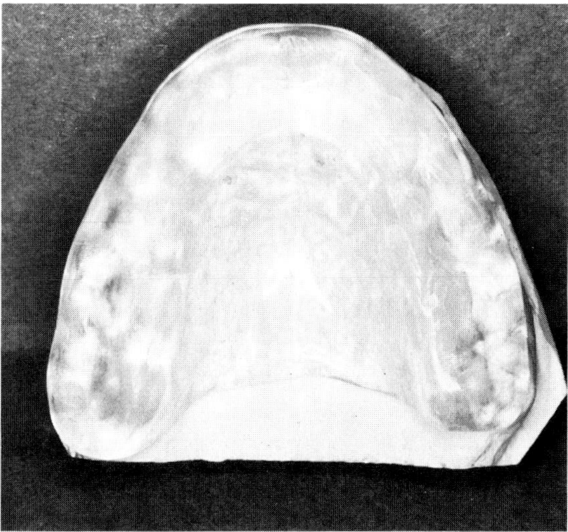

FIG. 9-11. An acrylic splint covering the palate and the occlusal surfaces of the maxillary teeth.

the catalyst and initiate bruxism. Tishler[117] says:

> The habit of grinding or pressing the teeth together occurs so frequently in connection with such cases that the writer believes traumatic occlusion to be a contributing factor of major etiological importance.

Many patients do not know that they grind their teeth or, if they do, that this is a pathological condition. The patient will usually report tired jaw muscles upon awakening. During the taking of the patient's history, he should be questioned carefully about day or night grinding and should be asked to verify his statement by checking with members of his family. Usually one or more members of the family will be aware of the existence of the habit.

Tooth clenching and grinding or "tooth doodling" during the waking hours is a very common manifestation of an interfering occlusal contact. The patient tries literally to "wear off" the interfering contact by moving the mandible constantly. In the case of clenching and grinding habits the forces applied to the teeth are constant rather than intermittent. Under this constant pressure, some fibers of the periodontal ligament are under constant tension while others are under constant compression. This continuation of tension and compression usually will cause deleterious effects within the structure and the tissues of the periodontal ligament. Intermittent normal forces are physiological in their action on the periodontal ligament. The orthodontic researches of Oppenheim[90] and others[22,24,27,69,96,97] have proved that the excessive constant force will produce degeneration of the ligament. The forces used in these experiments were only a fraction of the forces that can be applied during the periods of the clenching habit. The results of these habits are constantly greater trauma to the teeth which in turn create emotional factors. The emotional factor of the patient is a predisposing agent to tooth clenching and grinding during the time the patient is awake or asleep.

Treatment. The patient who grinds or clenches his teeth during the day or the night undergoes therapy in three phases:

1. Occlusal equilibration to remove all interferences to centric-relation occlusion and all the ranges of articulation. After the occlusal disharmony has been corrected, the patient should be checked

regularly for occlusal changes and as often as he feels any occlusal changes himself. Grewcock[48] states that "adjustment to a centric position [centric-relation occlusion] will, in the majority of cases, cure the bruxism."

2. In treating the psychic factor, the patient is given the following instructions for autosuggestion. He is told to repeat ten times after each meal, "Lips together, teeth apart."[77] He is also to guard all day against tooth contact or clenching. He must try to maintain the position in which only the lips touch while the teeth are held apart. These two methods of treatment are the first line of defense against bruxism.

3. If night grinding persists, an upper acrylic appliance (Fig. 9-11) is constructed (see Chap. 11 for full discussion).

All habits caused by pathologic occlusion are interrelated and have a basically similar etiology. The treatment in all cases is to eliminate the cause—the pathologic occlusion initiated by the interfering occlusal contact—rather than to be led astray by the various methods of treating only the symptoms.

Manifestations of Pathologic Occlusion in Temporomandibular Joint Arthrosis

The manifestation of pathologic occlusion in the temporomandibular joint is termed temporomandibular joint arthrosis. In 1940, Foged[38] suggested the name *arthrosis temporomandibularis* for the disease entity. The lesion was first described by Cooper[31] in 1823. Annondale,[3] in 1887, rendered the first surgical treatment which consisted of surgically fixing the meniscus. Since 1929, Konjetzny, Stapelmohr, Dufourmentel, Axhausen and others have demonstrated the importance of the part played by pathologic occlusion in the production of temporomandibular joint arthrosis. The intrinsic trauma causing the arthrosis results in changes in all the tissues within the joint.

Temporomandibular joint arthrosis makes up 90 per cent of all dysfunctions of this structure. The remaining 10 per cent is accounted for by external trauma (i.e., fractures and contusions, and diseases which affect the joint). The low incidence of organic diseases of the temporomandibular joint points to a functional disorder. Bauer[13] and Steinhardt[108] verified histologically the relationship between pathologic occlusion and temporomandibular joint arthrosis. The disorder has been known by its symptoms: temporomandibular cracking, snapping joint, *machoir à resort, kiefergelenkknacken,* etc. It has also been known by its articular changes as subarthrosis, dysarthrosis and arthrosis.

Temporomandibular joint arthrosis is a noninfectious, trophic, degenerative affection of the joint tissues initiated by intrinsic trauma and causing abnormal changes in the function of the joint. It cannot be considered a disease of aging or senility, since it commonly occurs in patients between 20 and 40 years of age. Pyrexia does not occur, but swelling caused by joint effusion—the escape of fluid from blood vessels or lymphatics into the tissues or cavity—may be present. The trauma causes changes within the tissues of the joint which may result in joint effusion. The effusion is a noninfectious and noninflammatory swelling of the arthrotic lesion and is usually monarticular but may be bilateral. Although bilateral lesions seldom develop simultaneously, when they do so, they may be of equal severity. Konjetzny's[68] histological studies of temporomandibular joint arthrosis proved it to be a noninflammatory condition. The disorder is caused by chronic intrinsic microtraumata by the head of the condyle to the joint structures. The abnormal movements of the head of the condyle are caused by the pathologic occlusion.

The bone structure and the fibrocartilaginous covering of the joint are affected by mechanical influences reflected upon the joint by the occlusion of the teeth. The loss of posterior teeth causes structural changes in the joint by altering the force and the direction of stress within the joint. Changes through bone resorption and apposition and through degeneration and reorganization of the cartilage, and in the fibers that make up the articulating surfaces and the disc also occur.[91,109] Haupl and Posansky,[55] using a functional orthopaedic appliance on a monkey, produced bone changes and bone formation in the glenoid fossa and on the condyle. A. W. Bauer[9] and W. H. Bauer[14] both maintain that the diverse symptoms of temporomandibular joint dysfunction are the result of traumatic arthrosis of the temporomandibular joint.

The symptoms of temporomandibular joint arthrosis are caused most frequently by the nonosseous tissues within the structure. Frequently, the roentgenograms of the tissues of the joint areas will appear only slightly abnormal, and yet the patient may complain of marked discomfort in these areas. The importance and the necessity of thorough analysis of all related factors that could contribute to these temporomandibular joint symptoms cannot be overemphasized. The temporomandibular joint roentgenograms must be evaluated in the light of the patient's clinical symptoms and the concept of the multiple conditions that will produce these symptoms.

Temporomandibular joint arthrosis may be divided into three categories: manifestations produced within the joint, neuromuscular (motor) manifestations, and neural (sensory) manifestations.

Roentgenographic Manifestations

The manifestations produced within the joint may be divided further into roentgenographic and clinical symptoms. The roentgenographic manifestations should be determined on the basis of the oblique-lateral transcranial projection, midorbitomeatal-baseline, corner-of-the-mouth projection and the inner-canthus, articular-eminence projection (see Chap. 12). These projections are modified lateral and anteroposterior views of the temporomandibular joints in open and closed positions. The manifestations observed in these roentgenograms are:

1. Pathological positional relationships of the condyle heads in the glenoid fossae
   a. Deviations from normal on one or both sides
   b. Dissimilar positioning of the right and the left condyles
   c. Condyles in anterior, posterior, superior, inferior, medial or lateral position or in any combination of these positions
   d. Pathological hypomobility or hypermobility of the condyles as evidenced by different distances traversed by the condyles from the closed to the open position. These distances should be compared with the distance traveled by a normal condyle. The right and the left distances traversed will vary.
2. Any placement of the condyles in positions other than normal will cause the joint gap to seem asymmetrical or completely obliterated
3. Glenoid fossae and articular eminences
   a. Roughened, irregularly shaped articular eminence and fossa floor
   b. Erosion of the fossa floor and articular eminence
   c. Angle of inclination of posterior wall of the articular eminence may vary from right side to left side
4. Meniscus (not visible roentgenographically)
   a. Calcific deposits may appear in the meniscus
   b. Apparent erosion and destruction of the meniscus as seen by the obliteration of the joint gap relationship

5. Condyle
   a. Contour: flattened, irregular, misshapen, eroded
   b. Disharmony of size and contour of the condyle to the glenoid fossa
6. Tympanic plate—eroded area of the plate caused by retrusion of the mandible
7. Subluxation and dislocation—positions of one or both condyles

A contributing factor to temporomandibular joint arthrosis is the repeated condylar microtrauma within the joint causing interference with the nutrient supply which in turn interferes with the lubrication of the articular surfaces of the joint and the nutrition of the joint. It is this alteration of the synovial fluid in the joint that exacerbates the clinical symptoms as they occur.

Clinical Manifestations of Temporomandibular Joint Arthrosis

The clinical manifestations of temporomandibular joint arthrosis are listed in the order in which they usually appear: clicking, crackling noises, crepitation, tenderness, pain in and around the joint. The neuromuscular manifestations include limited mandibular movements with or without pain, difficulty on opening in the morning, mandibular lock in certain positions on opening, compensation of the contralateral joint by hypermobility, subluxation, irregular mandibular opening and closing movements, condylar hypermobility, muscular dysfunction, muscle tenderness and spasm and the infrequent symptom of swelling in the preauricular area. Inflammation occurs only in extremely complicated cases. In addition, other symptoms may occur. These will be discussed under muscular and neural manifestations (see pp. 179–193).

The course of the symptomatology of temporomandibular joint arthrosis usually follows this order: The patient first notes lack of smoothness in function with concomitant clicking and crepitation. Periods of tenderness occur during function and rest. These pains may disappear and then return with greater severity; finally, extreme pain and trismus occur.

Clicking. Many investigators[4,6,47,60,98] have reported various theories as to the causes of the clicking noises produced within the temporomandibular joint. The sagittal opening distance at which the first click occurs is peculiar to each case. There may be one or more clicks in one joint, or the clicking may occur in both joints. Pringle[93] believes that clicking of the joint may be caused by a sudden contraction of the external pterygoid muscle which dislocates the disc medially and anteriorly. Lotsch[74] believes that during function in the forward gliding movement it is possible for the disc to be caught and its anterior attachment ruptured, thus causing clicking.

The intermediate click is caused by an impingement in the upper temporomandibular joint which holds the disc and the condyle temporarily; after this obstacle is overcome, the condyle snaps forward with a clicking noise. The final clicking is a result of the excessive movement at the end of the opening movement. Dubecq[34] feels that the injury and the click are between the disc and the external pterygoid muscle or between the disc and the condyle attachment. Boman[20] states that the joint and the occlusion are a functional unit; therefore, where the joint is affected by changes in the occlusion, the clicking is the result of the pathologic occlusion.

Thompson[114] explained the click as a snapping into position caused by an impingement of the posterior margin of the disc between the anterior surface of the condyle and the posterior surface of the eminence as the condyle and the disc are moved. Other investigators[39,95] believe that the causes of the clicking noises during mandibular opening and closing movements are folding and wrinkling of the

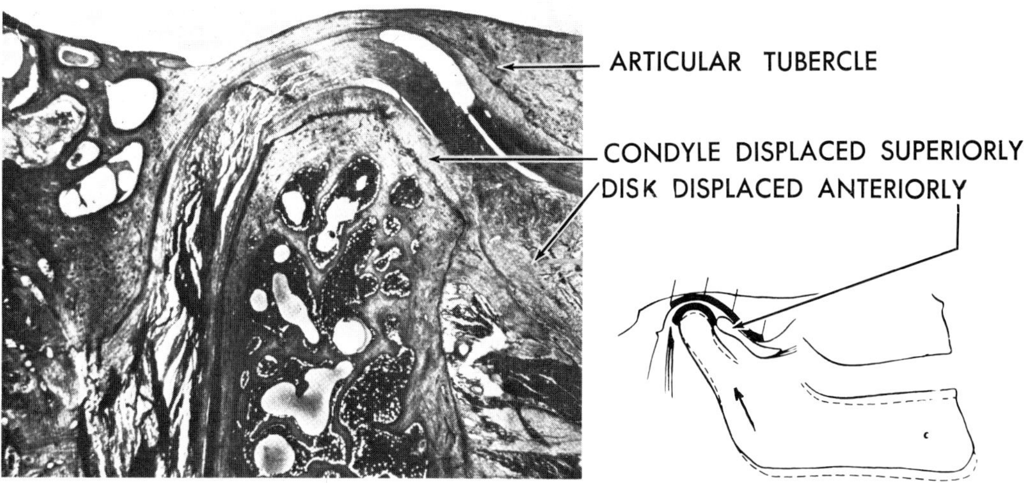

FIG. 9-12. Temporomandibular joint of a 45-year-old man. Section and diagram of a condyle, displaced posteriorly and superiorly, with the anterior surface of the condyle behind the posterior margin of the meniscus which has been displaced anteriorly. (Steinhardt, G.: Kiefergelenkerkrankungen, Die Zahn-, Mund- und Kieferheilkunde. vol. 3, Berlin, Urban, 1957)

meniscus, loose meniscus, muscle spasm, stretching of the joint ligaments by frequent subluxation, abnormal slippage of the disc attachment torn loose by the external pterygoid, loose periarticular structures, structural impediments to the movement of the disc, and irregularities of the condyle. It was the surgeons and the orthodontists who sought to explain the reasons for temporomandibular joint clicking. Axhausen[7] was one of the first to recognize the fact that more than one click can occur at various sagittal openings of the mandible. He noted two types of clicks—the intermediate and the final—and sought to correlate cause and effect. Boman[20] correlated pathologic occlusion and temporomandibular joint clicking. Hankey[50] in a study of 150 cases of temporomandibular joint arthrosis found that 57 per cent of the patients reported clicking of the joints as their main complaint. Approximately half of the clicking cases reported associated pain; 80 per cent of these reported unilateral painful clicking.

In the normal sagittal movements of the jaw, the structures of the temporomandibular joint move synchronously in their proper space relationships (see Chap. 5, the meniscus). The clicking or crackling noise that is made during the sagittal opening movements of the mandible is usually repeated during the closing movements. There are three types of clicking noises in the temporomandibular joint during the sagittal opening movements: the opening click, the intermediate click and the full opening click.

The opening click is associated with the Classes II and V pathologic occlusal relationships. It occurs because the condyle is positioned posteriorly and superiorly in the glenoid fossa with the anterior surface of the condyle behind the posterior margin of the meniscus (Fig. 9-12). As the jaw opens, the condyle must skip over the posterior surface of the meniscus. This results in the opening click.

The intermediate click, which makes up 75 per cent of the clicking cases, is associated with the Classes I, III and IV pathologic occlusal relationships. The convenience relationship of the teeth de-

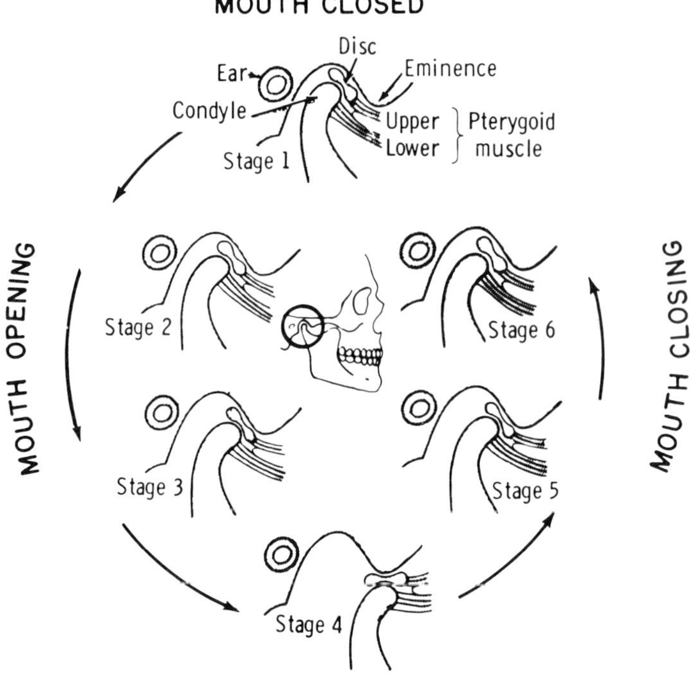

FIG. 9-13. Various stages of a normal right temporomandibular joint (area within the circle of center drawing of skull) as the jaw opens and closes the mouth. Stage 1: The components of the joint in the resting position with the mouth closed. Note that the condyle rests on the disc. Stages 2 and 3: The upper and lower parts of the external pterygoid muscle pulling the condyle and disc forward in coordination as the mouth opens slightly. Stage 4: The condyle, still resting on the center of the disc, is shown as it appears when the jaw is wide open. Stage 5 is similar to Stage 3, except that the jaw is now beginning to close. Stage 6 is like Stage 2 with the jaw closed further.

termines the convenience relationship of the condyles in the fossae. The meniscus is held in its position by the walls of the capsule and the tendon of the external pterygoid ligament. Prolonged convenience relationship damages and weakens the area of insertion of the tendon of the external pterygoid and the attachment of the anterior part of the meniscus to the condyle. Thus, the intimate spatial relationship of the condyle, the meniscus, the fossa and the external pterygoid tendon is disturbed. As the jaw opens, the external pterygoid muscles contract, and there is an erratic movement produced by the incoordinate pull of the upper head of the external pterygoid on the meniscus and the lower head of the external pterygoid on the neck of the condyle. The incoordinate movement plus the incorrect static relationship of the parts of the joint in the convenience relationship cause the mandible to function asynchronously in the opening movement.

Figure 9-13 diagrams the normal case, in which the disc and condyle slide forward together on the articular eminence. Figure 9-14 shows that in the spastic muscle the upper and lower fibers no longer contract coordinately, so that the condyle cannot remain in its normal place within the disc. As the malposed parts of the joint attempt to correct themselves during function, the condyle and

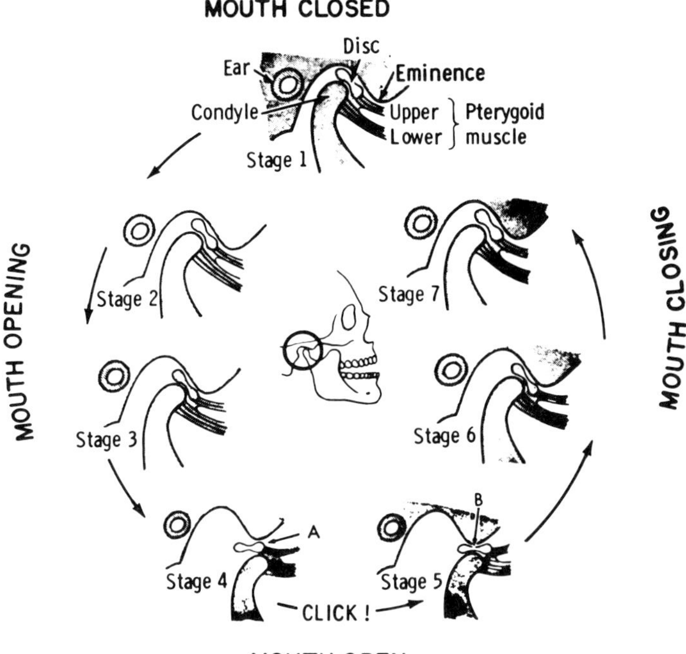

FIG. 9-14. Various stages of an abnormal (spastic) right temporomandibular joint as the jaw opens and closes the mouth. The upper and lower parts of the external pterygoid muscles are functioning incoordinately. Stage 4: The condyle is remaining in its place in the center of the disc, as in Stages 2 and 3, instead of riding on the thickened outer edge of the disc (*A*). Stage 5 (fully open position of the jaw): The disc snaps forward into place (*B*) producing the click. Stages 6 and 7 correspond to Stages 2 and 3 except that the jaw is closing.

the meniscus try to attain physiological positioning. In attempting this the various thicknesses of the meniscus come into play. It is the sudden snapping together of the parts as they ride over the varying thicknesses of the meniscus during function that causes the clicks in the various opening positions. The disc is thereby traumatized, and crepitation and pain eventually accompany the clicking sound as the disc becomes stretched, abraded, torn and subject to degenerative changes resulting from excessive wear and tear. Muscle spasms of the temporal, the masseter and the external pterygoid directly complicate and take part in the mechanism of the intermediate click.

The final click occurs in the full open position as the condyle passes over the anterior portion of the meniscus; the meniscus is pulled forward of the condyle; or both the meniscus and the condyle pass over the articular eminence. Pathologic occlusion can be the prime factor in all of these cases, causing hypermobility of the meniscus and/or the condyle and thus resulting in the click in the wide-open position.

Clicks Produced by Eccentric Movement. In addition to clicks produced during sagittal movements of the mandible, there are clicks produced by eccentric movements. Interferences on the nonfunctioning side will often cause a click as the patient functions in the functioning ranges of articulation. The click is produced in a manner similar to that which has been explained previously, by the incoordinate functioning of the parts of the joint.

Possible Etiology. It is the author's theory that the etiology of most of the clicking in the joint is caused by muscular incoordination which in turn is caused by pathologic occlusion. In the author's experience, this is verified by the disappearance of clicking in many cases after occlusal equilibration.

In Class V cases, restoration of the occlusal level is also necessary. If the temporomandibular joint arthrosis has been present over a long period, degenerative changes will have occurred within the meniscus owing to the strains of improper function. The cartilage and the meniscus may have been loosened from their attachment, roughened, atrophied, absorbed or may have undergone degeneration and destruction. Articular cartilage has poor regenerative power, and it is also recognized that slight trauma to the articular cartilage may produce damage and chronic degenerative changes which gradually increase in severity with function.[37]

Crepitation and Rubbing. The causes of crepitation and rubbing are articular surface injuries to the cartilage of the fossa, the condyle and the meniscus. The injuries are caused by the repeated microtrauma of the condyles. The uncoordinated muscular action of the condyle and the meniscus causes the grating and rubbing sounds during mandibular movements.

According to Bauer,[14] lesions occur in the cartilage of the condyle, the cartilage of the glenoid fossa and in the meniscus in that order. In time, as the trauma to the joint continues, the stretching of the capsule will irritate the nerve endings within the capsule and cause pain. This is followed by painful movement within the joint, especially during mastication. Gradually, the pain becomes worse and is accompanied by reduction of mobility caused by pain in the joint and muscle spasm induced by the dysfunction of the joint. Pain in the joint may be reported as occurring at a particular position of mouth opening or closing and associated with joint clicks, crepitus, etc. The pain may also be related to a particular function, such as chewing, yawning, swallowing, etc. The character of the pain may be described as lancinating, paroxysmal or dull.

Kellgren[65] found that noxious stimuli to fascia and tendons result in sharp localized pains. As the condition of the joint progresses, the character of the pain becomes steadier and duller, but distribution of the pain changes from a local to a diffuse area about the temporomandibular joint as muscle spasm develops. The patient may report varying periods of remission of the pain symptoms.

Hypermobility of the structures of the temporomandibular joint can be brought about by intrinsic trauma within the joint. The result of this intrinsic trauma is a stretching and tearing of the tissues that maintain the relationship of the parts of the joint to each other. The convenience relationship of the mandible causes a stretching of the capsule and the other related mandibular ligaments whose function it is to maintain physiological limitation of condylar excursions. The attachments of the meniscus and the soft tissues of the bilaminar zone also undergo stretching and strain. It is usually these structures that offer most resistance to excessive condylar movement. The important point is that the limiting structures have undergone changes. Pain may or may not accompany the hypermobile movements of the joint structure.

Endotracheal Intubation. Unfortunately, endotracheal intubation may serve as an antecedent to temporomandibular joint dysfunction. When a patient presents with pain and crepitation in the temporomandibular joints, he should be questioned as to the possibility of having had surgery involving endotracheal intubation—this may well be a clue to the source of the problem. When a patient is prepared for intubation, the mouth is first opened halfway by the hinge action of the temporomandibular joints. In order for the mouth to be opened wide enough to allow for positioning of the airway, the condyles must be positioned anterior to the articular eminences. This procedure is generally easily accomplished with the use of succinylcholine, a muscle relaxant. However, even in apparently normal persons, there may be damage (clicking, crepitation, etc.) to the meniscus and to the muscles and ligaments supporting the temporomandibular joints as a result of surgery involving intubation. Succinylcholine renders endotracheal intubation a relatively simple process, but joint damage due to unskilled management is not readily corrected.

Trends and Patterns of Temporomandibular Joint Arthrosis

Other investigators[10,39] in the field of temporomandibular joint arthrosis have observed definite trends and patterns. Foged, for instance, found the following pathological changes during operations on patients suffering from temporomandibular joint arthrosis:

1. In many cases the meniscus showed evidence of altered mobility either in abnormal looseness or, more often, in too firm fixation to the capitulum by fibrous adhesions.
2. Sometimes the lower joint cavity was more or less obliterated.
3. The articular cartilage showed macroscopic and microscopic signs of degeneration, sometimes with deformity of the capitulum.

Foged investigated 94 patients with 138 instances of the disease. He found that 18 per cent of the total were men, and 82 per cent were women. In 73 per cent of the cases, the symptoms were unilateral. Sixty per cent of the patients were between 10 and 30 years of age. The duration of the disease was 2 to 14 years before admission to the clinic. Pain was present in 82 per cent, reduction of mobility in 63 per cent, difficulty in mastication in 84 per cent and noises in the joint in 82 per cent of the cases.

Staplemohr's[107] report on 69 cases involving temporomandibular joint surgery showed that in every case the disc and its attachments were found to be altered. Sixty-seven per cent of the cases were women, 70 per cent had unilateral involvement, while 30 per cent had bilateral symptoms. In 91 per cent of the cases, the symptoms appeared before the age of 30. Staplemohr divided his cases into three groups. Group I clicked in one joint; Group II clicked in at least one joint, and mandibular movements were difficult; Group III clicked in the temporomandibular joints and also suffered from intermittent locking at the joints. Twenty per cent of the patients reported that the symptoms occurred after hard mastication, yawns, convulsive laughter and external trauma. Fifty-two per cent of the cases reported that the symptoms were spontaneous. Only 6 per cent of the cases were due to systemic diseases, such as mental debility, Parkinson's disease, arthritis deformans, influenza and others.

Boman[20] investigated 1,350 persons to determine what percentage had temporomandibular joint disorders. He found that the earliest that symptoms usually appeared was between the ages of 15 and 20, that most cases showed first symptoms before the age of 40 and that symptoms rarely appeared after the age of 50. He found that 1,007 (75%) of the cases he studied were free of symptoms and that 343 (25%) had symptoms of crackling, pain, etc.

Hankey,[50] in a survey of 150 cases of temporomandibular joint arthrosis, found that one-third developed symptoms between the ages of 20 and 30, during the years when the natural teeth were present. It is revealing to find that roughly 70 per cent involve females. In 63 per cent of the cases the onset was gradual. In fact, in many cases the onset was so insidious that the patient was unaware of the symptoms until they actually became disablingly painful.

Moyers[80] found that in 150 cases of temporomandibular joint disturbance, approximately 40 per cent had a history of previous orthodontic therapy. Brussell[25] pointed out that symptoms involving the temporomandibular joint are not uncommon.

His examination of 76 unselected persons comprising members of the 1938 senior dental class of the University of Minnesota revealed that 63 per cent of those examined had two or more clinical progressive symptoms involving the joint. In a more recent study and analysis of the data on 83 members of the 1947 dental class, the same investigator found that 57 per cent had two or more clinical symptoms involving the joint. When he examined 50 children between the ages of 10 and 14 with malocclusion necessitating orthodontia, Brussell found that 18 (36%) had at least two symptoms involving the temporomandibular joint. These were characterized by crepitus and luxation in one or both joints with the beginning of jerky movements of the mandible on opening wide. In the former report Brussell points out that in the typical patient with temporomandibular disability, more pronounced and advanced stages of malocclusion, muscular imbalance and resultant degenerative and alterative changes are apparent.

Lindblom's[72] classic report of 58 cases of temporomandibular joint arthrosis showed that when dental causes have been established by functional analysis and temporomandibular joint roentgenograms, and corrected, the arthrosis will disappear.

In an examination of 2,218 new college students at the Helsinki colleges, who averaged 21 years of age, Rantanen[94] found that 30 per cent of women and 18 per cent of men had symptoms of temporomandibular joint dysfunction. Clicking occurred in 15 per cent of the group.

Temporomandibular joint dysfunction produces, in varying degrees, compression, stretching, tearing and degeneration of the joint tissues which are among the least regenerative in the human body. Tissue changes within the joint are rarely revealed except by surgery.

Norgaard,[89] using his arthrographic technique, roentgenographed a large number of patients who complained of temporomandibular joint symptoms. He injected Per-Abrodil first into the lower joint cavity and then into the upper joint cavity, making it possible to visualize these changes and their relations to the meniscus, the glenoid fossa and the condyle. Displacement of the fluid by movements of the condyle revealed further information concerning the joint. Thus, it was possible to detect a perforated meniscus, adhesions between the various structures within the joint, obliteration of portions of the joint cavities and other pathological conditions.

Pathologic occlusion may exist without causing subjective symptoms. Injuries to the structures of the joint owing to pathologic occlusion can heal through changes within the occlusion and still not evidence any subjective temporomandibular joint symptoms. Therefore the temporomandibular joint must be possessed of great adaptability and tolerance. The determining factor is the resistance of the patient. It is at the stage when symptoms are first reported that the greatest degree of success can be achieved with proper therapy. If not corrected at this stage, serious conditions may develop. Temporomandibular joint arthrosis due to pathologic occlusion is a chronic disease that is reversible if the cause is corrected in time. The equilibration of the occlusion is the treatment which removes the causes—interfering contact, mandibular malposition and pathologic occlusion. Temporomandibular joint arthrosis can be prevented by maintaining the dentition in normal function.

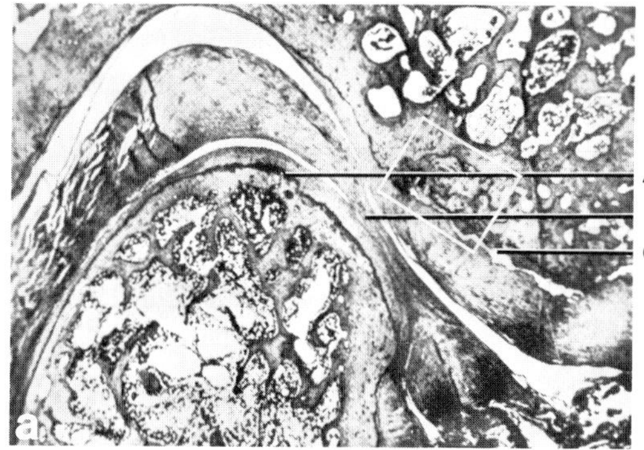

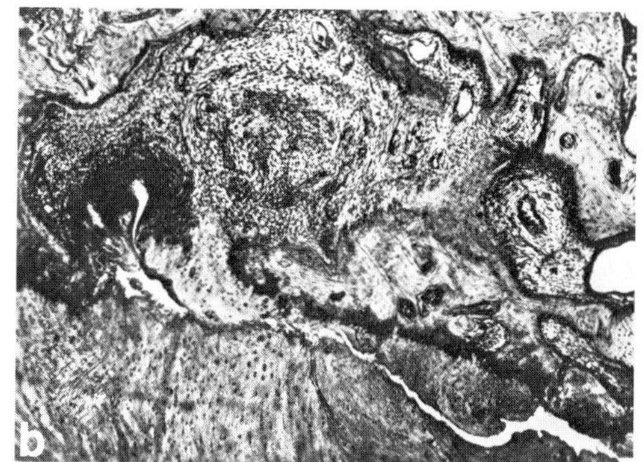

FIG. 9-15. Temporomandibular joint of a man 43 years of age with considerable overbite. On the condyle the cartilage is torn with exposure of the subchondral bone at A (*a*). The intermediate zone of the meniscus at B is rather thin. The cartilage at C, on the articular eminence, is torn, and vascularization of the subchondral bone and marrow can be seen. A microscopic section (*b*) of the inset (in *a*) is evidence of vascularization of the subchondral bone. (Steinhardt, G.: Kiefergelenkerkrankungen, Die Zahn-, Mund- und Kieferheilkunde. vol. 3, Berlin, Urban, 1957)

Temporomandibular Joint Arthrosis Deformans

When temporomandibular joint arthrosis evidences extreme change in the structure of the joint or joints, the disease is known as temporomandibular joint arthrosis deformans. The symptoms of arthrosis deformans are basically the same as those of temporomandibular joint arthrosis; however, the former are extremely severe. According to Steinhardt and Langen,[112] one can distinguish between physiological deformation of the joint (normal aging process of joints) and pathological deformation of the joint. Changes within the joint that are symptomless are part of the normal aging process, as opposed to temporomandibular joint arthrosis and arthrosis deformans as diseases.

The macroscopic and microscopic histopathology of temporomandibular joint arthrosis deformans consists of changes in the structures of the joint.[5,11,14,26,59,64,92,104,110,111,116] The changes that take place within the glenoid fossa and the articular eminence are:

1. Flattening and widening of the fossa floor (Fig. 9-15)
2. Change of the slope of the posterior wall of the articular eminence from a greater to a lesser angulation.

The bone which was formerly in the shape of a sine curve becomes flattened. This is illustrated in Figure 9-16 and actually in temporomandibular joint sections in Figures 9-17, 9-18, and 9-19. The flattening of the posterior wall of the articular eminence may vary from partial to total destruction of the eminence.

3. Roughening and exostosis of the articular eminence are characteristic (Figs. 9-17 and 9-18).
4. Eburnation of the articular surface appears as a sclerotic subchondral marginal zone (Figs. 9-15 and 9-18).
5. Destruction or tears of the articular cartilage expose the subchondral bone marrow spaces (Fig. 9-20).
6. Hyalinization and calcification develop (Figs. 9-15 and 9-19).

The changes that take place within the meniscus are those of position and structure. The changes in position consist of displacement of the meniscus anteriorly, posteriorly, medially, laterally or in any combination of these positions. In Figures 9-15 and 9-19, the meniscus is displaced anteriorly. The structure of the meniscus evidences external and internal changes.

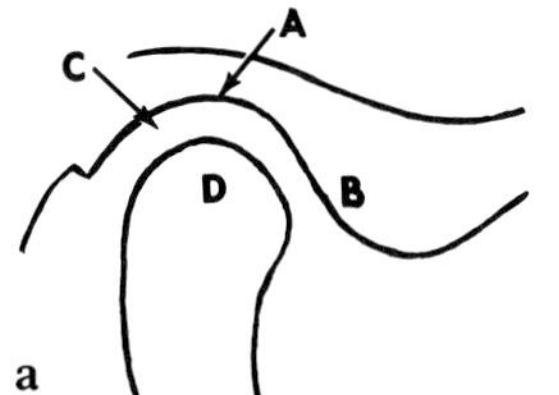

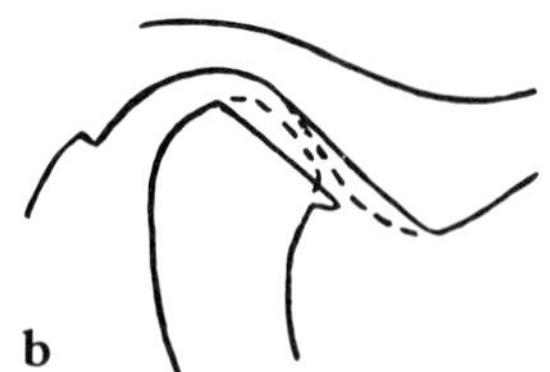

FIG. 9-16. Diagram (*a*) of the normal contours of the glenoid fossa, A, the posterior wall of the articular eminence, B, the joint gap, C, and the condyle, D. The arthrotic gliding joint (*b*). The dotted lines represent the former contours of the posterior wall of the articular eminence and superior surface of the condyle, indicating that the condyle has shifted into a superior-anterior position within the fossa. The glenoid fossa and the posterior wall of the articular eminence are flattened and widened. The joint gap is narrow superiorly and anteriorly and wide posteriorly due to condylar displacement. The anterosuperior surface of the condyle is flattened, and marginal lip formation is present. (After Steinhardt, G.: Zur arthopathia deformans des kiefergelenkes [Arthritic deformans of the temporomandibular joint]. Ztschr. Laryng. Rhin. Otol., *30:*475)

External changes

1. Tearing or stretching of the ligaments and the soft tissues which hold the meniscus in position

2. Extreme wear of the meniscus which includes hollowing, perforation, shredding, tearing and rupture (Figs. 9-15, 9-18, 9-19 and 9-21).

Internal changes

3. Calcific deposits

4. Degeneration of the cartilage[16] (Figs. 9-20 and 9-21).

The changes that occur in the condyle are:

1. Pronounced flattening on the anterosuperior surface (Figs. 9-15 and 9-19).

2. Exostosis, surface erosion and roughening of the articular surface (Figs. 9-18, 9-19 and 9-21).

3. Marginal lip formation and forma-

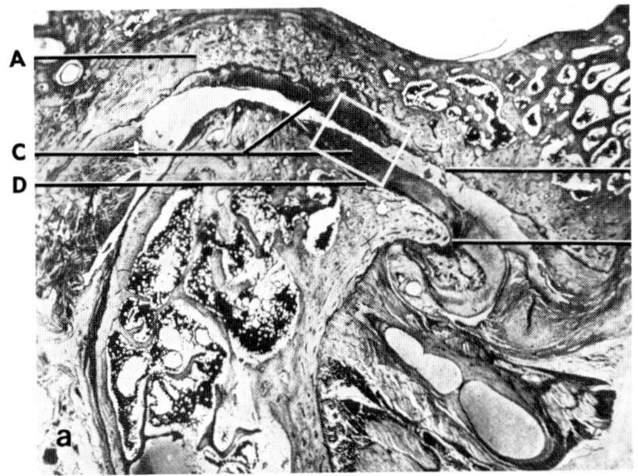

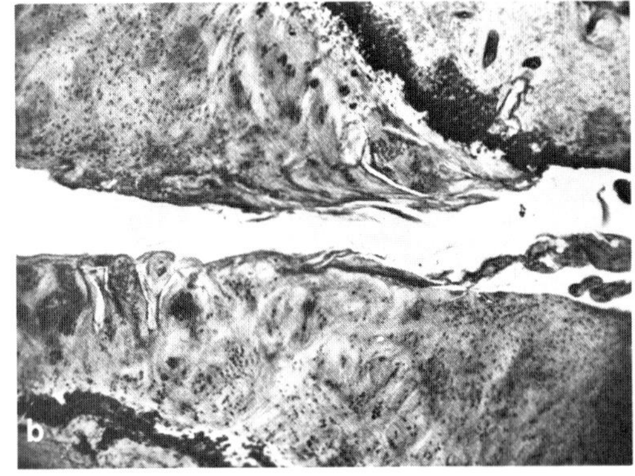

FIG. 9-17. Temporomandibular joint (*a*) of an edentulous woman aged 68. The glenoid fossa is filled in with new bone at A. The posterior wall of the articular eminence is flattened at B. Cartilage formation is present at C. The flattening and the concave structure of the superior surface of the condyle are evident at D, and lipping is present at E. The meniscus has been ruptured and is displaced anteriorly. In this microscopic section (*b*) of the inset in the view to the left, there is evidence of the irregular articular cartilage formation in the glenoid fossa and on the articular surface of the condyle. The meniscus is absent. (Steinhardt, G.: Kiefergelenkerkrankungen. Die Zahn-, Mund- und Kieferheilkunde. vol. 3, Berlin, Urban, 1957)

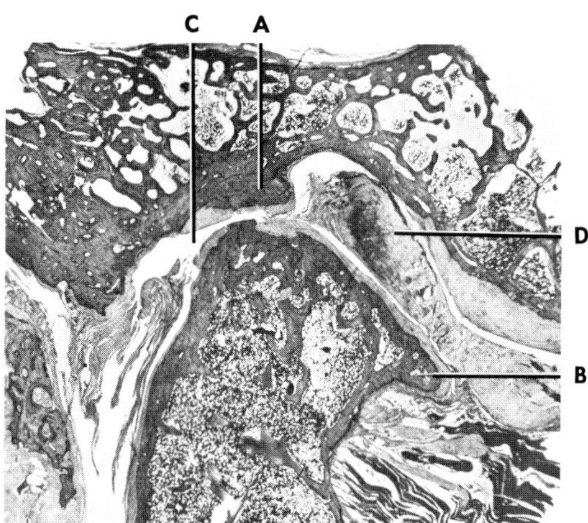

FIG. 9-18. Temporomandibular joint of an edentulous woman 81 years of age. Exostosis of the glenoid fossa is present at A, and of the condyle at B. The meniscus is torn at C and displaced anteriorly to D. Note the flat plane of the posterior wall of the articular eminence and the superior surface of the condyle to form flat arthrotic gliding surfaces. (Steinhardt, G.: Kiefergelenkerkrankungen, Die Zahn-, Mund- und Kieferheilkunde. vol. 3, Berlin, Urban, 1957)

tion of sharp anterior portions of the condyle (Figs. 9-15, 9-17 and 9-18).

4. Eburnation of the articular surface appearing as a sclerotic subchondral marginal zone (Fig. 9-18).

5. Destruction or tears of the articular cartilage, exposing the subchondral bone marrow spaces (Figs. 9-17, 9-20 and 9-21).

6. Hyalinization and calcification (Figs. 9-15, 9-19 and 9-21).

The widening and flattening of the fossa, in cases of arthrosis deformans, indicate changes due to mechanical destruction of the meniscus, articular cartilage and subchondral bone. Because of the changes of the interposed meniscus, the superior surface of the condyle rubs and grinds against the floor of the fossa and the posterior wall of the articular eminence. The tendency of the joint is to form arthrotic gliding surfaces with flattening of the posterior wall of the articular eminence and the superior surface of the condyle. This is illustrated best in Figures 9-15, 9-18 and 9-19. It should be observed that lesions occur at the periphery of the cartilage because that is the at-

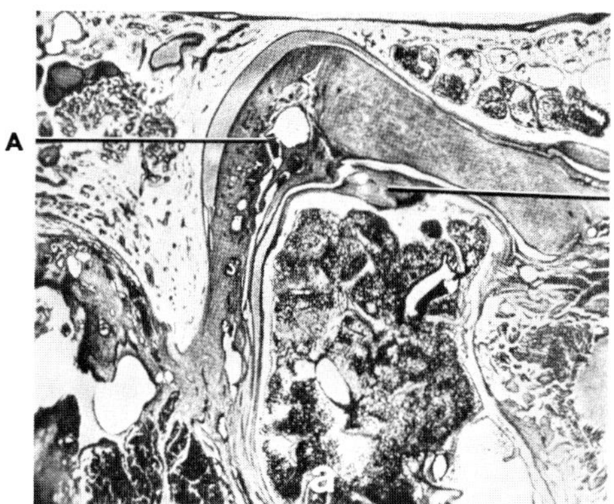

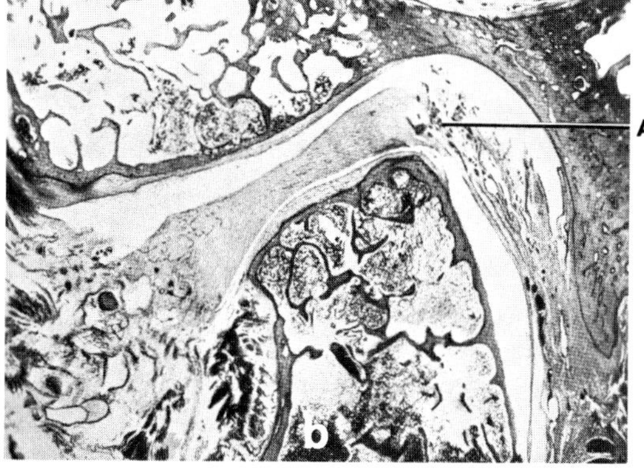

FIG. 9-19. Left and right temporomandibular joints of a man 64 years of age. Due to extreme lateral movements of the mandible there are cellular changes in the soft tissue posterior to the meniscus at A. The excessive lateral movements of the condyles caused a shifting of the cartilage from the posterior edge of the condyle to the middle of the condyle head at B. Both condyle heads are irregular in shape. (Steinhardt, G.: Kiefergelenkerkrankungen, Die Zahn-, Mund- und Kieferheilkunde. vol. 3, Berlin, Urban, 1957)

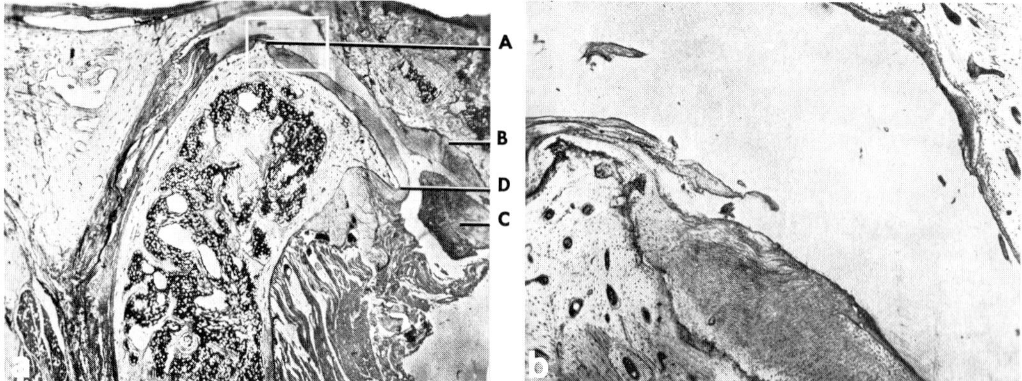

FIG. 9-20. Temporomandibular joint of an edentulous woman 63 years of age. An exostosis at A, and change of the condylar convex surface at B to a concave surface (*a*). The ruptured meniscus can be seen at C. Marginal lipping of the condyle is present at D. Flattening of the articular planes of the condyle and the posterior wall of the articular eminence can be observed. In this microscopic section (*b*) of the inset (in *a*), there is evidence of the exostosis, A, the concave surface, B, and the absence of the meniscus. (Steinhardt, G.: Kiefergelenkerkrankungen. Die Zahn-, Mund- und Kieferheilkunde. vol. 3, Berlin, Urban, 1957)

tachment area of the capsule. When the elasticity of the cartilage has been destroyed, the protection for the subchondral bone is lost, and deformation of the condyle takes place with marginal enlargements and exostoses. Exostoses may damage and sometimes destroy the meniscus.

Roentgenographically, arthrosis deformans evidences the following: (a) haziness and clouding of the outline of the bone; (b) flattening and irregularity of the articular surfaces; (c) possible irregular appearance of the joint gap and variation from a wide space to complete obliteration; (d) hypertrophic changes of the

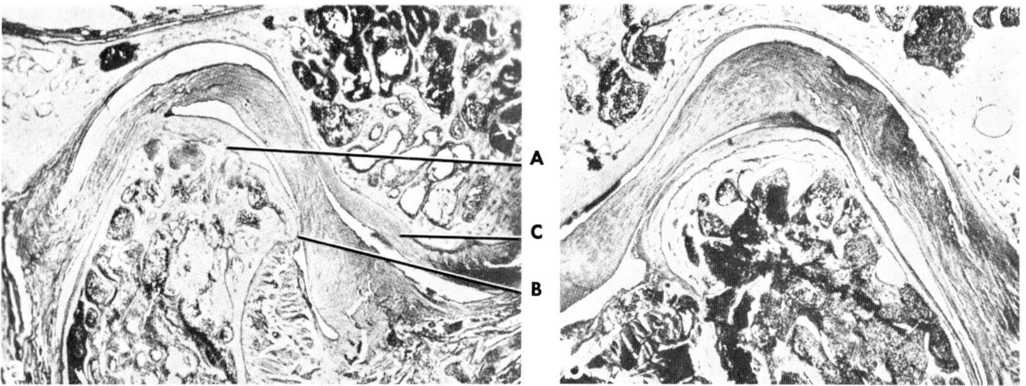

FIG. 9-21. Left and right temporomandibular joints of a man 76 years of age with considerable overbite. Torn cartilage and exposure of the subchondral bone and marrow spaces are seen at A, and the beginning of marginal lip formation on the condyle is seen at B. The convex surface of the posterior wall of the articular eminence at C has changed to a concave eroded area. This is the beginning of the flattening of the posterior wall. (Steinhardt, G.: Kiefergelenkerkrankungen, Die Zahn-, Mund- und Kieferheilkunde. vol. 3, Berlin, Urban, 1957)

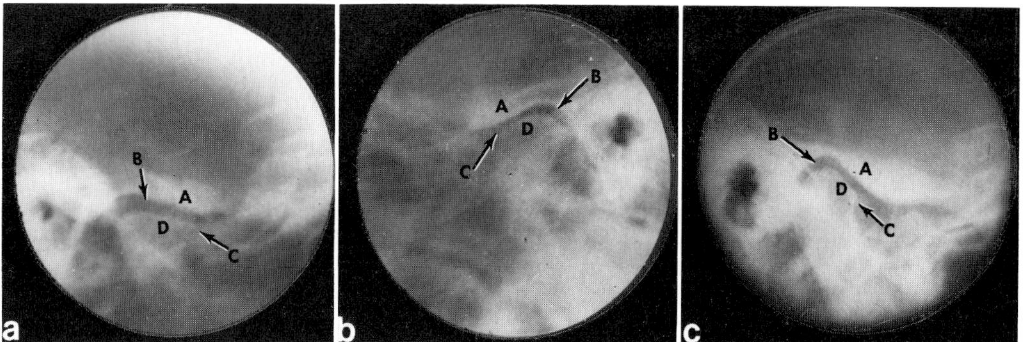

FIG. 9-22. Roentgenographic appearance of temporomandibular joint arthrosis deformans.

marginal bone (exostoses, marginal lipping, etc.); (e) increased or decreased density of the subchondral bone; and (f) variations in density of the trabeculated bone.[137]

Figure 9-22 is an example of temporomandibular joint arthrosis deformans. The floor of the glenoid fossa is irregular (*a*), the sine curve has been reduced to a flat arthrotic gliding surface with complete destruction of the eminence at A. The bone of the glenoid fossa appears almost solid (disappearance of trabeculated layer of bone). The joint gap, B, is wide posteriorly and superiorly and is narrower anteriorly. The condyle at C is eroded, flattened, lipped anteriorly and not very dense. The floor of the glenoid fossa is regular (*b*), but the posterior wall and crest of the articular eminence at A have been flattened and are very dense. Signs of erosion appear near the crest of the eminence. The joint gap is wider superiorly and posteriorly and is very narrow anteriorly. The condyle is irregular anteriorly with lip formation present at the anterior margin. The condyle does not appear to be dense. The floor of the glenoid fossa is fairly regular (*c*), but the posterior wall of the articular eminence A is flattened. The joint gap, B, is fairly normal. The beginning of marginal lipping is seen at C, on the condyle, which is flattened anteriorly at D.

Neuromuscular (Motor) Manifestations of Pathologic Occlusion

The direct effect of pathologic occlusion on various structures of the stomatognathic system have been described previously. In this section other motor effects of pathologic occlusion will be considered. Pathologic occlusion causes neuromuscular dysfunction by initiating pathological position and function of the mandible, the two temporomandibular joints and the muscles of the stomatognathic system. The manifestations of a disturbed neuromusculature are limited mandibular movement or excessive mandibular movement accompanied by crepitation, clicking, muscle spasm, tenderness and pain. The character and the range of the symptoms vary with each patient.

Muscle Spasm

A cause of dysfunction, tenderness and pain within the temporomandibular joint may be muscle spasm. A concomitant characteristic is almost always restricted mandibular movement. Muscle spasm is a reversible state of shortening which is no longer under voluntary control but usually is associated with neural reflex action. Owing to protective splinting, muscles that are affected can cause other

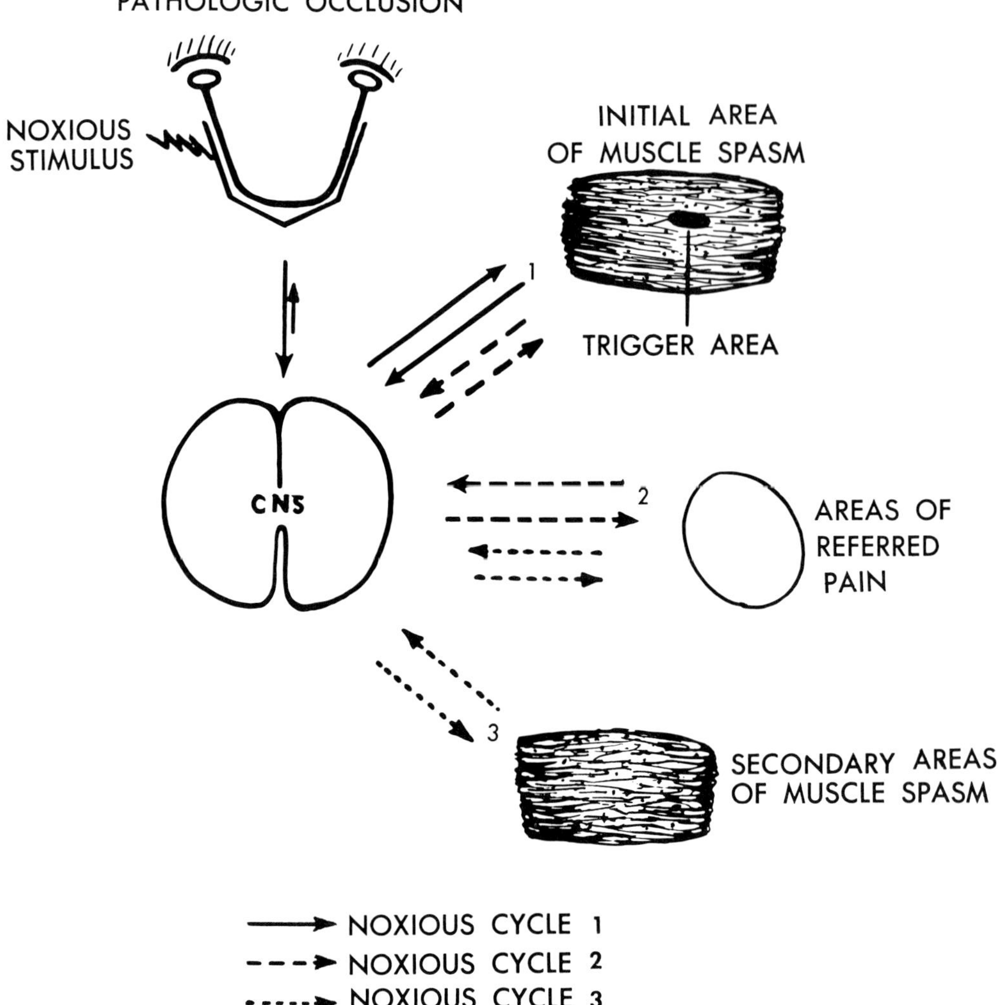

FIG. 9-23. The direct neural relationship between pathologic occlusion, as the noxious stimulus, and the resulting feedback cycles of muscle spasm, trigger areas, and referred pain, distant from the primary noxious stimulus.

muscles or other sections in the same muscle to go into spasm. In this manner, the effect and the area of the spasm are greatly increased. In the acute stage muscle spasm appears to be a neurophysiological disorder, but with the passage of time the spasm becomes chronic, and the tissues undergo organic changes. The cycle—muscle spasm, pain, spasm—can be initiated by pathologic occlusion which creates neuromuscular dysfunction.

When a patient closes in centric relation and strikes an interfering contact, stimulation of the proprioceptors and pain receptors initiates mandibular movement to avoid the interference. The mandible then assumes an unphysiological convenience relationship, and the coordination of the neuromuscular system is thrown out of balance. The condyles, the rami and the body of the mandible are now in an unphysiological position. The muscles, the tendons and the ligaments attached to these parts are also in a convenience

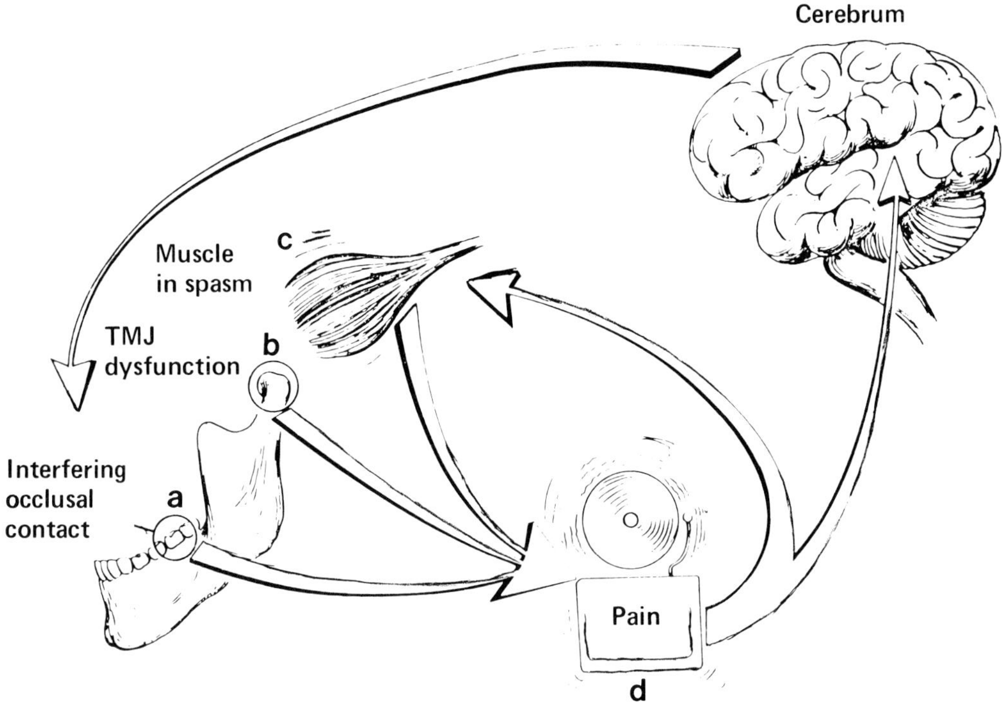

FIG. 9-24. Three different pathways producing pain in the temporomandibular joint and surrounding areas: interfering occlusal contact (*a*); malposition of the condyle and disc in the fossa (*b*), resulting in abnormal function; and spasm of the lateral pterygoid (*c*), caused by improper jaw relation. In every case a reflex arc is established at the spinal cord level while simultaneously a message is sent to the cerebrum. The result in both cases is a message to the muscle to disengage.

relationship. The convenience relationship has taken over the placement of the mandible, and the teeth do not permit the muscles to return the mandible to its centric-relation position. However, the normal reflex control of the muscles is constantly attempting to return the mandible to centric relation. This continuous stimulation causes the muscles to remain in a state of sustained contraction without movement. The effect of this incoordinated neuromuscular activity is dysfunction, pain and muscle spasm (Fig. 9-23). The primary hyperactivity of those muscles that are in convenience mandibular relationships is added to secondarily by the hyperactivity of the musculature that retracts the mandible, and thus the incoordinated function results in primary and secondary muscle spasm.

Duchenne[35] observed that "Muscles surrounding a joint would go into a state of hypertonus when the joint was injured, dislocated, or inflamed and may even go into a state of spasmodic contraction." Another investigator[61] states: "Though muscle spasms can be initiated reflexly within the periodontium of the teeth, they can also come from the sensory stimuli having their origin in the capsule of the joint." The interfering occlusal contact, pathologic occlusion and resulting incoordinated musculature produce primary noxious stimuli that travel to the central nervous system, which in turn produces other areas of muscle spasm (Fig. 9-24).

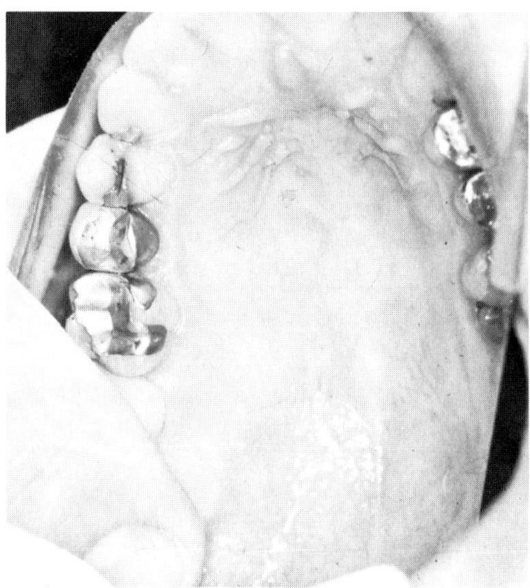

FIG. 9-25. Palpation of the lateral pterygoid for spasm.

The initial area of muscle spasm sends forth its own noxious impulses (cycle 1) which give rise to areas of referred pain, thus setting up a cycle between the muscle spasm area and the area interpreted as referred pain. The initial focus maintains a perpetual feedback cycle, and the referred pain it incited may be felt long after the original stimulus from the occlusion has passed. Noxious stimuli from the structures in the reference zone may also set up a cycle (cycle 2) of spasm in other muscles.[123] The secondary source or stimulus for the muscle-spasm-area, referred-pain pathway may be within the tissues of the joints, the muscles, the fascia, the tendons, etc. A third cycle (cycle 3) is created in secondary areas of muscle spasm.

Within the area of muscle spasm is what Travell and others have called a trigger area.[119] Travell[120] cites the trigger areas as points of exquisite tenderness within the muscle in spasm, from which impulses bombard the central nervous system and give rise to referred pain.

Whatever its origin, pain can cause vasoconstriction and ischemia of muscles and nerves. It is well known that nerves will fire in the presence of ischemia, and that muscles become tender and painful when used under ischemic conditions.[70] Travell[122] says, "A clinically active trigger area is revealed by three things: circumscribed deep hyperalgesia, localized fasciculation, and the capacity to set

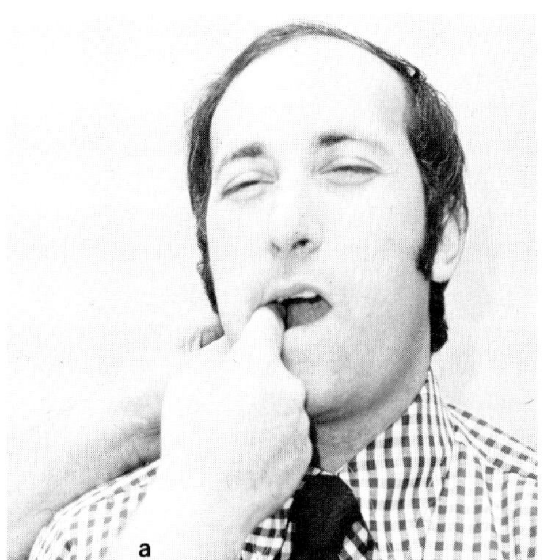

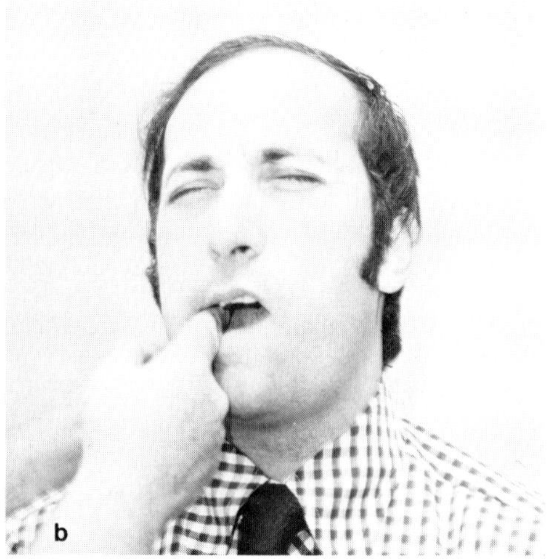

FIG. 9-26. Slight palpation reveals subacute pain in right lateral pterygoid muscle (*a*). Heavier palpation of the same muscle evokes severe pain response, as evidenced by patient's wincing (*b*).

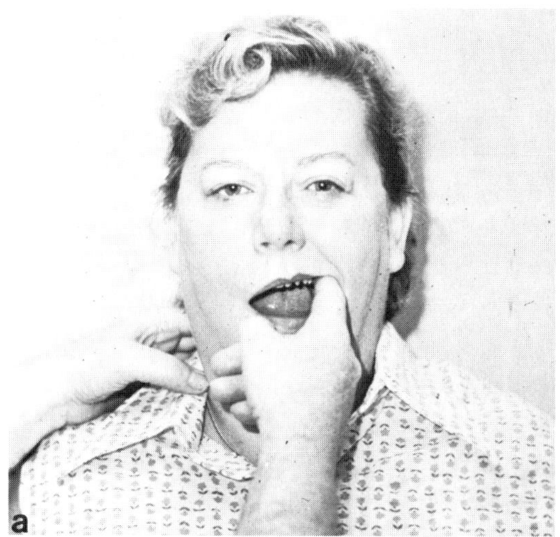

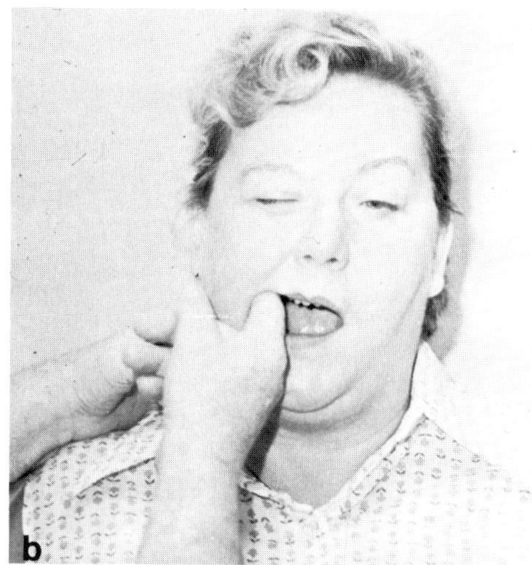

FIG. 9-27. When normal left lateral pterygoid is palpated, there is no pain (*a*). Palpation of patient's right lateral pterygoid evokes response of severe pain (note eyes) (*b*).

off referred pain." The trigger area sets off pain when it is stimulated by: movement that stretches the structure in which the trigger area is located, extreme heat or cold, or pressure.[125] It is the resistance of the muscle to stretching that provokes pain and leads to the protective device of apparent shortening, weakness and limited motion of the affected muscle.

> In the case of trigger areas located in fibrous structures about a joint, pain usually is not referred to any great distance from the trigger area in question. Trigger areas in the muscles are more likely to refer pain to a considerable distance, though not always; sometimes the reference zone [referred pain area] surrounds the trigger area.[123]

Treatment of the trigger area is an important adjunct to treatment of the pathologic occlusion. The need for eliminating the trigger area directly will be elaborated in the section on treatment.

Spasm is produced within the mechanism of the temporomandibular joint and within the muscles of other parts of the head and the neck. Patients with an apparently asymptomatic pathologic occlusion who suffer from temporomandibular joint dysfunction may actually have dormant muscle spasm of a subclinical nature. For example, such spasm and lack of coordination in one external pterygoid muscle will produce mandibular deviation on opening. Palpation will often reveal deep tenderness in the muscle of which the patient was previously unaware (Figs. 9-25, 9-26 and 9-27).

Other patients with an asymptomatic pathologic occlusion and temporomandibular joint dysfunction may present themselves with muscle spasm, tenderness, pain and limited mandibular motion initiated by overstretching of the ligaments and the muscles of the masticatory organ. The initiating mechanisms may be wide yawn, extra large bite, mouth open and under tension during a long operative procedure, or extensive oral surgery, etc.

Emotionally tense people and those with a history of general musculoskeletal spasm are predisposed to spasm of the muscles of the stomatognathic system. Other predisposing causes are nutritional deficiencies, syndromes of the menopause, male climacteric and hypometabolism.[122] The symptomatology of muscle tenderness, pain and spasm varies with the class and the severity of the patho-

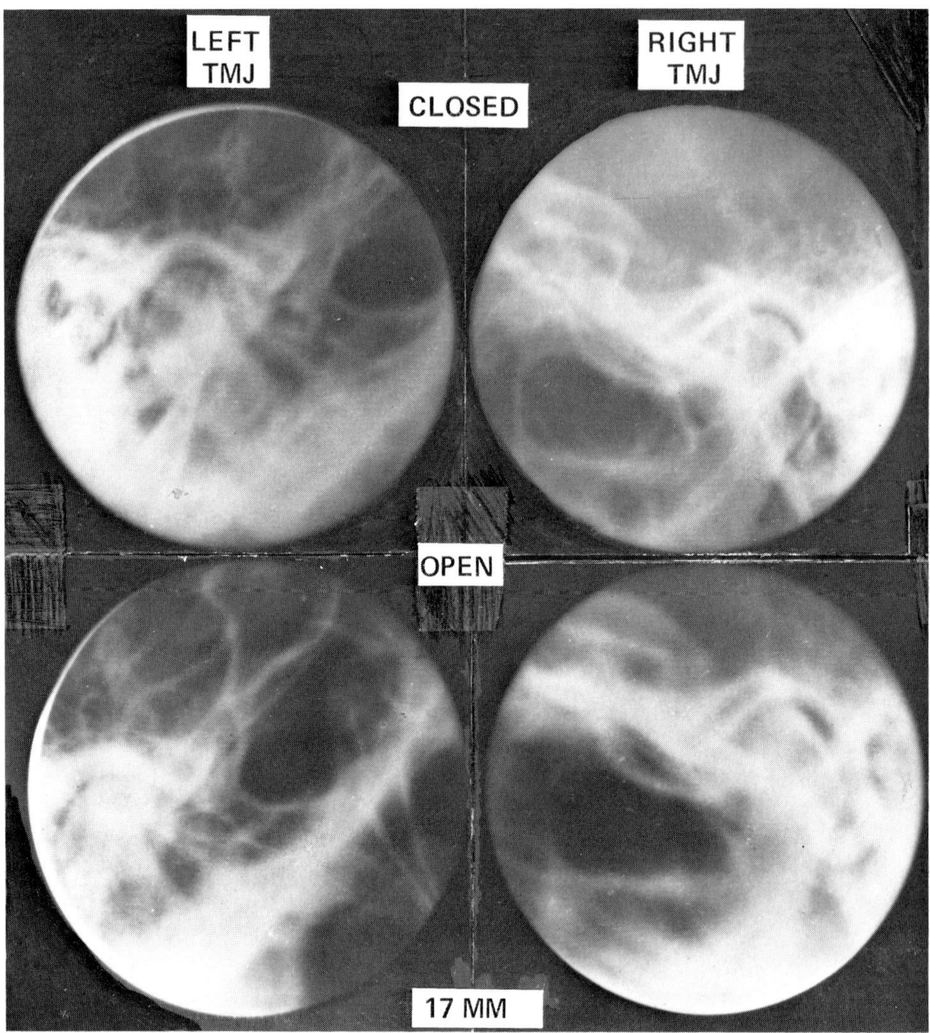

FIG. 9-28. Restricted sagittal-plane mandibular movement illustrating limited rotation and translation of the condyles as seen in the lower circles of the roentgenogram. The interincisal distance is 17 mm. (see Chap. 12).

logic occlusion. The relationship of pathologic occlusion and muscle spasm with their attendant symptoms is extremely complex. Drum[33] and Travell[123] have shown that muscles can be a source of pain. It is only by palpation of the musculature that these conditions are brought to light during the temporomandibular joint examination outlined in Chapter 6.

Associated with symptoms of muscle spasm are limited mandibular movements accompanied by pain. The pain acts as a warning signal and also as a protective mechanism to inform the patient that function should be curtailed. Patients may report that mandibular movements in the morning are "rusty" and difficult to perform, and that it sometimes takes from 15 minutes to an hour before any movement is possible. Such patients clench their teeth nocturnally and so produce spasm of the masticatory musculature.

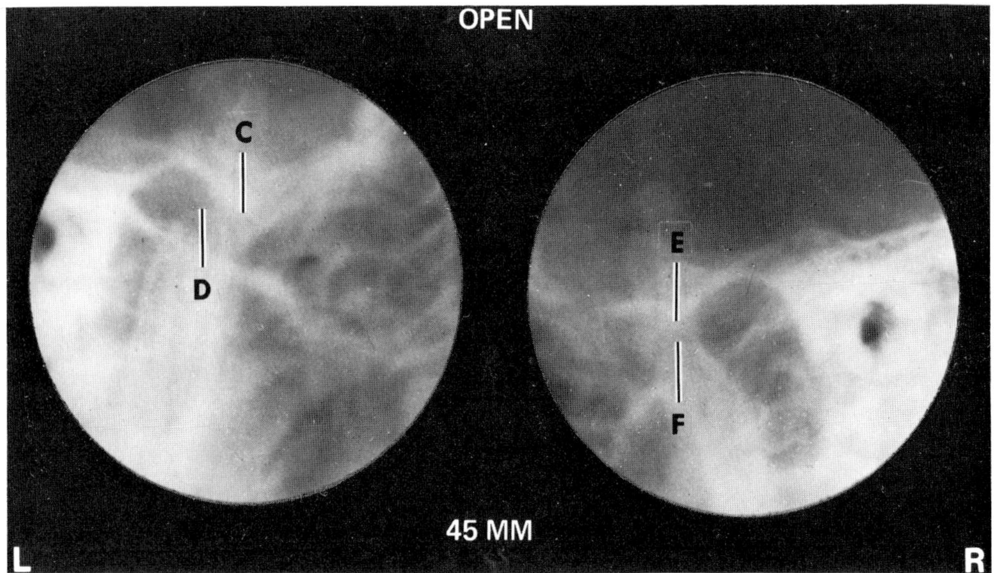

FIG. 9-29. Lateral roentgenograms in the open position, illustrating normal condylar movement in the right joint, E to F, and limited condylar movement in the left joint, C to D.

Restriction of mandibular movement in the sagittal-plane opening movement is of two types. The first type involves dysfunction of both joints with limited ability to open. Both condyles rotate and may translate to a limited degree (Fig. 9-28). The sagittal movement may be anywhere from 5 to 25 mm. and is accompanied by spasm and pain. The second type involves dysfunction within one joint during mandibular movement. One condyle achieves approximately normal position in the full opening movement, E to F, while the other rotates and translates to a limited degree, C to D, thus producing mandibular deviation as well as limited opening (Fig. 9-29).

Abnormal Sagittal Mandibular Movements Excluding Tooth Contact

The discussion of pathological sagittal mandibular movements has concentrated on the mandibular movement from the interfering occlusal contact (E in Fig. 8-5) to the habitual convenience relationship, H. In this section, the movement of the mandible from H to full sagittal opening will be discussed. A conspicuous and characteristic sign of temporomandibular joint dysfunction is deviation of the mandible, usually toward the symptomatic side, when the patient opens the mouth widely. This is the result of asynchronous muscular movement which produces unequal condylar advance.[20]

The distance E to Y in Figure 9-30*a* represents the normal sagittal mandibular plane opening and closing movements. The movement E to H is the cause of neuromuscular imbalance and temporomandibular joint dysfunction; both of

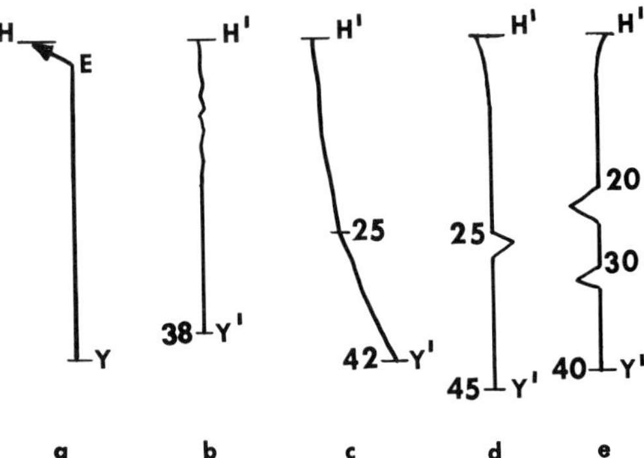

FIG. 9-30. Pathological sagittal-plane opening and closing mandibular movements.

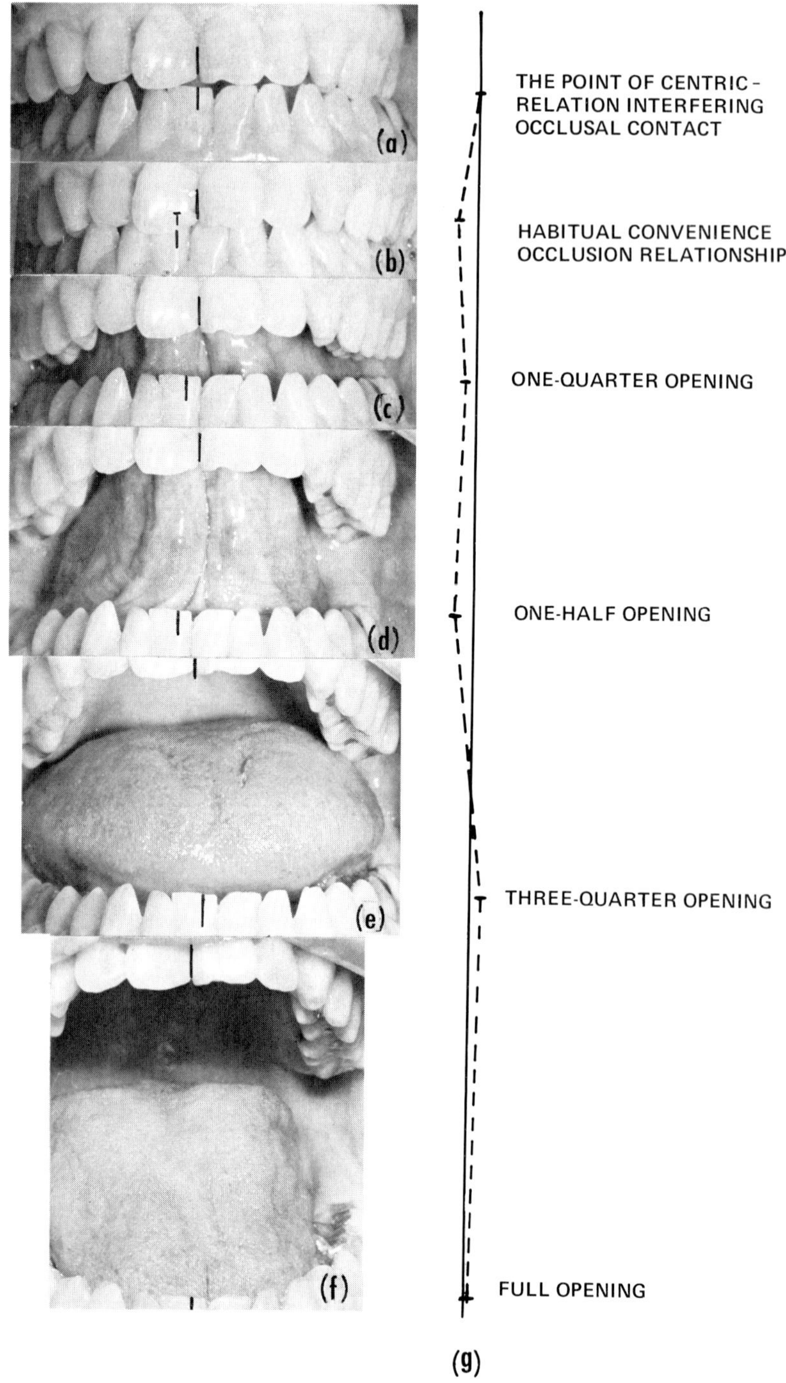

FIG. 9-31. A case of abnormal sagittal mandibular opening, illustrating the centric-relation interfering contact position, the habitual convenience-relationship occlusion and the erratic mandibular behavior approximately at the quarter, the half, the three-quarters and the full opening stages.

these conditions result in muscle spasm. The muscle spasm in turn results in incoordinate muscular movements between the muscle groups on the same side and on the opposite sides of the head. These incoordinate muscle movements result in erratic sagittal opening and closing movements, H′Y′. In (*b*) the mandible opened and closed with a wavy side-to-side motion, but the general trend was a straight line. In (*c*) the general trend of opening was on a curve with a decided change in direction at 25 mm. The patterns of sagittal movement (*d*) and (*e*) were accompanied by clicks at the points of sharp deviation from the general trend of movement.

Figure 9-31 demonstrates a case of abnormal sagittal mandibular movement. In (*a*), the patient is at the first point of interference on the centric-relation arc. The contact point between the upper central incisors and its extension on the lower central incisors is the reference point. The convenience relationship is illustrated in (*b*), in which is seen a 4-mm. mandibular deviation to the right. Figures 9-31*a* and *b* illustrate the shift E to Y in Figure 9-30*a*. It is this habitual mandibular shift in closure that creates neuromuscular dysfunction and its attendant symptoms which result in erratic sagittal mandibular movements. The one-quarter open position (Fig. 9-31*c*) shows a mandibular movement to the left of 2mm. The half-open position (*d*) shows a mandibular movement toward the right of 1½ mm. The three-quarter open position (*e*) shows a mandibular movement to the left of 6 mm. The full-open position (*f*) shows a mandibular movement to the right of 1½ mm. The solid and the dotted lines in (*g*) are the graphic illustrations of the solid reference line of the upper centrals and the dotted-line pattern of mandibular sagittal opening movement in (*a*) through (*f*).

Clicking was present in the right and the left temporomandibular joints and the mandible shifted from one side of the solid reference line to the other. In the full-open position the mandible returns to the solid reference line. It is the erratic mandibular behavior between the habitual convenience-relationship occlusion and the full-open position that reflects the effects of temporomandibular joint dysfunction.

Other causes of sagittal-plane deviations may be disease or external trauma which can be verified readily by roentgenography.

Compensatory Hypermobility of the Temporomandibular Joint

The definition of normal condylar excursion depends upon the comparison of condylar movement in right and left temporomandibular joints. It is fairly common to find both condyle heads ahead of the crest of the articular eminence in the open position. This positional relationship, a subluxation without symptoms, is normal for that patient (Fig. 9-32). However, if one condyle is positioned ahead of the eminence and the other condyle did not advance a similar distance, hypermobility of the advanced condyle can be said to exist. The hypermobile condyle has compensated by means of excessive movement, C to D, for the sluggish movement of the contralateral condyle, E to F (Fig. 9-33).

Referred Neural (Sensory) Manifestations of Pathologic Occlusion

In the previous sections, pain directly within the parts of the stomatognathic system was fully elaborated upon. In this section, the referred neural (sensory) manifestations of pathologic occlusion are traced from the teeth, the muscles and

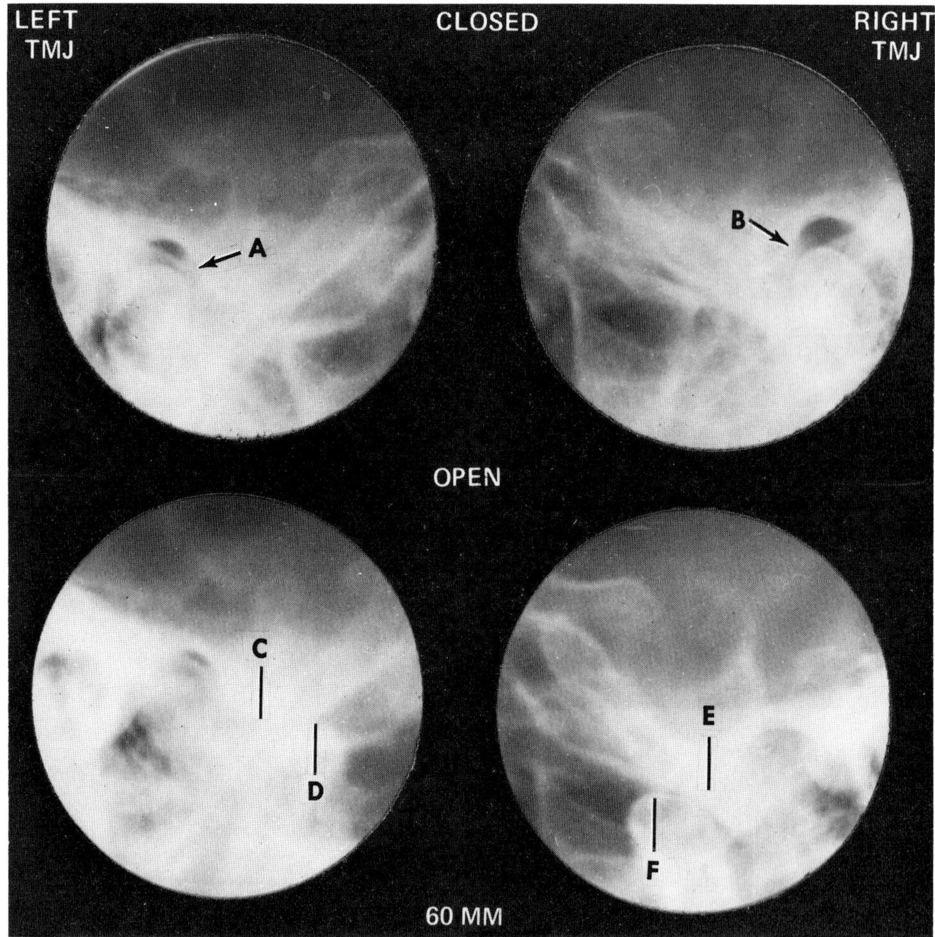

FIG. 9-32. Lateral roentgenograms illustrating normal condylar relationship in the closed position at A and B; and an equal positional relationship of C to D and E to F, subluxation in the open position.

the joint to other areas of the head and the neck where they result in head pains, headaches and other neural manifestations.

Referred Pain from the Teeth

Occlusal trauma can be the noxious stimulant that causes pain; locally, then in the tissue innervated by the nearest division of the 5th cranial nerve and, finally, diffusely throughout the tissue supplied by the other divisions of the 5th nerve. Often the site at which pain is felt is remote from the source of the noxious stimulus.

Figure 9-34 outlines on the face the areas of referred pain caused by noxious stimulation of the teeth. The remote symptoms of noxious stimuli to the teeth are surface hyperalgesia and tenderness to the areas illustrated.

It is generally thought that referred pain caused by noxious stimulation to the teeth is found only about the face. How-

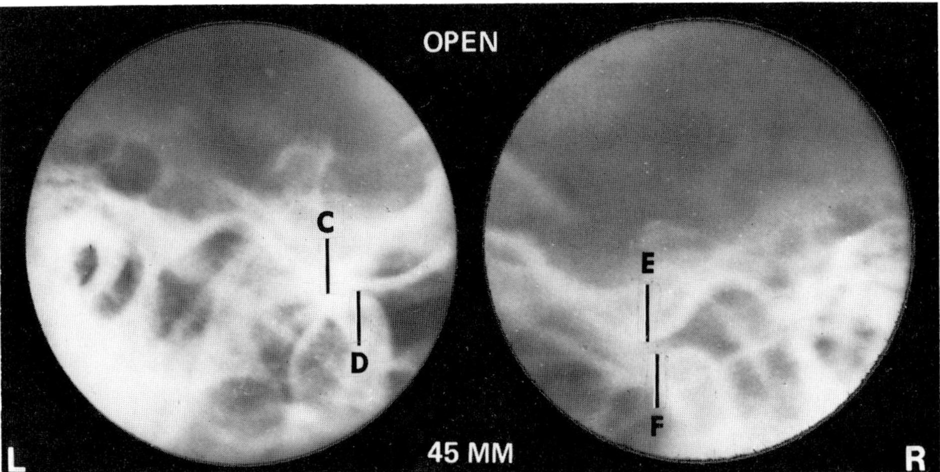

FIG. 9-33. Compensatory hypermobility of the left condyle as evidenced by its position anterior to the crest eminence, D to C, while the right condyle remains at the posterior aspect of the eminence, F to E.

ever, owing to the neural relationship of the first two cervical nerves and portions of the 5th cranial nerve, pain is referred also to areas about the back of the head and the neck. Figures 5-11, and 5-13–15 demonstrate the anatomical relationship of the referred pain areas and their zones of stimulation.

Referred Pain from the Muscles

As Lewis has demonstrated,[71] muscular dysfunction can give rise to referred pain. This author described the pain as disagreeable, diffuse and difficult to locate. It was continuous and wavered slightly in intensity.

The pain reference patterns of muscles can be used to locate the muscle that is the source of pain because these patterns are constant and similar in all people. Figure 9-35 illustrates the pain reference patterns of temporal, masseter and sternocleidomastoid muscles as well as their trigger areas, which are marked by an X. The pain patterns and the trigger areas of the external and the internal pterygoid muscles are difficult to illustrate.

Kellgren[65] reports that fascia and tendon sheaths give rise to sharp, localized pain, whereas muscle pain can be confused with that arising from other structures, such as the joints.

Noxious impulses occurring over long periods are apt to set up secondary trigger areas in the reference zone. These secondary areas are the most recent and therefore are more evident than the primary trigger area. Therefore, the usual procedure is to take care of the most recent trigger area first. Under such circumstances, it is difficult to identify the primary trigger area.

The trigger areas of muscular spasm can produce referred neural manifestations concomitant with the referred pain. Trigger areas can produce the following effects in the zone of reference:[118,121,123,124,126] (a) hyperalgesia; (b) cutaneous hyperesthesia; (c) deep tenderness [(a), (b) and (c) may persist in the zone of reference after the referred pain is gone]; (d) skeletal muscle contraction in the area of reference; (e) vasomotor and other autonomic effects, such as pilomotor stimulation (gooseflesh) and sweating, occurring only in the reference

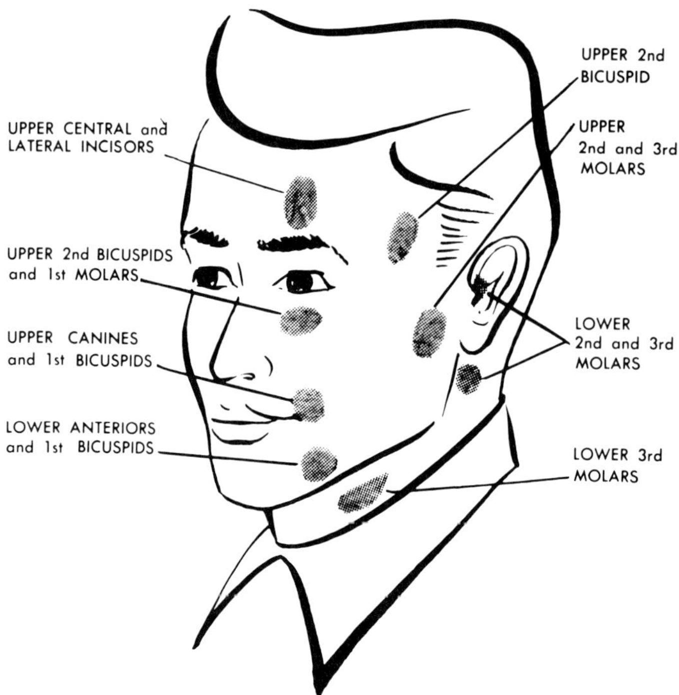

FIG. 9-34. Areas of referred pain on the face related to noxious stimulation of the teeth. (After Head and Shapiro, H. H.)

area. The skin temperature in the reference zone is lowered 1 or 2 degrees during cutaneous pain.[123]

Referred Pain from the Temporomandibular Joint

In any disturbance or functional change within the temporomandibular joint, one may expect referred pains from the joint. The perceived pain is caused by nerve stimulation rather than by nerve impingement as had been assumed. Head and neck pains associated with temporomandibular joint dysfunction are generally considered to be referred. These pains are dull, constant and unrelenting

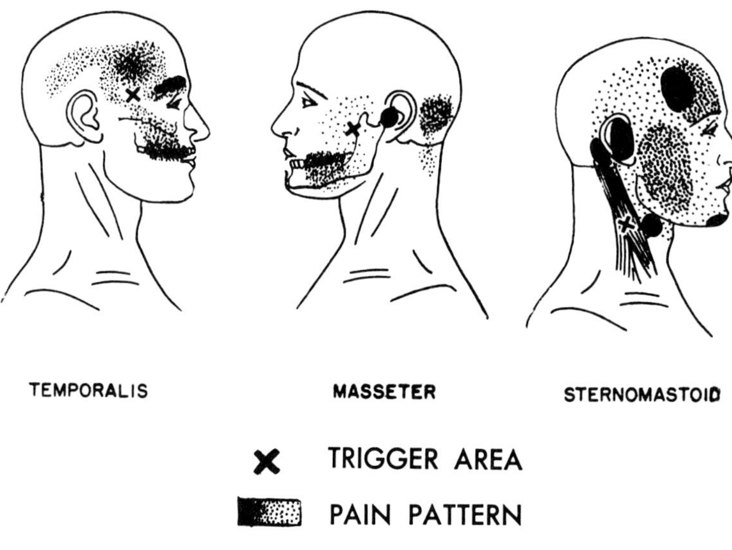

FIG. 9-35. Pain reference patterns associated with specific trigger areas of the muscles. (After Travell. *In* Travell, J., and Rinzler, S. H.: The myofacial genesis of pain. Postgrad. Med., *2*:425, 1952)

and are aggravated by mandibular movement. The pain is not limited to the distribution of the trigeminal nerve; other nerves may be involved. Regardless of the mechanism, direct and referred pain symptoms are associated with temporomandibular joint arthrosis. The pain symptoms are reported in various groups and combinations, depending upon the patient. Patients with temporomandibular joint arthrosis may complain of pain in any of the following areas (Fig. 9-36): frontal, temporal, vertex, occipital, parietal, nuchal, supraorbital, infraorbital, zygomatic, nasal, angle of the mandible, mental, preauricular, ear, postauricular and cervical.

Other areas of pain which are reported but are not illustrated in the diagram are: the soft and the hard palates, the throat, the maxillary and the mandibular teeth, the submaxillary gland region and the maxillary sinus.

All pains other than those at X, the temporomandibular joint, are referred from this area. Temporomandibular joint arthrosis causes superficial referred pain and, at the same time, causes various muscles of the stomatognathic system to go into spasm. The muscles which go into spasm become hyperalgesic and, in turn, cause referred pains which are superimposed upon those referred from the joint and other areas. The areas of referred pain caused by muscle spasm, such as those illustrated in Figure 9-35, may also occur in the throat, the cervical region, the suprahyoid and the infrahyoid regions, other areas of the head, the base of the neck, the shoulder, the arm and the fingers.

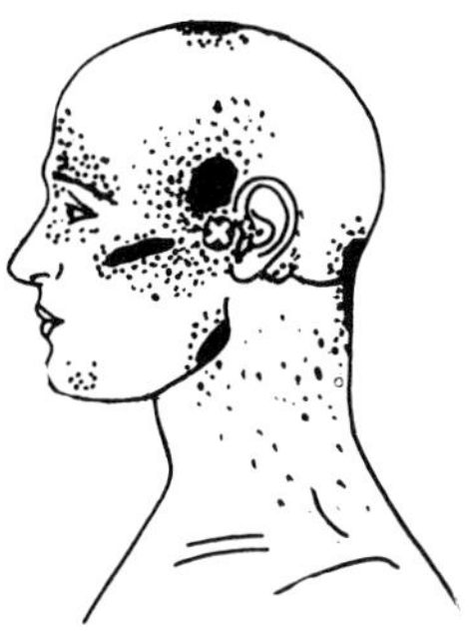

FIG. 9-36. Areas of referred pain from the temporomandibular joint, excluding those of muscle spasm. (After Travell)

Other Referred Neural Manifestations

Other referred neural manifestations that may accompany temporomandibular joint arthrosis must be considered in the light of their neural pathways. Many of these manifestations appear with the Class V reduced vertical relationships. Neural manifestations in the ear, such as tinnitus, buzzing and whooshing noises, stuffiness and blockage, may have their source in vascular dystrophy, as demonstrated by the work of Thonner.[115] His anatomical investigation demonstrates a hitherto unreported vascular connection from the internal maxillary artery to the inner ear.

Others[17,18,19,44,51,52] have claimed similar symptoms for temporomandibular joint arthrosis. Ronkin[99] and others[53,78,136] have claimed improvement of low-tone deafness through mandibular repositioning.

Excessive formation of earwax often accompanies temporomandibular joint dysfunction. This is not surprising if one keeps in mind the close relationship, from both an evolutionary (see Chap. 1) and an anatomical standpoint, of the temporomandibular joint and the ear. The skin of the external auditory canal is lined with tiny hairs and sebaceous glands. The deeper portion of the dermis contains the ceruminous glands, the relatively large lumina of which store the whitish secretion until some stimulus causes its release to the epidermis. Earwax is formed from a mixture of the secretions of the sebaceous and ceruminous glands. The ceruminous glands may be stimulated by both emotional and mechanical causes.[8] Thus, both the pain and anxiety, as well as the impairment of masticatory function resulting from temporomandibular joint dysfunction, can easily trigger increased formation of wax in the ear.

Increased salivation also may be a symptom of temporomandibular joint arthrosis, though a small percentage of patients have reported decreased salivation. The neural relationship between the auriculotemporal nerve and the otic ganglion, with its postganglionic fibers to the parotid gland, makes these effects possible.[102] The anatomical relationship between the auriculotemporal nerve, the otic ganglion, the sensory portion of the facial nerve which supplies the capsule, and the chorda tympani could influence the secretion of the submaxillary and the sublingual glands. Noxious impulses along the sensory portion of the facial and the auriculotemporal nerves from the joint, if strong enough, could stimulate the chorda tympani and affect the flow of saliva from these glands. This same neural relationship could be the basis for the aberrations of taste because of the relationship of the chorda tympani, which mediates taste. The lingual nerve, as part of the trigeminal, and in close anatomical relationship with the chorda tympani, can serve as the route for referred pain to the tongue.

Costen[32] and others[40] have reported glossodynia and taste aberrations as reflex manifestations of Class V pathological mandibular relationships. The author has also seen many patients who manifest a reduced vertical relationship and have metallic taste aberrations. Those patients with glossodynia seem to be beyond 50 years of age, mainly women and have a high incidence of other psychoneurotic symptoms.

The neural manifestation of vertigo is based upon Wolff's[131] reasoning that:

> Vertigo as an accompaniment of head pain . . . probably does not stem from derangements within the semicircular canals. To explain such vertigo it is unnecessary to assume damage to the eighth cranial nerve or brain stem, or fundamental derangements in brain stem circulation. It is probable that noxious impulses arising within the muscles and their attachments cause a widespread excitation of the brain stem near the vestibular nuclei and thus produce the vertigo.

Although its exact mechanism is unknown, a disturbance of the patient's sense of equilibrium ranks among the most serious consequences of temporomandibular joint dysfunction. As Groves states,

> Maintenance of equilibrium depends upon coordinated interaction of many senses. Sight, touch, and proprioception are all of high importance, but the vestibular apparatus is perhaps the most vital. Its normal function is so unobtrusive that it might be termed a "sixth sense," and yet its derangement is so dramatic and incapacitating an event that activities essential to life may become impossible.[49]

DIFFERENTIAL DIAGNOSIS OF TEMPOROMANDIBULAR JOINT DISEASES

Differential diagnosis involves consideration of the many conditions that cause symptoms simulating those of temporomandibular joint arthrosis. The questionnaire that is presented in Chapter 6 will enable the dentist to elicit and record the history and the symptoms on which the diagnosis may be based. The questionnaire will make it possible to classify the symptoms and to differentiate among the various disease entities that simulate temporomandibular joint arthrosis. Only after every organic cause for pain has been eliminated should a diagnosis of psychogenic pain be made. Our knowledge of pain and its mechanism is limited. Care must be observed in avoiding a diagnosis of psychogenic pain simply because the origin of the pain cannot be determined by present diagnostic procedures. Neurotic patients have a lower pain threshold than normal patients. This psychogenic overlay must be understood and taken into account; then the organic basis for the original disturbance may become evident.

Dental Disease and Minor Neuralgias

Dental infections, such as acute pericoronitis, impacted molars and pericementitis, may cause symptoms which are confused with those of temporomandibular joint arthrosis. Acute pericoronitis is accompanied by pain, pyrexia, swelling at the angle of the jaw and lymph node involvement. The distal inflammation about the retromolar tissue may result in partial or complete trismus. The diagnosis is made on the basis of the clinical and roentgenographic examinations.

Impacted molars may induce headaches and cause referred pain to the temporomandibular joint. The onset of pain is gradual and will diminish in time. Pain in the molar area can cause spasms of the masticatory musculature with resultant limited mandibular movement. Roentgenographic and clinical examinations form the bases for diagnosis.

Pericementitis of the two most posterior teeth in the upper and lower arches can also refer pain to the region of the temporomandibular joint and cause muscle spasm with resultant limited mandibular opening. Diagnosis is made on the basis of clinical and roentgenographic examinations.

Temporomandibular Joint Diseases

Temporomandibular joint diseases, such as dislocations, ankylosis, fractures and congenital malformations, may cause symptoms that are confused with those of temporomandibular joint arthrosis.

Dislocation of the temporomandibular joint is more common than is generally realized. The subluxation or self-reducing dislocation is a common phenomenon. According to Dufourmental[36] and Axhausen,[4] there are two kinds of habitual subluxations which the patients themselves learn to adjust by a special jaw movement or with the hand. These are luxation in the upper joint cavity (meniscotemporal) and luxation in the lower joint cavity (meniscocondylar). The presence of a habitual luxation usually presents hindrances to a favorable prognosis.

The luxation or dislocation of the temporomandibular joint is a forward displacement of the head of the condyle in front of the eminence. The forward dislocation sometimes occurs in connection with a fracture. The treatment of luxation consists of reduction and immobilization for a week, using interdental arch wires and rubber bands, to permit tissue repair. Treatment of acute dislocation should be reduction and immobilization for 2 to 3 weeks to prevent secondary hemorrhage and to permit tissue repair.

The surgical treatment for habitual subluxation[63] and recurrent dislocation[76] consists in creating an increase inferiorly of the articular eminence (bone block by arthroplasty). Results in these cases have not proved to be successful; resorption of the artificial spur has occurred. Annondale's[3] treatment for a case of displacement of a meniscus was suturing the meniscus to the tissues of the outer margins of the joint.

There are two types of ankylosis—fibrous and bony. Fibrous ankylosis, also called partial ankylosis, is the result of fibrotic changes in the joint following hemorrhage caused by external trauma. A slight space can be seen between the condyle and the fossa in the roentgenogram.

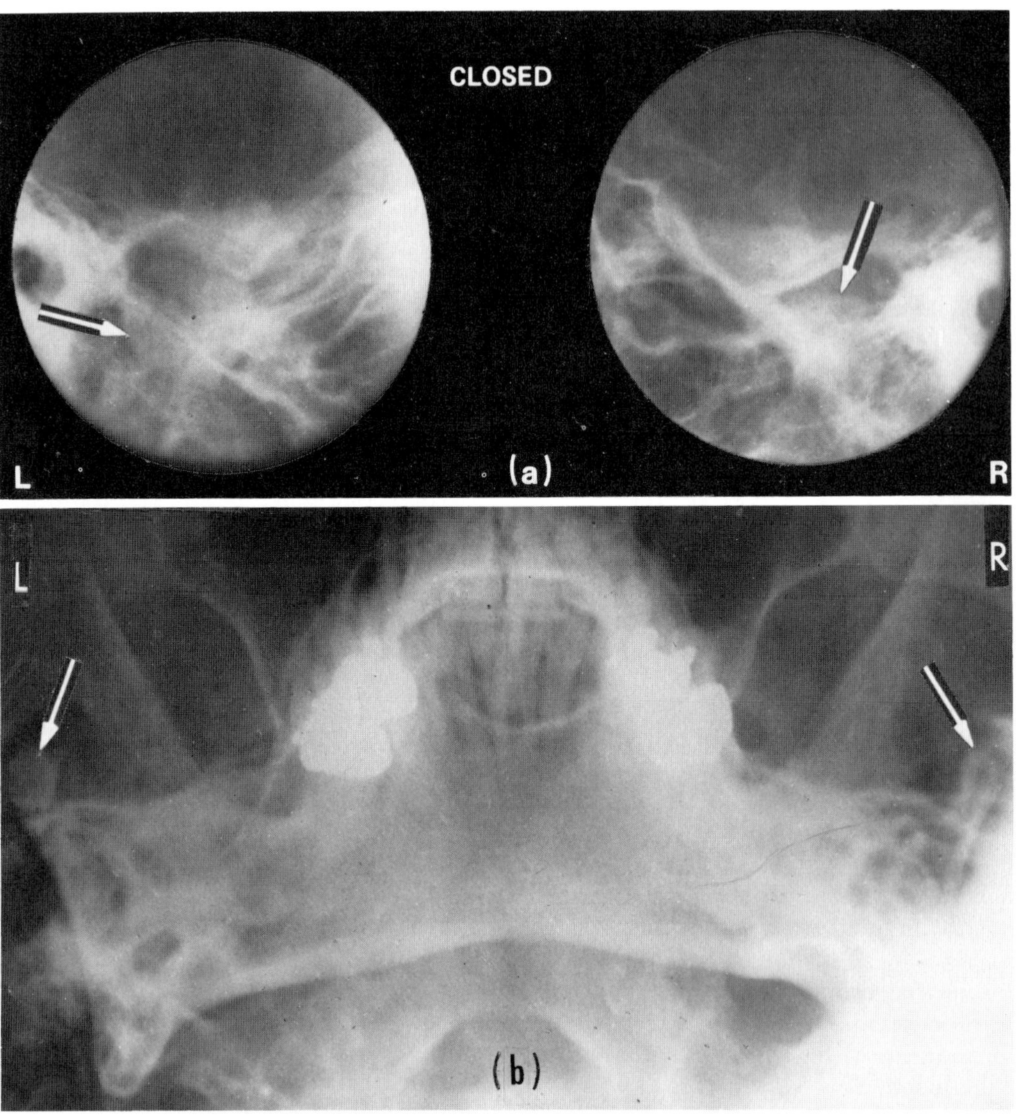

FIG. 9-37. Congenital malformation of the condyles as demonstrated in the lateral and anteroposterior roentgenographs of the same patient. The arrows point to the misshapen condyles.

The joint may have slight and limited movement.

Bony ankylosis is generally the result of infections or suppurative diseases. Complete bony union between the condyle and the fossa can be seen in the roentgenogram. The joint is completely immobile. Ankylosis may follow septicemic and rheumatic diseases of the temporomandibular joint. Congenital ankylosis occurs very rarely. The result of ankylosis during childhood is usually a retruded and malformed mandible.

Fractures of the neck of the condyle may be difficult to diagnose. The patient usually presents a history of severe trauma to the symphysis or directly to the joint. Symptoms are swelling, altered occlusion and pain in the area of the joint. When the dentist places a finger in the external auditory meatus while the patient moves his mandible, no condylar movement is felt. The diagnosis should be verified by roentgenogram.

Congenital malformations of the temporomandibular joint are not easily demonstrable except when they occur in gross form. Malformed condyles coupled with a pathologic occlusion give rise to a great many of the symptoms of temporomandibular joint arthrosis. Figure 9-37 demonstrates the necessity for roentgenography of the joint in more than one plane. In (*a*) the condyles are indistinct because of their size and shape; in (*b*) their true shape and relationship to the fossa become apparent. These cases should be treated for temporomandibular joint arthrosis, but the prognosis depends upon the degree of malformation.

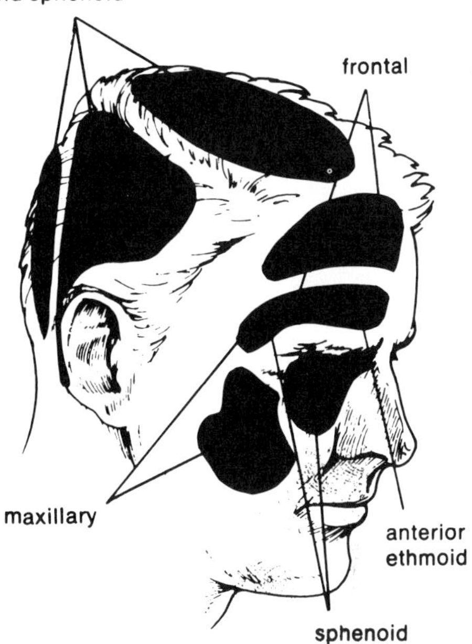

FIG. 9-38. Acute sinusitis. (After Shore, N.A., *et al.*: Symposium on Facial Pain: Patient Care. p. 38. Miller and Fink Publishing Corp., 1972)

Head Infections

Among the head infections that reflect pain and other symptoms to the head, and particularly to the temporomandibular joint, are osteomyelitis, epidemic parotitis, sinusitis, furunculosis of the ear, middle ear infections, and herpes zoster infection.

Osteomyelitis. The usual presenting symptoms of osteomyelitis are sudden pain, a sharp rise in temperature and leukocytosis. When it occurs in the upper or lower second and third molar region it will also affect the muscles of mastication and the temporomandibular joint by means of referred pain and trismus. The history, the clinical and roentgenographic examination (which shows no change in the acute stage of the disease for 10 to 20 days) and the biopsy will establish the diagnosis. In the advanced stages, sequestra surrounded by an area of dense bone can be seen roentgenographically.

Epidemic parotitis can be differentiated by the characteristic swelling which occurs just anterior to and below the ear. Jaw movements produce pain which will diminish if the affected part remains at rest. Other symptoms are malaise, increased irritability, anorexia, headache, muscular pain, lymphocytosis and pyrexia.

Sinusitis. The onset of the pain of sinusitis may be sudden or gradual and may be accompanied by pyrexia, anorexia, vertigo, periorbital edema and dull, boring pain. The pain is of the "phantom" type, and the areas are tender to palpation.

Acute frontal sinusitis causes pain over the sinus and may also involve pain in the eye, root of the nose, temple, occiput and vertex. Acute maxillary sinusitis often results in pain referred to the frontal area, cheek and jaw; whereas sphenoid and ethmoid sinusitis cause pain between and behind the eyes, over the vertex and occasionally suboccipitally (Fig. 9-38). In acute frontal sinus disease the pain generally is less when the patient has been lying down and so is felt more during the day when he is up and around. In acute maxillary sinusitis, the pain may also be less when the patient

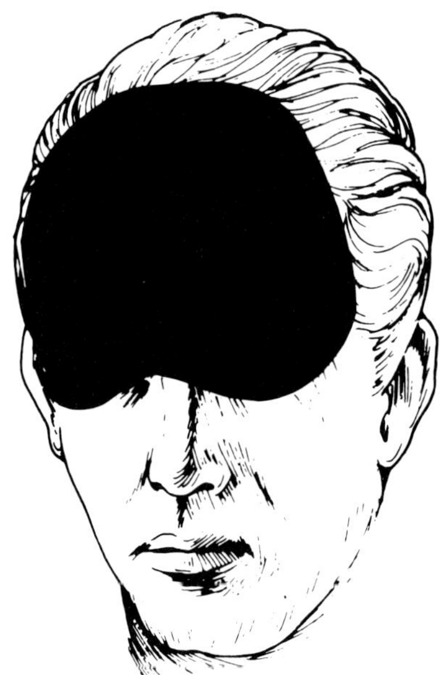

FIG. 9-39. Postherpetic neuralgia. (After Shore, N.A., *et al.*: Symposium on Facial Pain: Patient Care. p. 38. Miller and Fink Publishing Corp., 1972)

lies on the side opposite to the affected side. Usually there is a history of previous head cold. Roentgenographic verification by the Waters' projection is a most important diagnostic aid, the sinus appearing cloudy.

Furunculosis is a painful infection of the ear. The auricle and the canal are frequent sites of purulent skin infections. The onset may consist of acute pain, fullness in the ears, impaired hearing and postauricular swelling. Rigidity of the masseter and the temporal muscles may be caused by furuncles on the floor of the canal and this will result in impaired mandibular masticatory movements.

Middle ear infections present symptoms of impaired hearing, a feeling of fullness in the ears, tinnitus and dizziness. The pain varies in intensity with the type of infection; therefore, the radiation of the pain from the ear to other parts of the head will vary with the severity of the middle ear disease. Otoscopic examination will reveal the cause of the pain to be the ear and not the joint.

Herpes zoster is an acute infection of the central nervous system involving primarily the dorsal root ganglia. Clinically, it is characterized by a vesicular eruption and neuralgic pain in the cutaneous areas supplied by the peripheral sensory nerves arising in the affected root ganglia. Geniculate herpes results from the involvement of the geniculate ganglion. Manifestations include pain in the ear; vesicular eruptions in the external auditory canal, on the auricle, the soft palate and the anterior pillar of the fauces; and facial paralysis on the involved side. Infection of the gasserian ganglion results in ophthalmic herpes, manifested by vesicular eruptions in the distribution of the ophthalmic division of the 5th nerve. Postherpetic neuralgia may persist for years after the acute attack has subsided (Fig. 9-39).

Musculoskeletal Disease

Musculoskeletal diseases that must be considered in the differential diagnosis of temporomandibular joint diseases are external traumatic arthritis, infectious arthritis, rheumatoid arthritis and degenerative joint disease or osteoarthritis.

External Traumatic Arthritis. The patient presents a history of a blow to the joint. The symptoms are pain, which may radiate about the ear, swelling, crepitation, redness, limitation of movement and muscle spasm. Mandibular movement produces joint pain which is relieved by rest of the part. This is a monarticular disturbance, and treatment consists in systemic therapy, sedation, immobilization and rest.

Infectious Arthritis. This may be caused by tuberculous, gonococcal, luetic, septicemic or other organisms which invade the temporomandibular joint. Pain, swelling, redness and leukocytosis are among the symptoms. The diagnosis is verified by culture of the joint fluid. Tuberculous invasions may

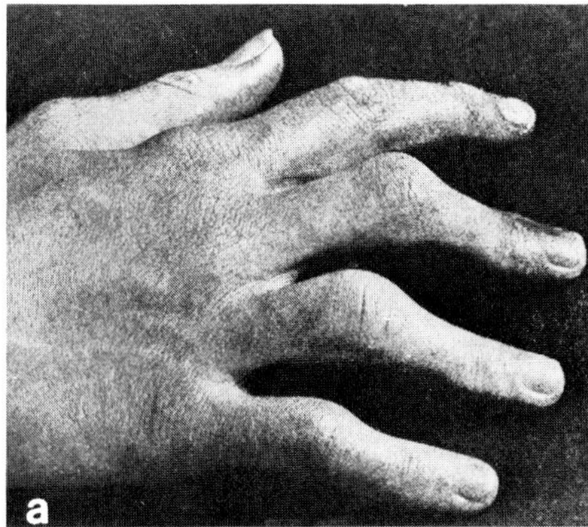

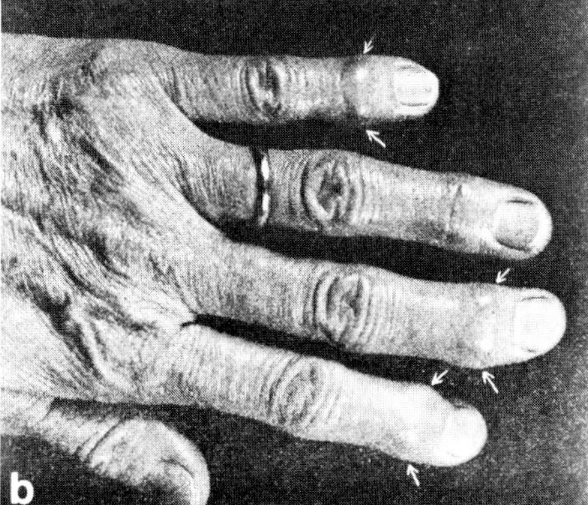

FIG. 9-40. Rheumatoid arthritis (*a*), demonstrating swelling and deformities at proximal interphalangeal joints. Heberden's nodes of osteoarthritis are characteristically at the bases of the terminal phalanges, while the proximal phalangeal joints are not usually involved (*b*). (Hollander: Comroe's Arthritis and Allied Conditions. Philadelphia, Lea & Febiger, 1960)

produce joint destruction which can be visualized roentgenographically. These diseases are systemic and should be treated by a physician. Local palliative treatment such as rest and immobilization of the joint should be prescribed by the dentist.

Rheumatoid arthritis is a systemic disease that may be manifested in the temporomandibular joint by limited motion, local pain, warmth and swelling. The joint and muscle symptoms are severest when the patient awakens in the morning, and they usually diminish with the day's activities. Pain in the joint is accompanied by splinting of the adjacent muscles with resultant muscle spasm.

Symptoms of Rheumatoid Arthritis. There are three groups of symptoms: transitory, acute, and chronic. Transitory symptoms are limitations of motion, referred pain to the teeth, the mandible and the maxilla, the neck, and the ear. The interincisal distance may be limited to roughly 25 mm. for the first days. Acute symptoms consist of the transitory symptoms plus local temporomandibular joint pain, swelling and warmth. The interincisal distance may be limited to 10 mm. These symptoms usually last for 6 to 10 weeks. Chronic symptoms are characterized by severe pain, limitation of interincisal distance to 25 mm., and they continue for over 4 months.[15,28] Another diagnostic feature of chronic rheumatoid arthritis is the swelling and the deformation of proximal interphalangeal joints (Fig. 9-40*a*). Diagnosis is based upon history, roentgenographic changes that are demonstrable and laboratory findings.

Treatment of Rheumatoid Arthritis. Treatment consists mainly in therapy of the involved soft tissues rather than of the bony and cartilaginous joint elements. Muscles, tendons, fasciae and skin are implicated, and these can be treated quite successfully. The steps in therapy are:

1. Eliminate trauma to the joint.
2. After inflammation has subsided, treat muscle spasm.
3. Administer subcutaneous injections of 0.5 mg. to 1.0 mg. of neostigmine.[135]
4. Prescribe corrective exercises to restore mandibular movement.

Since rheumatoid arthritis is a systemic disease which usually involves other areas, treatment should be carried out in cooperation with a physician.

Degenerative Joint Disease or Osteoarthritis. This has been confused with temporomandibular joint arthrosis. The relationship between temporomandibular joint arthrosis due to pathologic occlusion and osteoarthritis is the connecting link between normal aging, incipient degeneration and active degeneration of the temporomandibular joint. The purpose of this classification is to separate temporomandibular joint arthrosis from osteoarthritis. The latter can be distinguished by the presence of Heberden's nodes (Fig. 9-40*b*) about the terminal interphalangeal joints. There is frequent involvement of the weight-bearing joints. There are no systemic symptoms such as fever, and the patients are usually over 40 years of age and frequently overweight. Those joints that receive the greatest trauma during life are most affected.

It is very important to distinguish between the terms *arthritis* and *arthrosis* as they apply to the temporomandibular joint. True arthritis is an inflammatory, degenerative, nonreversible disease. Conversely, temporomandibular joint arthrosis is a dysfunction, not a disease, and as such, under proper treatment, it can be reversed.

Symptoms of Osteoarthritis. The clinical onset is gradual, with mild symptoms. The dull pains in the temporomandibular joint are vague, and limited motion and stiffness are present. Stiffness follows periods of rest and disappears as motion is resumed. The only evidence of the disease may be a grating sound or crepitation when the joint is moved. At the onset, the symptoms are short-lived, but as degeneration progresses they occur more frequently and last longer. The joint becomes stiffer, pain more frequent, and motion more limited. Marginal lipping or spurs may be seen roentgenographically.

Treatment of Osteoarthritis. Analgesics, graded exercises, massage, local heat, diathermy and ultrasonic vibration comprise the treatment. Improvement generally follows intra-articular injection of 0.5 to 1.0 ml. of hydrocortisone. In the more severe cases of rheumatoid arthritis or osteoarthritis, hydrocortisone injections may have to be repeated at intervals varying from several weeks to several months. Occasionally, however, a second injection is not necessary for 12 to 18 months. Advanced bony changes within the joint may necessitate arthroplasty with joint debridement.

Major Neuralgias

Although the neuralgias present an extraordinary problem in differential diagnosis, Bonica[21] provides a comprehensive picture of all of them. In the diagnosis of the neuralgias, it may be very difficult to differentiate between the pain symptoms that result from temporomandibular joint arthrosis and those that result from trigeminal neuralgia. Due to incorrect diagnosis, the wrong treatment may be initiated.

Frequently, patients with symptoms of pain have been mistakenly diagnosed as suffering from tic douloureux and have not been relieved by alcohol block of the primary divisions of the trigeminal nerve. Cases have been reported[128] in which partial or complete section of the sensory root did not abolish the pain. However, when the "bite" of these patients was altered, most, if not all, of the distressing symptoms were relieved. Relief occurred after the occlusion was reoriented after the methods of nerve block and surgery had failed.[128] Therefore, it is obvious that more than the distribution of the 5th nerve is involved in this pain complex.

Four major neuralgias must be considered in the differential diagnosis of neuralgic pains of the head: major trigeminal neuralgia (tic douloureux), glossopharyngeal neuralgia, atypical facial neuralgia and sphenopalatine neuralgia.

Major Trigeminal Neuralgia

McMurtry[75] has given a fascinating description of the history of trigeminal neuralgia:

The first complete description of the disease was by John Locke in 1677. This physician and philosopher was called upon to examine the wife of the English ambassador to France, the Countess of Northumberland. After examining her he wrote in detail a description of his findings and treatment, to four physician friends in England, asking them for their advice. Another opinion solicited was that of the not yet famous Sydenham. Some quotes removed from the texts of these letters demonstrate an accurate and timely portrayal of the disease, and the search for various avenues of therapy which has remained a problem through the following centuries.

LOCKE STATES THAT "On Thursday night last I was sent for to my Lady Ambassadise, whom I found in a fit of such violent and exquisite torment, that it forced her to such cries and shrieks as you would expect from one upon the rack, to which I believe hers was an equal torment, which extended itself all over the right side of her face and mouth. When the fit came there was, to use My Ladys own expression of it, as it were a flash of fire all of a sudden shot into all of those parts, and at every one of those twitches which made her shriek out, her mouth was constantly drawn to the right side towards the right ear by repeated convulsive motions, which were constantly accompanied by her cries. . . . These violent fits terminated on a sudden and then My Lady seemed to be perfectly well. . . . Speaking was apt to put her into these fits: sometimes opening her mouth to take anything, or touching her gums. . . . At night when I was called, I present ease by topical anodyn applications to those parts of her gums where the first beginnings of her fits appear. . . . I thought it necessary to purge her . . . . but I saw no indication for bleeding." It appeared that she was somewhat relieved by medicinal applications and in a subsequent letter to Dr. Mapletoft, Locke describes the application of a "blistering plaster" to her neck.

ONE REPLY TO LOCKE'S letters was from Dr. John Mecklethwaite, President of the Royal College of Physicians. He states, "Upon consideration of the case of the most excellent lady so very well stated, it seems clear that the blood is not at fault, but some pungent vapor which affects the nerve. . . . But because the pain is most urgent it will be necessary to give opiates inwardly and apply little sponges or linen dipped in syrup of castor and liquid laudanum to the part pained and apply large blisters under the ear and under the armpit of the side affected. . . ."

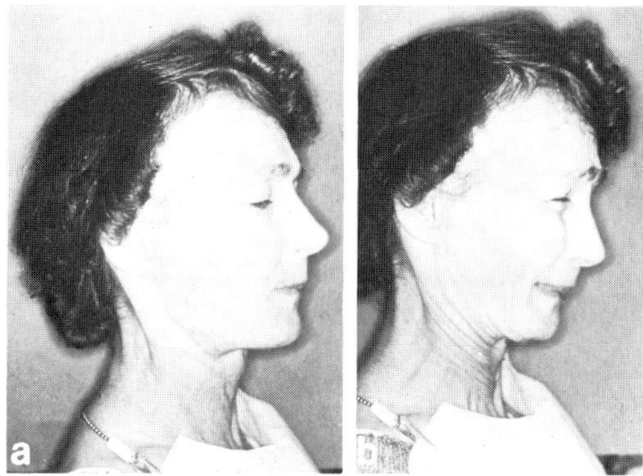

FIG. 9-41. The patient's facial expression before (*a*) and during (*b*) a paroxysm of pain in trigeminal neuralgia.

DR. EDMUND DICKINSON noted that, "From the history of the symptoms I conceive the distemper . . . is not a sanguinous but a nerval kind. . . . The weakness of the nerves seems to have its origin from the tearing of some nerves in the drawing of a tooth on that side." He recommended "strengthening of the nerves" by the use of Queen of Hungary's water. Sir Charles Scarburgh wrote and recommended leaches to the gum itself or cauterizing the gum to the very bottom. The unfortunate lady seems to have improved with, or in spite of, the various treatments.

NICOLAS ANDRE IN 1756 described the disease as *tic douloureux*. He believed the problem to be of the nature of convulsions (centuries later our most effective medical treatments are of the anti-convulsive nature). Seventeen years later John Fothergill described fourteen cases in such detail that the disease was then known as Fothergill's disease. Fothergill mentions that the disease was often seen in elderly people. He states, "From imperceptible beginnings, a pain attacks some part or other of the face or side of the head; sometimes about the orbit of the eye, sometimes the ossa malarum, sometimes the temporal bones are the parts complained of. The pain comes suddenly, and is excruciating; it lasts but a short time, perhaps a quarter or half a minute, and then goes off; it returns at irregular intervals. . . . Eating . . . will bring it on some persons. Talking, or the least motion of the muscles of the face, affects others; the gentlest touch of a handkerchief will sometimes bring on the pain, while a strong pressure on the part has no effect." (See trigeminal neuralgia trigger zones, Fig. 9-43.)

SAMUEL FOTHERGILL, nephew of John Fothergill, felt the disease should be called "facies morbus nervorum crucians." Regarding the etiology of trigeminal neuralgia, he advanced a premise, true today "I do not even hazard a conjecture, but wait until greater experience and information should throw some light on a subject which opinion cannot explain nor hypothesis prove."

Characteristics of Trigeminal Neuralgia. The chief characteristics of major trigeminal neuralgia are lancinating paroxysms of pain in one of the divisions of the trigeminal nerve. These start suddenly and stop as suddenly. In the early stages, these attacks last no longer than a minute or two, and there are periods of freedom from pain for as long as a week, a month or a year. As time passes, the intervals of freedom from pain become shorter, and the attacks increase in severity. The patient lives in constant dread of another attack. The pain is rarely bilateral. Most patients describe specific areas as "trigger zones" which excite an attack when they are lightly touched. The most common of these zones are the upper lip lateral to the ala nasi, the upper lip near the angle, the gingiva, the mental area and the infraorbital area. Secondary trigger points may occur in other areas at the peripheral nerve endings. The pain frequently radiates to the temporomandibular joint. The pain pattern remains constant, but as the disease progresses the pattern becomes larger. It is characteristic that analgesics and narcotics seldom relieve the pain.

Attacks are precipitated by cold, washing, talking, eating and drinking. Sensation is not impaired. The patient's history is usually typical enough to be diagnostic in itself. The facial expression is usually distorted during the paroxysms of pain. Figure 9-41 illustrates the facial expression of a patient suffering from trigeminal neuralgia before and during a paroxysm. Tumors and nerve lesions produce persistent pain and sensory impairment and must be considered in the diagnosis. An aid in the confirmation of a diagnosis of trigeminal neuralgia is the use of trial procaine nerve block in the affected area.

If there is any doubt as to whether a patient is actually suffering from trigeminal neuralgia, the following simple office test can be performed.

1. Place a tongue blade between the patient's cheek and teeth on the painful side.
2. Have the patient close his mouth, and start to gently rotate the tongue blade.
3. Gradually increase the force and speed of movement until a brief attack of trigeminal pain is produced.

This test will never cause pain in any disorder that might be confused with trigeminal neuralgia.

Treatment of Trigeminal Neuralgia. Medical treatment for trigeminal neuralgia cannot be considered satisfactory because the effects are transient, and frequently the pain is only partially relieved. Diathermy, roentgen-ray therapy and thiamine chloride have been administered to patients with very little success in relieving the pain. Thiamine chloride is used because these patients often have a vitamin deficiency, since they cannot eat properly. Temporary relief is afforded by the inhalation of amyl nitrite;[129] the oral administration of nicotinic acid, 100 to 200 mg. before meals and at bedtime;[79] the inhalation of trichlorethylene, which seems to be specific to the trigeminal nerve, several times a day; ferrous carbonate in doses of 4 g. daily with meals;

and vasodilators and antihistamines[130] have proved to be somewhat beneficial. Smith and Miller[106] have reported success in the relief of pain after using stilbamidine. Daily injections of 1,000 μg. of vitamin B_{12} for 2 to 14 days have been effective in relieving the pain.[101]

Recently, carbamazepine has come into use in the treatment of trigeminal neuralgia, but the results have been far from ideal. Although some patients report complete relief from pain, others are not helped at all, and serious side effects can occur. Strict guidelines are provided for the administration of the drug, together with a clear warning of its possible dangers:

> Fatal cases of aplastic anemia have been reported following treatment with carbamazepine. Agranulocytosis, thrombocytopenia and transitory leukopenia have also been observed. Complete blood and platelet counts should be done prior to and at regular intervals during treatment with the drug to help in the early detection of serious bone marrow injury. Abnormalities in initial blood tests should rule out use of the drug. Also, patients should be made aware of such early toxic signs of a potential hematological problem as fever, sore throat, mouth ulcers, easy bruising and petechial or purpuric hemorrhage. Should such signs appear, the patient should be advised to discontinue the drug and to report to the physician immediately.

There have been reports that even in cases in which the drug has proved helpful in eliminating or reducing the pain of major trigeminal neuralgia, prolonged usage may diminish or abolish its effectiveness.[73]

Patients who suffer from trigeminal neuralgia also need psychological support while awaiting definitive therapy. The intense pain may lead to mental depression and even to suicide. Early diagnosis and therapy are most important. Definitive therapy consists of alcohol nerve blocking or of surgical interruption of the nerve. The alcohol block produces a period of relief varying from 6 months to 3 years.[54]

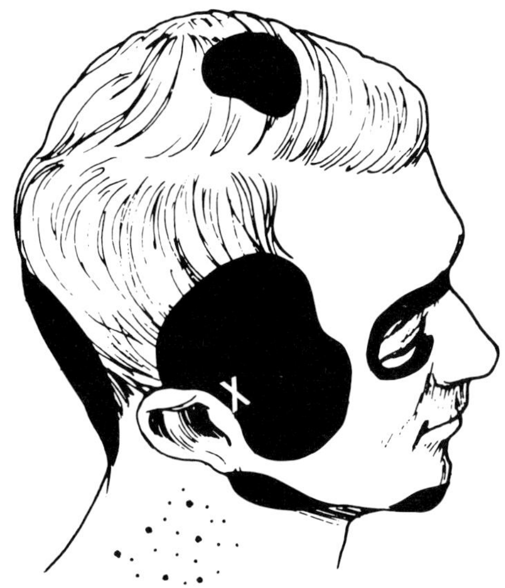

FIG. 9-42. Temporomandibular joint dysfunction. (After Shore, N.A., *et al.*: Symposium on Facial Pain: Patient Care. p. 38. Miller and Fink Publishing Corp., 1972)

The advantages of the alcohol nerve block are that pain is relieved immediately and that there is less risk than is involved in surgery. In cases of facial pain when the cause cannot be removed, such as carcinoma of the jaw, the block may assist in confirming the diagnosis and may enable the patient to be restored to good physical condition before surgery is undertaken. The disadvantages of alcohol block are discomfort, varying with the skill of the operator; diminishing relief with each successive injection; complications such as cranial nerve palsies and hematomas; and partial or complete failure to relieve pain. Finally, alcohol nerve block almost never produces a complete cure of the disease.

Surgical intervention for trigeminal neuralgia consists of the following operations: nerve evulsion, retrogasserian neurotomy, decompression procedures, resection of the sensory root of the trigeminal nerve, the subtotal resection of Frazier, mesenphalic tractotomy and med-

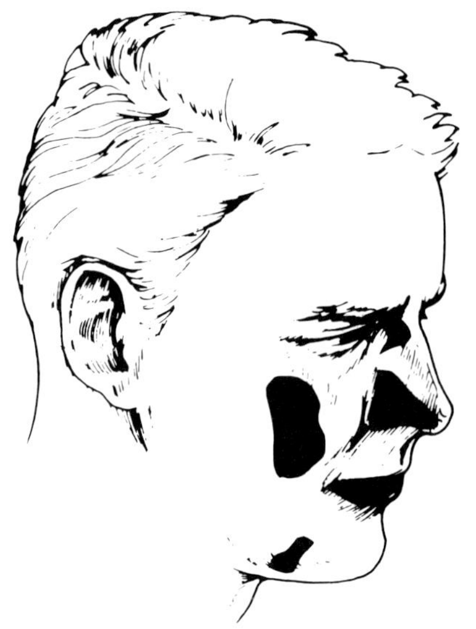

FIG. 9-43. Trigeminal neuralgia trigger zones. (After Shore, N.A., *et al.*: Symposium on Facial Pain: Patient Care. p. 38. Miller and Fink Publishing Corp., 1972)

dullary tractotomy. Surgery is the one method of relieving trigeminal neuralgia.

Differences Between Tic Douloureux and Temporomandibular Joint (TMJ) Dysfunction. Because tic douloureux is likely to be confused with temporomandibular joint dysfunction, it would be well to review the differences between the two. The pain in the latter usually has the quality of a dull ache, either superficial or deep, in the joints and associated muscles (Fig. 9-42). This pain does not start and stop suddenly. It may last for long periods, then disappear for weeks or months at a time, only to return with greater severity. The lancinating pain of tic, set off by light pressure on a trigger zone as in Figures 9-36 and 9-43, is definitely not characteristic of temporomandibular joint arthrosis. Although there may be "trigger areas" associated with the muscle spasm of temporomandibular joint arthrosis (see p. 179), considerably greater stimulation of these zones (e.g., direct palpation) is needed to invoke exquisite pain. In tic, even a gentle breeze may set off an episode of pain; this would rarely occur in temporomandibular joint arthrosis. In fact, the muscle spasm itself, which gives rise to the so-called trigger areas in temporomandibular joint arthrosis, is not observed in tic douloureux. Also, while the pain of tic may radiate along the mandibular branch of the trigeminal nerve *to* the temporomandibular joint, the pain of temporomandibular joint dysfunction always radiates *from* the temporomandibular joint. The extreme facial distortion accompanying an episode of tic is rarely seen in those suffering from the pain of temporomandibular joint dysfunction.

Although not definitive in the diagnosis, it is important to remember that major trigeminal neuralgia very rarely affects both sides of the face. Bilateral involvement is much more common, however, in temporomandibular joint arthrosis. Also, there are distinctive physical signs of temporomandibular joint arthrosis such as clicking and crepitation in the joints, mandibular deviation upon mouth opening, and limited or excessive mandibular movement in all ranges of articulation: none of these signs is observed in tic. Finally, it has been noted that the pain of temporomandibular joint arthrosis can be relieved by the ingestion of alcohol—a couple of ounces of whiskey, for example—along with aspirin. Such relief is not available to those afflicted with tic douloureux.[134].

Glossopharyngeal Neuralgia

This rare syndrome is characterized by recurrent attacks of severe pain identical to major trigeminal neuralgia. These pains occur in the middle ear, the base of the tongue, the tonsils, the neck and the throat (Fig. 9-44). This condition is often termed tic douloureux of the 9th cranial nerve. The disease is most common in men after the age of 40. This disease must be distinguished from trigeminal neuralgia involving the mandibular division. This is done by location of the pain, precipitation of an attack by touching the tonsils, and causing the disappearance of the pain by anesthetizing the affected area with Pontocaine. Alcohol injection does not yield satisfactory results, and the treatment of choice is intracranial division of the 9th nerve.[29]

Sphenopalatine Neuralgia

Also known as Sluder's headache, this type of neuralgia causes episodic, recurrent pain lasting from a few minutes to several days. The pain occurs unilaterally in the orbit and nose and in the temporal bone behind the mastoid process. It may extend just beyond the auditory canal and cause earache (Fig. 9-45). During an attack the pain is continuous and may be very intense. Episodes are marked by swelling of the nasal mucosa with concomitant copious nasal secretions and blockage. The causes of this condition are not known; however, immediate relief is obtained by cocainization of the sphenopalatine ganglion on the affected side.[132]

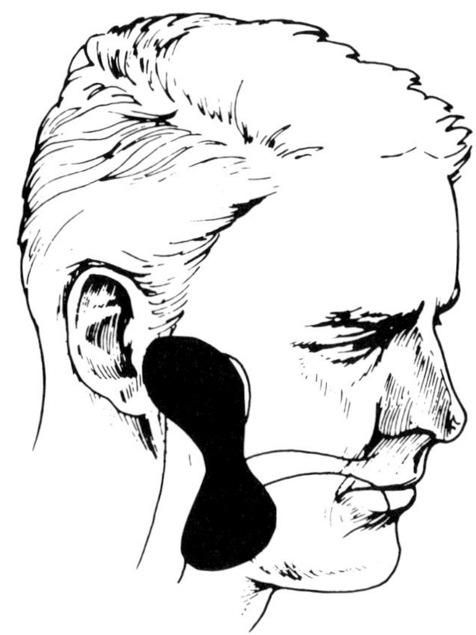

FIG. 9-44. Glossopharyngeal neuralgia. (After Shore, N.A., *et al.*: Symposium on Facial Pain: Patient Care. p. 38. Miller and Fink Publishing Corp., 1972)

Atypical Facial Neuralgia

This neuralgia causes deep, poorly localized, continuous, aching pain. Episodes usually last for periods of a few hours to several days, with pain-free periods of several days to 9 months. It is Wolff's opinion that this condition is analogous to migraine headache and results from dilatation of one or more parts of the external carotid artery. The pain can be terminated by intramuscular administration of ergotamine tartrate. Wolff distinguishes between this periodic facial neuralgia and chronic atypical facial neuralgia. The latter causes continuous pain which may endure for months or years. Because there is a high correlation between this pain and depression, anxiety, or hysteria in the patient, it has been speculated that chronic atypical facial neuralgia is psychogenic. No form of drug therapy has proved successful in treating this condition.[133] The etiology of the syndrome is so obscure that one investigator has described chronic atypical facial neuralgia as "a true example of a 'wastebasket' diagnosis."[100]

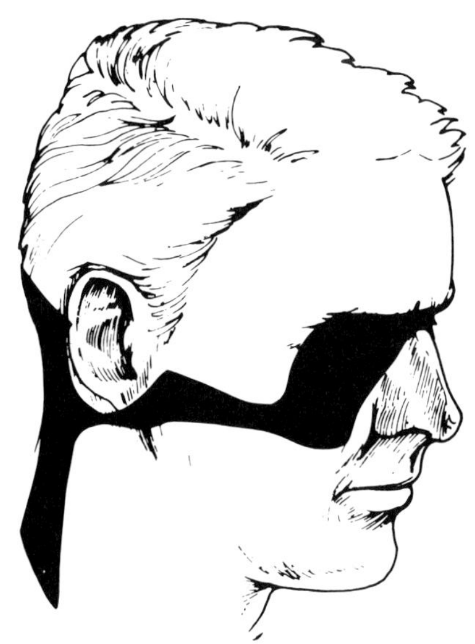

FIG. 9-45. Sphenopalatine neuralgia. (After Shore, N.A., *et al.*: Symposium on Facial Pain: Patient Care. p. 38. Miller and Fink Publishing Corp., 1972)

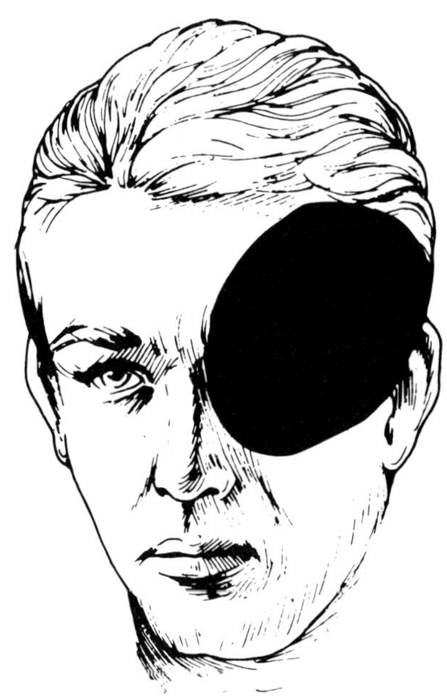

FIG. 9-46. Cluster head pain. (After Shore, N.A., *et al.:* Symposium on Facial Pain: Patient Care. p. 38. Miller and Fink Publishing Corp., 1972)

In the major neuralgias, confirmation of the diagnosis should be sought from a neurologist or a neurosurgeon.

Vascular Disease

Temporal arteritis presents a distinctive pattern of head pain. Wolff[130] states that painful mastication was the first symptom in half the patients. Persistent headaches of a deep, aching, throbbing nature and of high intensity are present. The headaches appear when the patient is in a prone position and disappear when he is upright. Often before all definitive diagnostic symptoms of temporal arteritis are present, there is pain in the teeth, the ear, the zygoma, the nuchal region and the occiput.[130] Among the diagnostic features generally present are anorexia, prostration, fever, sweating, loss of weight and leukocytosis. The area over the artery evidences pain, heat, swelling, tenderness and redness. The only treatment that seems at all effective is arterial resection. Other vascular lesions that may produce minor trigeminal neuralgias are aneurysms of the internal carotid and basilar arteries, cavernous angioma and lesions of the petrosal vein.

Cluster and Migraine Headache

Both cluster and migraine headache are of vascular origin and produce pain primarily in the frontal and orbital regions of the face. Pain may also be referred to other parts of the face and the neck.

Cluster headaches are paroxysmal and usually are felt as intense, boring pain in the eye (Fig. 9-46). If the pain occurs in the lower face instead, it may be confused with trigeminal neuralgia. However, unlike tic, an attack usually takes 5 to 10 minutes to develop and continues for 45 minutes to a couple of hours. Onset is usually at night, and there may be as many as six attacks in 24 hours. The headaches occur in a series over about 6 to 8 weeks, followed by a trouble-free period of months to years.

Migraine typically causes pain in the

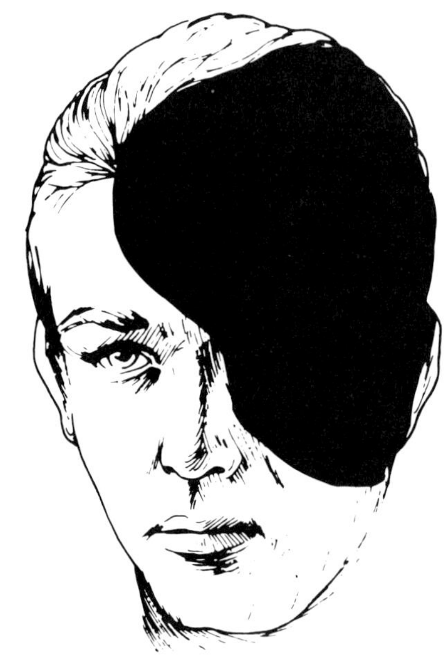

FIG. 9-47. Migraine headache. (After Shore, N.A., *et al.:* Symposium on Facial Pain: Patient Care. p. 38. Miller and Fink Publishing Corp., 1972)

supraorbital, retroorbital and temporal regions (Fig. 9-47) though the pain may also be localized in the cheek and jaw. It is especially in the latter case that migraine can be a problem in the differential diagnosis of temporomandibular joint dysfunction. A migraine attack usually lasts 1 or 2 days (sometimes longer). It is characterized by a throbbing pain which may be replaced by a steady, intense ache as the episode progresses, and it is accompanied by nausea and vomiting.

Neoplasms

Neoplasms have been known to affect the temporomandibular joint. Benign tumors result in swelling and impaired function but usually do not cause pain. Spontaneous bone fracture and destruction of the underlying bone may take place. Any neoplastic lesion proximal to the gasserian ganglion may give rise to minor trigeminal neuralgia. Neoplasms of the larynx and the pharynx may refer pains to the head and the face, causing symptoms resembling those of temporomandibular joint arthrosis. An early neoplasm in the arytenoid region of the larynx will refer severe pain to the region of the ear and to the angle of the mandible. Neoplasms of the nasopharynx cause severe pains to the maxillary area and to the side of the head.

Other symptoms may be deafness, asymmetry of the palate, either tingling or a sensation of numbness along the side of the jaw or the face, paralysis of the external and the internal pterygoids, and the masseter and the temporal muscles because of compression of the motor fibers of the trigeminal nerve and paralysis of the muscles of the soft palate.[103] Tumors invading the floor of the skull from the nasopharynx and tumors involving the cerebellopontine angle produce pain similar to that which occurs with trigeminal neuralgia. Clinical and roentgenographic examinations and biopsy confirm diagnosis.

REFERENCES

1. Agnew, R. G.: Pain problems in the practice of dentistry. JADA, *53:*517, 1956.
———: The management of obscure pain by the general practitioner. JADA, *53:*532, 1956.
2. Alkory, *In* Ackermann, F.: Le mécanisme des machoires. Paris, Masson, 1953.
3. Annondale, T.: Displacement of the interarticular cartilage of the lower jaw and its treatment by operation. Lancet, *1:*411, 1887.
4. Axhausen, G.: Pathologie und therapie des kiefergelenkes (Pathology and therapy of the temporomandibular joint). Fortschr. Zahn. *6:*177, 1930; *7:*199, 1931; *8:*201, 1932.
5. Ibid.: *6:*177, 1930.
6. ———: Die operative freilegung des kiefergelenkes (The exposure of the temporomandibular joint by operation). Chirugie, *16:*713, 1931.
———: Erfahrung über die retroaurikulare freilegung des kiefergelenkes (Experiences concerning the retroauricular exposure of the temporomandibular joint). Dtsch. Zahn-Mund-Kieferhk., *5:*255, 1938.
7. ———: Das kiefergelenkknacken und seine behandlung (Clicking temporomandibular joint and its treatment). Dtsch. Ztschr. Chir., *232:*238, 1931.
8. Ballantyne, J.: Anatomy of the ear. *In* Ballantyne, J. and Groves, J. (eds.): Scott-Brown's Diseases of the Ear, Nose and Throat. ed. 3, vol. 1, pp. 3–4. Philadelphia, J. B. Lippincott, 1971.
9. Bauer, A. W.: Osteo-arthrosis. Br. J. Phys. Med., *16:*199, 1953.
10. Bauer, W.: Anatomische und mikroskopische untersuchungen über das kiefergelenk (Anatomic and microscopic researches concerning the temporomandibular joint). Z. Stomatol., *20:*1136 (No. 18), 1932.
11. ———: Anatomische und mikroskopische untersuchungen über das kiefergelenk mit besonderer berucksichtigung der veranderung bei osteoarthritis deformans (Anatomic and microscopic examination of the tem-

poromandibular joint with special consideration of changes in cases of osteoarthritis deformans). Z. Stomatol., *19:*1273, 1932.
12. Ibid.: *20:*1334 (No. 18), 1932.
13. Ibid.: *30:*1136, 1932.
14. Bauer, W. H.: Osteoarthritis deformans of the temporomandibular joint. Am. J. Pathol., *17:*129, 1941.
15. Bayles, T. B., and Russell, L. A.: The temporomandibular joint in rheumatoid-arthritis. JAMA, *116:*2842, 1941.
16. Behan, R.: Loose cartilage in the temporomaxillary joint; subluxation of the inferior maxilla. Ann. Surg., *67:*536, 1918.
17. Bleiker, R. F.: Ear disturbances of temporomandibular origin. JADA, *25:*1390, 1938.
18. Block, L. S.: Diagnosis and treatment of disturbances of the temporomandibular joint especially in relation to vertical dimension. JADA, *34:*259, 1947.
———: The temporomandibular syndrome as related to full denture prosthesis. JADA, *42:*428, 1951.
———: Discussion of the physiology of the muscles of mastication. J. Pros. Dent., *1:*708, 1951.
———: Muscular tensions in denture construction. J. Pros. Dent., *2:*198, 1952.
———: Preparing and conditioning the patient for intermaxillary relations. J. Pros. Dent., *2:*559, 1952.
———: The prosthodontist and the temporomandibular joint syndrome. JADA, *46:*671, 1953.
———: Tensions and intermaxillary relations. J. Pros. Dent., *4:*204, 1954.
19. Block, L. S., and Harris, E.: An approach to a rational study and treatment of temporomandibular joint problems. JADA, *29:*349, 1942.
20. Boman, K.: Temporomandibular joint arthrosis and its treatment by extirpation of the disc. Acta Chir. Scand., *95* (Suppl. 118):21, 1947.
21. Bonica, J. J.: Management of Pain. Philadelphia, Lea & Febiger, 1953.
22. Box, H. K.: Studies in Periodontal Pathology (No. 7). Canadian Research Foundation, Toronto, 1927.
———: Twelve Periodontal Studies. Toronto, University of Toronto, 1940.
23. Boyens, P. J.: Value of autosuggestion in the therapy of "Bruxism" and other biting habits. JADA, *27:*1773, 1940.
24. Breitner, C.: Experimentelle veranderung der mesiodistalen beziehungen der oberen und unteren zahnreihen, (Experimental changes of the mesiodistal relation between the upper and the lower arches), Ztschr. Stomatol., *28:*134, 620, 1930; *29:*343, 1931.
———: Bone changes resulting from experimental orthodontic treatment. Am. J. Ortho., *26:*521, 1940.
———: Further investigations of bone changes resulting from experimental orthodontic treatment. Int. J. Ortho., *27:*605, 1941.
———: The tooth-supporting apparatus under occlusal changes. J. Periodont., *13:*72, 1942.
———: Alteration of occlusal relations induced by experimental procedure. Am. J. Ortho., *29:*277, 1943.
25. Brussell, J.: Temporomandibular joint diseases: differential diagnosis and treatment. JADA, *39:*532, 1949.
26. Buchman, J.: Lesions of the temporomandibular joint. Am. J. Ortho., *25:*355, 1939.
27. Bunting, R. W.: Oral Hygiene and Preventive Dentistry. Philadelphia, Lea & Febiger, 1950.
28. Burket, L. W.: Oral Medicine. Philadelphia, J. B. Lippincott, 1971.
29. Ibid.: p. 301.
30. Coolidge, E. D.: The thickness of the human periodontal membrane. JADA, *34:*1260, 1937.
———: Traumatic and functional injuries occurring in the supporting tissues of human teeth. JADA, *25:*343, 1938.
———: Periodontia. J. Wisconsin D. Soc., *23:*173, 1947.
———, and Hine, M. K.: Periodontia. Philadelphia, Lea & Febiger, 1954.
31. Cooper, A.: A Treatise on Dislocations and Fractures of the Joints. London, 1823.
32. Costen, J. B.: Glossodynia: reflex irritation from the mandibular joint as the

principal etiologic factor. Arch. Otolaryngol., *22:*554, 1935.

Costen, B., Clare, M. H., and Bishop, G. H.: The transmission of pain impulses via the chorda tympani nerve, Ann. Otol. Rhinol. Laryngol., *60:*591, 1951.

33. Drum, W.: Erwiederung auf die arbeit von Iskraut: kaumuskelspasmus und neuralpathologie (Response to Iskraut's: muscle spasms and neuropathology). Zahn. Welt, *6:*155, 1950.
34. Dubecq, X. J.: L'appareil moteur du menisque mandibulaire. Semaine Dent., 1934.

———: Recherches morphologiques, physiologiques et cliniques sur le menisque mandibulaire. Rev. Odontostomatol., *1:*1, 1937.

———: Morphologie du menisque mandibulaire. Arch. Anat. Histol. Embryol., *34:*187, 1952.

35. Duchenne: Recherches électoniques et pathologiques sur les proprietés et les usages de la corde des tympani. Arch. Gen. Med., *24* (Series *4*):385, 1850.
36. Dufourmentel, L.: Chirurgie de l'articulation temporo-maxillaire. Paris. Masson, 1920.
37. Durman, D. C.: Arthritis and injury, J. Michigan M. Soc., *54:*301, 1955.
38. Foged, J.: Om kaebeledsknapen og lignende sygdomme i kaebeleddet. Tandlaegebladet., *45:*605, 1941.
39. ———: Temporomandibular arthrosis. Lancet, *257:*1209, 1949.
40. Gilpin, S. F.: Glossodynia. JAMA, *106:*1722, 1936.
41. Glickman, I.: Clinical Periodontology. p. 372. Philadelphia, W. B. Saunders, 1953.
42. Ibid.: p. 383, 1953.
43. Ibid.: p. 386, 1953.
44. Goodfriend, D. J.: Dysarthrosis and subarthrosis of the mandibular articulation. D. Cosmos, *74:*523, 1932.

———: Symptomatology and treatment of abnormalities of mandibular articulation. D. Cosmos, *75:*844, 947, 1106, 1933.

———: Abnormalities of the mandibular articulation. JADA, *21:*204, 1934.

———: Role of dental factors in the cause and treatment of ear symptoms and disease. D. Cosmos, *78:*1292, 1936.

45. Gordon, S. M.: Dental Science and Dental Art. Philadelphia, Lea & Febiger, 1936.
46. Gottlieb, B., and Orban, B.: Die veranderungen der gewebe bei ubermassiger beanspruchung der zahne (Changes of the tissue due to excessive use of the teeth). Leipzig, Thieme, 1931.

———: The Biology and Pathology of the Tooth and Its Supporting Mechanism. New York, Macmillan, 1938.

47. Grewcock, R. J. G.: Occlusal equilibration in general practice. D. Pract. D. Rec., *5:*313, 1955.
48. ———: Oral rehabilitation. Br. D. J., *98:*41, 1955.
49. Groves, J.: Physiology of equilibration. *In* Ballantyne, J., and Groves, J. (eds.): Scott-Brown's Diseases of the Ear, Nose and Throat. ed 3, vol. 1, p. 109. Philadelphia, J. B. Lippincott, 1971.
50. Hankey, G. T.: Arthrosis of the temporomandibular joint. Br. D. J., *97:*249, 1954.

———: Pain of temporomandibular origin. Lond. Hosp. Gazette, *59:* June 1955.

51. Harris, H. L.: Anatomy of the temporomandibular articulation and adjacent structures. JADA, *19:*584, 1932.
52. ———: Diagnosis in closed bite conditions. JADA, *26:*964, 1939.
53. ———: Effect of loss of vertical dimension on anatomic structures of the head and neck. JADA, *25:*127, 1938.
54. Harris, W.: An analysis of 1433 cases of paroxysmal trigeminal neuralgia and the end results of gasserian alcohol injection. Brain, *63:*209, 1940.
55. Haupl, K., and Posansky, R.: Studies in the transformation of the temporomandibular joint. Dtsch. Zahn-Mund-Kieferh., *6:*7, 1939.
56. Held, A. J.: Pathogeny of parodontolyses of diseases characterized by a progressive atrophy of the paradontium. Paradontologie, *61* (2), 1952.
57. Herzog, H.: Zahnbeweglichkeitsverhaltnisse bei asymmetrischer kaufunktion (Relations of dental mobility in asymmetric masticatory function). Zurich, Thesis, 1956.
58. Hirt, H., and Muhlemann, H. R.: Diag-

nosis of bruxism by means of tooth mobility measurements. Paradontologie, *9:*47, 1955.

59. Humphreys, H.: Age changes in temporomandibular joint and their importance in orthodontics. Int. J. Ortho., *18:*809, 1932.
60. Ireland, V. E.: The problem of the clicking jaw. Proc. R. Soc. Med. (Sec. Odont.), *44:*363, 1951.
61. Jarabek, J. R.: The adaptability of the temporal and masseter muscles; an electromyographical study. Angle Ortho., *24:*193, 1954.
    ———: An electromyographic analysis of muscular and temporomandibular joint dysfunction due to imbalances in occlusion. Angle Ortho., *26:*170, 1956.
62. Jozat, R.: Uber veranderungen des periodontiums durch entlasting (Changes in the periodontal tissues caused by changes in occlusion). Dtsch. Zahn. Wchnschr., *36:*155, 1933.
63. Kallenberger, K.: Habitual subluxation of the temporomandibular joint. Rev. Mens. Suisse Odont., *57:*403, 1947.
64. Keller, R.: Le problème de l'occlusion traumatissante. Rev. Mens. Suisse Odont., *49:*349, 1939.
65. Kellgren, J. H.: On the distribution of pain arising from deep somatic structures with charts of segmental pain area. Clin. Sci., *4:*35 (No. 1), 1939.
66. Kellner, E.: Das verhaltnis der zement und periodontal breiten zur funktionellen beanspruchung der zahne (The relation of the thickness of cementum and the periodontal membrane to the functional condition of the teeth). Z. Stomatol., *29:*44, 1931.
67. ———: Histologische befunde an antagonistenlosen zahnen (Histologic findings on teeth without antagonists). Z. Stomatol., *26:*271, 1928.
68. Konjetzny, G. E.: Habitual dislocation of the lower jaw. Arch. Klin. Chir., *116:*681, 1921.
69. Kronfeld, R., and Boyle, P. E.: Histopathology of the Teeth and Their Surrounding Structures. ed. 2. Philadelphia, Lea & Febiger, 1949.
70. Lewis, T.: Pain. New York, Macmillan, 1942.
71. Ibid.: p. 80.
72. Lindblom, G.: Disorders of the temporomandibular joint, causal factors and the value of temporomandibular radiographs in their diagnosis and therapy. Acta Odont. Scand., *11:*61, 1953.
73. Lloyd-Smith, D. L., and Sachdev, K. K.: A long-term low dosage study of carbamazepine in trigeminal neuralgia. Headache, *9:*64, 1969.
74. Lotsch, F.: Diskusschadigungen des kiefergelenkes einschliesslich der sog. unterkieferverrenkungen, (Damages of the disc of the temporomandibular joint including the so-called dislocations of the mandible). Arch. Klin. Chir., *149:*40, 1927.
75. McMurtry, J. G.: The history of medical and surgical interests in facial pain. Headache, *9:*1, 1969.
76. Mayer, L.: Recurrent dislocation of the jaw. J. Bone Joint Surg., *15:*889, 1933.
    ———: Recurrent dislocation of the jaw. Dtsch. Zahn. Wchnschr., *38:*96, 1935.
77. Miller, S. C.: Oral Diagnosis and Treatment. London, Lewis, 1946.
78. Monson, G. S.: Impaired function as result of closed bite. JADA, *8:*833, 1921.
    ———: Case histories. JADA, *11:*55, 1924.
79. Moore, M. T.: Treatment of multiple sclerosis with nicotinic acid and vitamin B. Arch. Int. Med., *65:*1, 1940.
80. Moyers, R. E.: Lecture to the Soc. of Oral Physiology and Occlusion, 1955.
81. Muhlemann, H. R.: Tooth mobility. J. Periodont., *25:*22, 125, 202, 1954.
82. ———: Tooth mobility. Tooth mobility changes through artificial alterations of the periodontium. J. Periodont., *25:*198, 1954.
83. Muhlemann, H. R., and Fehr, C.: Zur beurteilung des paradonts vermittels zahnbeweglichkeitsmessungen (Diagnosis of periodontosis by measuring tooth mobility). Dtsch. Zahn. Ztschr., *11:*634, 1956.
84. Muhlemann, H. R., Herzog, H., and Rateitschak, K. H.: Okklusion und artikulation im atiologiekomplex parodontaler erkrankungen (Occlusion and articulation in the etiologic complex of periodontal diseases). Paradontologie, *11:*20, 1957.

———: Quantitative evaluation of the therapeutic effect of selective grinding. J. Periodont., *28:*11, 1957.

85. Muhlemann, H. R., Herzog, H., and Vogel, A.: Occlusal trauma and tooth mobility. Schweiz Monatschr. Zahn., *66:*527, 1956.
86. Muhlemann, H. R., Hirt, H., and Herzog. H.: ARPA Int., *14:*1, 1955.
87. Muhlemann, H. R., Wortman, P., and Marthaler, T. M.: Zahnbeweglichkeit (tooth mobility). Parodontologie, *9:*24, 1955.
88. Muhlemann, H. R., and Zander, H. A.: Tooth mobility III. The mechanism of tooth mobility. J. Periodont., *25:*128, 1954.
89. Norgaard, F.: Arthrography of mandibular joint. Acta Radiol., *25:*679, 1944.
90. Oppenheim, A.: Bone changes during tooth movement. Int. J. Ortho. Oral Surg. Radiog., *16:*535, 1930.
91. Orban, B.: Oral Histology and Embryology. p. 332. St. Louis, C. V. Mosby, 1944.
92. Pommer, G.: Über die mikroskopischen kennzeichen der arthritic deformans, (Microscopic symptoms of arthritic deformans). Virchows Arch. (Pathol. Anat.), *263:*434, 1927.
93. Pringle, J. H.: Displacement of the mandibular meniscus and its treatment. Br. J. Surg., *6:*385, 1918.
94. Rantanen, A. V.: Leukanivelen fysiologisen subluksaation yleisyydesta nuorilla (The frequency of physiologic subluxation in the temporomandibular joint of young people). Suom. Hammasläák. Toim., *50* (No. 2):133, 1954.
95. Rees, L. A.: Structure and function of the temporomandibular joint. Br. D. J., *96:*125, 1954.
96. Reitan, K.: The mechanical and histologic problems in the rotation of teeth. Nor. Tannlaegeforen. Tid., *50:*1, 1940.

———: Tissue changes following rotation of teeth in dogs. Northwestern Univ. Bull., *40:*8, 1940.

97. ———: Om de teoretiske vetningslinjer for beh. av dypt bitt og deres betydnin i proksis (About the theoretical directions for treating deep bite and its importance in practice). Nor. Tannlaegeforen. Tid., *59:*41, 1949.

———: The initial tissue reaction incident to orthodontic tooth movement as related to the influence of function. Acta odont. scand., Oslo, (Suppl. 6), 1951.

———: Grunntrekk fra stottevevets omfromning ved eksperimentell tannforskyvning (Fundamentals concerning the tissue reaction in experimental tooth movement). Odont. Tidskr., *61:*293, 1953.

———: Tissue changes following experimental tooth movement as related to time factor. D. Rec., *73:*559, 1953.

98. Riesner, S. E.: Temporomandibular reaction of occlusal anomalies. JADA, *25:*1938, 1938.
99. Ronkin, S. H.: Improvement of low-tone deafness and tinnitus by mandibular repositioning. Arch. Otolaryngol., *57:*669, 1953.

———: Repositioning the mandible in cases of obstructive (low tone) deafness and tinnitus. Ann. Dent., *13:*8, 1954.

100. Rushton, J. G.: Patient Care, *6:*32, 1972.
101. Ruskin, S. L.: The role of coenzymes of the complex enzymes and amino acids in muscle metabolism and balanced nutrition. Am. J. Dig. Dis., *13:*110, 1946.
102. Sarnat, B. G.: The Temporomandibular Joint. p. 86, Springfield (Ill.), Charles C Thomas, 1951.
103. ———: Oral and facial cancer. D. Radiogr. Photogr., *27:*(1) 1, 1954.
104. Schwartz, J.: Arthritic deformans des kiefergelenkes (Arthritic deformans of the temporomandibular joint). Dtsch. Monatsschr. Zahn., *47:*959, 1929.
105. Shore, N. A.: Examination for temporomandibular joint dysfunction. New York State D. J., *24:*397, 1958.
106. Smith, G. W., and Miller, J. M.: The treatment of tic douloureux with stilbamidine. Bull. Johns Hopkins Hosp., *96:*146, 1955.

———: Stilbamadine and tic douloureux. J. D. Med., *11,* 232, 1956.

107. Staplemohr, V.: Sur les craquements de l'articulation temporomaxillaire et les luxations habituelles de la machoire (Noises and habitual luxations of the temporomandibular joint). Acta Chir. Scand., *65:*1, 1929.

108. Steinhardt, G.: Uber den kaudruck und dessen bedeutung fur die prothetische versorgung des luckengebisses, Zahn. Welt, *6:*291, 1951.

———: Neuere erfahrungen uber verlauf und behandlung des kiefergelenk-knackens (The course and treatment of the clicking jaw). Dtsch. Zahn-Mund-Kieferh. *16:*27, 1952.

———: Uber die bei behandlung von bissanomalien mittels intermaxillarer verbande moglichen gelenkveranderungen und deren erkennung im rontgenbild (Possible changes of the joint in the treatment of anomalies of the bite through intermaxillary bands and their recognition in the x-ray picture). Zahn. Welt, *7:*15, 1952.

———: Die bedeutung der kiefergelenkforschung fur die totale prothese, insbesondere fur die forderung nach indibidueller gelenkbahnregistrierung (The importance of temporomandibular joint research in the field of full dentures, in relationship to individual joint path registration). Dtsch. Zahn. Ztschr., *11:*833, 1956.

———: Kiefergelenkerkrankungen (Temporomandibular joint diseases), Dtsch. Zahn-Mund-Kieferh., *3:*517, 1957.

109. ———: Die beanspruchung der gelenkflachen bei verschiedenen bissarten (Investigation into the stresses in the mandibular articulation and their structural consequences). Dtsch. Zahn., *91:*1, 1934.

———: Zur pathologie und therapie des gelenkknackens bei kieferschliessbewegung (Pathology and therapy of temporomandibular joint clicking in closing movement). Zahn. Wchnschr., *43:*1043, 1934.

110. ———: Über die gegenseitige abhangigkeit zwischen paradentium und kiefergelenk beim kauvorgang (The interdependence of paradentium and temporomandibular joint during mastication). Dtsch. Zahn. Ztschr., *5:*1157, 1950.

111. ———: Die bedeutung der form und funktion der kiefergelenke fur die herstellung der totalen prothese (The importance of form and function of the temporomandibular joint), Dtsch. Zahn-Mund-Kieferh., *5:*24, 1938.

112. Steinhardt, G., and Langen: Vergleichende rontgenologische und anatomische untersuchungen am kiefergelenk (Comparative roentgenologic and anatomic examinations of the temporomandibular joint). Fortschr. Geb. Röntgenstr. Nauklearmed., Vol. *48,* 1933.

113. Thielemann, K.: Biomechanik der Paradentose (Biomechanics of Periodontosis). Munich, Barth, 1956.

114. Thompson, J. R.: Lectures to graduate class in orthodontics. Northwestern Univ., 1952.

115. Thonner, K. E.: Ett behandlat kakledsarthrosfall med horselforbattring (Therapy in temporomandibular joint arthrosis). Sven. Tandlak. Tidskr., *38:*751, 1945.

———: Nagot om karlanatomien i kakledsregionen och oat (The aural anatomy in the region of the temporomandibular joint). Sven. Tandlak, Tidskr., *39:*751, 1946.

———: Aural symptoms in relation to the temporomandibular joint. Acta Odont. Scand., *10:*180, 1953.

116. Thouren, G.: Om kakleden. Odont. Tidskr. *5:*112, 1941.

117. Tishler, B.: Occlusal habit neurosis. D. Cosmos, *70:*690, 1928.

118. Travell, J.: Early relief of chest pain by ethyl chloride spray in acute coronary thrombosis. Circulation, *3:*120, 1951.

119. ———: Factors affecting pain of injection. JAMA, *158:*368, 1955.

120. ———: Ethyl chloride spray for painful muscle spasm. Arch. Phys. Med., *33:*291, 1952.

121. ———: Rapid relief of acute "stiff neck" by ethyl chloride spray. J. Am. M. Women's Assoc., *4:*89, 1949.

122. ———: Referred pain from skeletal muscle. The pectoralis major syndrome of breast pain and soreness and the sternomastoid syndrome of headache and dizziness. New York State J. Med., *55:*331, 1955.

123. ———: *In* Ragan, C.: Connective Tissues. p. 86. New York, Macy, 1951.

124. Travell, J., and Bigelow, N. H.: Role of somatic trigger areas in the patterns of hysteria. Psychosom. Med., *9:*353, 1947.
125. Travell, J., and Rinzler, S. H.: The myofascial genesis of pain. Postgrad. Med., *11:*425, 1952.
126. Travell, J., and Weeks, V. D.: Postural vertigo due to trigger areas in the sternocleidomastoid muscle. J. Pediatr., *47:*315, 1955.
127. Warnekros, L.: Über die ursachen des fruhzeitigen verlustes der zahne (The causes of early loss of teeth). Berl. klin. Wchnschr., *25:* 1906.
128. White, T. C., Campbell, J., and Anderson, H.: An investigation into temporomandibular joint dysfunction. D. Rec., *72:*49, 1952.
129. Wolff, H. G.: Cerebral circulation, the action of amyl nitrate. Arch. Neurol. Psychiat., *22:*686, 1929.
130. ———: Headache and Other Pain. New York, Oxford, 1948.
131. Ibid.: p. 539.
132. ———: Headache and Other Head Pain. p. 499. New York, Oxford, 1963.
133. Ibid.: pp. 502–503.
134. Ibid.: p. 530.
135. Wrammer, T.: Studies on the effect of neostigmine on muscular symptoms in rheumatoid arthritis. Acta Med. Scand. (Suppl.), 242, 1950.
136. Wright, W. H.: Deafness as influenced by malposition of the jaws. JADA, *7:*979, 1920.
———: Some observations of jaw relationships to be considered during full denture construction. JADA, *9:*209, 1922.
137. Zimmer, E. A.: Die roentgenologie des kiefergelenkes (Radiography of the temporomandibular joint). Rev. Mens. Suisse Odont., *51:*949, 1941.

Additional Basic References

Manifestations of Pathologic Occlusion and Temporomandibular Joint Dysfunction

Alpert, R. L.: The temporomandibular joint pain dysfunction syndrome. J. South Carolina Med. Assoc., *68:*379–382, 1972.

Atwood, D. A.: A critique of research of the posterior limit of the mandibular position. J. Pros. Dent., *20:*21–36, 1968.

Boyle, P. E.: Traumatic occlusion in periodontics and as an etiologic factor in periodontal disease. New York J. Dent., *23:*316, 1953.

Chasen, A. I.: Occlusal disharmony and temporomandibular joint disturbances as a source of pain. J. D. Med., *12:*107, 1957.

Cobin, H. P.: The temporomandibular syndrome and centric relation. New York J. Dent., *18:*393, 1952.

Costen, J. B.: The mechanism of trismus and its occurrence in mandibular joint dysfunction. Ann. Otol. Rhinol. Laryngol., *48:*499, 1939.

———: Diagnosis of mandibular joint neuralgia and its place in general head pain, Ann. Otol. Rhinol. Laryngol., *53:*655, 1944.

Dawson, P. E.: Temporomandibular joint pain-dysfunction problems can be solved. J. Prost. Dent., *29:*100, 1973.

Dechaume, M., Poggioli, J. A., and Rouot, J.: The part played by a sympathetic nervous system in the pathogenesis of disorders resulting from dental malocclusion. Oral Surg., *6:*1047, 1953.

DeVanna, A.: Facial pain. New York State D. J., *54:*1684, 1954.

Eisenman, M.: Occlusal dysharmonies as related to cranial nerve syndromes, J. Am. Osteopath A., *54:*114, 1954.

Fleetwood, C. T.: The general physical improvement and soft tissue resulting from correction of traumatic occlusion and establishment of proper direction of functional forces. J. Can. D. A., *9:*543, 1943.

Friedman, A. P., Frazier, S. H., Jr., and Schultz, D. (ed.): The Headache Book. Dodd, Mead & Co., 1973.

Gerry, R. G.: Traumatic injuries of the temporomandibular joint. J. Oral Surg., *13:*232, 1955.

Hankey, G. T.; Ballard, F. C., and Storey, G. O.: Affection of the temporomandibular joint. Proc. R. Soc. Med., *49:*983, 1956.

Held, A. J.: Equilibration fonctionelle de la dentition par meulage (Functional equilibration of the dentition by grinding), Paradontologie., *66:*(2), 1948.

Kallenbach, T. E.: Effect of functional disorganization of the mouth and teeth: operative factors in reestablishment to normal. D. Cosmos *73:*759, 1931.

Loos, S.: Mechanik des Kiefergelenkes (Mechanics of the Temporomandibular Joint). Vienna, Urban, 1946.

Markowitz, H. A., and Gerry, R. G.: Temporomandibular joint disease. Oral Surg., *2:*1309, 1949.

Moulton, R. E.: Psychiatric considerations in maxillofacial pain. JADA, *51:*408, 1955.

Nadler, S. C.: Detection and recognition of bruxism. JADA, *61:*473, 1960.

Raginsky, B. B.: Psychosomatic dentistry, J. Can. D. A., *9:*914, 1954.

Ramfjord, S. P.: Bruxism, a clinical and electromyographic study. JADA, *62:*21, 1961.

———: Dysfunctional temporomandibular joint and muscle pain. J. Pros. Dent., *11:*353, 1961.

Riesner, S. E.: Head and facial pains associated with disturbances of the temporomandibular joints. New York J. Dent., *13:*65, 1947.

Russell, L. A., and Bayles, T. B.: The temporomandibular joint in rheumatoid arthritis. JADA, *28:*533, 1941.

Salman, I.: Traumatic injuries to the temporomandibular joint. J. Oral Surg., *7:*277, 1949.

Sicher, H.: Structure and functional basis for disorders of the temporomandibular articulation. J. Oral Surg., *13:*275, 1955.

Staz, J.: Disturbances of the temporomandibular articulation. J. D. A. South Africa, *3:*15, 1948.

Travell, J.: Temporomandibular joint pain referred from muscles of the head and neck. J. Prost. Dent., *10:*745, 1960.

Differential Diagnosis of Temporomandibular Joint Disease

Behrman, S.: Facial neuralgias. B. D. J., *86:*197, 1949.

Couch, C. D., Jr.: Facial pain. J. Oral Surg., *14:*216, 1956.

Friedman, A. P.: Modern Headache Therapy. St. Louis, C. V. Mosby, 1951.

Glaser, M. A.: Facial neuralgia, its etiology and treatment. JADA, *26:*1483, 1939.

Grant, F. C., Groff, R. A., and Levy, F. H.: Section of descending spinal root of fifth cranial nerve. Arch. Neurol. Psychiatr., *43:*493, 1940.

Harrigan, W. F.: Facial pain. Oral Surg., *5:*563, 1952.

Papper, E. M., and Rovenstine, E. A.: Pain syndromes of the face. Oral Surg., *1:*542, 1948.

Raney, R., Raney, A. A., and Hunter, C. R.: Treatment of major trigeminal neuralgia through section of the trigeminal tract in the medulla. Am. J. Surg., *80:*11, 1950.

Shapiro, H. H.: Differential diagnosis of oral pain. Oral Surg., *4:*1353, 1951.

10 Treatment of Temporomandibular Joint Arthrosis

The treatment of temporomandibular joint arthrosis requires simultaneous therapy to three major areas: the temporomandibular joint, the muscles and the teeth. The therapy consists of combinations of pharmaceutical, mechanical and other treatments to these areas as necessary. The treatment of each major area consists of direct and complementary therapy to the specific part.

The diagnosis of malfunction of any part in the major area forms the basis of the choice of therapy. In this section each therapy is discussed individually as to its administration, application, efficacy, precautions, etc.

Direct Therapy to the Joint

The direct drug therapy to the joint consists of the intra-articular injection of hyaluronidase, hydrocortisone acetate and sclerosing solutions, as needed in each particular case. Intra-articular injections of the temporomandibular joint require special procedures for each drug used.

Precautions for Temporomandibular Joint Injections

The capsule of the temporomandibular joint lies about 5 mm. below the skin, and the joint cavity extends beyond, to a depth of about 20 mm. Extreme precautions must be taken during intra-articular injections because of the curvature of the articulating surfaces and the presence of the superficial temporal branch of the external carotid artery. The artery lies about 5 mm. anterior to the auricle, immediately beneath the skin and on the temporal fascia. Care must be taken not to deposit the drug of choice periarticularly or into the superficial temporal branch of the external carotid artery. Pseudoparesthesia of areas supplied by the 7th nerve may occur because of the anesthetic that was infiltrated into the preauricular area. The signs of pseudoparesthesia on the affected side are facial asymmetry, paralysis of the muscles of expression and the lower eyelid, drooping of the corner of the mouth and tearing of the eye. The patient should be told that the affected side will return to normalcy as soon as the anesthetic has worn off.

As seen in Figure 10-1, the facial nerve can be found in many different positions, ranging from the masseter to the temporomandibular joint. It is important to understand that the injection of Xylocaine without epinephrine spreads quickly. If the nerve is affected, the palpebral muscles are anesthetized and the patient cannot blink his eyes. Seat the patient so anesthetized in a darkened room with a piece of facial tissue over the affected eye. If he leaves the office and the muscles are not permitted to close and protect it, the eye is vulnerable to injury.

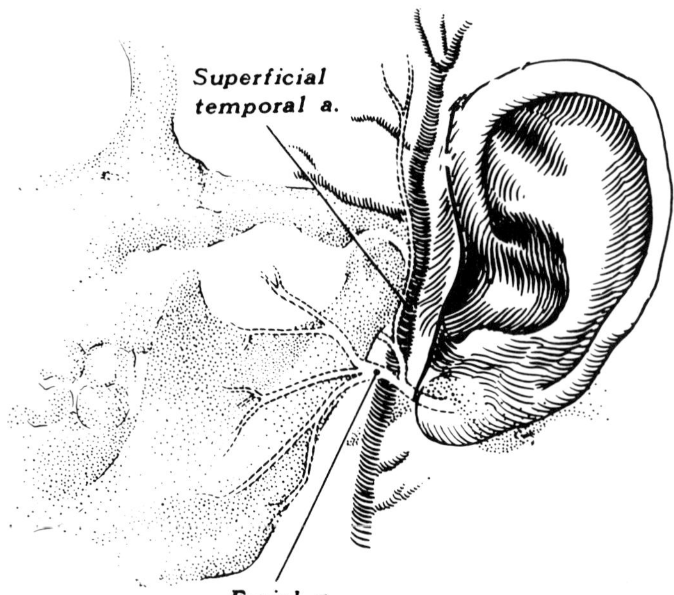

FIG. 10-1. Distribution of the facial nerve.

General Instructions

A preparatory sterile surgical technique is of paramount importance because of the possibility of infection to the joint and the other tissues in this area. The possibility of infection is minimized by careful observance of sterile procedure. For all intra-articular injections, no matter which drug is used, prepare the area of the temporomandibular joint that is to be injected as follows: shave, wash with germicidal soap and sterile water, sponge with colorless Zephiran chloride and drape with sterile linen. Use sterile gloves and autoclaved syringes and needles. The intra-articular joint injection can be rendered practically painless by preceding it with an injection of a local

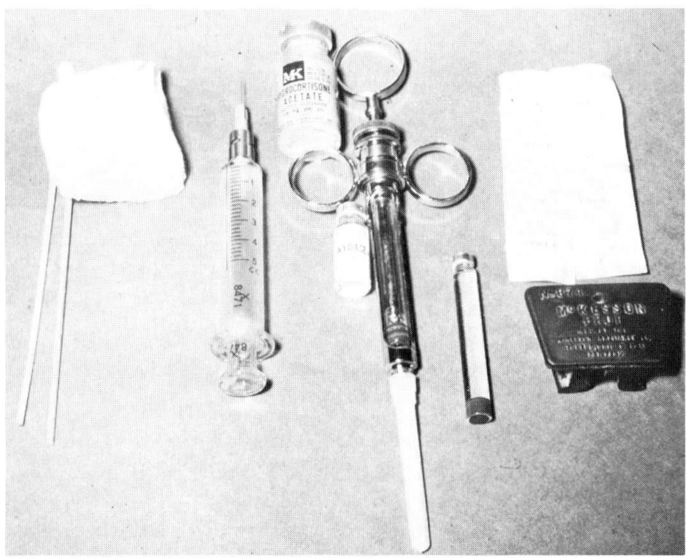

FIG. 10-2. The armamentarium necessary for injections of the temporomandibular joint are (*left to right*) sterile gauze pads; syringe with short needle for Xylocaine without epinephrine; ampule of hydrocortisone acetate; ampule of Wydase; Luer-lok syringe; carpule of Xylocaine; McKesson bite block.

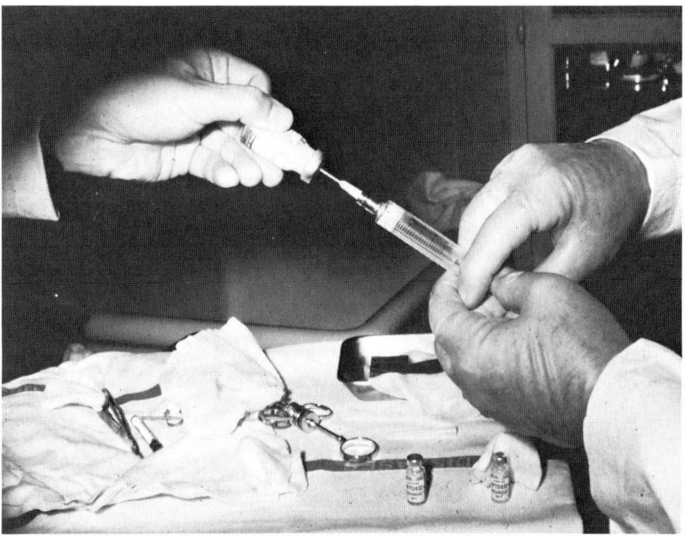

FIG. 10-3. Injecting hydrocortisone acetate into a vial of Wydase.

anesthetic without epinephrine into the soft tissues in the area around the joint. The specific injection technique of each drug is elaborated upon under the discussion of the drug. The armamentarium used in the injection process is shown in Figure 10-2.

Selection of Drugs for Injection

Hyaluronidase. Hyaluronic acid is a component of synovial fluid and the ground substance of connective tissue and is believed to be responsible for the increased viscosity of synovial fluid in pathologically involved joints.[13] It is believed that this alteration of the synovial fluid balance either influences or results from the pathological conditions within the joint. Hyaluronidase is a mucolytic enzyme which acts specifically on the hyaluronic acid portion of the intercellular ground substance and of the synovial fluid, depolymerizing and hydrolyzing it. Its action is purely local, and no systemic side effects attend its use.[9]

The use of hyaluronidase is indicated in temporomandibular joint arthrosis because its action within the joint: increases synovial permeability, lyses excessively viscous hyaluronic acid,[10] aids in reestablishing proper fluid balance in the synovial fluid and in the joint tissues and allows the tissues to return to a physiological state. Proper diagnosis is important because hyaluronidase must not be injected into tissue in the presence of bacterial infection. The use of hyaluronidase will institute and facilitate the retarded reconstruction of the synovial fluid and the damaged joint tissues. Hyaluronidase alleviates factors that delay healing but it does not itself cause healing. Relief of many of the symptoms of temporomandibular joint arthrosis, such as clicking noises, crepitus, pain in joints and muscles, decreased mandibular mobility, etc., may result from the intra-articular use of hyaluronidase.

Hyaluronidase is stable indefinitely in the dry state at room temperature or refrigerated, but in the soluble state it must be refrigerated. The dosage is 150 to 300 turbidity reducing units (TRU) per injection, depending upon the severity of the pain, the capacity of the upper chamber and the mobility of the joint. The patient experiences a slight warm to burning sensation during the injection.

It was found that 1 ml. of hyaluronidase and 1 ml. of hydrocortisone acetate in a double-injection technique produced

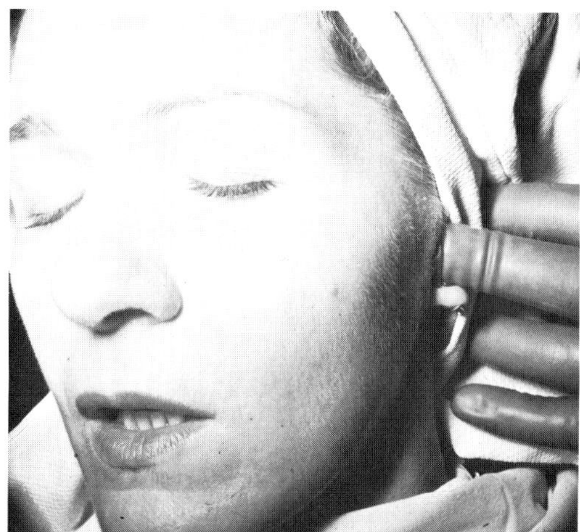

FIG. 10-4. The condyle is pushed out of the fossa prior to injection.

internal pressure to the capsule and resulted in postinjection pain. Injecting 1 ml. of hydrocortisone acetate into a 150 TRU vial of lyophilized hyaluronidase (Wydase) powder results in a total of 1.2 ml. of injectable material, which does not cause internal pressure within the joint (Fig. 10-3).

Xylocaine. The 2 per cent Xylocaine that is infiltrated into the area to provide anesthesia should not contain a vasoconstrictor, because vasoconstrictors are believed to counteract the effects of the enzyme. In addition to providing anesthesia for the hyaluronidase injection, it is used to break up the trigger zone in the capsule of the joint. Accidental injection of hyaluronidase directly into the bloodstream is quite harmless because its toxicity is minimal.[11] Others[13] have used a combination of procaine and hyaluronidase intra-articularly as the therapy.

Injection Technique. The injection, an exacting procedure, is as follows:

1. Have the patient open wide and close his mouth a few times, and note the movements of the condyle within the joint.
2. Wearing sterile rubber gloves, place your forefinger over the surgically prepared preauricular area as the patient opens and closes his mouth (Fig. 10-4).
3. Press inward and have the patient open wide.
4. Maintain finger pressure on this area for a minute or so and a depression will be evident which definitely locates the posterior portion of the capsule of the temporomandibular joint.
5. Infiltrate about ½ ml. of 2 per cent Xylocaine solution into the area (Fig. 10-5). Wait about 15 minutes before proceeding further.
6. Have the patient open wide, palpate as before and insert a mouth prop to keep the jaws apart and prevent reflex closure.
7. Using a 24-gauge, 1⅝-inch needle on a Luer-Lok syringe, insert the needle about 10 mm. in front of the external auditory meatus into the depressed area.
8. Direct the needle upward, inward and forward at an angle of approximately 45° (Fig. 10-6).
9. Insert the needle gently about 10 mm. into the joint capsule until resistance is met.
10. Withdraw the needle slightly and aspirate. If blood does not appear in the syringe, slowly inject the hyaluronidase.

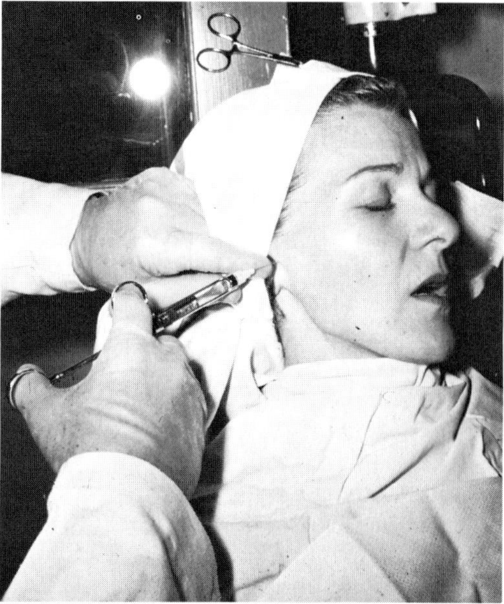

FIG. 10-5. Injection of Xylocaine into the joint.

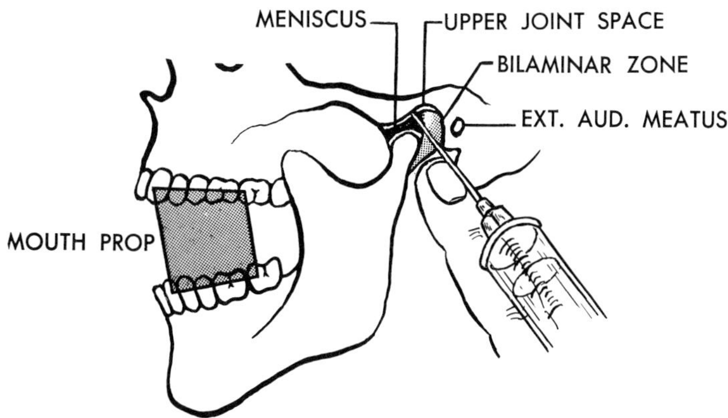

FIG. 10-6. The temporomandibular joint injection technique. (After Henny and Ivory)

11. Remove the needle and place a dressing over the puncture point.

12. Maintain pressure against the injected joint for 5 minutes. The extraoral pressure is necessary to increase and maintain the interstitial pressure within the joint.

The technique of this injection places the hyaluronidase in the upper joint space. A lower joint space injection is not necessary because of the "spreading factor" property of the enzyme.

The postinjection sequelae are slight to deep pain within the joint for a period of about 5 minutes, persistence of a feeling of tenderness and fullness for a day or two, complaint of a slight alteration in the occlusion, an absence of swelling, temperature and erythema. Sensitization to hyaluronidase occurs infrequently. The directions to the patient are to maintain soft diet until advised otherwise, and restrict mandibular movements during mastication, speech, yawning and laughing, for example.

Hydrocortisone Acetate. Injections of hydrocortisone acetate are effective for all noninfectious, inflammatory conditions of the temporomandibular joint. Besides its specific action for reducing the inflammation, it also reduces pain and trismus. If the condition of temporomandibular joint arthrosis is superimposed upon rheumatoid arthritis, hydrocortisone acetate is the specific drug of choice. Its action is temporary, and, if chronic irritations from occlusal disharmony persist or if other areas of arthritic conditions are not controlled, the pain is certain to return.

The treatment with hydrocortisone acetate consists of 0.5 to 1.0 ml. (10 to 25 mg.) sterile hydrocortisone acetate suspension U.S.P. injected with 150 TRU lyophilized hyaluronidase (Wydase) into the joint. A second or third injection at varying intervals is sometimes necessary to give full relief. Injection locally into the joint is the treatment of choice because the action is directed solely to the affected area, and all side effects from systemic administration are avoided. Intra-articular injections of the drug give relief of joint symptoms in rheumatoid arthritis for 4 to 7 days or more, but when osteoarthritis is present, one or two injections at weekly intervals may produce relief for 6 months.[3] Hydrocortisone acetate should be stored at room temperature since it may agglomerate at low temperature.

It is imperative to use a sterile injection technique because the joints to be injected are diseased and are less resistant to infection than normal joints. Contraindications for the intra-articular use of hydrocortisone acetate are the presence of active or questionably healed infectious diseases, such as tuberculosis and any of the infectious arthritides.

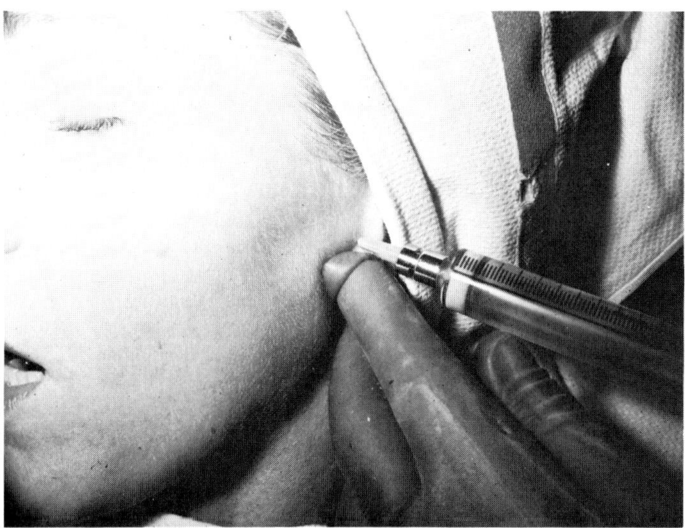

FIG. 10-7. Injection of hydrocortisone acetate and Wydase into the joint. *Note:* The condyle has been pushed forward.

The accuracy of the injection determines the efficacy of the treatment. The drug must enter the synovial cavity in order to affect the inflamed synovial tissue.

The injection technique is as follows:

1. Prepare the patient surgically as described previously in the hyaluronidase injection technique.
2. Create the depression which locates the posterior portion of the capsule.
3. After testing for possible blood vessel puncture, infiltrate 1 ml. of 2 per cent procaine at a depth of 3 mm. into the depressed area. Wait about 15 minutes before proceeding further.
4. Have the patient open wide, palpate as before and insert a mouth prop to keep the jaws apart and prevent reflex closure.
5. Using a 24-gauge, 1⅝-inch needle on a Luer-Lok syringe, insert the needle into the depressed area.
6. Direct the needle upward, inward and forward at an angle of approximately 45°.
7. Insert the needle about 10 mm. until the roof of the glenoid fossa is struck.
8. Withdraw the needle 1 mm., aspirate, and if blood does not appear in the syringe, inject 0.5 ml. of hydrocortisone acetate (Fig. 10-7).
9. Withdraw the needle, place a dressing on the puncture point, and maintain pressure on the site of the injection for a minute or so as the patient gently moves the mandible.

Complementary Therapy to the Joint

The complementary therapy to the direct treatment of the joint is heat and rest.

Heat. The application of moist heat to the joint area will dilate the blood vessels, thus bringing more blood to the area and hastening healing. The heat will also aid in the relief of pain. The heat application is carried out as follows:

1. Dip a heavy towel in boiling water; wring out well and apply to the painful area.
2. After the loss of the original heat, reprepare and reapply the towel.
3. Keep the water as hot as possible.
4. Carry out the procedure for 5 minutes every half hour, for 2 hours (i.e., 4 times in 2 hours). After an interval of 4 hours, repeat, if necessary.

Rest. As has been mentioned, rest after injection therapy is important. The patient should avoid strain to the area by elimi-

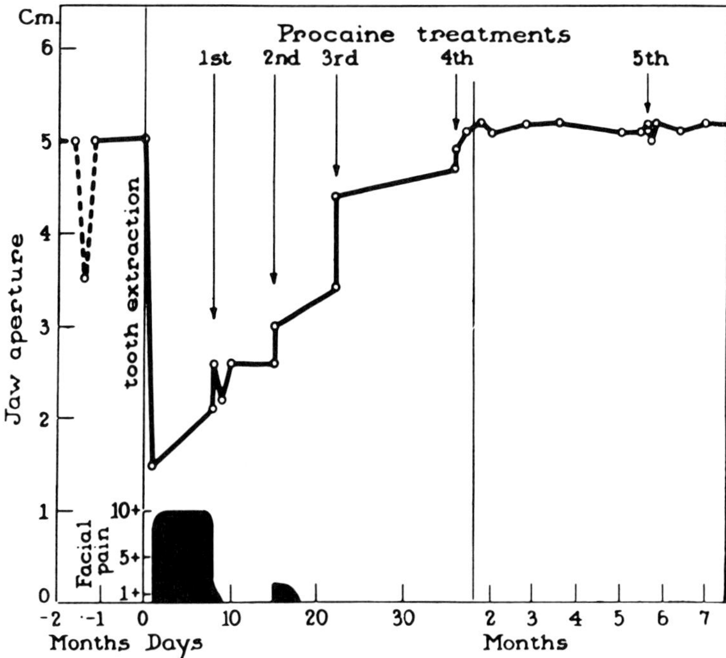

FIG. 10-8. Response of pain (*black*) and limited motion (*heaviest line*) to procaine infiltration of trigger areas in a case of acute trismus following tooth extraction. (Travell, J.: *In* Ragan, C.: Connective Tissues. p. 114. New York, Macy, 1951)

nating excessive mandibular movements and excessive masticatory forces.

Direct Treatment to the Muscles

The direct treatment of the spastic musculature is the injection of Xylocaine without epinephrine (Xylocaine with epinephrine causes muscle contraction) and the external use of ethyl chloride spray.

Xylocaine. As explained previously, Xylocaine infiltration into the areas of muscle spasm and trigger areas will interrupt the cycles of noxious stimuli, muscle spasm and referred pain and therefore result in symptomatic relief. Xylocaine is infiltrated into the trigger areas of the muscles in spasm which cause limited mandibular movement and local and referred pain. To avoid ischemia to the muscles the Xylocaine solution should not contain vasoconstrictors. The advantages of Xylocaine are that minimal strength and concentration produce beneficial effects, and practically no toxic effects result from its use.

Figure 10-8 illustrates the typical effects following local block of trigger areas in the masseter muscle of a patient with acute trismus. Note that the infiltration was repeated at intervals of several days and that there was an immediate slight increase in the interincisal distance and total relief of pain. The case proceeded in a stepwise manner, as indicated in the figure. The clinical results were the relief of pain and improvement in the range of motion.

Trigger areas may also be blocked by infiltration with normal saline and by thorough peppering of the area with a dry needle. However, Travell has stated, ". . . that in clinical experience, the order of efficiency would be procaine first, saline next and needling last."[22] Xylocaine, saline and dry needling all cause an intense momentary pain in the trigger

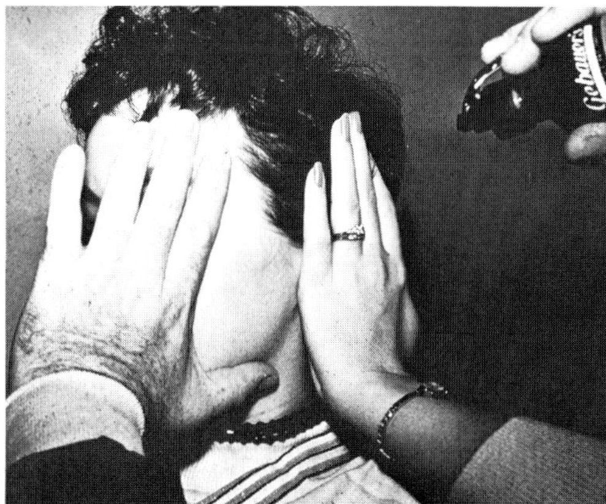

FIG. 10-9. The proper method of spraying ethyl chloride. (After Travell, J.)

area when one of these is used to break the neural cycle from the trigger area to the reference zone.

The temporal, masseter, and the internal and the external pterygoid muscles are the muscles of mastication which may contain trigger areas that necessitate blockage in order to ameliorate trismus and gain rapid relief from pain. The technique for each muscle is specific. After the patient is prepared surgically, use a 25-gauge, 1⅝-inch needle in a Luer-Lok syringe for the injection (as for all injections). Instruct the patient to move his jaw repeatedly and gently after the injection.

The temporal muscle injection is performed with the mouth closed and with the teeth in contact. Palpate for the trigger point and inject upward and inward at a 45° angle a distance of 5 to 10 mm., depending on the thickness of the tissues.

The masseter presents three possible trigger sites that may need blocking: the origin, the body and the insertion. All blocking is performed with the mouth closed and the teeth touching. The depth of needle penetration is 5 to 10 mm. The trigger zone at the origin is injected upward and inward at an angle of 45°. The trigger zone in the body is grasped between the thumb and the forefinger and infiltrated in the same manner. The trigger zone at the insertion is injected in the same manner as the trigger zone at the origin.

The internal pterygoid injection is performed with the mouth closed and the teeth touching. The forefinger of the free hand is pressed on the neck below the angle of the mandible. The needle is inserted at the medial side of the angle of the mandible and is directed upward at an angle of 45° to a depth of 10 to 15 mm., depending on the thickness of the tissues.

The external pterygoid injection is performed with the mouth kept open by a rubber bite block inserted on the side opposite the muscle to be injected. Insert the needle into the mucosa 10 mm. posterior to the hamular notch. Direct the needle upward and backward so that the procaine is deposited in the body of the muscle. The possible postinjection sequel is a feeling of fullness within the muscles.

Ethyl Chloride. Ethyl chloride spray is used as a counterirritant to interrupt and block muscle spasm and referred pains. It is often effective in producing blockage of the spasm and the pain without itself producing the pain that can occur with Xylocaine. The ethyl chloride spray technique may be used for pain and spasm in the temporal, the masseter and the sternocleidomastoid muscles and in the temporomandibular joint trigger area.

The technique of application is based upon the procedures as outlined by Travell, Kraus, and others.[14,19,21,22,24] It is imperative to control the application of the ethyl chloride so that only the relevant structures are sprayed. The seated patient places the hand of the side to be sprayed on one side of the muscle to be sprayed, and the operator places a towel on the other side of the muscle, in this manner limiting the area to be sprayed and protecting the rest of the head. Hold the container at an acute angle to the patient at a distance of 2 feet (Fig. 10-9). Apply the spray very lightly with rhythmic movements in a sweeping manner that should produce very little cooling. Start the spray on the trigger area and lightly sweep over the reference zones as the patient repeatedly moves his jaw. If the pain is not diminished, spray the area again. Do not frost the sprayed area, because a frosted area on the skin will produce pain, erythema and possibly a dermatitis. Travell emphasizes that "there are two features in the mechanism of action of ethyl chloride spray, used in this manner: intermittent cold, and intermittent touch."[23] Both features tend to break up the cycle of noxious impulses.

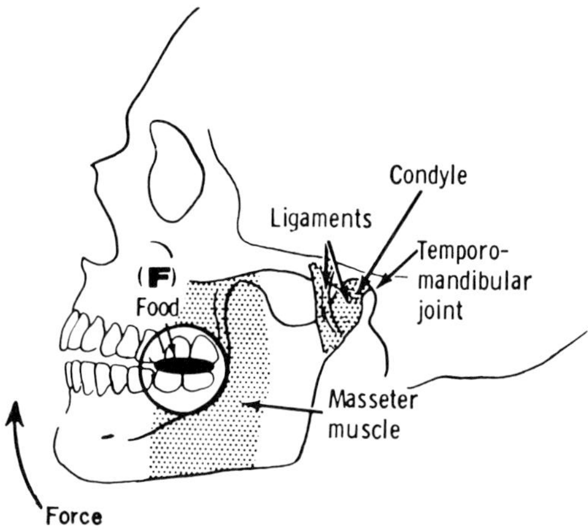

FIG. 10-10. The left side of the skull with the jaws slightly open. Note the temporomandibular joint and its components, and the relationship of the joint to the masseter muscle. The large arrow indicates the direction in which the masseter muscle pulls upward when chewing a piece of food (*F*).

Complementary Treatment to the Muscles and Ligaments

The complementary therapy to the muscles and ligaments consists of alterations in dietary and mouth-opening habits, exercises, and the use of muscle relaxants and heat.

Mastication and Mouth-Opening Habits

Almost invariably, patients with temporomandibular joint dysfunction suffer from stretched, and bruised joint ligaments (See Chap. 5 for a discussion of the anatomy of the ligaments associated with the temporomandibular joint). Restoration of normal function to the ligaments is aided by the avoidance of hard, chewy foods. Patient cooperation in making a drastic change in eating habits can be secured only through a full explanation of the rationale behind the request.

When a patient with a weakened temporomandibular joint mechanism tries to chew a piece of hard food, as the masseter pulls up, normal mastication cannot take place. Instead, because the joint is weak, the food acts as a fulcrum, forcing the joint open. The result of this temporary subluxation is severe and intense pain throughout the face and head. This process is diagrammed in Figure 10-10.

In explaining this situation to the

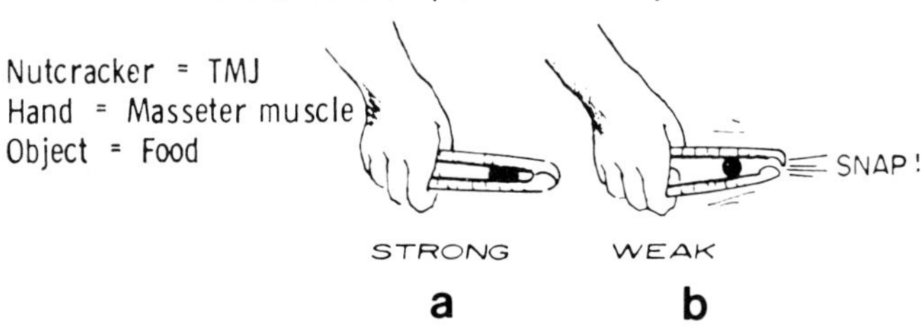

FIG. 10-11. The way in which the temporomandibular joint (*TMJ*) works when chewing a piece of hard food can best be illustrated by its comparison with a nutcracker. The nutcracker is strong and crushes the nut (*a*). The mechanism (nutcracker) is weak. Instead of cracking the nut, the nutcracker itself comes apart (*b*).

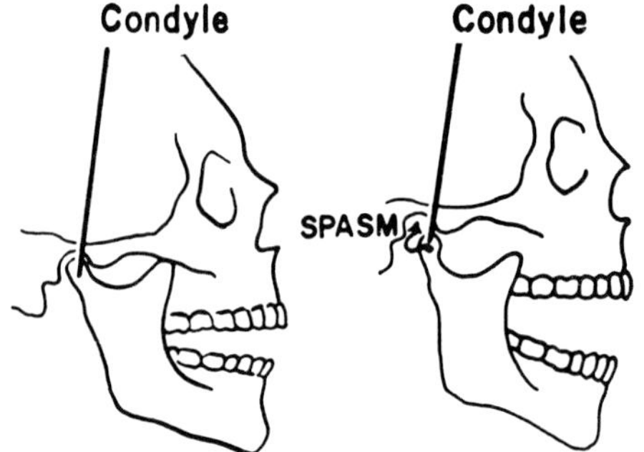

FIG. 10-12. Muscle spasm takes place when a person with stretched (abnormal) ligaments bites off a piece of food with the front teeth. Note that the condyle is brought to the front of the eminence. Because of uncoordinated contraction, the lateral pterygoids go into spasm.

patient it may be valuable to draw an analogy between the mechanism of the temporomandibular joint and that of a nutcracker (Fig. 10-11). The strong nutcracker crushes the nut; but the weak one comes apart at the hinge. Tell the patient that in the temporomandibular joint this kind of process entails a progressive stretching, weakening, and bruising of the supporting ligaments.

A similar situation arises when a person with temporomandibular joint dysfunction bites off a piece of hard food with his front teeth. Because his ligaments are badly stretched, they cannot help to guide the condyle back into the glenoid fossa in a smooth, coordinated

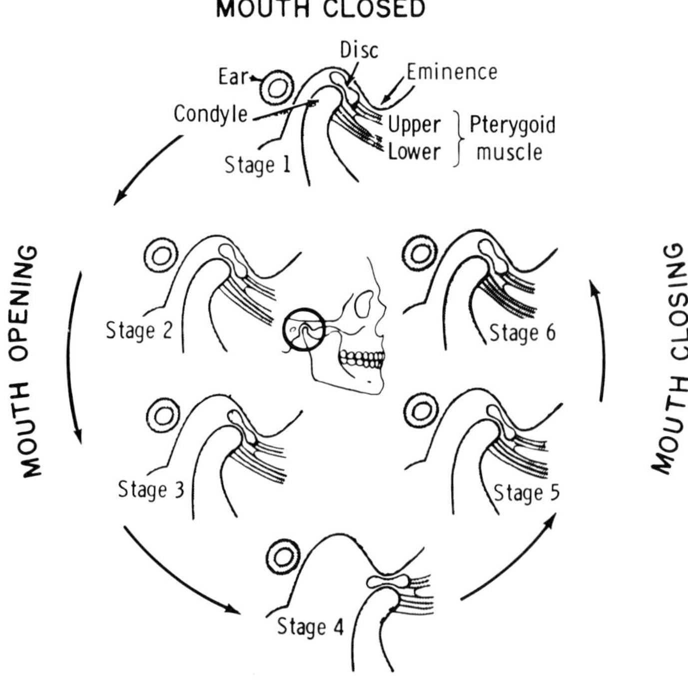

FIG. 10-13. Various stages of a normal right temporomandibular joint (area within the circle of center drawing of skull) as the jaw opens and closes the mouth. Stage 1: The components of the joint are in the resting position with the mouth closed. Note that the condyle rests on the disc. Stages 2 and 3: The upper and lower parts of the external pterygoid muscle pull the condyle and disc forward in coordination as the mouth opens slightly. Stage 4: The condyle, still resting on the center of the disc, is shown as it appears when the jaw is wide open. Stage 5: This is similar to Stage 3, except that the jaw is now beginning to close. Stage 6: This is like Stage 2 with the jaw closed further.

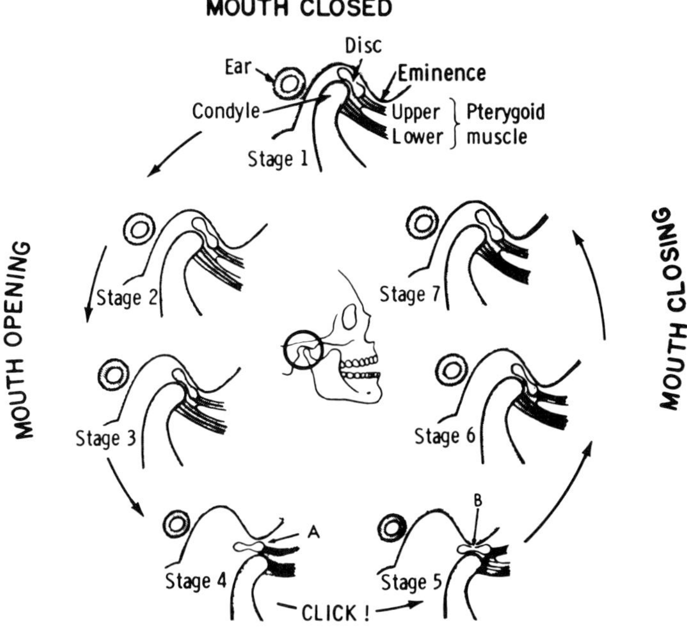

FIG. 10-14. Various stages of abnormal (spastic) right temporomandibular joint as the jaw opens and closes the mouth. The upper and lower parts of the external pterygoid muscles are functioning incoordinately. Stage 4: The condyle is remaining in its place in the center of the disc, as in Stages 2 and 3, instead of riding on the thickened outer edge of the disc (*A*). Stage 5: (Fully open position of the jaw) The disc snaps forward into place (*B*) producing the click. Stages 6 and 7: These correspond to Stages 2 and 3 except that the jaw is closing.

fashion. As shown in Figure 10-12, the lateral pterygoids go into spasm and the condyle returns to the fossa accompanied by an erratic, wavy movement of the jaw, often associated with clicking and intense pain. Thus, advise the patient to avoid all hard, brittle or chewy foods, to cut his food into bite-sized pieces, and to chew slowly and carefully with his back teeth. If he is conscientious in following the prescribed change in diet, the result will be a marked diminution of pain and spasm, and the ligaments will gradually regain their elasticity.

Chapter 8 provides a detailed discussion of the mechanisms contributing to the clicking, crepitation and muscular spasm observed in temporomandibular joint dysfunction. Again, sound patient education in the mechanics of the problem provides the key to successful treatment. Clicking results from incoordinate contraction of the two bodies of the lateral pterygoids (see p. 141), so that the disc snaps over the condyle rather than following its movements smoothly and coordinately. Figures 10-13 and 10-14 contrast the relationship of condyle, disc, and pterygoid during mouth opening in the normal or in the abnormal case. At Stage 3 (Fig. 10-14), the condyle and disc still bear the correct relation to each other. At Stage 4, the condyle slides over the articular eminence, but because of incoordinate contraction of the lateral pterygoids, the disc lags behind. It is in the progression from Stages 4 to 5 that clicking occurs,

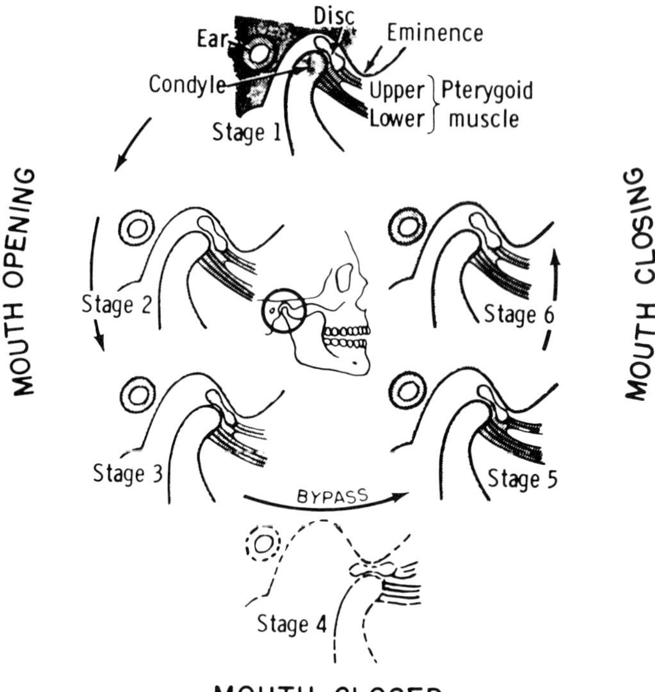

FIG. 10-15. Modified stages of opening and closing the mouth to avoid clicking. By bypassing Stage 4, the upper and lower parts of the lateral pterygoid muscle move in harmony with one another and, thus, prevent the condyle from riding on the thickened edge of the disc and producing the click.

as the spastic pterygoid causes the disc to snap forward into its proper place over the center of the condyle. Therefore, if Stage 4 is bypassed (Fig. 10-15), the disc will remain in contact with the condyle and clicking will be prevented. Explain the entire sequence of events to the patient (diagrams such as the ones in this text are extremely helpful), and instruct him never to open his mouth wider than the thickness of his thumb.

Muscle Exercises

As an adjunct to the injection therapy for the purpose of increasing limited mandibular movement, exercises involving the muscles of mastication are employed. They are used, on the one hand, to help break up the muscle spasm and, on the other hand, to maintain and increase the limited jaw movement to full physiological function, whenever muscle spasm or trismus has been a part of the joint arthrosis symptoms.[14,19] Muscle exercise may be employed for two basic reasons: to increase or maintain physiological elasticity of the muscles, and to increase the power ability of a muscle. In joint arthrosis, the interest lies first with restoring physiological elasticity, then with restoring muscle power. Exercise should be performed under painless conditions. As mentioned previously, local anesthetics and other drugs may be injected into muscles and into the joint area whenever muscle spasm, trismus and joint pain occur. These therapeutic measures free the functioning areas from pain and permit freer muscle movement.

Two exercises have proved particularly

effective in increasing the extent of mouth opening in cases of severely limited mandibular movement. The first is the finger–thumb exercise, prescribed for the patient who can barely open his mouth.

> ***Finger-Thumb Exercise***
>
> Place your thumb on the biting edge of the upper incisors and your forefinger on the biting edge of the lower incisors.
>
> With slight pressure, force the teeth and jaws apart until minimal pain is encountered.
>
> Repeat the exercise for 30 seconds every 2 hours (especially during times of relaxation such as when watching television or reading).

If this program is followed consistently, the extent of jaw opening gradually increases.

When the patient is able to open his mouth painlessly to the extent of 12 mm., initiate another regimen, the cork exercise. Cut a cork about 3 cm. long so that its upper and lower surfaces are flat and it tapers from a width of 30 mm. at the wide end to 15 mm. at the narrow end (Fig. 10-16).

Instruct the patient in the procedure for the cork exercise.

> ***Cork Exercise***
>
> Gradually insert the small end of a tapered cork into your mouth until your jaws are separated and you begin to feel pain in the jaw joints and muscles.
>
> Leave the cork in place for 30 seconds before removing it. Repeat this procedure every 2 hours.

When the initial pain disappears, the patient places the cork farther into his mouth, thus opening the jaws slightly wider—again, only to the point of invoking slight pain. Eventually, if the routine is carried out in accord with instructions, the total range of jaw opening will be increased to the extent of 30 mm. (Fig. 10-17).

The author does not advocate the forceful spread of the jaws because of the possibility of inducing fractures of the teeth and sprains and tears in soft tissues, the muscles and the joints; nor does he advocate that the exercises be performed to the point of inducing more than slight pain.

Once acute pain and spasm have lessened, more direct therapy to the muscles can be initiated. When the temporomandibular joint and its associated ligaments and musculature are functioning harmoniously, the mandible is automatically retruded during mouth opening. When the muscles and ligaments are weakened, the patient can be taught to retrude the mandible consciously through training and exercise of the suprahyoid muscles (see Chap. 5 for the anatomy of this group of muscles). The therapy proceeds as follows.

Instruct the patient to first do the exercise in front of a mirror. He must keep his mouth closed with his teeth touching lightly, and the supraphyoids flexed (Fig. 10-18). The patient will be able to see the actual contraction if he is doing the exercise properly. If the procedure is followed accurately, the jaw will be retruded. The patient is told to repeat the exercise 3 times every hour.

When the patient has mastered this exercise, tell him to try contracting the suprahyoids in the same manner but with the mouth slightly open. Each day he should gradually increase the extent of mouth opening. If the procedure is followed accurately, the condyle will remain in its normal place in the center of the disc. Eventually the practice will become second nature and the patient will be able to open his mouth to the normal extent of 35 to 45 mm.

The advantage of these exercises is that

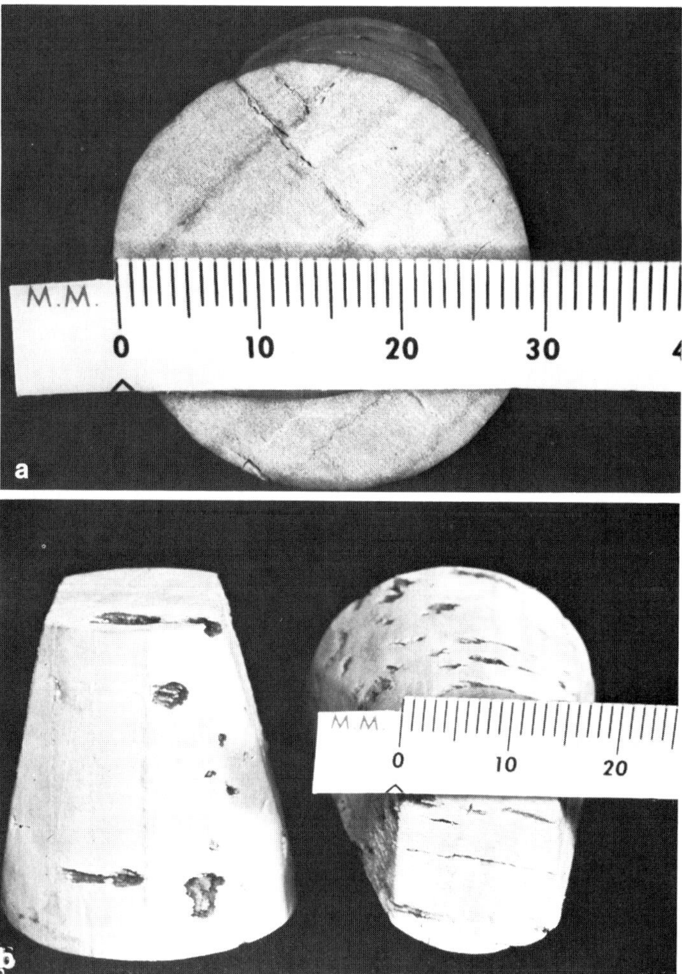

FIG. 10-16. For the cork exercise, the cork is 30 mm. at its widest end (*a*); it is 15 mm. at its narrowest (*b*).

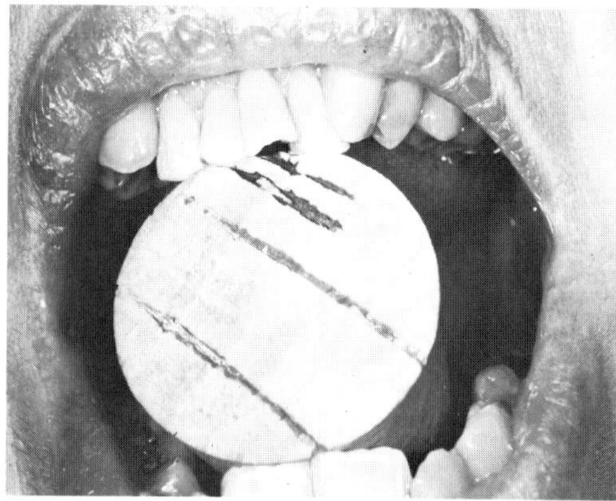

FIG. 10-17. Total range of jaw opening has been increased to 30 mm.

the spastic muscles are permitted to rest and clicking is eliminated; consequently, there is no strain on the lateral pterygoid muscles. The lateral pterygoids then function in neuromuscular harmony, as they were intended to do, and the pathological neuromuscular pattern of function is replaced by a normal pattern.

Pharmacological Agents

The emotional stress induced by physical illness is far more important than is realized. Every illness is a stress situation which potentially can traumatize and threaten the psychological equilibrium of

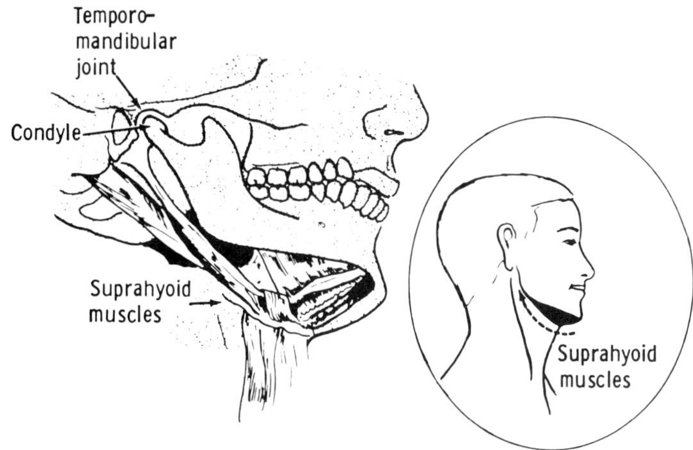

FIG. 10-18. The suprahyoid muscles, showing their location under the chin, and their relationship to the temporomandibular joint.

the patient. The anxiety of the patient can aggravate and heighten the symptomatology of temporomandibular joint arthrosis and can create additional somatic disturbances. This self-induced state sometimes incapacitates the patient far more than the original symptoms of the arthrosis (see Chap. 7). A muscle relaxant which can be used in ambulatory treatment for neuromuscular hypertension and can exert its therapeutic effect without hindering the daily activities of the patient has its proper place as an adjunct to the other therapy for temporomandibular joint arthrosis. Control of emotional stress, because it can check night grinding, clenching and other neurotic habits, appreciably extends the dentist's therapeutic scope. The duration of treatment for temporomandibular joint arthrosis makes optimal control of emotional stress vitally important.

The management of facial pain, in particular temporomandibular joint pain due to muscular spasm, has been greatly advanced with the advent of the ataraxics. These drugs merit careful consideration by the dental profession.

However, some general cautionary procedures must be followed. It is absolutely necessary to take a careful history of the patient. Know exactly what medication he is currently taking and elicit such information as his drinking habits (ingestion of alcohol may be very dangerous if a CNS-acting drug is being taken simultaneously). Since any ataraxic may cause confusion or drowsiness, caution the patient receiving such a drug against driving a car or operating machinery. If long-term therapy is indicated, take liver function tests and complete blood counts periodically.

Thoroughly familiarize yourself with the action, side effects, and possible adverse reactions of all analgesics, sedatives, and muscle relaxants. Such information can be found in detail in any good textbook of pharmacology or therapeutics, as well as in the appropriate section of the *Physicians' Desk Reference*. As L. E. Francis observes, "It must be kept in mind that all drugs are dangerous substances, but the dangers are lessened when the clinician is completely cognizant of the facts of both his drugs and his patients."[6]

Muscle Relaxants. Muscle relaxants or lissives are drugs that alleviate muscle spasm, anxiety and tension. A muscle relaxant that has proved useful in dentistry is diazepam (Valium).

Valium is a minor tranquilizer of the benzodiazepine group. It apparently acts on the thalamus and hypothalamus, and does not exhibit peripheral autonomic blocking effects. It has the property of reducing muscle spasm while alleviating underlying emotional components such as anxiety, tension and fear. This twofold action makes it a particularly effective adjunct in the treatment of temporomandibular joint arthrosis. Side effects are usually minimal but may include fatigue, drowsiness and ataxia. The drug is contraindicated in patients with acute narrow angle glaucoma. Occasionally, paradoxical adverse reactions have been encountered, such as hyperexcited states, anxiety, rage, sleep disturbances, or increased muscle spasticity. If any of these occur, the drug should be discontinued immediately.

Valium should not be administered in conjunction with drugs that may potentiate its action, such as phenothiazines, narcotics, barbiturates, and the antidepressant drugs known as MAO (monoamine oxidase) inhibitors.

Dosage: The initial dose of Valium is usually 1 mg. after each meal and 2 mg. before retiring—a total of 5 mg. per day. The clinical response of the patient determines whether the dose shall be adjusted up or down. For instance, if the initial dose is too small, it is increased to 2.5 mg. three times a day and 5 mg. at bedtime.

Chlorzoxazone with acetaminophen (Parafon Forte) is useful in providing relief of pain, stiffness, and limitation of motion associated with muscle spasm. Unlike Valium, it does not have a tranquilizing effect. Chlorzoxazone is a centrally acting skeletal muscle relaxant, apparently acting at the spinal cord level and in the subcortical areas of the brain, where it inhibits multisynaptic reflex arcs involved in producing and maintaining skeletal muscle spasm. Acetaminophen provides an analgesic effect supplementing the pain relief due to muscle relaxation.

Dosage: The usual dose is 1 tablet after each meal and before retiring.

Valium and Parafon Forte are usually prescribed simultaneously for temporomandibular joint patients. The two act synergistically extremely well, providing a greater measure of relief than either is capable of producing alone.

Chlorphenesin carbamate (Maolate) may be used if Valium and Parafon Forte prove ineffective, or if the patient reacts adversely to either drug. It has been shown in double-blind clinical trials to be effective in relieving the discomfort associated with skeletal muscle trauma and inflammation. Generally it is very well tolerated; adverse reactions such as dizziness or nausea are both rare and mild. Maolate should not be administered in conjunction with any barbiturate.

Dosage: The starting dose is 400 mg. four times daily; this dose can be increased if necessary to 800 mg. (2 tablets) three times daily until a positive response is effected; the patient can then be continued on a lower, maintenance dosage.

Meprobamate (Equanil) is not as widely used as it once was in dentistry, but, like Maolate, it may be valuable in treating patients who do not tolerate or respond to Valium treatment. It has a selective action on the thalamus and a blocking action on the spinal interneurons, action which influences neuromuscular coordination and lessens psychic tension.[2] It does not affect the autonomic functions.[1] Muscle spasm and rigidity are reduced, and nervous tension is allayed.[4,5,8] Meprobamate is well tolerated, non-habit forming and usually free from side effects. The only side effect frequently reported is drowsiness. If the dosage is reduced, the drowsiness will disappear with continued use. In a few cases excitement rather than relaxation has occurred.[16] A rare allergic reaction has been reported which may be associated with fever, angioneurotic edema, faintness or bronchospasm, and use of the drug should be discontinued immediately. For those patients who are to receive long-term therapy, complete blood counts should be performed.

Dosage: Meprobamate is administered orally in tablets of 400 mg. each. The starting dose is 1 tablet three times a day and, if indicated, 1 before retiring. The clinical response of the patient determines whether the dose shall be adjusted up or down.

Carisoprodol, or isopropyl meprobamate (Soma) is a potent skeletal relaxant which acts specifically on interneurons to relieve muscle spasm, pain and stiffness. The only usual side effect is drowsiness. Like Maolate and Equanil, it is used only for those patients who do not tolerate or respond to Valium.

Dosage: 350 mg. (1 tablet) four times a day.

Other muscle relaxants occasionally used as adjuncts in the treatment of temporomandibular joint dysfunction include Robaxin and Trancopal.

Methocarbamol (Robaxin) is a skeletal muscle relaxant that exerts a selective action on the CNS, resulting in a diminution of skeletal muscle hyperactivity without alteration of normal muscle tone. Side effects are rare and usually minor, but may include drowsiness and mild nausea.

Dosage: An initial oral daily dose of 6 g. for 2 or 3 days is suggested; thereafter, a maintenance dose of 4 g. (in divided doses).

Chlormezanone (Trancopal) is a nonhypnotic muscle relaxant and tranquilizer that acts on the CNS and peripherally on the neuromusculature. Side effects are rare (occurring in less than 3 per cent of patients), but may include drowsiness, drug rash, nausea, and depression.

Dosage: The usual adult oral dose is 200 mg. three or four times daily, but some patients can obtain relief of symptoms from half that dose.

Imipramine hydrochloride (Tofranil) is a potent antidepressant with mild muscle relaxant properties. It is primarily a psychotherapeutic drug and is used in the treatment of the muscle spasm of temporomandibular joint dysfunction only in the rare event that other specific muscle relaxants are ineffective or cause serious adverse reactions. Obtain the advice of the patient's physician before initiating Tofranil therapy.

Dosage: 25 mg. (1 tablet) after each meal and before retiring.

Other Tranquilizers. Two very commonly prescribed tranquilizers are chlordiazepoxide hydrochloride (Librium) and chlordiazepoxide hydrochloride and clidinium bromide (Librax). The latter combines the antianxiety effects of Librium with the gastrointestinal antispasmodic effects of clidinium bromide (Quarzan), but is contraindicated in patients with glaucoma. Adverse reactions include dizziness, drowsiness, ataxia and confusion, especially in elderly patients. Less common side effects are skin eruptions, edema, nausea and constipation. Occasional cases of blood dyscrasias, including agranulocytosis, jaundice and hepatic dysfunction have been reported.

Analgesics. In addition to the muscle relaxants, various analgesics are valuable in treating the pain associated with temporomandibular joint arthrosis.

Throughout the history of man's attempt to relieve pain and its associated suffering, probably the most consistently effective, widely used, and least dangerous drug yet discovered is acetylsalicylic acid: aspirin. It acts as an antipyretic and anti-inflamatory agent as well as an analgesic. Francis states: "It may raise the threshold for pain stimuli relayed from the thalamus to the cerebral cortex. There is also much evidence that acetylsalicylic acid may be effective in modifying the cause of pain at the site of origin. Edema and pain are reduced at the same time. There are some people who may have an idiosyncrasy to acetylsalicylic acid; upon ingestion of the drug they show an allergic response such as edema of the lips, tongue and eyelids, or skin rash. The main side effects are nausea, vomiting and diarrhea. These are caused mainly by local irritation of gastric mucosa.

Dosage: Orally, 300–600 mg. (i.e., one

or two 5 gr. tablets) every 3 hours as necessary. No greater analgesic effect is achieved by a dose greater than 600 mg."[7]

Acetaminophen (Tylenol) is recommended for the individual who exhibits an idiosyncratic reaction to aspirin, or whose medical history is one of gastric ulcer, past or present. Many physicians also feel that aspirin is contraindicated if the patient is taking a corticosteroid.

Dosage: 2 tablets (325 mg. each) every 4 hours.

A similar and also frequently used analgesic is the coal-tar derivative phenacetin. Its effects are similar to those of aspirin; however, it is thought to be more toxic.

Codeine phosphate, aspirin, phenacetin, and caffeine (Empirin with codeine) is useful in the management of pain that cannot be relieved by aspirin or phenacetin alone. Codeine is a narcotic agent effective in relieving moderate pain; its analgesic action is supplemented by the calming effect which it exerts on the patient. The drug may be habit forming, and long-term therapy is not advisable.

Dosage: 1 tablet (either ⅛ or ¼ gr. codeine, depending on severity of pain) three times daily, as needed.

Propoxyphene hydrochloride (Darvon) is a mild analgesic structurally related to methadone. It is commonly prescribed for the relief of mild to moderate pain. Although related to the narcotic analgesics, it is considerably less potent. Darvon has the potential for creating psychological and, occasionally, physical dependence and tolerance, and should be used with care. Adverse reactions may include dizziness, sedation, nausea and vomiting.

Dosage: The usual adult dose is 65 mg. orally every 4 hours as needed.

Oxycodone hydrochloride, oxycodone terephthalate, aspirin, phenacetin, and caffeine (Percodan) is an analgesic and sedative that may be used to relieve moderate to moderately severe pain. The principal analgesic agent, oxycodon, is a semisynthetic narcotic with qualitative effects similar to those of morphine (more potent than codeine). It should be used with caution in patients receiving other narcotic analgesics, tranquilizers, sedatives, the phenothiazines, or any CNS-depressant agent. Adverse reactions may include light-headedness, dizziness, nausea and vomiting. As with any narcotic agent, long-term therapy is inadvisable because of the risk of establishing tolerance as well as physical and psychological dependence on the drug.

Dosage: The usual adult dose is 1 tablet every 6 hours as needed to relieve pain.

Meperidine hydrochloride (Demerol) is a synthetic narcotic analgesic and sedative useful in alleviating moderate to severe pain. As with Percodan, extreme caution must be exercised if the drug is administered to patients receiving other narcotic analgesics, tranquilizers, phenothiazines, sedatives or any other CNS depressant. It should not be administered to patients who have received MAO inhibitors. Demerol should not be used on a long-term basis, again because of the potential for developing dependence (physical and psychological) and drug tolerance. Respiratory depression, light-headedness, dizziness, dryness of the mouth, sweating, nausea, vomiting and constipation may occur; however, if present, these adverse reactions usually disappear with smaller doses.

Dosage: The usual adult dose is 50 to 150 mg. orally every 3 to 4 hours, depending on the severity of the pain.

Butalbital, caffeine, aspirin and phenacetin (Fiorinal) tablets are used for the treatment of nonlocalized headache pain. Butalbital is a mild sedative and supplements the action of aspirin and phenacetin. Because butalbital may be habit forming, prolonged therapy with Fiorinal is not recommended.

Dosage: The usual adult dose is 1 tablet every 4 hours, as needed.

Phenobarbital, ergotamine tartrate, and levorotatory alkaloids of belladonna (Bellergal Spacetabs) may be used to alleviate recurrent, throbbing head pain. Bellergal has an inhibitory effect on the sympathetic and parasympathetic nervous systems, as well as on the cortical centers. Although it may be highly effective in relieving head pain, it can be habit forming, and long-term therapy is not advised.

Dosage: The usual adult dose is ½ tablet twice a day and 1 tablet before retiring, or as needed.

Indomethacin (Indocin) possesses specific advantages in the symptomatic treatment of pain associated with joint inflammation in rheumatoid arthritis, ankylosing spondylitis, degenerative joint disease of the hip and gout. It has anti-inflammatory, antipyretic, and analgesic properties; and, when indicated, is suitable for long-term therapy. Adverse reactions may include headache, dizziness, nausea, diarrhea and abdominal pain. It is *not* a simple analgesic and should not be used for conditions other than those listed; thus, it is rarely needed as an adjunct to the treatment of temporomandibular joint dysfunction.

Dosage: 25 mg. after breakfast and again after dinner.

Phenylbutazone (Butazolidin Alka) like Indocin, is not an ordinary analgesic, and its use is contraindicated except in diseases such as gout, rheumatoid arthritis, osteoarthritis, rheumatoid spondylitis and psoriatic arthritis. The drug is an anti-inflammatory, antipyretic analgesic agent and usually affords prompt relief of pain, fever and swelling. It should not be used whenever edema, a history of drug allergy, blood dyscrasia, or renal, hepatic, or cardiac damage are present. Also, the probability of toxic side reactions (such as edema, due to alterations in electrolyte balance, nausea and drug rash) increases with the age of the patient. Since the drug may cause serious blood dyscrasias, patients treated with Butazolidin Alka should be given regular hematograms—once a week initially, and thereafter either weekly or once every 2 weeks. Again, it must be emphasized that, like Indocin, Butazolidin Alka is indicated primarily in arthritic conditions and usually has no place in the treatment of temporomandibular joint dysfunction. However, when a patient suffers from deep, intractable pain in the temporomandibular joints, the drug may be used for a maximum of 1 week to alleviate the pain.

Dosage: 100 mg. (1 tablet) after each meal.

Sedatives. These may be used as adjuncts to analgesics in pain management. The most common are the barbiturates; of these the ones generally employed are phenobarbital, pentobarbital and secobarbital. The three differ in time of onset and duration of action. All barbiturates may be habit forming and should be administered with caution. Because these drugs are detoxified in the liver, particular care must be exercised if a barbiturate is administered to a patient with impaired hepatic function. In all cases, seek the advice of the patient's physician before initiating therapy with a barbiturate.

Sodium phenobarbital (Luminal) in small doses has a pronounced sedative and antispasmodic effect; large doses are hypnotic. Sleep usually occurs within 30 to 60 minutes and lasts 6 to 10 hours following a dose of 100 to 200 mg. Side effects with doses up to 200 mg. are rare; however, larger doses may result in vertigo, headache, and nausea on the following day.

Dosage: The usual adult dose is 16 to 32 mg. to achieve a sedative effect, or 100 to 350 mg. to induce sleep. Larger doses may sometimes be needed to obtain the desired effect but should never exceed 600 mg. in 24 hours.

Sodium pentobarbital (Nembutal) takes effect within 15 to 30 minutes, and its duration of action is usually 3 to 6 hours.

Dosage: The adult daytime dose is 30 mg. three or four times a day; the hypnotic dose is 100 mg.

Sodium secobarbital (Seconal) is short acting and has a very rapid onset of effect. It is thus used primarily to treat insomnia, rather than as a daytime sedative.

Dosage: The usual adult dose is 100 mg. at bedtime.

Hyoscyamine sulfate, atropine sulfate, hyoscine hydrobromide, and phenobarbital (Donnatal) provides a prompt peripheral antispasmodic effect as well as central sedation. Its primary use in dentistry is for tense patients who are prone to anxiety about dental visits. Administration approximately ½ hour before the patient is to see the dentist will facilitate a far more effective examination and treatment.

Heat

The application of moist heat to the spastic muscles of the head and the neck (i.e., masseter, temporal, sternocleidomastoid and other neck muscles) may aid the relief of pain and of the spasm by bringing more blood to the area. The method of application is described in the section on therapy of the joint.

Vitamin Adjuncts

Allbee with vitamin C is a vitamin supplement containing thiamine mononitrate, riboflavin, calcium pantothenate, pyridoxine hydrochloride, niacinamide, and ascorbic acid. It is used to treat the pain symptoms and as a dietary supplement in temporomandibular joint arthrosis. The latter use is especially important since many temporomandibular joint patients suffer nutritionally because of restricted mouth opening and masticatory ability.

Dosage: A 100 mg. tablet of thiamine chloride orally, and 1,000 mg. of vitamin B_{12} intramusculary, administered daily for 10 to 14 days, have been used for relief of pain due to minor neuralgias of the 5th cranial nerve. [12,18] Sinclair[20] claims to have relieved temporomandibular joint pain by large doses of ascorbic acid. He prescribed daily doses of 500 mg. for a period of 2 weeks.

The treatment of minor neuralgias of the 5th nerve with vitamins has not yet been definitely established, and their use is empiric.

Surgical Treatment of Temporomandibular Joint Arthrosis

Surgical treatment in arthrosis of the joint is indicated only after all the conservative treatments have failed and the patient continues to suffer. Consultation with the surgeon is advised before a decision is made as to what the final course will be—extirpation of the disc or removal of the condyle.

Treatment of the Dentition

The treatment of the temporomandibular joint and muscles, as discussed previously, is mainly the treatment of the symptoms of temporomandibular joint arthrosis. If the results of the treatment of the temporomandibular joint and the muscles are to be lasting, the basic cause must be removed. The cause of these symptoms is occlusal disharmony and its resultant pathologic occlusion. Therefore, it is necessary to integrate the treatment of the dentition in the plan of treatment as soon as practical. In many cases it is impossible to treat the dentition until a major portion of the joint and muscle symptoms is alleviated, and this is accomplished as discussed previously. The treatment of the dentition consists in eradicating the etiological factors as listed in the beginning of Chapter 8, and the performance of occlusal equilibration as soon as practical. The treatment of the dentition is separated into the treatments of the five classes of pathologic occlusion.

The precise and exacting technique of occlusal equilibration is basic to the treatment of all the classes of pathologic occlusion. It is merely mentioned in the plan of treatment but fully elaborated in Chapters 13 through 16.

Treatment of Pathologic Mandibular Protrusive Relationship (Class I). The treatment of Class I cases consists of:

1. Equilibration of the occlusion in centric relation and in all the ranges of articulation
2. If the existence of an unopposed, erupting upper third molar is the cause of the pathologic occlusion, then three modes of treatment are possible: extraction, splinting to the upper second molar or restoration of an opposing tooth in the lower arch.
3. Occlusal rehabilitation, if necessary

Infrequently, cases of Class I pathologic occlusion present themselves with deeply imbedded mandibular convenience-relation habit patterns. The construction of a palatal acrylic biteplate to remove the noxious stimulus of the interfering occlusal contact will upset the pathological pattern in a short period of time and allow equilibration of the occlusion in centric relation to be performed. The Shore Mandibular Autorepositioning Appliance (see Chap. 11) will relieve traumatic stresses and give the temporomandibular joint time for rest and repair. The joint tissues are particularly vulnerable because of their avascular cellular nutrition and inability to obtain complete immobility.

Treatment of Pathologic Mandibular Retrusive Relationship (Class II). The treatment of Class II cases consists of:

1. Equilibration in centric relation and in all the ranges of articulation
2. If the existence of an unopposed, erupting lower third molar is the cause of the pathologic occlusion, three modes of treatment are possible: extraction, splinting to the lower second molar or restoration of an opposing tooth in the upper arch.
3. Occlusal rehabilitation, if necessary

Treatment of Increased Vertical Relationship (Class III). The treatment of Class III cases consists of equilibration in centric relation and and in all the ranges of articulation.

Treatment of Pathological Medial or Lateral Shifts of the Mandible Due to Crossbite Relationships (Class IV). The treatment of Class IV conditions consists of occlusal equilibration in centric relation and in all the ranges of articulation and occlusal rehabilitation, when necessary.

Treatment of Reduced Vertical Relationship (Class V). Class V cases are of two types: those which occur owing to the loss of posterior tooth support; those in which loss of posterior teeth has not occurred. In the latter case the decreased vertical dimension may be due to excessive wear or failure of the dentition to erupt to the proper level of occlusion. The treatment of Class V cases due to loss of posterior tooth support consists of a temporary upper and/or lower partial denture with acrylic saddles and acrylic teeth to restore the vertical dimension to a level proper and comfortable for the individual patient. The temporary dentures must be equilibrated in centric relation and in all the ranges of articulation.

The treatment of the Class V cases due to wear of the posterior teeth and lack of proper occlusal development consists of covering as many segments of the arches as are necessary with temporary occlusal splints constructed of acrylic or metal. The vertical dimension is restored to the proper level for the patient. Figure 10-19*a*

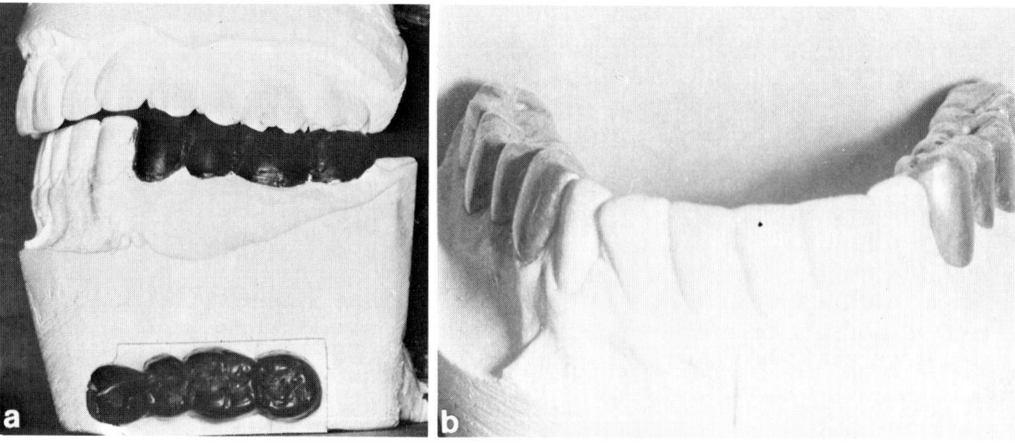

FIG. 10-19. Wax patterns for metal or acrylic occlusal splints (*a*). Metal splints on cast (*b*).

illustrates the wax patterns of an occlusal splint; (*b*) illustrates the metal occlusal splints on the cast. Similarly, a partial denture with acrylic teeth may be constructed and acrylic added or removed from the occlusal surfaces of the teeth as needed to establish proper vertical dimension. After a sufficient trial period, permanent restorations are made to the established comfortable vertical dimension. Occlusal equilibration in centric relation and in all the ranges of articulation is the final step in the treatment.

REFERENCES

1. Berger, F. M.: Meprobamate, its pharmacologic properties and clinical uses. Int. Rec. Med. & Gen. Pract. Clin., *169:*184, 1956.
2. Berger, F. M., and Schwartz, R. P.: Oral myanesin in the treatment of spastic and hyperkinetic disorders. JAMA, *137:*772, 1948.
3. Blackburn, C. R. B.: Cortisone—a review. D. J. Australia, *27:*1, 1955.
4. Borrus, M. D.: Study of the effect of miltown on psychiatric states, JAMA, *157:*1596, 1955.
5. Dickel, H. A., Dixon, H. H., Wood, B. A., and Shanklin, J. G.: Electromyographic studies of patients treated with meprobamate. West. J. Surg., *64:*197, 1956.
6. Francis, L. E.: Clinical applications; analgesics. *In* Alling, C. A. (ed.): Facial Pain. p. 228. Philadelphia, Lea & Febiger, 1968.
7. Ibid: p. 233.
8. Gillette, H. E.: Relaxant effects of meprobamates in disabilities resulting from musculoskeletal and central nervous system disorder. Int. Rec. Med. & Gen. Pract. Clin., *169:*453, 1956.
9. Goodman, L. S., and Gilman, A.: The Pharmacological Basis of Therapeutics. ed. 2, p. 1026. New York, Macmillan, 1955.
10. Held, A. J.: Pathogeny of parodontolyses of diseases characterized by a progressive atrophy of the paradontium. Paradontologie, *61*(2), 1952.
11. Henkel, G. H.: The role and applicability of hyaluronidase in clinical dentistry. Oral Surg., *9:*463, 1956.
12. Hill, A. V. (As quoted in Ruskin, S. L.): The role of coenzymes of the complex enzymes and amino acids in muscle metabolism and balanced nutrition. Am. J. Dig. Dis., *13:*110, 1946.
13. Kochan, E.: Treatment of temporomandibular joint disturbances with hyaluronidase. Oral Surg., *9:*513, 1956.
14. Kraus, H.: Therapeutic Exercises. Springfield (Ill.), Charles C Thomas, 1949.
15. Maddox, W. D., Gibilisco, J. A., and Steinhilber, R. M.: Movement disorders

of the jaw and tongue following prochlorperazine therapy. J. D. Med., *17:*10, 1962.

16. Ostrander, F. D.: New drugs useful in dentistry. JADA *54:*461, 1957.
17. Panuska, H. W.: Dilantin hyperplasia—surgical management. D. World, *19:*(2nd quarter) 1964.
18. Ruskin, S. L., Merrill, A. T.: Nutrition, newer studies of iron ascorbate. Am. J. Dig. Dis., *16:*386, 1949.
19. Schwartz, L. L.: Ethyl chloride treatment of limited painful mandibular movement. JADA, *48:*497, 1954.
    ———: Pain associated with the temporomandibular joint. JADA, *51:*394, 1955.
    ———: Temporomandibular joint syndromes. J. Pros. Dent. *7:*489, 1957.
20. Sinclair, J. A.: Vitamin C deficiency—a factor in producing subluxation, pain in the temporomandibular area and other dental involvement. D. Items Int., *63:*313, 1941.
21. Travell, J.: Basis for the multiple uses of local block of somatic trigger areas (procaine infiltration and ethyl chloride spray). Mississippi V. Med. J., *71:*13, 1949.
22. ———: *In* Ragan, C.: Connective Tissues. New York, Macy, 1951.
23. Ibid., p. 119.
24. Travell, J., and Rinzler, S. H.: The myofascial genesis of pain. Postgrad. Med., *11:*425, 1952.

Additional Basic References

Manifestations of Pathologic Occlusion and Temporomandibular Joint Dysfunction

Boyle, P. E.: Traumatic occlusion in periodontics and as an etiologic factor in periodontal disease. N. Y. J. Dent., *23:*316, 1953.

Chasen, A. I.: Occlusal disharmony and temporomandibular joint disturbances as a source of pain. J. Dent. Med., *12:*107, 1957.

Cobin, H. P.: The temporomandibular syndrome and centric relation, N. Y. J. Dent., *18:*393, 1952.

Costen, J. B.: The mechanism of trismus and its occurrence in mandibular joint dysfunction, Ann. Otol. Rhinol. Laryngol., *48:*499, 1939.

———: Diagnosis of mandibular joint neuralgia and its place in general head pain, Ann. Otol. Rhinol. Laryngol., *53:*655, 1944.

Dechaume, M., Poggioli, J. A., and Rouot, J.: The part played by a sympathetic nervous system in the pathogenesis of disorders resulting from dental malocclusion, Oral Surg., *6:*1047, 1953.

DeVanna, A.: Facial pain. N. Y. State D. J. *54:*1684, 1954.

Eisenman, M.: Occlusal dysharmonies as related to cranial nerve syndromes. J. Am. Osteop. Ath. Assoc., *54:*114, 1954.

Fleetwood, C. T.: The general physical improvement and soft tissue resulting from correction of traumatic occlusion and establishment of proper direction of functional forces. J. Can. D. A., *9:*543, 1943.

Gerry, R. G.: Traumatic injuries of the temporomandibular joint. J. Oral Surg., *13:*232, 1955.

Hankey, G. T.; Ballard, F. C., and Storey, G. O.: Affection of the temporomandibular joint. Proc. Roy. Soc. Med., *49:*983, 1956.

Held, A. J.: Equilibration fonctionelle de la dentition par meulage. (Functional equilibration of the dentition by grinding). Parodontologie, *66*(No. 2): 1948.

Kallenbach, T. E.: Effect of functional disorganization of the mouth and teeth: operative factors in reestablishment to normal. D. Cosmos, *73:*759, 1931.

Loos, S.: Mechanik des Kiefergelenkes (Mechanics of the Temporomandibular Joint). Vienna, Urban, 1946.

Markowitz, H. A., and Gerry, R. G.: Temporomandibular joint disease. Oral Surg., *2:*1309, 1949.

Moulton, R. E.: Psychiatric considerations in maxillofacial pain. JADA, *51:*408, 1955.

Raginsky, B. B.: Psychosomatic dentistry. J. Can. D. A., *9:*914, 1954.

Riesner, S. E.: Head and facial pains associated with disturbances of the temporomandibular joints. N. Y. J. Dent., *13:*65, 1947.

Russell, L. A., and Bayles, T. B.: The temporomandibular joint in rheumatoid arthritis. JADA, *28:*533, 1941.

Salman, I.: Traumatic injuries to the temporomandibular joint. J. Oral Surg., *7:*277, 1949.

Sicher, H.: Structure and functional basis for disorders of the temporomandibular articulation. J. Oral Surg., *13:*275, 1955.

Staz, J.: Disturbances of the temporomandibular articulation. J. D. A. South Africa, *3:*15, 1948.

Differential Diagnosis of Temporomandibular Joint Disease

Behrman, S.: Facial neuralgias. Br. D. J., *86*:197, 1949.

Couch, C. D., Jr.: Facial pain. J. Oral Surg., *14:*216, 1956.

Friedman, A. P.: Modern Headache Therapy. St. Louis, C. V. Mosby, 1951.

Glaser, M. A.: Facial neuralgia, its etiology and treatment. JADA, *26:*1483, 1939.

Grant, F. C., Groff, R. A., and Levy, F. H.: Section of descending spinal root of fifth cranial nerve. Arch. Neurol., *43:*498, 1940.

Harrigan, W. F.: Facial pain. Oral Surg., *5:*563, 1952.

Papper, E. M., and Rovenstine, E. A.: Pain syndromes of the face. Oral Surg., *1:*542, 1948.

Raney, R., Raney, A. A., and Hunter, C. R.: Treatment of major trigeminal neuralgia through section of the trigeminal tract in the medulla. Am. J. Surg., *80:*11, 1950.

Shapiro, H. H.: Differential diagnosis of oral pain. Oral Surg., *4:*1353, 1951.

Treatment of Temporomandibular Joint Arthrosis

Bailey, E. E.: A method of diagnosing and treating cases requiring repositioning of the mandible and rebuilding of the occlusal surfaces of the teeth. JADA, *24:*33, 1937.

Benzer, P., and Schaffer, A. B.: The use of hyaluronidase in the treatment of traumatic swelling. Oral Surg., *5:*1315, 1952.

Benzer, P., and Thornwood, A.: A preliminary report on the use of hyaluronidase in the treatment of traumatic swellings. Oral Surg., *4:*1515, 1951.

Berten, F.: Beitrage zur therapie des kiefergelenkes (Studies of the therapy of the temporomandibular joint). Dtsch. Zahn. Wchnschr., *17:*234, 1942.

Boman, K., Lindblom, G., Sundberg, S.: Kakledsarthrosen, dess kikrurgiska och tandorto pediska behandling. Sven. Tandlak Tidskr., *36:*441 (5), 1943.

Bonnet-Roy o. Deliberos: Subluxation temporo-maxillary posttraumatique recidivante, reduite sans intervention sanglante parraitement prothetique (Prosthetic treatment of temporomandibular joint subluxation). Mem. Acad. Chir., *67:*134, 1941.

Good, M. C.: The problem of rheumatism. Br. J. Phys. Med., *14:*56, 1951.

Henny, F. A.: Intra-articular injection of hydrocortisone into the temporomandibular joint. J. Oral Surg., *12:*314, 1954.

———: The painful temporomandibular joint J. Oral Surg., *13:*341, 1955.

Horton, C. P.: Treatment of arthritic temporomandibular joints by intraarticular injection of hydrocortisone. Oral Surg., *6:*826, 1953.

Morgan, D. H.: Temporomandibular Joint Surgery—Correction of Pain, Tinnitus and Vertigo. Dental Radiog. Photog., *46:*2, 1973.

Ragan, C., and Meyer, K.: The hyaluronic acid of synovial fluid in rheumatoid arthritis. J. Clin. Invest., *28:*56, 1949.

Schweitzer, J. M.: Oral Rehabilitation. St. Louis, C. V. Mosby, 1951.

Stream, L. P.: Cortisone in Dentistry, New York, Dental Items of Interest, 1957.

11 *The Shore Mandibular Autorepositioning Appliance*

IMPORTANCE OF DIAGNOSING TEMPOROMANDIBULAR JOINT DYSFUNCTION

Ninety-five percent of all instances of temporomandibular joint (TMJ) dysfunction evidence the following four factors, singly or in combination:

1. Neuromuscular spasm of the external pterygoid and associated muscles
2. Habitual convenience relationship of the mandible (caused by interfering occlusal contacts in centric relation)
3. Negative occlusal proprioception that results in abnormal "mandibular gait"
4. Stress, and its effect on the muscles of the stomatognathic system (see Chap. 7)

Any one or combination of these four factors will position the mandible incorrectly.

Depending on the anatomical location of nagging head pain, internists, otolaryngologists, neurologists and orthopaedists often are called upon for consultations. In addition, patients with temporomandibular joint dysfunction—"the great mimicker" of head pain—also are referred to the psychiatrist, who is asked to determine whether the pain is of psychosomatic origin.

Some patients are told, by psychiatrists or other medical specialists, that they are psychosomatically ill and must simply learn to live with pain that has no physical basis. However, it may be that such patients are not psychosomatically ill, but somatopsychically ill. It is the pain that makes them neurotic, not the neurosis that causes the pain—which does have a physical origin in dysfunction.

The temporomandibular joint dysfunction problem can be so perplexing, and the pain so intense, that some persons have been driven almost to the brink of suicide. Others in whom the etiology of head pain was mistakenly diagnosed as tic douloureux (trigeminal neuralgia), have had condylectomies, minisectomies, cranial nerve sections, alcohol injections into the trigeminal nerve, and other drastic attempts at therapy such as complete extraction of perfectly sound teeth.

The stresses of today's society—and the related nocturnal grinding and other problematic oral habits—are responsible for a growing incidence of persons with temporomandibular joint dysfunction. Another cause is the amount of rehabilitation by dentists that is improperly coordinated with the rest of the stomatognathic system.

When occlusal registrations are being taken, some patients continually bite in different patterns because they cannot position the mandible correctly. This condition is negative proprioception. And the resulting habitual placement of the mandible is an engram—defined as "a lasting mark or trace left by a stimulus (a habit)."

The concept of the engram is basic to the understanding of habitual pathologic occlusion. The dentist has no way of checking the accuracy of the occlusal registrations.

Because of their "oral acrobatics," these patients have a variety of seemingly unrelated symptoms. Such patients go from dentist to dentist, unsuccessfully seeking help. Even though they may have their occlusion ground in by three or four dentists, new, painful symptoms inevitably appear and the old ones are not alleviated.

When there is improper placement of the mandible, muscle spasm, convenience relationship, and negative proprioception must be eliminated before occlusal registrations are attempted and before restorative treatment is initiated.

A patient in spasm can be compared with a person whose gait is abnormal because he is suffering from a charleyhorse or muscle strain. Because of spasms of the external pterygoid, masseter, and temporal muscles, which are responsible for movement of the mandible in centric relation, such a patient cannot give a normal centric-relation mandibular placement (normal mandibular gait).

If pain exists because of noxious impulses to and from the temporomandibular joints, normal neuromuscular placement of the mandible is impossible. The patient with negative proprioception cannot position his mandible correctly. In such circumstances, the teeth position the mandible and the muscles are stretched, pulled, and squeezed. This is a result of the pathologic occlusion, which must be unlocked. Unlocking the occlusion is necessary in order to free the mandible from the dominance of the abnormal occlusion, and thereby bring the muscles into a normal resting position. The mandible and condyles can then assume physiological placement within the temporomandibular joints, thus facilitating normal physiological function with positive proprioception.

BITEPLANES, BITEPLATES AND SPLINTS

For many years, biteplanes and Hawley biteplates have been used in the treatment of temporomandibular joint dysfunction and so-called bad bites. The purpose of these devices is to free the mandible from pathologic occlusion. Biteplanes and Hawley biteplates should not be used in treating temporomandibular joint dysfunction because they permit occlusal contact only on the anterior teeth, thereby allowing the temporal and masseter muscles to pull the condyles up into the fossae of the sore and aching temporomandibular joints. In addition, iatrogenic extrusion of posterior teeth is common with these devices.

In many instances, hard acrylic splints with smooth occlusal planes have, indeed, been known to unlock the occlusion. But too often these devices have created new occlusal problems, because the smooth occluding surface of the biteplane was determined by the dentist—rather than by the physiological mandibular gait of the patient.

SHORE MANDIBULAR AUTOREPOSITIONING APPLIANCE

The basic principle of the Shore Mandibular Autorepositioning Appliance (SMAA), developed 15 years ago, is one of self-determination. The patient alone gradually determines the physiological placement of his mandible in centric relation, by going through the functional movements while the autorepositioner is being made. In freeing the mandible from malocclusion, the Shore Mandibular Autorepositioning Appliance transmits the force of mandibular closure through the teeth to the maxilla, thus removing pressures from the traumatized joints.

The Shore autorepositioner eliminates neuromuscular spasm of the external pterygoids and associated muscles, habitual convenience relationship of the mandible, and negative occlusal proprioception. It simultaneously enables the mandible and the temporomandibular joints to position themselves physiologically; that is, by eliminating the neuromuscular dysfunction and the habitual convenience relationship of the occlusion, the negative occlusal proprioception is converted to positive proprioception. Positive proprioception helps the mandible to return gradually to its physiological position.

In fabricating the Shore Mandibular Autorepositioning Appliance, a temporarily incorrect functional occlusion is created in acrylic. Initially, the occlusal path of the mandibular repositioner is about 50 per cent inaccurate, because of the patient's habitual incorrect mandibular gait. But by gradually changing the occlusal pattern (functional generated path) and equilibrating the occlusal surfaces of the appliance, the muscle spasm, habitual convenience relationship, and negative occlusal proprioception are eliminated.

The old method of grinding in the occlusion without consideration of neuromuscular spasm, convenience mandibular relationship and negative proprioception resulted in many failures. Because of inaccuracies and hit-or-miss results, the procedures of occlusal equilibration and the treatment of temporomandibular joint dysfunction acquired a bad reputation.

The Shore Mandibular Autorepositioning Appliance has been used by hundreds of practitioners during the past 15 years with remarkably good results.

Technique of Fabricating the SMAA

To construct a Shore Mandibular Autorepositioning Appliance proceed as follows:

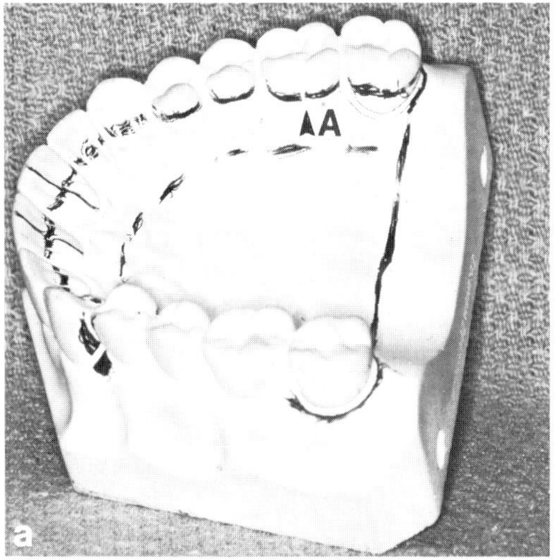

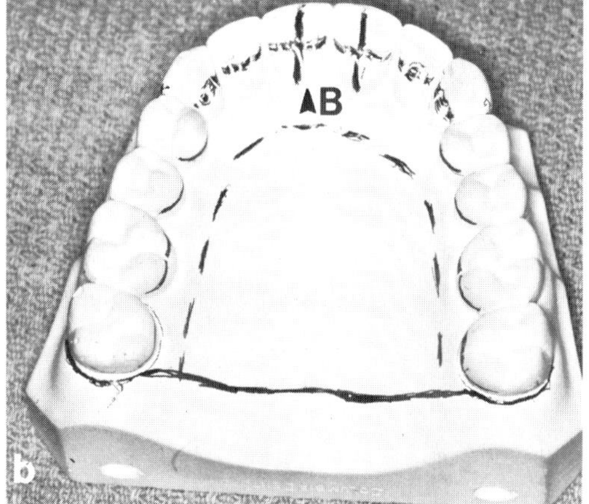

FIG. 11-1. The upper cast (*a*) with a pencil mark on the linguo-occlusal surfaces of the teeth (A), as well as a mark (B) for the anterior ramp (*b*). Using the pencil marks as a guide, an acrylic palate is fabricated. The technician should make a palatal relief.

1. Make an upper cast from an alginate or hydrocolloid impression.

2. Mark the linguo-occlusal surfaces of the upper cast (Fig. 11-1).

3. Make an acrylic palate, covering the palate and the linguo-occlusal tooth surfaces. For fixation the acrylic palate has two buccal arm clasps distal to the most posterior teeth, two ball clasps posterior to the cuspids, and an acrylic ramp 3 mm. thick on the lingual aspect of the central incisors (Fig. 11-2). Figure 11-3 depicts the acrylic palate and clasps.

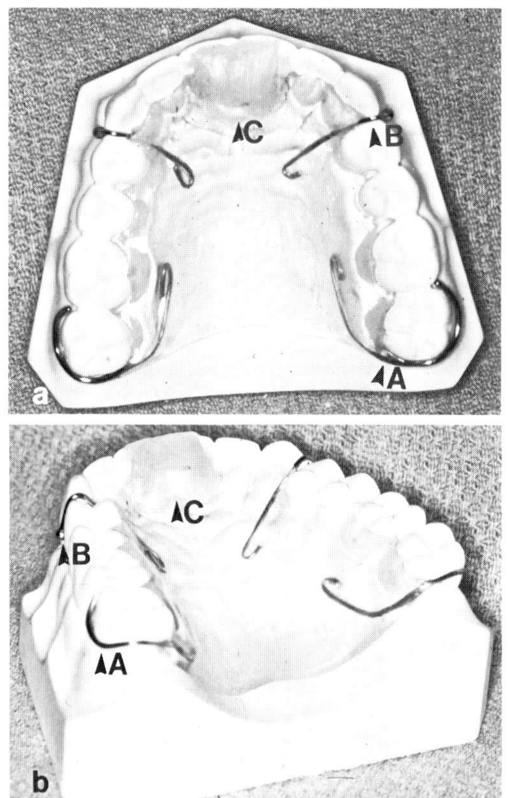

FIG. 11-2. The acrylic palate covers the palatal surface and the linguo-occlusal surfaces of the teeth (*a*,*b*). There are two buccal arm clasps distal to the most posterior teeth (A), two ball clasps posterior to the upper cuspids at (B), and the small acrylic ramp, about 3 mm. thick, on the lingual surface of the central incisors (C).

4. Check the appliance in the patient's mouth for overextension and any other possible discrepancies in fit (Fig. 11-4). Subsequently, trim the anterior stop (*arrows*, Fig. 11-4) to allow 1- to 2-mm. clearance between the upper and lower posterior teeth.

5. Apply cocoa butter or petrolatum to the cast (Fig. 11-5*a*) and to the dentition (*b*) to prevent the union of fresh acrylic to temporary acrylic bridgework, old facings, acrylic crowns, etc. Nothing is so embarrassing as the inadvertent removal of an acrylic facing or an acrylic jacket.

Figure 11-6 depicts Caulk orthodontic powder and liquid, and a dappen dish.

6. While the plastic palate is out of the patient's mouth, apply liquid monomer to its occlusal edges (Fig. 11-7).

7. Mix liquid and resin in the deep side of a dappen dish (Fig. 11-8*a*). Figure 11-8*b* shows a soupy mix being prepared for later use, in the shallow side of the dappen dish. The primary mix (Fig.

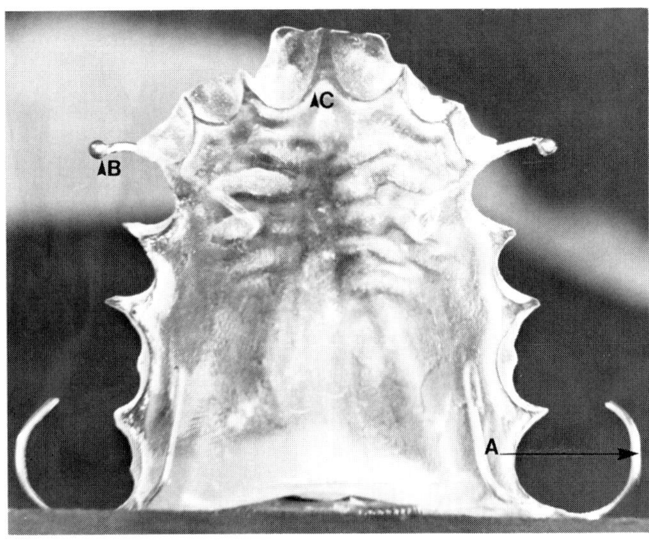

FIG. 11-3. The appliance is depicted off the cast showing the buccal arms (A), the ball clasps (B) and the anterior ramp (C).

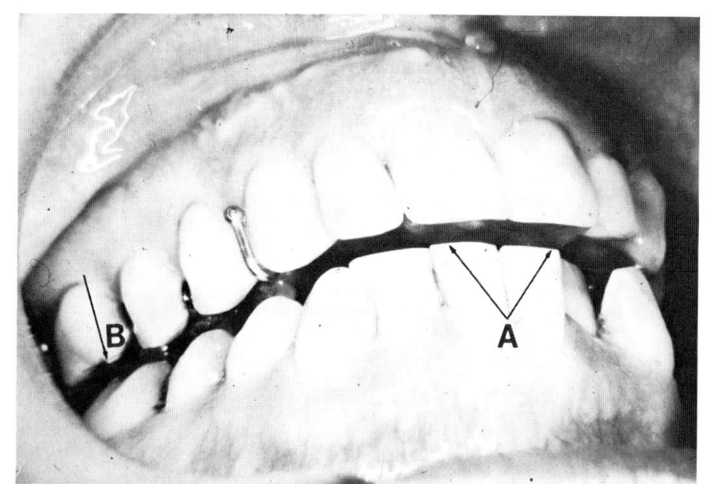

FIG. 11-4. The appliance is tested in the patient's mouth; it is checked carefully for discrepancies in fit, such as rocking and overextension. The importance of the ramp cannot be overemphasized. The ramp (A) is trimmed until there is a 2 to 3 mm. clearance between the upper and lower posterior teeth (B).

11-9), should approximate the consistency of soft caramel. Scrape the mix from the dappen dish into the petrolatum-covered palm of the hand (Fig. 11-10*a*). Knead the soft resin (*b*) under cold running water to remove excess liquid resin.

8. Roll the acrylic into a cigarette shape (Fig. 11-11*a*). Add the "cigarette roll" of acrylic to the palate's edges (*b*). Place a few drops of monomer at a time (Fig. 11-12) between the lingual surfaces of the Shore Mandibular Autorepositioning Appliance and the soft acrylic. By pressing gently on the area, the resin adheres better.

9. Return the appliance to the patient's mouth (Fig. 11-13), instruct him to close his mouth in centric relation, onto the trimmed acrylic stop, and to perform all functional mandibular movements for 1 minute (Fig. 11-14). He then moves his jaw from side to side many times, then forward and back, again many times, ending by biting in the most retruded position. As the patient moves through a functionally generated path, prepare a "soupy" resin mix (Fig. 11-15) in the small end of the dappen dish. At this point, trim the excess acrylic flash from the device (Fig. 11-16) with a steel spatula.

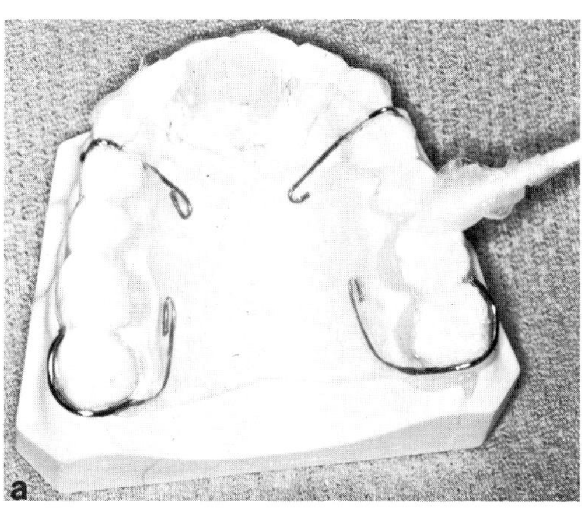

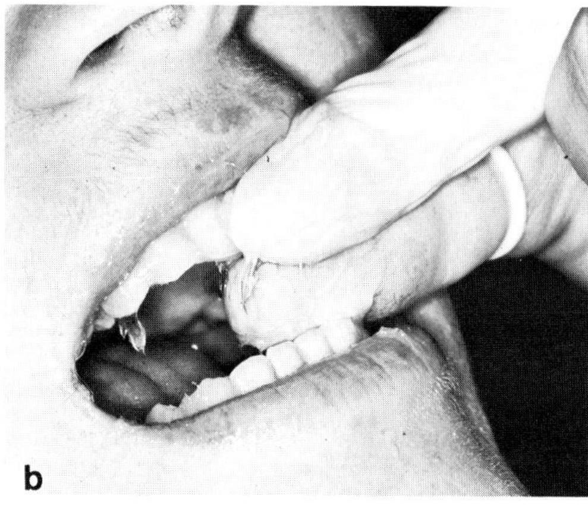

FIG. 11-5. The appliance is removed from the mouth and placed on a petrolatum-covered cast (*a*). Using finger cots, petrolatum is applied to all areas of the patient's teeth (*b*).

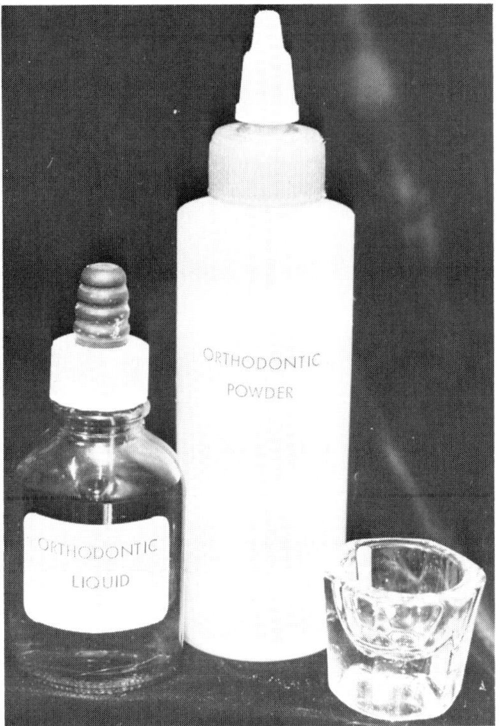

FIG. 11-6. The Caulk orthodontic powder and liquid are very strong resins.

10. Remove the autorepositioner (Fig. 11-17) to permit the patient to rinse with cold water. While the appliance is out of the patient's mouth, fill any small openings in it with the soupy acrylic mix.

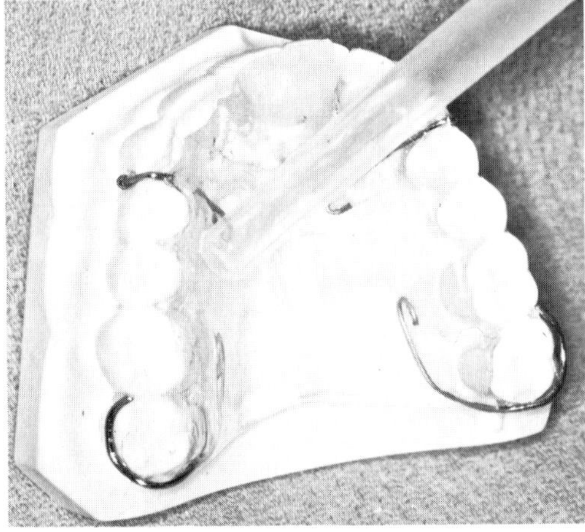

FIG. 11-7. The appliance is placed on the petrolatum-covered model. The borders of the appliance are wetted with liquid monomer.

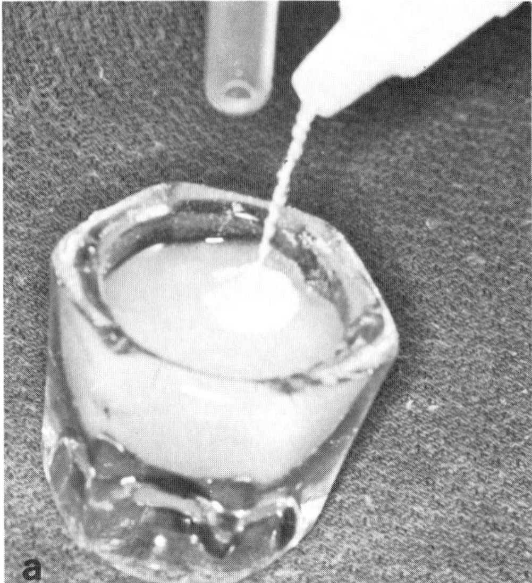

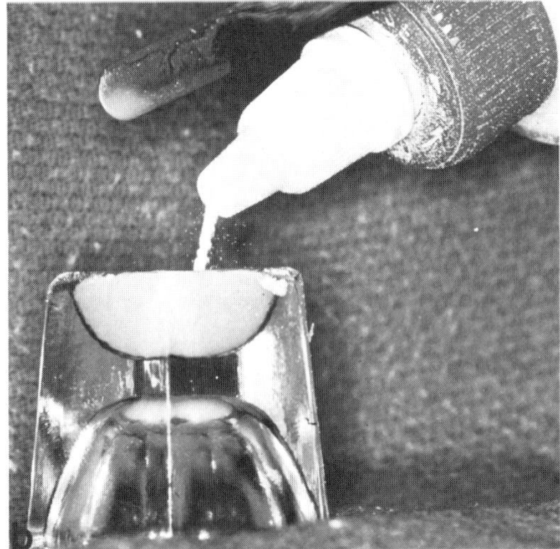

FIG. 11-8. The larger side of the dappen dish (*a*) is used for making the primary mix and the smaller side is used for the secondary or "soupy" mix (*b*).

11. Reinsert the appliance repeatedly, at approximately 15-second intervals, to prevent "drag" of the acrylic, which cures in about 6 minutes.

12. When the resin cures, remove the Shore Mandibular Autorepositioning Appliance from the patient's mouth (Fig. 11-18), and trim the excess acrylic without disturbing the occlusal surfaces (depressions) that make contact with the lower teeth.

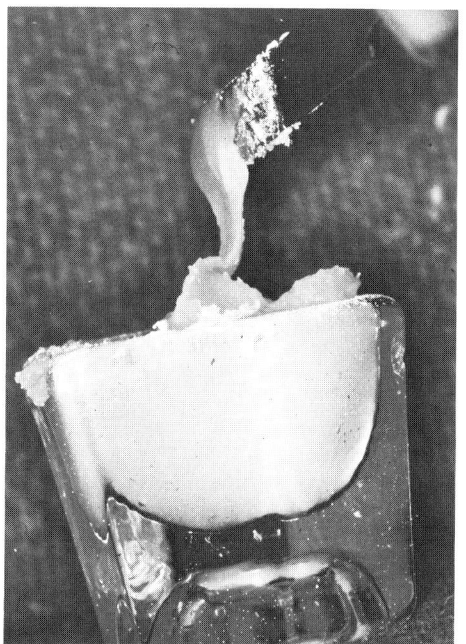

FIG. 11-9. The dappen dishes, filled with the acrylic mixes, are ready for use. The primary mix should approximate the consistency of soft caramel.

13. The Shore Mandibular Autorepositioning Appliance is equilibrated in centric-relation occlusion, using green 22-gauge casting wax, red ribbon, and blue paper.

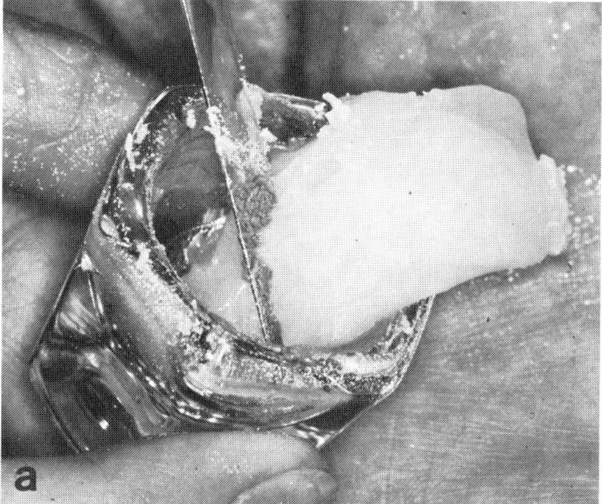

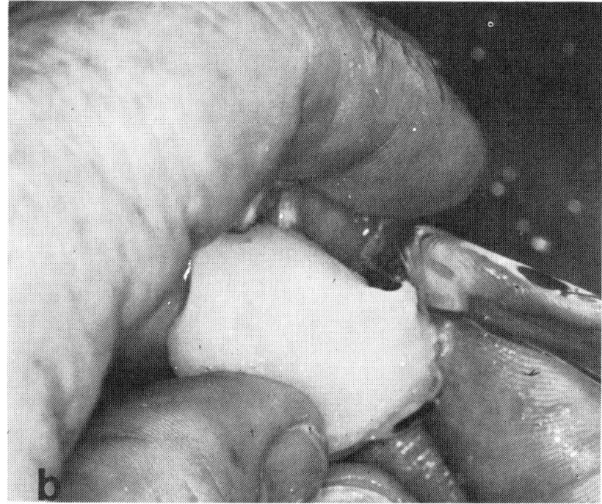

FIG. 11-10. Mixture is scraped from the dappen dish, into the petrolatum-covered palm of the hand (*a*). The soft resin is kneaded, under cold running water, to remove excess liquid resin (*b*).

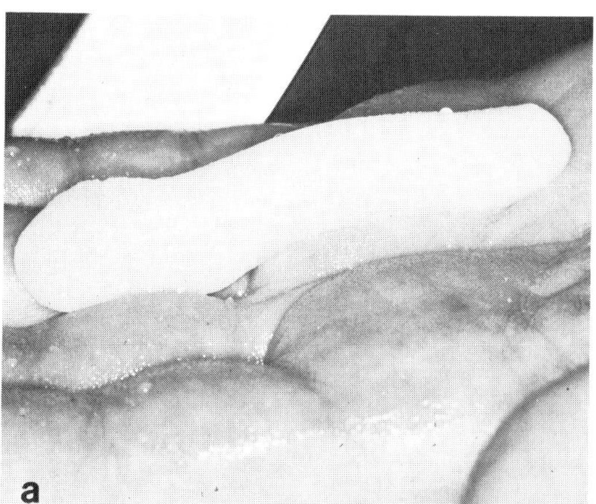

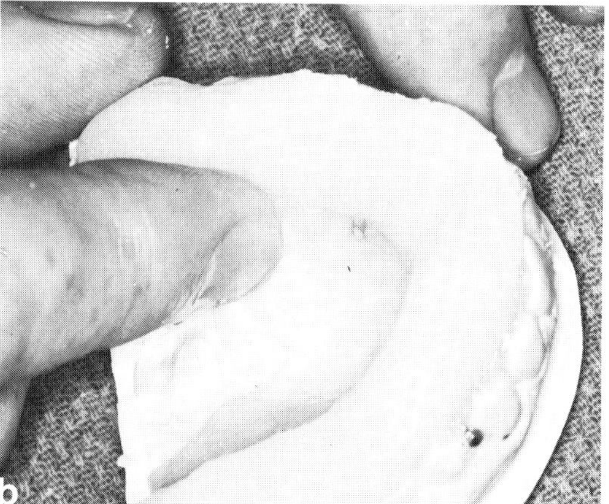

FIG. 11-11. The resin is rolled into a cigarette shape (*a*) and placed around the linguo-occlusal surfaces of the appliance (*b*), on the petrolatum-covered cast.

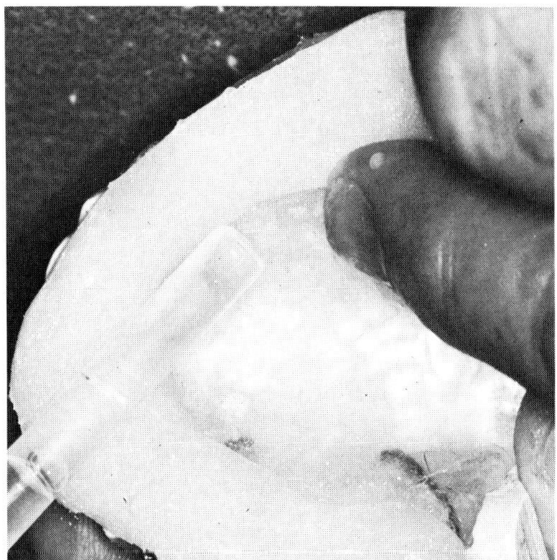

FIG. 11-12. Applying monomer to "cigarette roll" of acrylic.

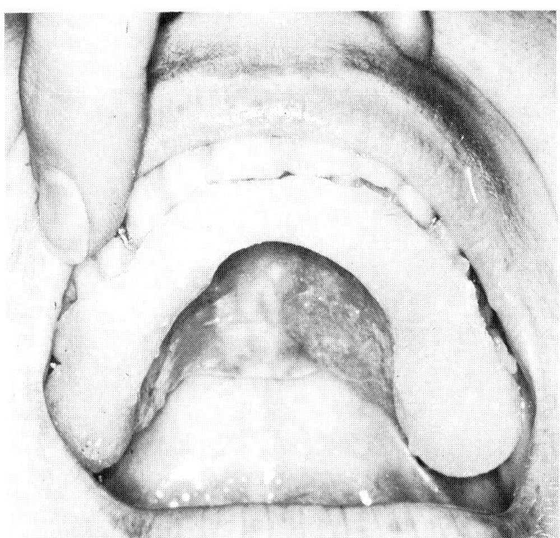

FIG. 11-13. The Shore Mandibular Autorepositioning Appliance is removed from the petrolatum-covered cast and inserted in the patient's mouth.

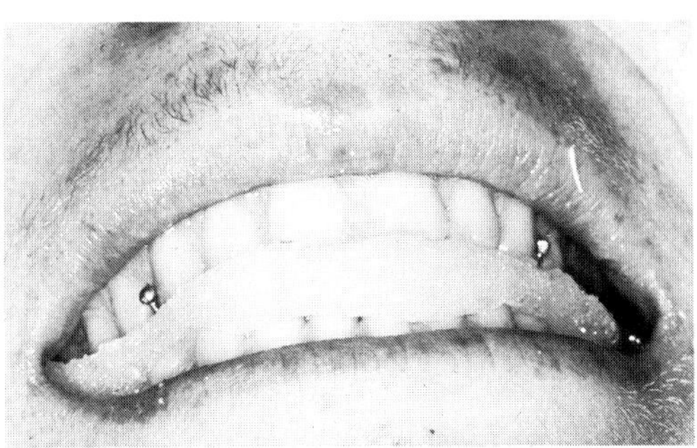

FIG. 11-14. The patient bites into the soft acrylic.

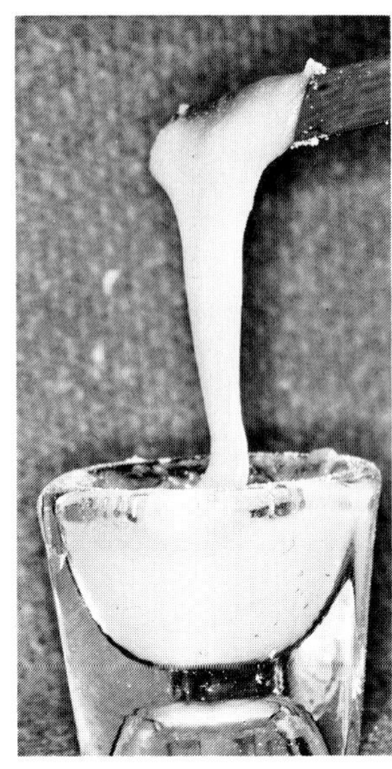

FIG. 11-15. A soupy resin mix is prepared.

14. After the occlusion is freed in the eccentric ranges of articulation, buff the occlusal surfaces to a high polish (Fig. 11-19).

In Figure 11-20, a finished appliance is

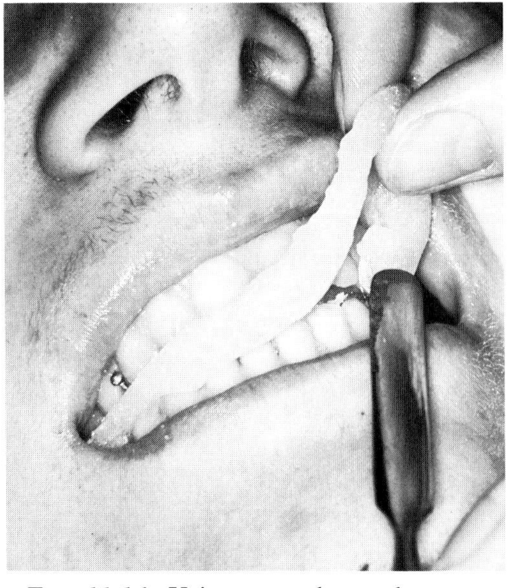

FIG. 11-16. Using a steel spatula, excess flash is quickly removed from the Shore Mandibular Autorepositioning Appliance.

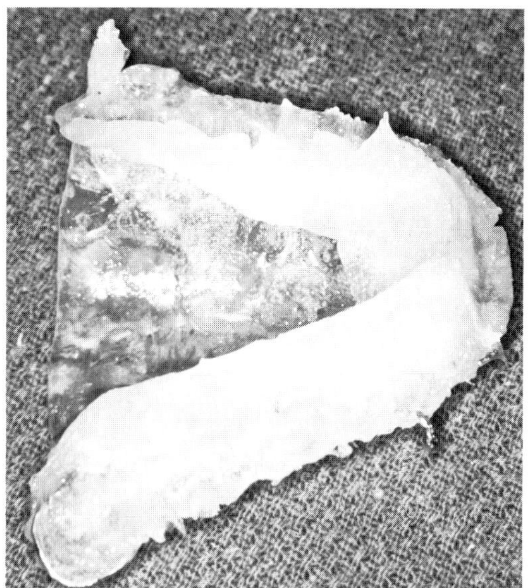

FIG. 11-17. The appliance is removed from the patient's mouth and the excess acrylic is removed.

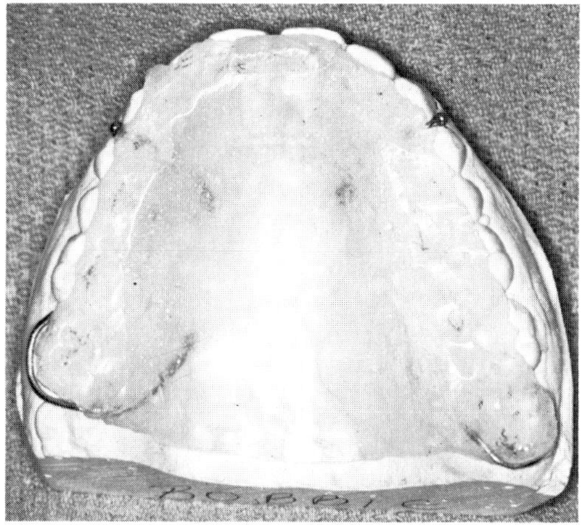

FIG. 11-18. Trimming the appliance.

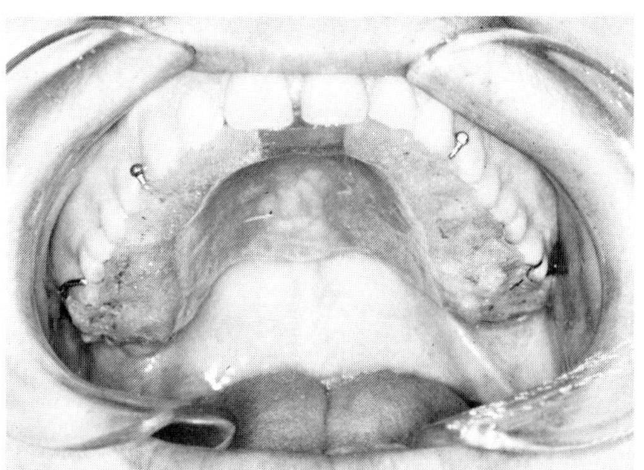

FIG. 11-19. The appliance is reinserted in the patient's mouth, then is equilibrated.

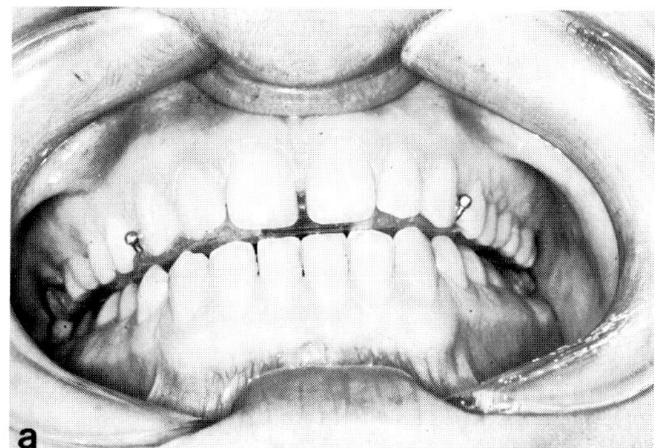

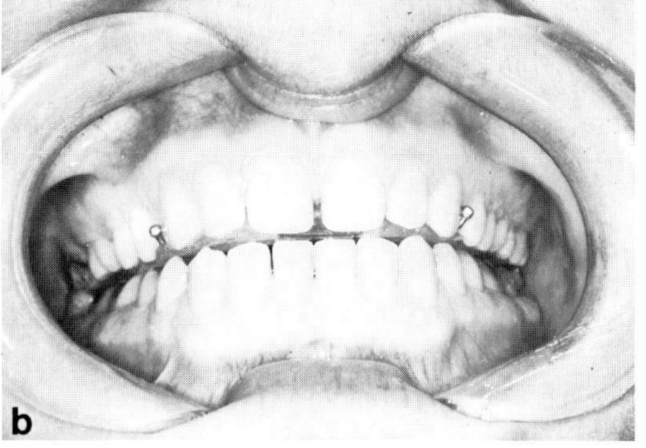

FIG. 11-20. Very little of the appliance is seen in the patient's mouth (*a,b*).

present in the patient's mouth although very little can be seen.

The autorepositioning appliance must be adjusted weekly or biweekly. Abnormal mandibular gait initially makes the occlusal path of the appliance 50 per cent inaccurate. Gradually, though, the unfavorable occlusal pattern is corrected

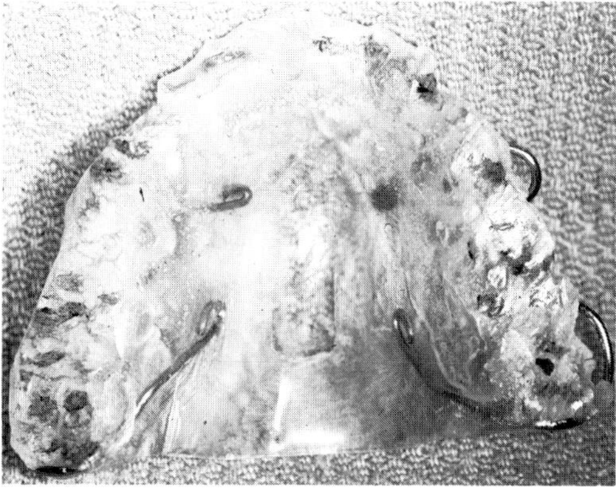

FIG. 11-21. The centric-relation equilibration of the Shore Mandibular Autorepositioning Appliance.

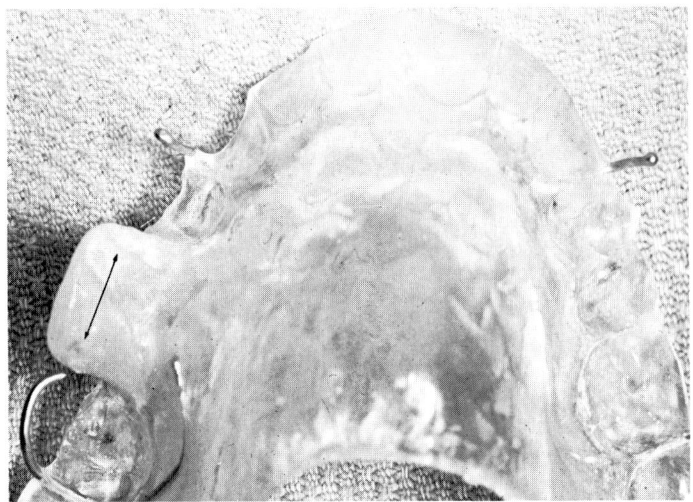

FIG. 11-22. A block of acrylic (*arrow*) is added to area of missing teeth.

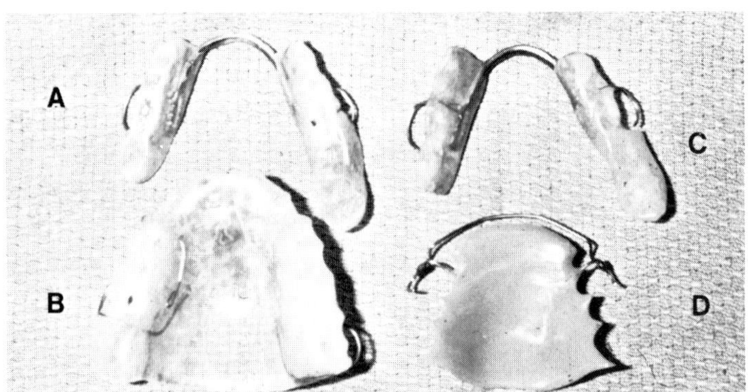

FIG. 11-23. Weak appliances. A, B and C fell apart under stress. The Hawley appliance (D) creates pressure only on the anterior teeth.

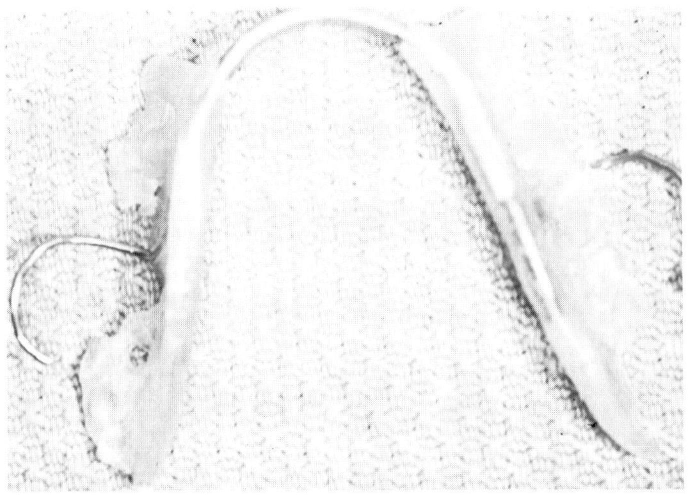

FIG. 11-24. The acrylic in this appliance lacked strength in the lower molar region.

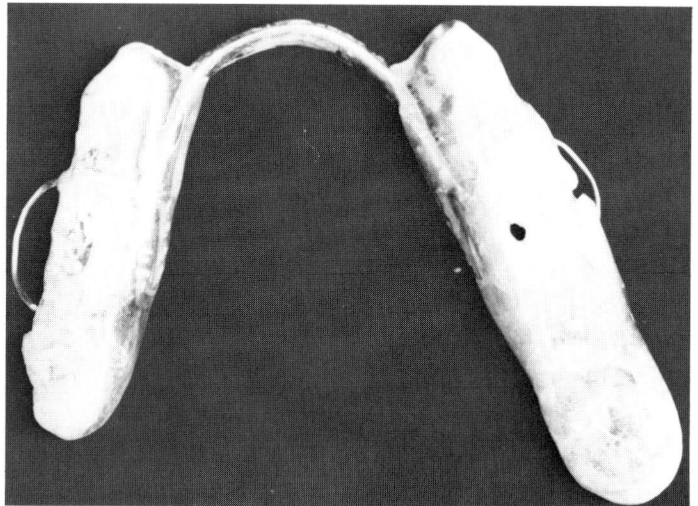

FIG. 11-25. Lower appliance without an anterior stop.

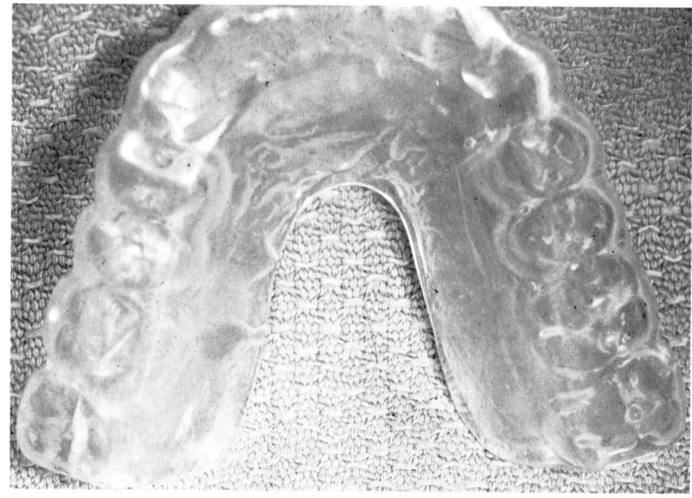

FIG. 11-26. Hard acrylic upper appliance without clasps.

by equilibrating the appliance during weekly or biweekly appointments.

An occlusal view of the SMAA (Fig. 11-21) demonstrates a finished case of occlusal equilibration of the appliance. The marks are both blue and red and contact all of the lower teeth in centric relation. There are no holes in the occlusal surfaces. If the patient is symptom-free at this point, he is in centric relation and is ready for occlusal equilibration of his dentition.

Only after all symptoms are eliminated, including head pain, clicking, crepitation, nocturnal grinding, and mandibular deviation, can occlusal equilibration of the teeth be performed with accuracy.

In the event that the patient has missing teeth in the posterior region, add an acrylic block in the edentulous area (Fig. 11-22).

Certain appliances are contraindicated in the treatment of temporomandibular joint dysfunction. Figure 11-23 demonstrates four different types of such appliances: *A*, *B* and *C* are appliances that fell apart under stress and were repaired repeatedly. The Hawley appliance (*D*)

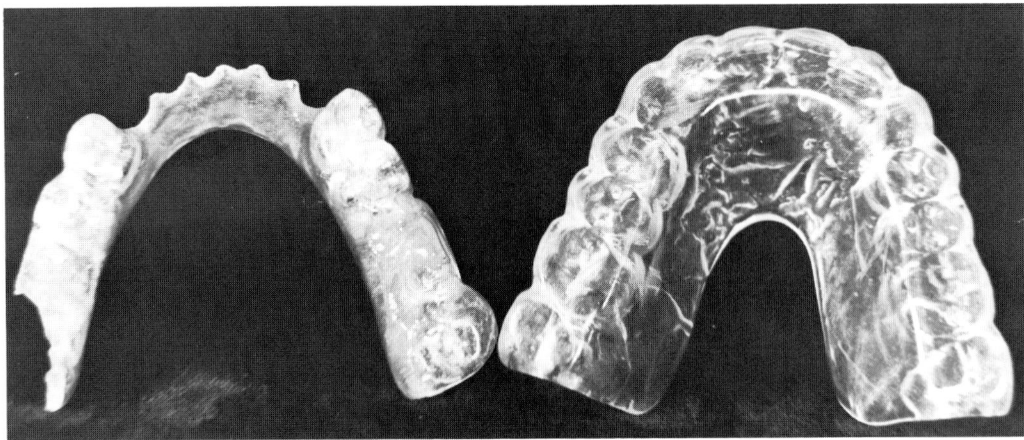

FIG. 11-27. Upper and lower block appliances.

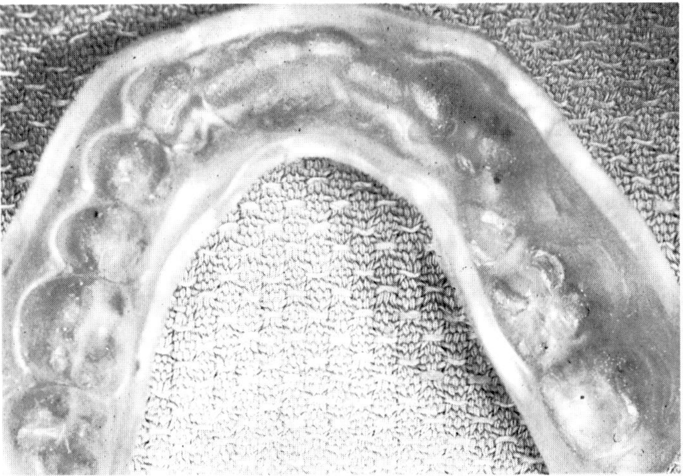

FIG. 11-28. Lower arch bruxism appliance is made of soft rubber.

creates pressure only on the anterior teeth and is accompanied by extrusion of the posterior teeth.

Another type of appliance (Fig. 11-24) illustrates a lack of strength of acrylic in the lower molar region. Lower appliances are undesirable because they usually break in the molar occlusal region, fracture in the anterior region, and allow the upper teeth to extrude. If made too thick in the posterior region, in an attempt to minimize breakage, lower appliances encroach on the freeway space. In many cases, appliances of the type seen in Figure 11-25 are fabricated for the lower arch. Such appliances encroach on the vertical dimension and open the bite, because there is no contact in the anterior region.

The solid block appliance is another type that is sometimes improperly used. It is made of hard acrylic and has no clasps. Appliances of this type (Fig. 11-26) are used in the upper arch as night guards. These devices should not be used in attempting to reorient the mandible by au-

FIG. 11-29. Soft rubber appliance, chewed through by patient, in turn acts as orthodontic appliance.

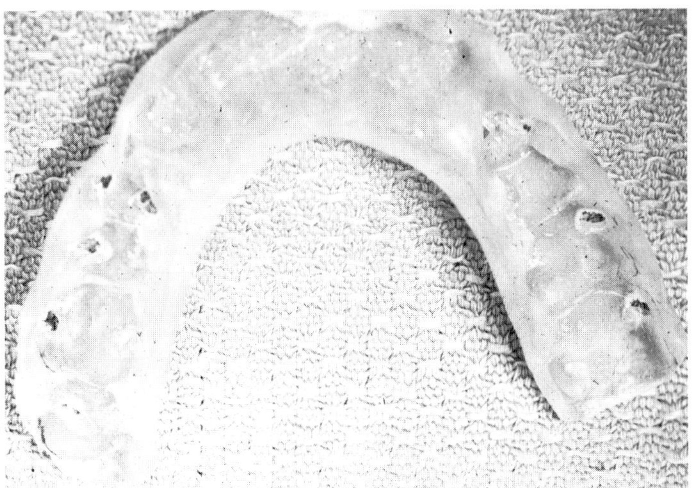

torepositioning. The basic problem is that the highly polished occlusal surfaces allow the mandible to skid on its interfering occlusal contact. Figure 11-27 depicts upper and lower block appliances, which cannot be successfully equilibrated.

Also contraindicated in the treatment of temporomandibular joint dysfunction are soft rubber appliances of the type shown in Figure 11-28. These appliances are intended to serve as night guards. However, patients readily bite through the soft rubber appliance (Fig. 11-29) which then acts as an orthodontic appliance.

BASIC REFERENCES

Goldman, H.: Seminar. University of Pennsylvania, 1961.

Karolyi, M.: Beobachtungen uber Pyorrhea Alveolaris. Oesterr.-Ungar Vierteljhrschr. Zahnh. *17*:259, 1901.

Shore, N. A.: Mandibular Autorepositioning Appliance. JADA, *75*:908, 1967.

———: TMJ stress alleviated by autorepositioning appliance. Clin. Dent., *3*:2, 1975.

———: The Shore mandibular autorepositioning appliance. J. Chicago D. Soc., 1975.

Travell, J., and Rinzler, S. H.: The myofascial genesis of pain. Postgrad. Med., *11*:425, 1952.

Wolff, H. S.: Headache and Other Pain. p. 622. New York, Oxford University Press, 1948.

12 *Roentgenography of the Temporomandibular Joint*

Functional roentgenography of the temporomandibular joint is a valuable adjunct in the complete dental examination. It will lead to a better understanding of dysfunction of this joint and of the temporomandibular joint syndrome. The chief value of this procedure is that the roentgenographic findings may be correlated with and corroborated by the clinical findings. Both in diagnosis of temporomandibular joint disorders and in roentgenography of the joint, the fact that there are two interdependent joints which act in concert must be borne in mind.

A minimum of two lateral views of each joint should be made: the first with the teeth clenched in the patient's habitual convenience relationship; the second with the mouth opened wide so that the maxillary and the mandibular teeth are separated as much as possible. The first of these views will demonstrate the condyle-to-fossa relationship, not in centric-relation occlusion, but in the habitual convenience relationship. This relationship should be compared with that in a normal joint, and any deviations should be noted. The second view will demonstrate the position of the condyle and its relationship to the articular eminence as well as the length and the inclination of the path that the condyle traverses. The practitioner must be thoroughly conversant with the normal path as well as with the normal relationship of the condyle to the articular eminence so that he may be aware of deviations from the normal.[31]

A cardinal consideration in interpreting all roentgenograms is that they are invariably two-dimensional representations of three-dimensional objects. The missing dimension is depth, which lies in the line of the central rays of the x-ray machine. The third dimension may be visualized by taking additional two-dimensional views at approximately 90° to the original view. It is for this reason that the dentist may have to take other roentgenograms in addition to the basic ones.

For further roentgenographic investigation into the structure and the position of the component parts of the joint, two mediolateral views are presented. One is the mediolateral view of the glenoid fossa, the joint gap and the condyles in the closed position; the other is the mediolateral view of the condyle in the open position, demonstrating the articular eminence, the joint gap and the head of the condyle.

Because of the complexity of the structure itself and the possibility of superimposition of extraneous structures, it is difficult to prepare a good roentgenogram of the temporomandibular joint. Three problems are involved. The first is the close proximity of many other osseous structures which makes interpretation

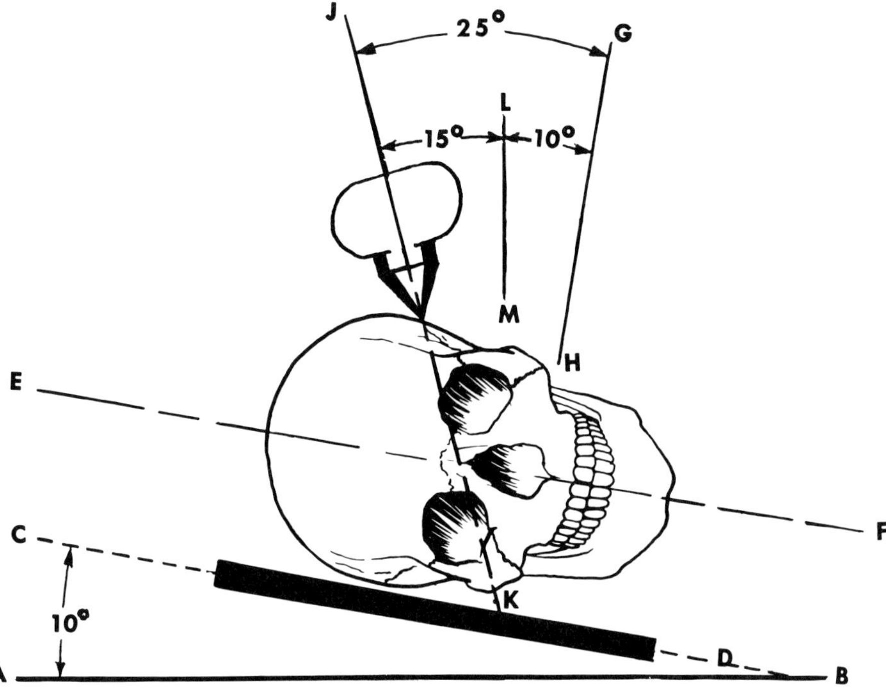

FIG. 12-1. Principles of the technique of the oblique-lateral transcranial projection.

very difficult. The second is the difficulty involved in duplicating the projection at various times during treatment for purposes of comparison and evaluation. This difficulty is caused by variations in the angle of the x-ray beam, the position of the patient's head and the position of the cassette. The third problem is the difficulty of securing a clear roentgenogram which accurately depicts the structures in the desired view. The value and the reliability of temporomandibular joint roentgenography depend upon the success with which the practitioner solves these three problems.[2,8,22,23,25,26]

OBLIQUE-LATERAL TRANSCRANIAL PROJECTION

The method of choice for the lateral view of the temporomandibular joint is the oblique-lateral transcranial projection. This projection makes possible the most accurate demonstration of the structures of the joint in any lateral position and condition. It also makes it possible to maintain the angle of the beam, of the patient's head and of the cassette on each side in either the closed or the open position. If utilized properly and accurately, the temporomandibular joint roentgenogram will be a valuable diagnostic aid and will provide confirmation of other accurately assessed data from the clinical examination.

A lateral roentgenogram of the skull parallel with the sagittal plane will result in a view in which one of the joints covers the other and produces a blurred and unclear picture of the area. Oblique-lateral transcranial roentgenography aimed at the joint nearest the cassette will avoid such superimposition and will provide a clear view of the area. The principles of this projection are illustrated in Figure 12-1. AB is the horizontal, CD is the position of the cassette at 10° from the horizontal, and EF is the sagittal plane of the skull parallel with CD. LM is perpendicular to AB, and GH is perpendicular to CD; therefore, GH forms a 10° angle with the vertical, LM. The central ray of

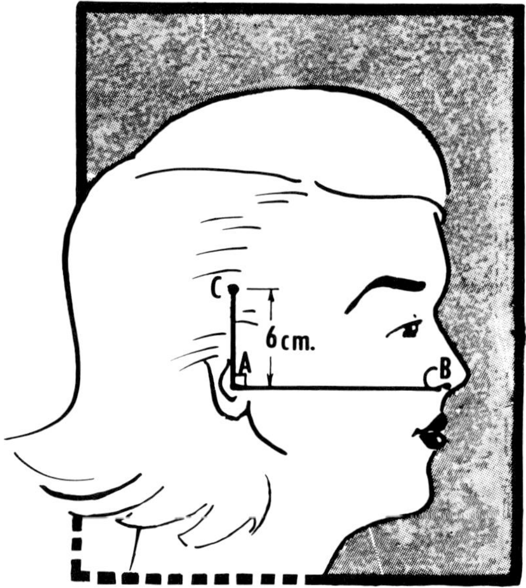

FIG. 12-2. Landmark for the entrance of the central ray for the oblique-lateral transcranial projection.

projection of the temporomandibular joint will produce an accurate lateral view of the structures of the joint and their relationships to each other, and, in addition, avoids the superimposition of the temporal bone, the basisphenoid and the dorsum sella on the joint structures.[1,7,11,19,24,27–29] All lateral-oblique transcranial roentgenograms represent a view of the lateral slope of the condyle and the glenoid fossa at A and B of Figure 12-3.

Equipment and Supplies

The technical equipment and supplies that are required for lateral-oblique transcranial roentgenography of the temporomandibular joint are:

1. Dental x-ray machine
2. Dental chair

the machine, JK, is set at 15°. This satisfies the 25° angle with the horizontal which is the basic principle of the oblique-lateral transcranial projection.

The landmark for the entrance of the central ray is 6 cm. above the superior edge of the external auditory meatus. As shown in Figure 12-2, AB is a line from the superior edge of the external auditory meatus to the ala of the nose. Point C is 6 cm. above point A and perpendicular to line AB. Point C is the central-ray landmark. Line AB on the patient is placed parallel with the upper border of the cassette. The cassette must be parallel with the sagittal plane of the skull, EF in Figures 12-1 and 12-3. It has been found that the superior surface of the condyle at A, in Figure 12-3, and the inclination of the glenoid fossa at B are at an average angle of approximately 25° to the horizontal. The cassette, CD, is set at 10° to the horizontal, and the patient places his head so that the sagittal plane, EF, is parallel with the cassette. The central ray, JK, enters at 15° to the vertical, thus satisfying the 25° angulation to the horizontal. This

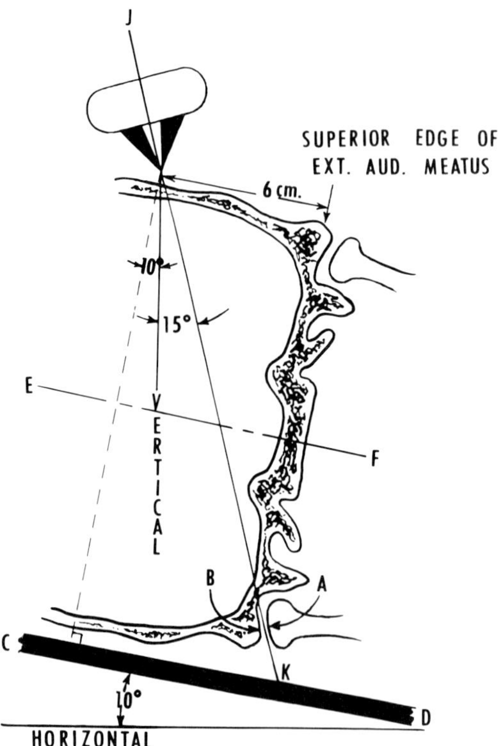

FIG. 12-3. The rationale for the mechanics of the oblique-transcranial projection. Relate to Figure 12-1. (After Grewcock)

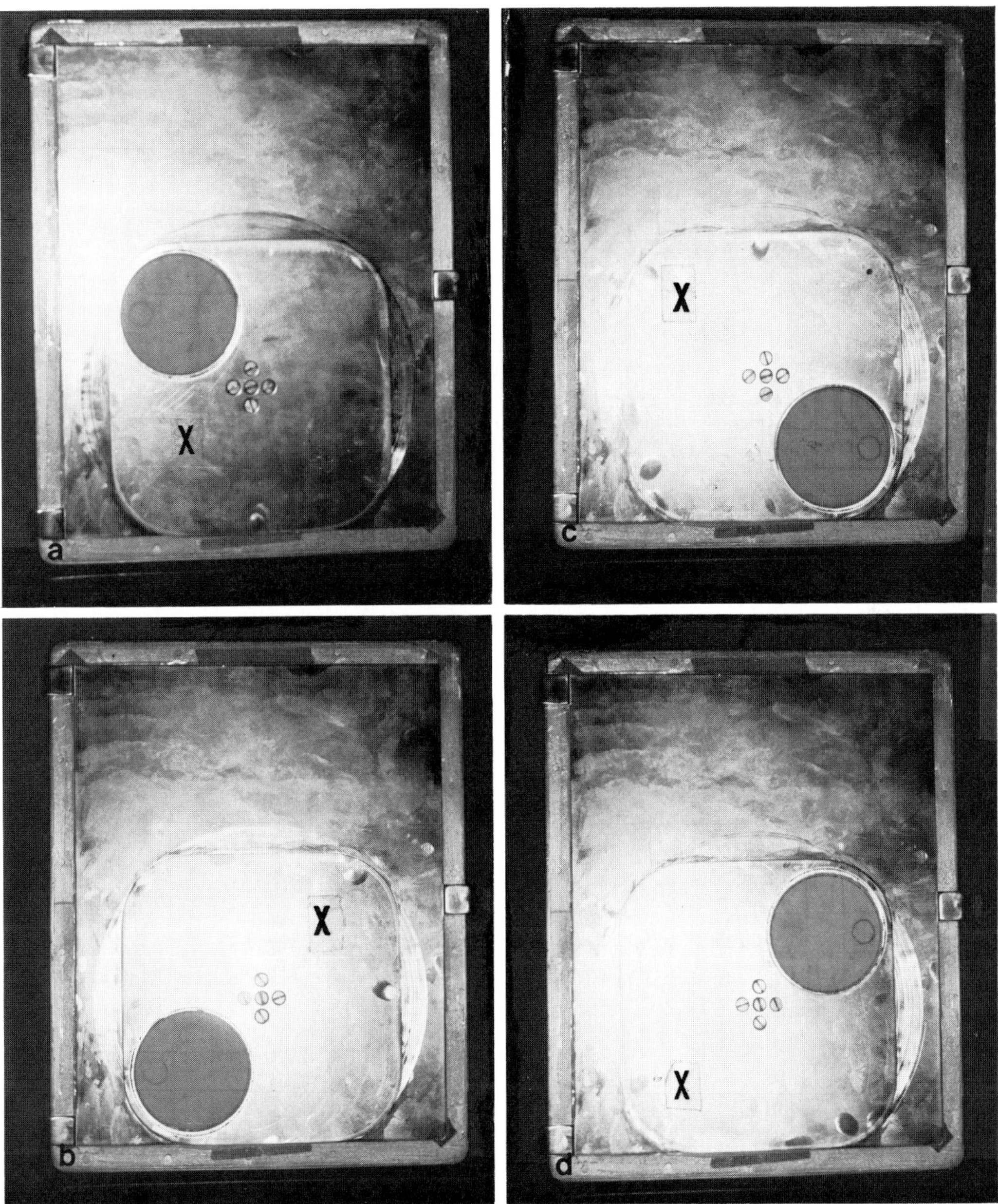

FIG. 12-4. The Martini evaluator mounted on an 8″ × 10″ cassette showing the four positions of film exposure.

3. Adjustable small stool
4. Large rubber bands for securing the cassettes to the headrest of the dental chair.
5. Cassette—8″ × 10″—with fast intensifying screens
6. X-ray film, 8″ × 10″
7. Martini evaluator or substitute
8. Mask for data printing
9. Lead letters, dates and suitable holding frame for imprinting identifying data
10. Rubber bite blocks
11. Cotton-tipped applicators, ½ inch

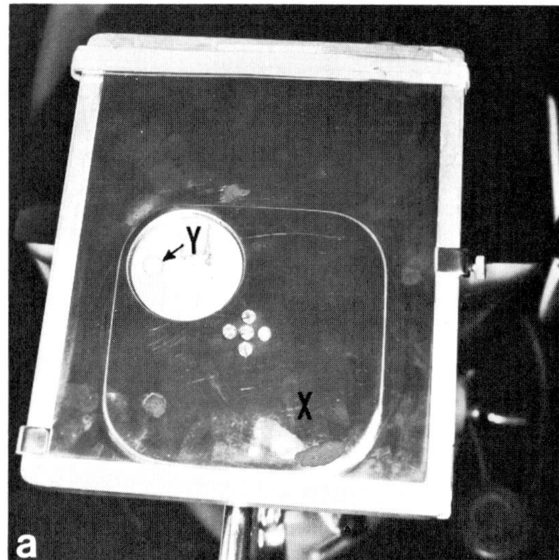

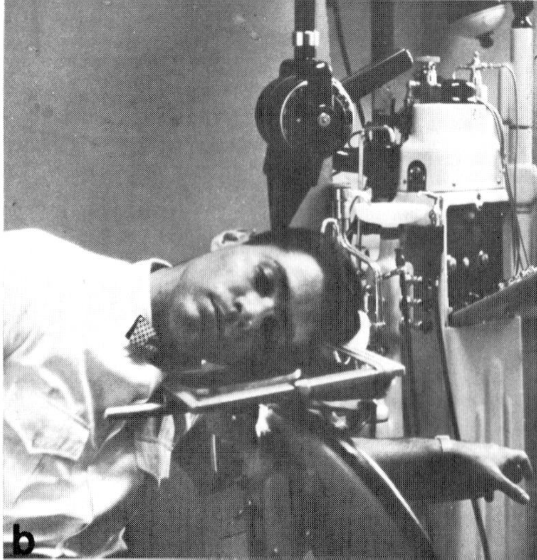

FIG. 12-5. Cassette, with attached evaluator in position A, fastened to the head-rest with rubber bands at a 10° angle (*a*). Patient and x-ray machine positioned for exposure of the film (*b*).

Procedure for Oblique-Lateral Transcranial Projection

Figure 12-4 illustrates the Martini evaluator fastened to an 8″ × 10″ cassette. The plate X of the evaluator can be rotated so that four circular exposures may be made on one film. As illustrated, the positions of the plate as it is rotated are used in the following manner:

Position A, left temporomandibular joint with teeth in habitual convenience relationship

Position B, left temporomandibular joint with teeth at greatest interincisal distance

Position C, right temporomandibular joint with the teeth at the greatest interincisal distance

Position D, right temporomandibular joint with the teeth in habitual convenience relationship

Figure 12-5*a* shows the placement of the cassette and the Martini evaluator which is fixed in position A. Both are held to the headrest of the chair by large rubber bands. These must be strong enough to secure both cassette and evaluator firmly. Using a 10° level, it is quite simple to set the headrest at an angle of 10° from the horizontal so as to create plane CD in Figure 12-1. To ensure proper centering of the relevant structures of the temporomandibular joint within the circle of the evaluator plate, insert a small cotton-tipped applicator in the external auditory meatus of the side that is to be roentgenographed. Note circle Y within the circle of the evaluator, X. Place the other end of the cotton-tipped applicator in the center of the circle, thus positioning all the relevant structures.

The first roentgenogram is taken of the left temporomandibular joint in convenience relationship, position A. Figure 12-5*b* shows the patient properly seated. Both feet are flat on the floor and the left arm is on the armrest for balance. Only his temple should touch the cassette. When the patient is positioned, grasp his chin with your left hand and place your right hand on top of the patient's head. Move the patient's head to loosen the neck muscles; then, with firm fingers on the patient's chin and holding it up, place

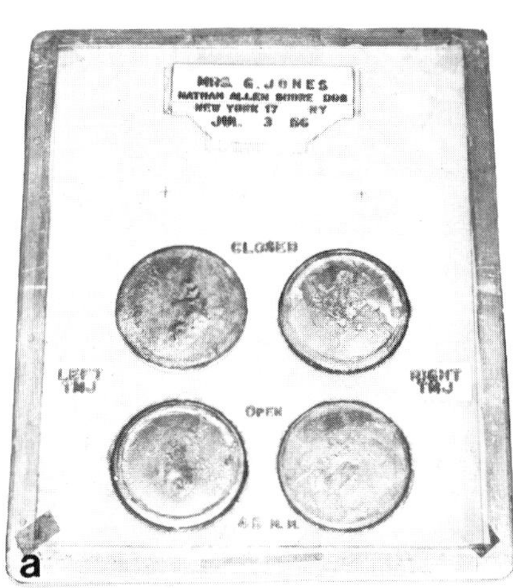

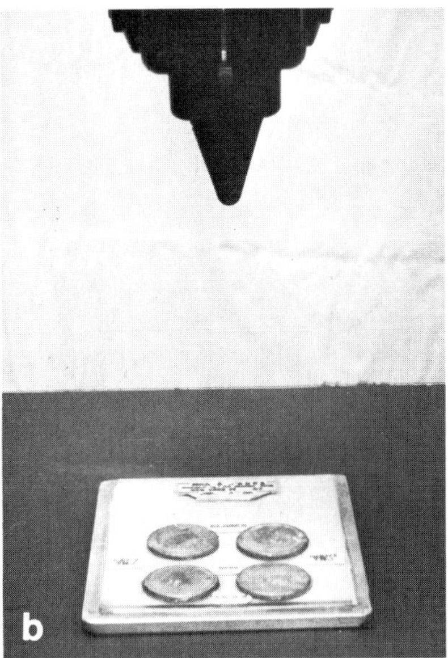

FIG. 12-6. The masking and data frame shown on the cassette (*a*) and in position for exposure of data to film (*b*). In Figure 12-7 the results of using this masking frame can be seen.

the patient's temple on the cassette. Then instruct the patient to look over your left shoulder. Position the cotton-tipped applicator in circle Y (Fig. 12-5*a*). The patient's teeth should be tightly clenched in convenience relationship. Note that the head is axially and sagitally parallel with the cassette (Fig. 12-1). Line AB of Figure 12-2 should be parallel with the base of the cassette.

The next step is to set up the x-ray machine. Point C of Figure 12-2 is the point at which the central ray must enter. Keep the horizontal bar of the frame holding the tube head of the machine parallel with the top of the cassette, and set the tube at a 15° angle, as in line JK of Figure 12-1. Figure 12-5*b* demonstrates the position of the tube head.

Caution the patient not to move and to look straight ahead at some fixed point. Separate the patient's lips to make certain that the teeth are clenched. Instruct him to take a deep breath and hold it while the film is being exposed. With a 45 kv-5 ma. machine expose the film for 4½ to 6 seconds, depending upon the age of the patient, the width of the patient's skull and the density of his body bone structure. With a 65 kv-10 ma. machine the exposure should last about 2 or 3 seconds. Rotate the evaluator to the lower position, B in Figure 12-4, to take the open-mouth view. Insert the proper bite block in the patient's mouth, measure the interincisal distance in millimeters and note it on the patient's chart. The average range is from 35 to 45 mm. With the bite block in place, position the patient and set the machine as was done in making the first exposure; then expose the film. Rotate the evaluator to position C for roentgenography of the right joint. Retain the bite block in the patient's mouth and insert a cotton-tipped applicator in his right ear. Seat him so that the right joint now rests against the evaluator. Expose the plate for the right position without removal and subsequent replacement of the bite block. After exposure of the film, remove the bite block, turn the evaluator to position D, and repeat the same proce-

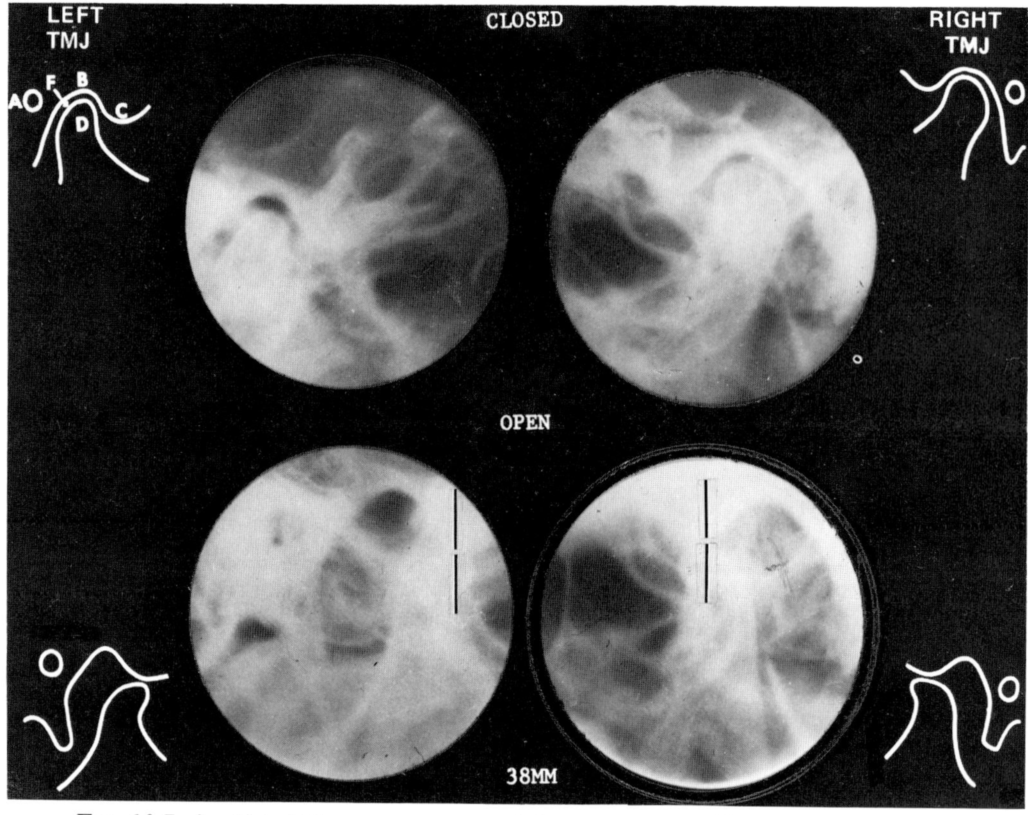

FIG. 12-7. An 8″ × 10″ roentgenogram of the temporomandibular joint produced by the oblique-lateral transcranial projection, demonstrating the closed and the open positions of each joint and their tracings. In the tracing, A represents the external auditory meatus; B, the glenoid fossa; C, the articular eminence; D, the condyle; and F, the joint gap.

dure described above for taking position A. Expose the film for the right closed position. Now, remove both the cassette and the evaluator from the headrest. After the evaluator has been removed, place the cassette upon a horizontal surface and place the masking and data frame in proper position (Fig. 12-6). This frame consists of an 8″ × 10″ sheet of clear plastic with four lead discs in position to mask the joint exposures just taken. Place appropriate identifying data upon the plastic sheet as shown. Position the head of the x-ray tube at 90°, 15 inches from the masking frame, and expose the film for 1 second. Carefully process the film.

The advantage of taking the temporomandibular joint roentgenogram in the manner described is that many factors remain constant:

1. All four views appear on one plate.
2. All identifying data and measurements are recorded in one place.
3. Processing factors are identical for all four views.
4. Cassette angulation is constant.
5. There is very little extraneous superimposition.
6. Detail is clear.[9,10]

Those who are interested in studying the position of the condyle in the fossa before the habitual convenience relationship shifts the condyles may do so by using a thin centric-relation Aluwax bite which shows no holes, indicating freedom from interfering occlusal contacts. Temporomandibular joint roentgenograms should be taken with this Aluwax bite in position in the patient's mouth. These roentgenograms will show the position of the condyle before it has been shifted by mandibular malposture caused by occlusal disharmony. This technique of roentgenography is based upon the work of Lindblom,[17] Grewcock,[13] Martini[21] and Updegrave.[31]

Interpretation of Roentgenograms

The interpretation of lateral roentgenograms of the temporomandibular joint depends upon the correlation of all available clinical data with the clinical symptoms. In the lateral roentgenogram of the normal temporomandibular joint (Fig. 12-7), note the floor of the glenoid fossa, the evenness of the joint gap and the relationship of the condyle to the anterior, superior and superoposterior walls of the glenoid fossa. The character of the bone and the shape of the condyle are also important details to observe. In the open position, note the new relationship and the condition of the structures.

As an aid in interpretation, make tracings for comparative measurements of condylar position and movement. Using a bright viewbox and tracing paper laid over the roentgenogram, trace the following structures with a sharp pencil: external auditory meatus; glenoid fossa and articular eminence; condyle head and neck (Fig. 12-7). The variables in contour, size, inclination and position of these structures will become apparent. In the open-position tracings, place a dot in the center of the condyle and another dot in the center of the articular eminence. Draw perpendicular lines through these dots. Use the vertical lines to determine the distances the condyle traveled and its relationship to the center of the eminence.

In examining the lateral view closed-position roentgenograms for defects and deformities within the joint, check the left and the right joints for differences. Observe the following:

1. The contour of the floor of the glenoid fossa for irregularity and defects
2. The density of the floor of the glenoid fossa
3. The contour of the articular eminence
4. The density of the articular eminence
5. The joint gap or space

In the last, the condyle apparently centered within the fossa, providing an almost equidistant joint gap or space anteriorly, superiorly and superoposteriorly between the condyle and the glenoid fossa. A comparison of the joint gaps of the left and the right views will usually reveal similar shapes. The joint gap may be irregular or partially obliterated. The condyle may be in an anterior, superior, posterior, inferior position or in any combination of these relationships to the floor of the glenoid fossa, thus causing irregularity of the joint gap. Observe the contour of the condyle for distortion of shape, pathological deformation, sprues, spurs and protuberances on the articular surfaces, as well as for flattening of the condyle eburnation and disharmony of shape of the condyle and of the shape of the fossa. Also observe the condyle for erosions of the osseous articular surface (infectious arthritis), generalized deossification (rheumatoid arthritis), cystic deossification beneath the subchondral cortex of the condyle, and condylectomy. Note the shape and the tilt of the neck of the condyle from the moderately forward tilt to an extreme tilt. Observe the density of the condyle, as well as the auditory meatus, the density of its surrounding bone and its proximity to the glenoid fossa.

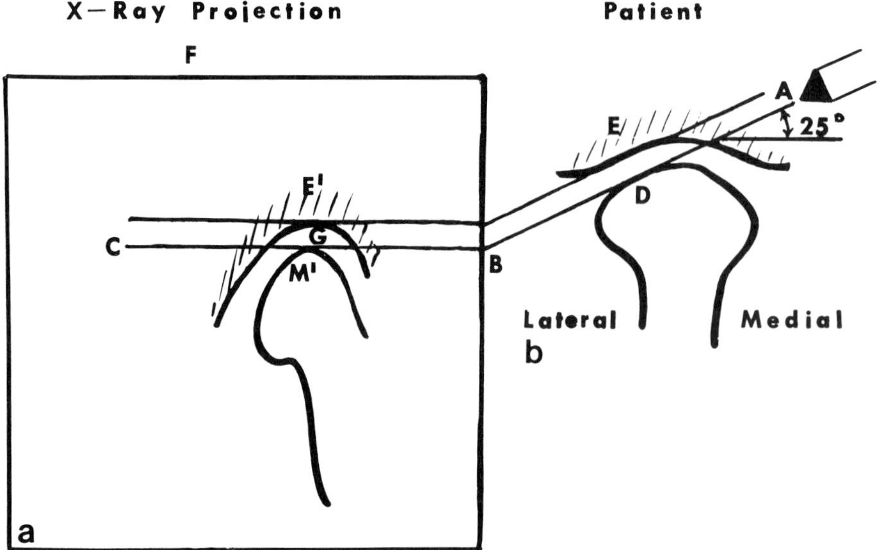

FIG. 12-8. The resulting projected view on a film (*a*) of the lateral-oblique transcranial projection of a normal temporomandibular joint of a patient (*b*). (After Norgaard)

In examining the lateral view of the open position, compare the left and the right plates and observe the following:

1. The condition and the shape of the floor of the glenoid fossa, the articular eminence and the head of the condyle
2. The angle of inclination of the posterior wall of the articular eminence
3. The distance the condyle has traveled from the closed position and possible unilateral excursion of the mandible
4. The joint space between the articular eminence and the condyle
5. The relationship of the center of the condyle to the center of the articular eminence

Hypermobility of the condyle is evident in the roentgenogram when the condyle will have passed slightly anterior to the normal position, moderately anterior to the point of self-reducing subluxation or extremely anterior to this point of dislocation. These conditions may occur unilaterally or bilaterally. In a true dislocation the condyle is anterior and superior to the articular eminence.

Hypomobility of the condyle will be evidenced in the roentgenogram by limited movement of one or both condyles in the open position (i.e., measured by the distance between the condyle center and the center of the eminence). This helps to determine whether the action of the condyle is rotary, translatory or both.

Other data obtainable from the roentgenogram will be developmental defects, calcific deposits, ankyloses, fractures, areas of osseous rarefaction and condensation, traumatic injuries and diseases such as tuberculosis; fibrous or bony ankylosis in stages of varying degree may appear within the joint; evaluation of treatment during use of treatment splints, thus confirming the treatment for restoration of vertical dimension.[4,5]

Pitfalls in Interpreting Oblique-Lateral Projections

The primary factor influencing interpretation of the roentgenogram is that the dimension of depth is lost in the lateral view. Because this dimension lies in the direction of the central ray, any move-

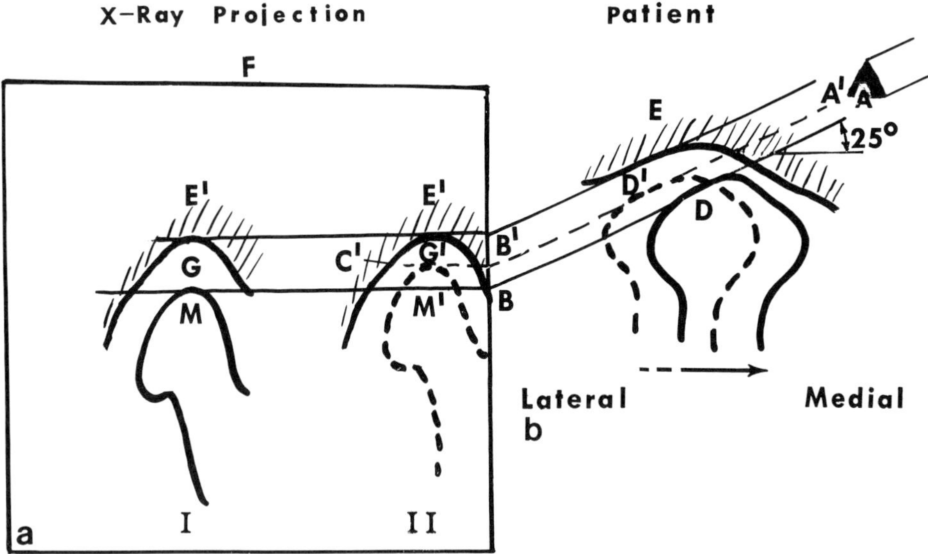

FIG. 12-9. The projection (*a*,I) of a medial shift of the condyle (*b*, *solid line*). The normal condyle (*dotted line*) in (*a*,II) and (*b*) is illustrated for comparison. Compare G with G′. A medial movement (*b*, *solid line*) is misinterpreted as an inferior movement. (After Norgaard)

ment along the line of that ray is not recorded on the lateral view. Mediolateral condylar movements in the line of the central ray may be confused with movements in the superoinferior direction because both directional movements produce similar profiles.

The problems of the interpretation of condylar position in the line of the central ray are demonstrated in the following discussion. Figure 12-8*a* shows the lateral-oblique transcranial projection of a normal right temporomandibular joint with the condyle in the glenoid fossa. Drawing (*b*) shows the mediolateral view of the right joint. The angle of the ray is 25°, and the x-ray line, ADB, is parallel with the lateral slope of the condyle and the floor of the glenoid fossa, E. This projection is superimposed on the film, F, as CB, with the joint gap at G, the floor of the glenoid fossa at E′ and the condyle in its normal position. The lateral slope of the condyle, D, of drawing (*b*) is labeled point M′ in drawing (*a*). It is important to understand that drawing (*a*) is not an actual lateral view but a projected view of the temporomandibular joint at an angle of 25° to the horizontal.

Figure 12-9 demonstrates a medial shift of the condyle of the right temporomandibular joint. The position of the condyle is represented by the solid line, D. The dotted line, D′, represents the normal position of the condyle. The angle of the x-ray at 25° produces the path, ADB, and the projection (*a*), I, on film F, with resulting joint gap G′ in (*a*), II. Therefore, a medial shift of the condyle without a change in the vertical position can produce an x-ray projection of a condyle head in an inferior position.

In Figure 12-10*b*, the dotted line condyle similar to D in Figure 12-9 represents a medial shift without vertical change. The solid-line condyle represents an inferior position without mediolateral change. The x-ray path, AB, projected on film, F, produces the joint gap, G. Thus, it can be seen that both a medial shift and an inferior shift of a condyle will produce similar images of a condyle in an inferior

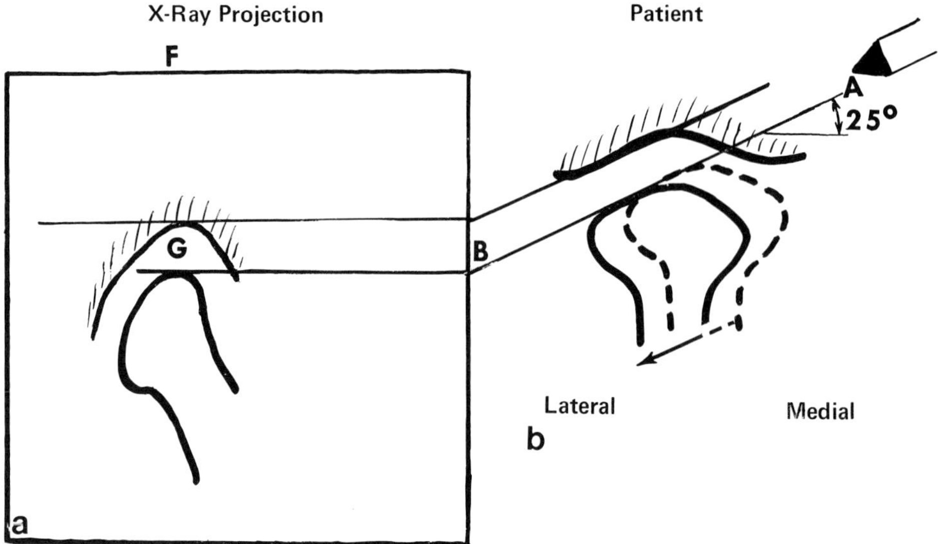

FIG. 12-10. The misinterpretation of the relationship of an inferior and a medial shift of the condyle in (*b*) and the similarity of their resultant projections in (*a*). (After Norgaard)

position on the film with a joint gap wider than normal. By similar reasoning, Figure 12-11 shows that a superior position of the solid-line condyle without mediolateral change, and a lateral position of the dotted-line condyle with vertical

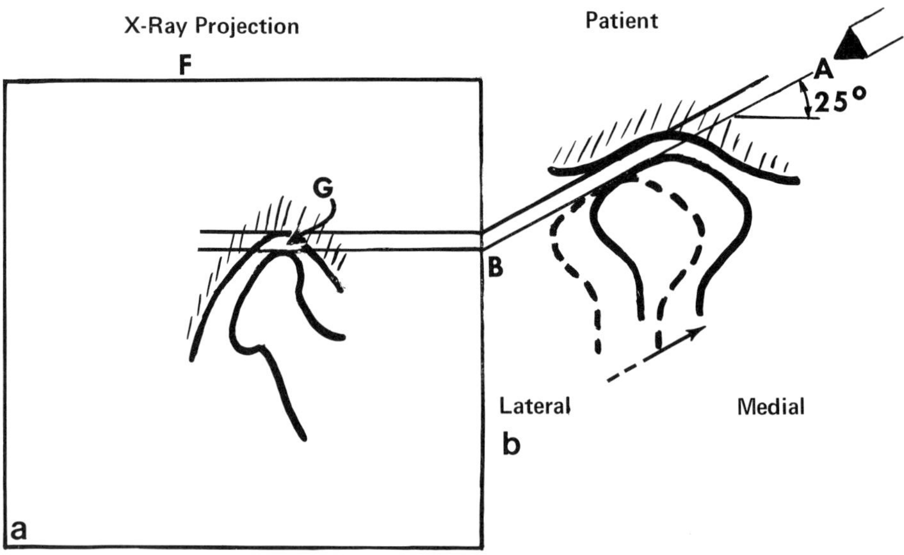

FIG. 12-11. The misinterpretation of the relationship of a superior and a lateral shift of the condyle in (*b*) and the similarity of their resultant projections in (*a*). (After Norgaard)

change produce similar images on the film—a condyle in a superior position with a joint gap narrower than normal.

Figures 12-8 to 12-11 serve to warn the unwary not to make snap diagnoses of temporomandibular joint disorders solely on the basis of oblique-lateral transcranial projection roentgenographic studies. To supply the third dimension so that roentgenographic visualization of the temporomandibular joint is possible, techniques for making mediolateral views must be considered. Two projections aid in producing roentgenograms of mediolateral views of the temporomandibular joint. They are the midorbitomeatal-baseline, corner-of-the-mouth projection with the teeth clenched and the inner-canthus, articular-eminence projection with the teeth at the maximum interincisal distance. These projections are generally considered as modified antero-posterior exposures.[6,15,16,20,30]

THE MIDORBITOMEATAL-BASELINE, CORNER-OF-THE-MOUTH PROJECTION

A mediolateral view of the floor of the glenoid fossa, the joint gap and the superior surface and neck of the condyles of the right and the left temporomandibular joints in the closed position may be roentgenographed on the same film and at the same time by using the midorbitomeatal-baseline, corner-of-the-mouth projection. This projection is based on the work of Waters and Waldron[32] and Whitehouse.[33]

Equipment and Supplies

The technical equipment and supplies that are required to make this projection are:

1. Dental x-ray machine
2. Dental chair
3. Adjustable stool or chair
4. Leveling device

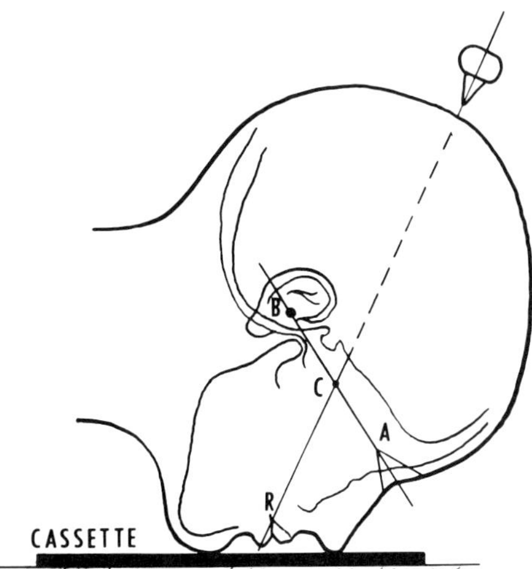

FIG. 12–12. Principle of the technique of the midorbitomeatal-baseline, corner-of-the-mouth projection. (After Whitehouse)

5. Large rubber bands for securing cassette to headrest
6. Cassette—8″ × 10″—with fast intensifying screens
7. X-ray film, 8″ × 10″
8. Flexible 12″ ruler
9. Skin-marking pencil
10. Mask for data printing with lead letters

Procedure for Midorbitomeatal-Baseline, Corner-of-the-Mouth Projection

The first step in the procedure is to draw on the patient's face the guide to the entrance point and the path of the central ray. Using a ruler and a skin pencil, mark the orbitomeatal baseline, AB. A is the outer canthus of the eye, and B is the superior border of the external auditory meatus (Fig. 12-12). Measure the distance from A to B and mark the midpoint with a dot at C; using the flexible ruler, draw a line upward connecting the corner of the mouth, R, with C, forming line CR. This is the line that creates the angulation for the central ray.

Fasten the cassette to the headrest, (Fig. 12-13*a*), and place it parallel to the

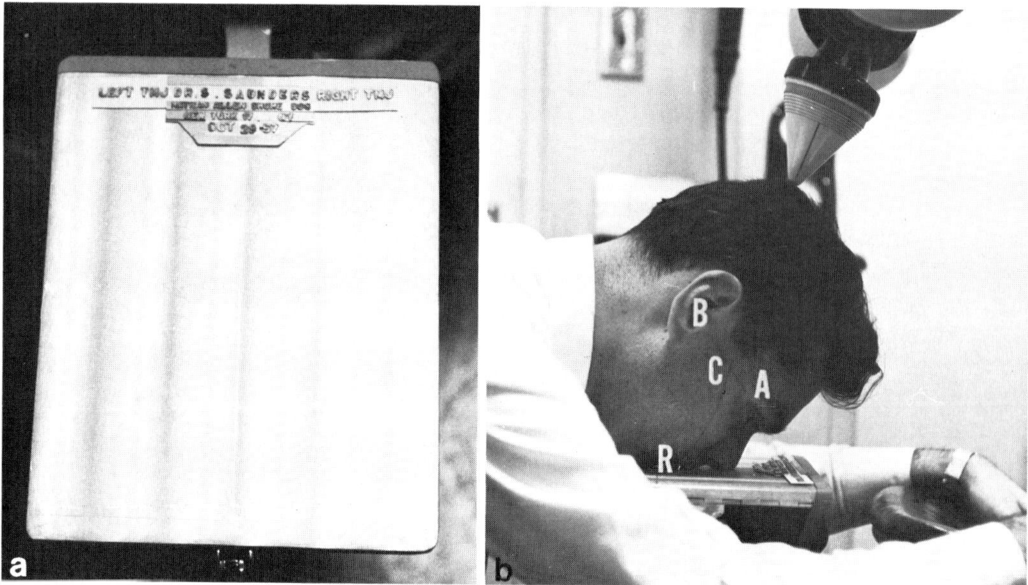

FIG. 12-13. The fastening of the cassette and the placement of the identifying data (*a*). The placement of the patient's head and arms, and the angulation of the central ray to the marked lines on the face (*b*) are illustrated; refer to Figure 12-12.

floor with the aid of a level. Place identifying data at the top of the cassette. Seat the patient on a stool behind the dental chair, as in (*b*), with both arms forward on the armrests, his nose and chin touching the center of the cassette and the teeth clenched. Adjust the central ray of the machine so that it passes along the line CR (Fig. 12-12). The tube head is parallel with the top of the cassette and centered directly over the patient, who holds his breath while the film is exposed. The exposure factor is 65 kv at 15 ma for 3 seconds.

Roentgenographic Interpretation

The projection of mediolateral views of both temporomandibular joints in the closed position on a single film permits study of the relationships of the component structures in a third dimension not shown in the lateral views.

In the mediolateral views of the closed-position temporomandibular joints (Fig. 12-14) observe the following:

1. The greatest value of this projection is the visualization of each condyle, glenoid-fossa relationship in the mediolateral direction. Any mediolateral movement is directly observed. The superoinferior or anteroposterior movement of the condyle is seen only as a relative movement which is observed by the variation in the widths of the joint gaps. For this reason this view must be correlated with and corroborated by the lateral view.
2. The mediolateral contour and density of the posterior wall of the articular eminence
3. The gap between the posterior wall of the articular eminence and the superior surface of the condyle
4. The mediolateral contour and density of the condyle
5. The mediolateral contour and density of the neck of the condyle
6. A mediolateral view of the coronoid process
7. Demonstration of osseous changes in a mediolateral view of the joint, the mandible, the nasal bones, the malar

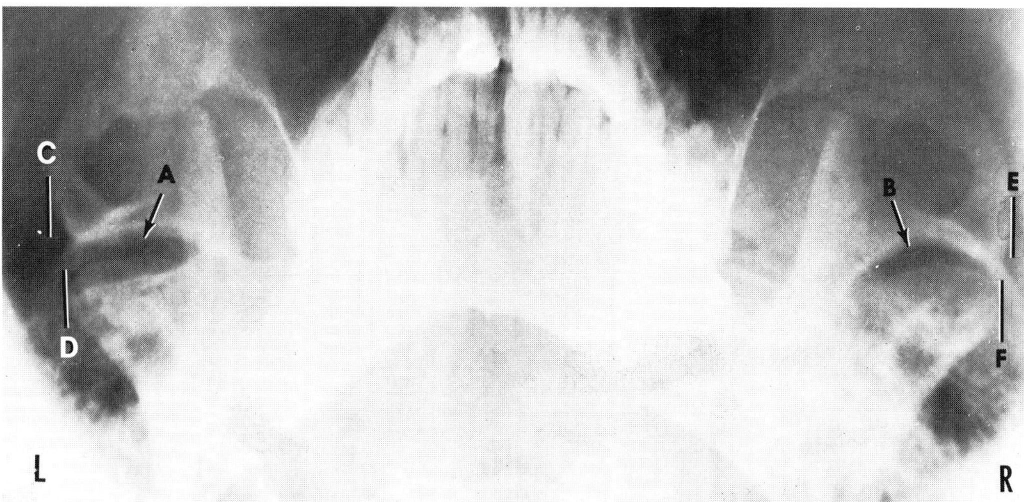

Fig. 12-14. Temporomandibular joint roentgenogram, an anteroposterior projection of normal joints. A and B indicate the left and right joint gaps. The distances between the lines C and D and E and F represent lateral shifts of the condyles, when present.

bones, the zygoma, the zygomatic arches and the antra

This view can also serve as a preoperative view for the surgeon to determine the areas of fractures, dysplasia, etc.

In the mediolateral view it is possible to verify the normal or pathological features as seen in the lateral views. It may also be taken with the teeth in the open position.[14,20]

Pitfalls in Interpreting the Midorbitomeatal-Baseline, Corner-of-the-Mouth Projection

As explained in the section on pitfalls in interpreting the oblique-lateral transcranial projection, the dimension of depth is lost in all roentgenographic two-dimensional views. The loss of depth creates a similar problem of interpreting condylar movement in this projection. Anteroposterior condylar movements in the line of the central ray may be confused with movements in a superoinferior direction because both directional movements in this view can produce similar profiles.

The mechanics of interpreting condylar position in the line of the central ray are demonstrated in the following discussion. Figure 12-15 shows the midorbitomeatal-baseline, corner-of-the-mouth projection of a normally positioned right temporomandibular joint (*a*), and its film projection, a mediolateral view (*b*). The x-rays pass parallel with the posterior wall of this eminence, E, and the anterior surface of the condyle, C, producing on the film, F, projection lines AB and DG, respectively. The distance between AB and DG is the projected joint gap. Figure 12-15*c*,*d* demonstrates that dissimilar positions of the condyle in the glenoid fossa can project similar images on the x-ray film. The solid-line condyle, S, represents a superior position with respect to normal, and the dotted-line condyle, T, represents an anterior position with respect to normal. The x-ray beam, AD, along the posterior wall of the articular eminence, E, projects the line AB on the film with E′ as the eminence. The superior position, condyle S, and the anterior position, condyle T, are both projected on the film as line DG.

The following conclusions may be drawn from the projected image on the

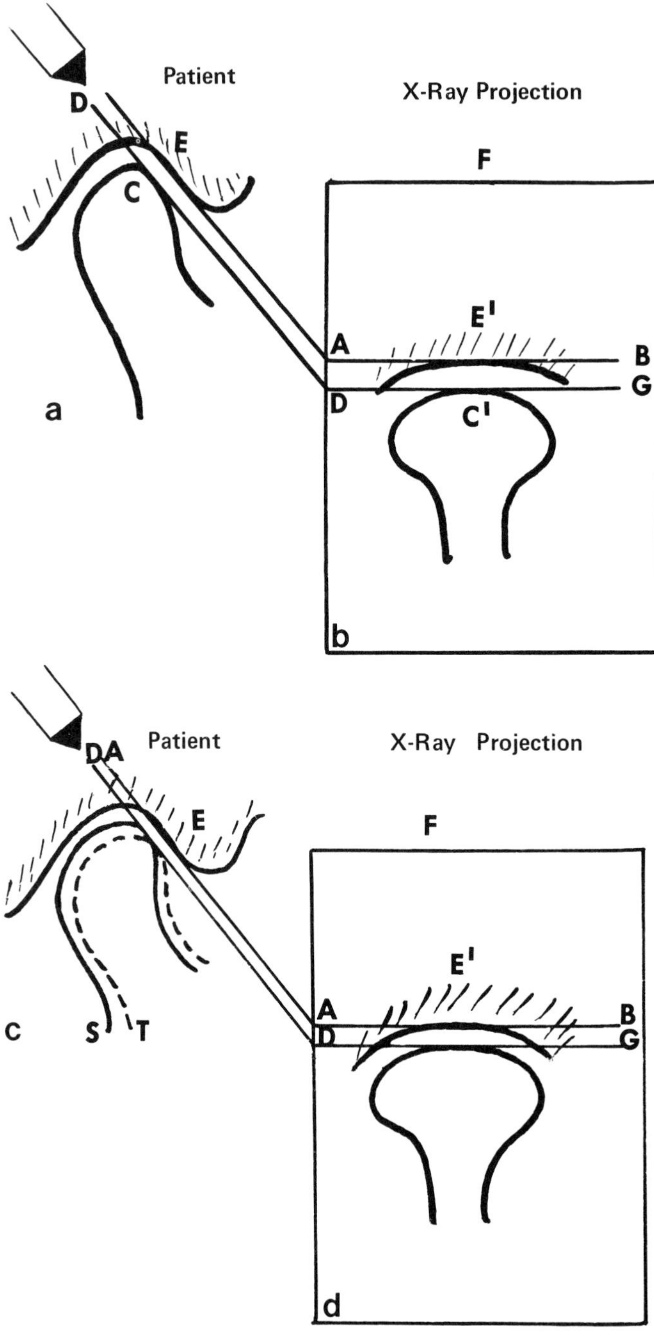

FIG. 12-15. The midorbitomeatal-baseline, corner-of-the-mouth projection of a normal positioned temporomandibular joint of a patient (*a*), and the resultant projected view (*b*) on a film. A superior and an anterior position of a patient's condyle (*c*) and the similar projection they both can give on the film in (*d*). The projection of the normal condyle level is shown as DG.

film. A superior or an anterior position of the condyle may yield similar images (Fig. 12-15*c*,*d*). Both condyle positions yield joint gaps that are narrower than normal. By the same reasoning, an inferior or a posterior position may yield similar x-ray images and joint gaps that are larger than normal. If Figure 12-15 is viewed again in the light of these conclusions, it will be seen that an apparently normal projection may not indicate a normal position, since any position along the line of the

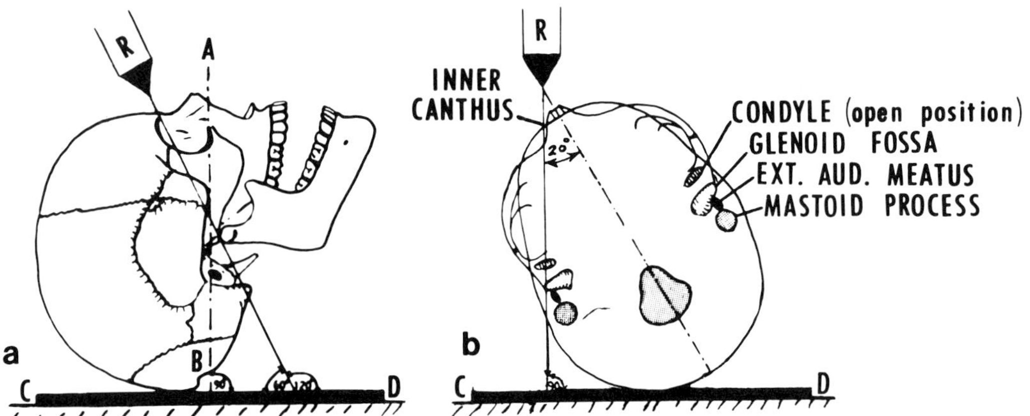

FIG. 12-16. Principles of the technique of the inner-canthus, articular-eminence projection. (After Zimmer, E. A.: Die Roentgenologie des Kiefergelenkes. Rev. Mens. Suisse Odont., *51:*949)

x-rays will produce a similar image. Therefore, it must be emphasized that one projection is not enough for correct interpretation. Both lateral and mediolateral views are necessary for correct orientation of the condyle in the glenoid fossa.

THE INNER-CANTHUS, ARTICULAR-EMINENCE PROJECTION

A mediolateral view of the articular eminence, the eminence-condylar gap, and the superior surface and the neck of the condyle in the open position may be roentgenographed by the inner-canthus, articular-eminence projection (Fig. 12-16). This projection is based upon the work of Zimmer[34] and of Grant and Lanting.[12]

Figure 12-17 depicts the placement of the head in relation to the central ray. In (*a*) the head is placed upon the cassette so that the Frankfort horizontal plane, AB, is perpendicular to the cassette, CD. Then the head is tilted 20° to the side, keeping plane AB perpendicular to the cassette (*b*). The mouth is opened wide. The tube is angled 60° caudad with the horizontal, and the landmark for the entrance of the central ray, R, is the inner canthus of the eye.

Equipment and Supplies

The technical equipment and supplies that are required for making this projection are:

1. Dental x-ray machine
2. Dental chair
3. Protractor and leveling device
4. Large rubber bands for securing cassette to the headrest of the dental chair
5. Cassette—8″ × 10″—with fast intensifying screens
6. X-ray film, 8″ × 10″
7. Leaded rubber sheeting—8″ × 10″—with one quarter, 4″ × 5″, cut out for masking
8. Plastic sheet—8″ × 10″—for data printing, lower half covered by leaded rubber sheeting, 5″ × 8″
9. Lead letters for printing

Procedure for Inner-Canthus, Articular-Eminence Projection

The procedure for roentgenographing the inner-canthus, articular-eminence projection is as follows.

1. Set the dental chair with the back

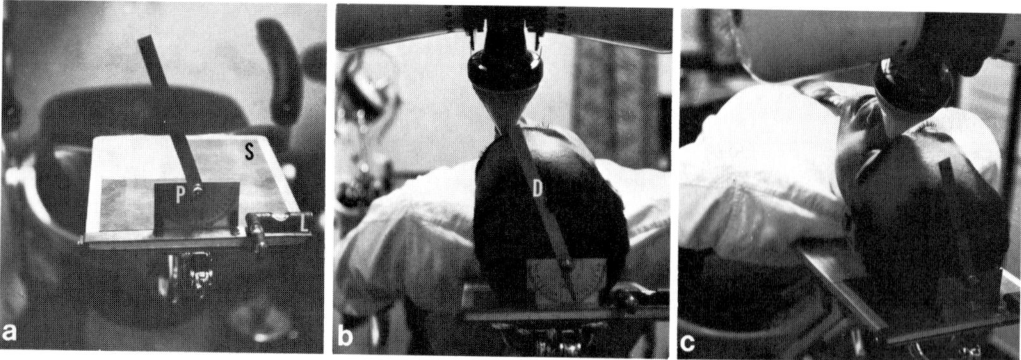

FIG. 12-17. Cassette, protractor, level assembly and rubber sheeting in position for the inner-canthus, articular-eminence projection (*a*). Sagittal plane of the patient's head parallel with D (*b*). Patient and x-ray machine positioned for the exposure of the film (*c*).

and the headrest so that the patient will be in a supine position.

2. Place and fasten the cassette to the headrest with the rubber bands (Fig. 12-17*a*).

3. Set the protractor, P, and level assembly, L, on the cassette and make the cassette level and parallel with the floor.

4. Turn the degree indicator, P, to 70° on the protractor, P, for roentgenography of the left temporomandibular joint.

5. Place the leaded rubber sheet, S, on

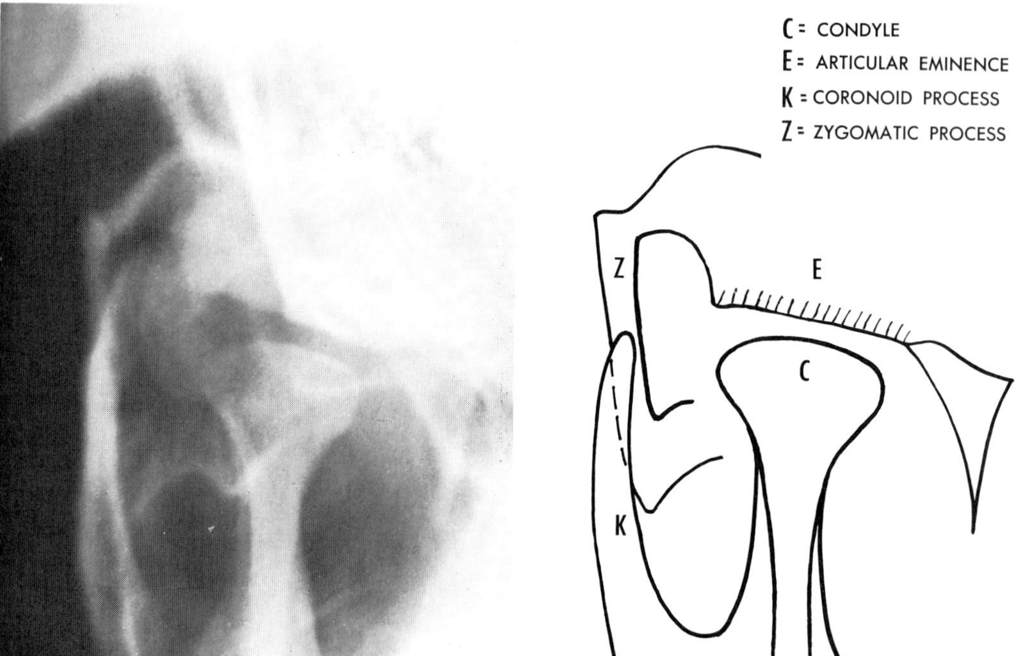

FIG. 12-18. Roentgenogram and tracing of the right temporomandibular joint produced by the inner-canthus, articular-eminence projection, demonstrating the joint structures mediolaterally in the open position. (After Zimmer)

the cassette so that the cut-out quadrant is on the lower left side.

6. Place the patient in the dental chair as in (*b*) and (*c*).

7. Check the cassette level to make certain that it is parallel with the floor.

8. Rotate the patient's head to the left with the sagittal plane of the skull parallel with the degree indicator, D, as in (*b*) and (*c*).

9. Direct the patient to open wide, and place the rubber bite block in the molar region.

10. Angle the x-ray machine 60° in the caudad direction and place at the inner canthus of the eye of the side being roentgenographed (*c*).

11. Tell the patient to hold his breath while the film is exposed.

12. Reverse the lead rubber sheeting, exposing the lower right quadrant of the cassette.

13. Set the protractor for 110°, and place the sagittal plane of the patient's head parallel with the degree indicator.

14. Using the technique described above, roentgenograph the right temporomandibular joint. The exposure factors are 65 kv at 15 ma for 1 second.

15. Place the cassette on a flat surface, place the printing and data mask upon it, and expose the film for 1 second.

Roentgenographic Interpretation

This view of the relationships and condition of the component structures of the temporomandibular joint in the open position (Fig. 12-18) is useful for the following reasons:

1. The condyle is oriented mediolaterally to determine mediolateral displacement in the open position.

2. This image supplies the third view for the open-position lateral projections for correlation and corroboration.

3. The mediolateral contour and density of the articular eminence may be observed in the anterior view, rather than the posterior view as with the midorbitomeatal-baseline, corner-of-the-mouth projection.

4. The gap between the articular eminence and the condyle may be observed.

5. The mediolateral contour of the condyle may be observed in the anterior view, rather than the posterior view as with the midorbitomeatal-baseline, corner-of-the-mouth projection.

6. The density of the condyle may be determined.

7. The contour and the density of the neck of the condyle may be evaluated.

8. Pathological condylar changes and pathosis in a mediolateral view (i.e., position, partial ankylosis, etc.) may be demonstrated.

9. Preoperative view enables the surgeon to predetermine the extent and the area of condylar surgery.

10. Postoperative views enable the surgeon to evaluate results of treatment.

Pitfalls in Interpretation

As explained in earlier sections, the conditions of dimensional confusion are always present in any projection, and this one is no exception. Therefore, the same precautions in interpretation must be taken.

Correlation of Temporomandibular Joint Roentgenograms and Clinical Symptoms

The factors which cause temporomandibular joint derangement are pathologic occlusion, systemic and local diseases and external trauma to the components of the joint. The analysis of the roentgenograms of the temporomandibular joint should corroborate the clinical symptoms. The correlation of pathologic occlusion and temporomandibular joint roentgenograms is based upon the displacement of the condyles in the fossae.

Figure 12-19 illustrates the position of

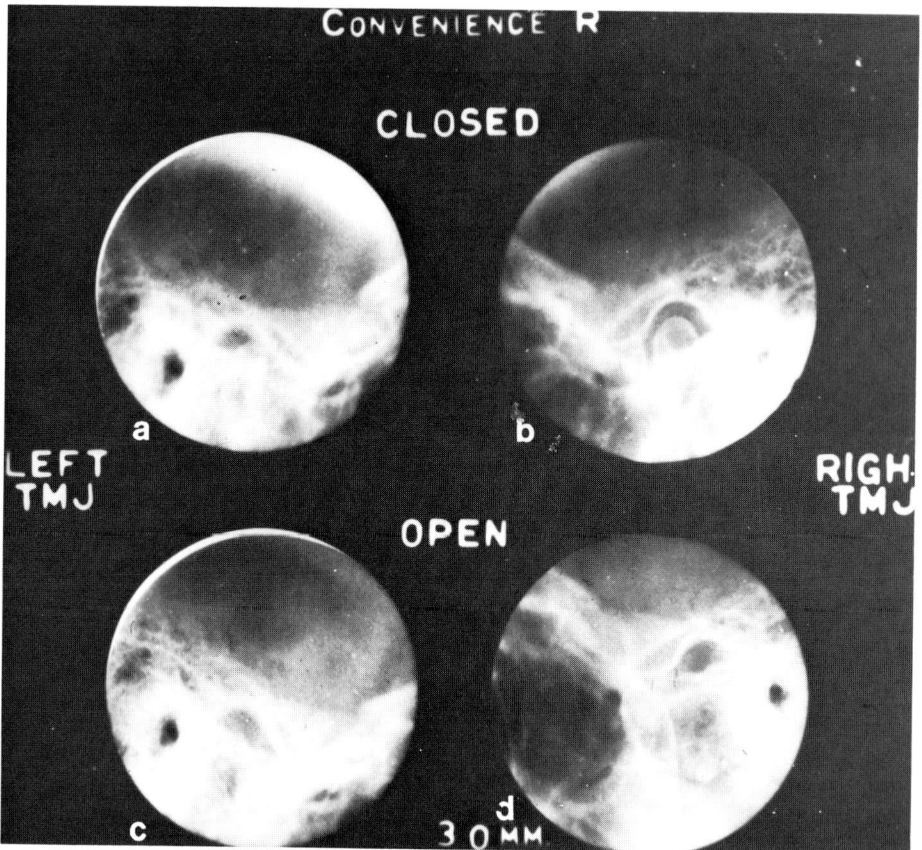

FIG. 12-19. Pathological convenience relationship prior to therapy (1959).

the condyles in the fossae when the mandible is in habitual pathological convenience relation in the right- and left-closed position. The condyle is displaced at (*a*) and (*b*). In the opened position the left condyle is 5 mm. short of the center of the eminence (*c*).

The factors of pathologic occlusion that result in displacement of the condyles are the interfering occlusal contact and the movement of the mandible which results from such a contact.

To illustrate the relationship of these factors, consider a hypothetical case. The temporomandibular joint roentgenogram, closed-position, lateral view, one side, exhibits a large joint gap. As was pointed out in the section on the interpretation of the roentgenogram of the lateral projection, the condyle is either in medial or in inferior position. To determine whether the position of the condyle is medial or inferior, the mediolateral, closed-position view should be roentgenographed. Clinically, the medial position of the condyle can be caused by an interfering occlusal contact on the buccal planes of the lower buccal or lingual cusps in a Class I mandibular protrusive relationship. The inferior position of the condyle can be caused by an interfering occlusal contact in a Class III increased vertical relationship. Thus the correlation of the interfering occlusal contact and the position of the condyle can be seen in this case. To complete the picture, the movement of the mandible must be observed from the interfering contact on the centric-relation

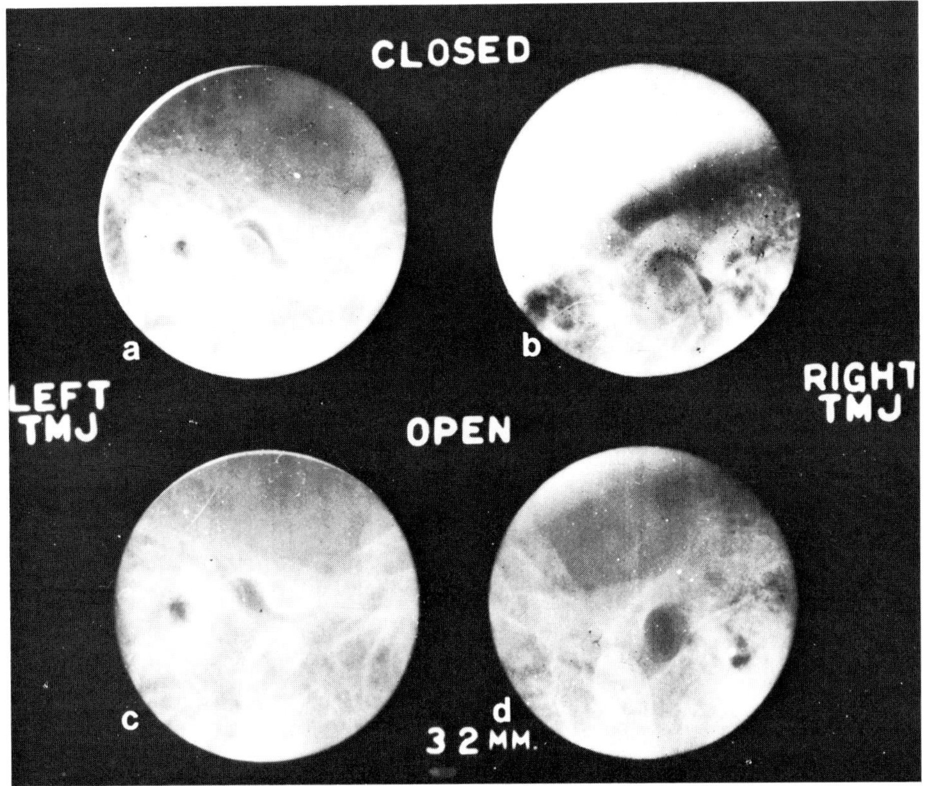

FIG. 12-20. The same patient as in Fig. 12-19 (1975) in correct centric-relation occlusion 16 years after therapy was started.

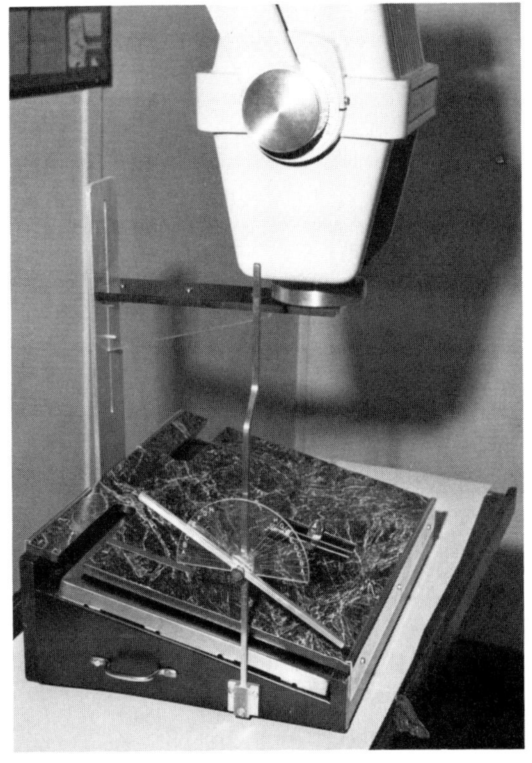

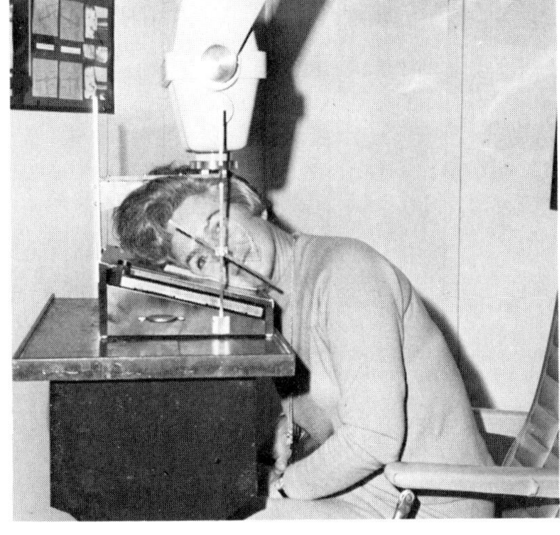

FIG. 12–21. The use of the Updegrave x-ray board. (Courtesy of Dr. W. J. Updegrave)

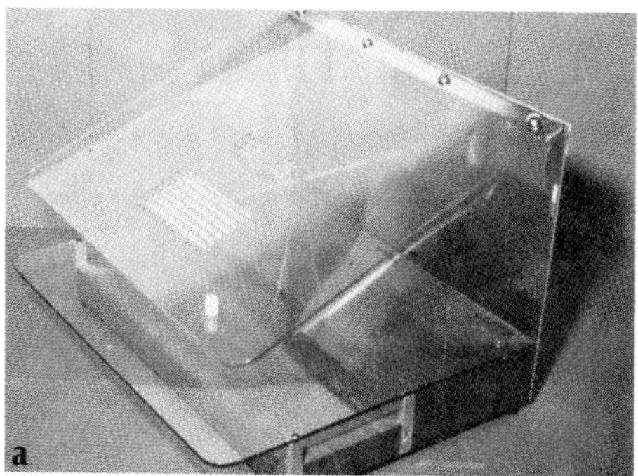

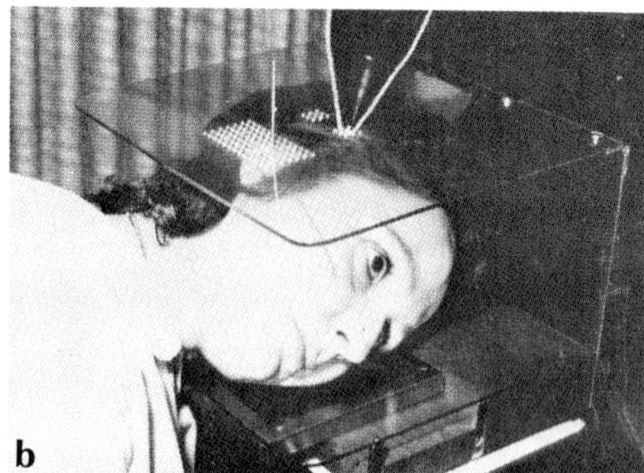

FIG. 12-22. Temporomandibular joint head positioner (*a*). The head positioner permits three-dimensional control of head position (*b*).

arc to the final stage of pathological closure. The Aluwax bite that is described in the next chapter establishes the exact contacting planes of the interfering occlusal contact that initiates this pathological mandibular movement.

The correlation of systemic disease, local disease and external trauma to the joint components with the temporomandibular joint roentgenographs is based upon the existing conditions of the osseous structures and the malposition of the condyle within the glenoid fossa.[3] The roentgenographic manifestations of these diseases are discussed in the section on differential diagnosis of temporomandibular joint disease in Chapter 9. For comparison, see roentgenograms of the same patient 16 years later (Fig. 12-20). This patient is still pain free. Notice the equidistant joint gap in the closed position at (*a*) and (*b*) and the correct placement of the condyle in the open position at (*c*) and (*d*).

The Updegrave TMJ board (Fig. 12-21) illustrates the placement of the head when taking roentgenograms of the temporomandibular joint. Further information can be obtained from the many articles written by W. J. Updegrave.[31]

Also depicted is the temporomandibular joint head positioner (Fig. 12-22), which permits three-dimensional control of head position.

REFERENCES

1. Altschul, W.: Die radiologische darstellung des kiefergelenkes (Radiography of the temporomandibular joint). Fortschr. Geb. Röntgenstr., *27:*23, 1919.
   ———: Studies on the temporomandibular joint. Am. J. Roentgenol. Radium Ther., *26:*452, 1931.
   ———: Some new methods in roentgenography. Am. J. Roentgenol. Radium Ther., *27:*659, 1927.
2. Amer, A.: Approach to surgical diagnosis of the temporomandibular articulation through basic studies of the normal. JADA, *45:*668, 1952.
3. Bender, T. J., Jr.: Mechanical Basis of Low Back Pain. Med. A. Mobile, Ala. 1954.
4. Bergman, S. A.: Importance of temporomandibular joint roentgenograms in mouth rehabilitation. New York State D. J., *20:*103, 1954.
5. Berry, H. M.: Cinefluorography with image intensification for observing temporomandibular joint movements. JADA, *53:*517, 1956.
6. Berry, D. C., and Chick, A. O.: Temporomandibular joint: interpretation of radiographs. D. Pract., *7:*18, 1956.
7. Bishop, P. A.: A roentgen consideration of the temporomandibular joint. Am. J. Roentgenol. Radium Ther., *21:*556, 1929.
8. Boman, K., Lindblom, G., and Sundberg, S.: Kakledsarthrosen, dess kirurgiska och tandortopediska behandling, Sven. Tandlak. Tidkskr., *36:*441, 1943.

9. Donovan, R. W.: A method of temporomandibular joint roentgenography for serial or multiple records. JADA, *49:*401, 1954.
10. Fuchs, A. W.: Radiography of the jaws, Part III, The temporomandibular articulation. Radiogr. Clin. Photogr., *9:*5, 1933.
11. Goldstein, M.: Instrument and method for radiography of the temporomandibular joint. D. Digest, *62:*536, 1955.
12. Grant, R., and Lanting, H.: An improved technic for roentgenographic examination of the temporomandibular joint and condyle. J. Oral Surg., *11:*95, 1953.
13. Grewcock, R. J. G.: A simplified technique of temporomandibular joint radiography. Br. D. J., *94:*152, 1953.
14. Helm, M.: Radiography of the paranasal and mastoid regions in the erect position. Med. Radiogr. Photogr. *30*(2)*:*40, 1954.
15. Husted, E.: Methods and problems in temporomandibular joint examination. D. World, *12*(1)*:*37, 1957.
16. King, W. A.: A radiographic analysis of a clinical determination of the transverse axis of the movement of the mandible. Thesis, Northwestern Univ., 1951.
17. Lindblom, G.: Technique for roentgenographic registration of the different condyle positions in the temporomandibular joint. D. Cosmos., *78:*1227, 1936.
18. Lundstrom, A.: Cephalometric registrations as an aid in diagnosing malocclusions, Acta Odont. Scand. *11:*100, 1953.
19. McGaha, W. R.: A localizing device for radiography of the mandibular articulation. Med. Radiogr. Photogr., *31*(3)*:*108, 1955.
20. Marolt, A.: Tatsachen und hypothesen, (Facts and theories). Schweiz. Monatsschr. Zahn., *63*(9)*:*880, 1953.
———: Experimentelle untersuchungen uber die gleitbewegungen des unterkiefers (Experimental studies regarding the gliding movements of the mandible). Odont. Rev., *7*(2)*:*167, 1956.
———: Rontgenologische untersuchungen uber die bewegung der kondylen beim seitbiss (Roentgenologic studies concerning the movements of the condyles in the sideward bite). Schweiz. Monatsschr. Zahn. *66*(3)*:*183, 1956.
21. Martini, J. J.: Maxillofacial radiography. Oral Surg., *3:*1540, 1950.
———: Personal communications, 1950.
22. Mayerson, M.: A radiographic and clinical study of the positions of the condyles in individuals exhibiting malfunctions of the temporomandibular joints. Northwestern Univ. Bull., *54:*14, 1953.
23. Norgaard, F.: Temporomandibular Arthrography. Copenhagen, Einar Munksgards, 1947.
24. Richards, A. G., and Alling, C. C.: Extra-oral radiography, mandible and temporomandibular articulation. D. Radiogr. Photogr., *28*(1)*:*1, 1955.
25. Ricketts, R. M.: Variations of the temporomandibular joint as revealed by cephalometric laminography. Am. J. Ortho., *36:*877, 1950.
26. Ruskin, R.: An evaluation of a technique and its implication in interpretation of radiographs of the temporomandibular articulation. Northwestern Univ. Bull., *54:*11, 1953.
27. Spear, L. B., and Grayson, A. J.: Making roentgenograms of temporomandibular articulation. JADA, *45:*209, 1952.
28. Speidel, L. D., and Maxon, A. S.: Reliability of method of orienting head for temporomandibular roentgenograms. Int. J. Ortho., *25:*250, 1939.
29. Sproull, J.: Technique of roentgen examination of the temporomandibular articulation. Am. J. Roentgenol., *30:*262, 1933.
30. Steinhardt, G.: Die praktische bedeutung der rontgenaufnahmen des kiefergelenkbereiches (The practical meaning of temporomandibular joint x-rays). Dtsch. Zahn. Ztschr., *10:*349, 1955.
31. Updegrave, W. J.: An improved roentgenographic technic for the temporomandibular articulation. JADA, *40:*391, 1950.
———: An evaluation of temporomandibular joint roentgenography. JADA, *46:*408, 1953.
———: Temporomandibular articulation. Dent. Radiogr. Photogr., *26:*41 (No. 3), 1953.
———: Roentgenographic observations of functioning temporomandibular joints. JADA, *54:*488, 1957.
32. Waters, C. A., and Waldron, C. W.:

Accessory nasal sinuses, describing a modification of occipito-frontal position. Am. J. Roentgenol. *2:*633, 1915.

33. Whitehouse, S. H.: Dental Radiography. DuPont Handbook, Wilmington, 1955.
34. Zimmer, E. A.: Die rontgenologie des kiefergelenkes (Radiography of the temporomandibular joint). Rev. Mens. Suisse Odont. *51:*949, 1941.

Additional Basic References

Updegrave, W. J.: Evaluation of TMJ roentgenography. JADA, *46:*408, 1963.

Weinberg, L. A.: Radiographic Investigations of TMJ Function, J. Pros. Dent., *33:*6, 1975.

———: Technique for temporomandibular joint radiographs. J. Pros. Dent., *28:*284, 1972.

13 Equilibration of the Occlusion in Centric Relation

One of the first to investigate, treat and report upon traumatogenic occlusion was Karolyi of Vienna. After his first report in 1901,[3] he delivered many lectures and four additional papers. He noted that there was usually no periodontal involvement in an abraded dentition with a zero vertical overbite. To provide the greatest freedom of movement, he ground the teeth in the lateral and protrusive ranges of articulation. Among other early workers in this field were Alkory[1] and Warnekros.[5] Since Karolyi, many investigators have advocated various principles and methods of equilibrating the occlusion through selective reshaping of the teeth. In the United States, Hutchinson[2] gave many demonstrations of occlusal equilibration about the year 1905. For many years, the large number of methods of occlusal equilibration was attended by various fads, fancies and opinions, but there were little factual data to support any of them, and there were no clear and detailed manuals of procedure. Many of the operative techniques were based upon the talent and the judgment of the individual operators; therefore, there was a great deal of room for error. In many cases, dentists were the prisoners of terms manufactured to suit a theory, but these were impractical in actual use. Consequently, it is necessary to clarify principles and definitions so that they are both understandable and practical.

This chapter will present a detailed step-by-step procedure for the determination of centric relation and for the equilibration of the occlusion in centric relation. The technique outlined can be followed by any dental practitioner, and it may be checked and tested at each step.

Many critics of occlusal equilibration feel that selective reshaping or grinding closes the bite. The author vehemently disagrees with this opinion. Actually, the interfering contact keeps the bite open in centric relation. When interfering contacts in centric relation are removed, the teeth are permitted to assume normal centric-relation occlusion. The removal of the interfering contact should not be interpreted as closing the bite but rather as the correct placement of the occlusal surfaces of the contacting teeth.

A traumatogenic occlusion is a pathological relationship of the occlusal surfaces of the teeth and may produce injury to the teeth, their supporting structures, the neuromuscular system and the temporomandibular joint. The result is an occlusal trauma, which is the injury or the result produced by the traumatogenic occlusion, that is, the occlusion produces the trauma. The trauma does not produce the occlusion; there is no such thing as a traumatic occlusion.

The only rules for equilibration that can be laid down categorically are those that will apply to teeth which are in ideal

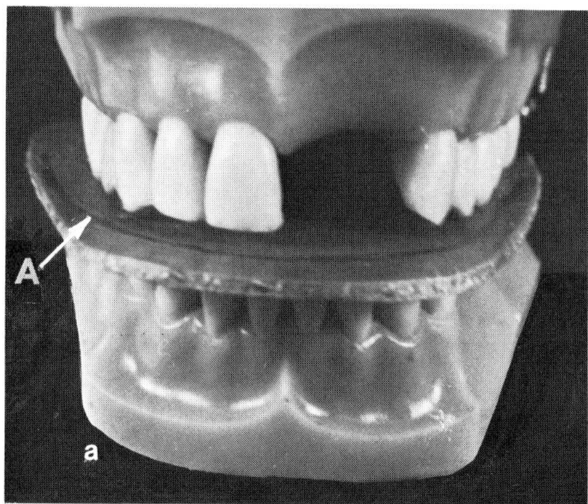

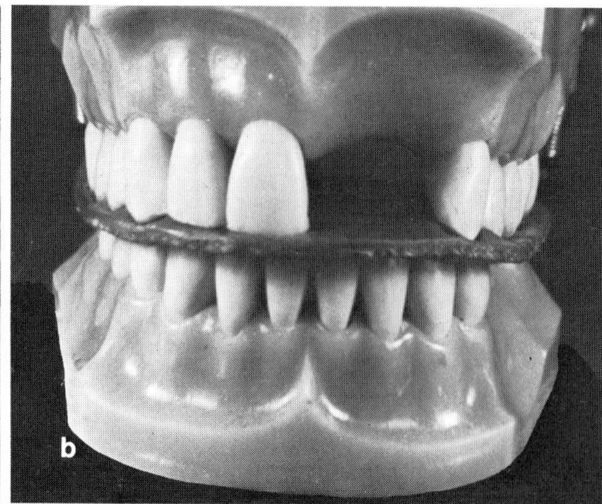

FIG. 13-1. The trim line, A, ⅛ in. buccal to the upper models is marked on the Aluwax form (*a*). The trimmed wax form (*b*) conforms to the upper arch. (Shore, N. A.: The equilibration of the occlusion of the natural dentition. JADA, *44*:414, 1952)

position. Such an occlusion is rarely found in practice. Therefore, it is extremely important to understand the general principles involved in grinding or reshaping the teeth rather than blindly to follow rules which may or may not apply to any individual patient. If the general principles of selective reshaping are thoroughly mastered, the plan for each case can be formulated.

Because all mandibular movements begin and end in centric-relation occlusion, the reshaping of the teeth in centric relation is the starting point for the equilibration of the natural dentition. Unless centric-relation occlusion is present, the dentition cannot be equilibrated properly in the ranges of articulation.

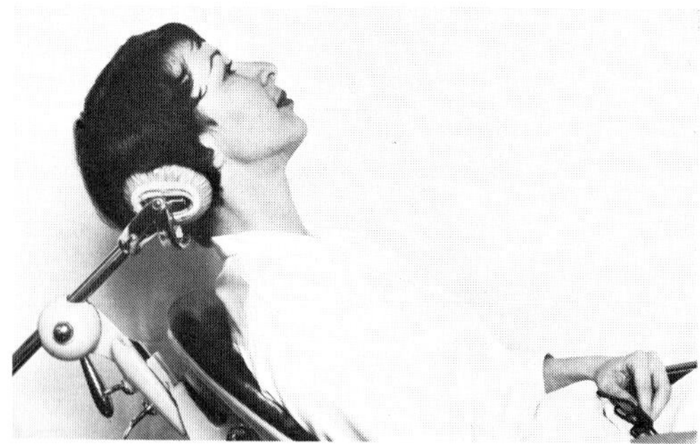

FIG. 13-2. Position for training the patient to give a centric-relation bite.

The procedure for equilibrating the occlusion in centric relation involves four steps:

1. Obtaining the centric-relation registration
2. Locating and marking the interfering contact surfaces of a pair of opposing teeth
3. Deciding where to grind or reshape the teeth
4. Actually reshaping the teeth

OBTAINING THE CENTRIC-RELATION REGISTRATIONS

Recording the Centric-Relation Wax Bite

The recording of the centric-relation wax bite is the most important procedure that must be accomplished in preparing a case for study on the articulator. It is the record of the patient's closure on the centric-relation arc which is established by the hinge-axis. Centric relation is a mandible-to-cranium, bone-to-bone relationship. It has nothing to do with the teeth. Despite the fact that there are no teeth present when a full denture is being constructed, a centric-relation wax bite is taken. It is also possible to take a centric-relation wax bite when the natural dentition is present. The accurate use of any restoration that is made on any instrument outside the mouth itself will depend basically upon the accuracy of the centric-relation wax bite. This wax bite orients the mandible to the maxilla in centric relation and will clearly reveal any occlusal interference to centric-relation occlusion. The centric-relation wax bite establishes two things—the position of the mandible in relation to the skull, and the relationship of the occlusal surfaces of the opposing teeth just before they make contact.

To obtain a centric-relation record, an Aluwax form is used consisting of two layers of wax separated by a layer of gauze. The wax form is measured on the upper study cast of the patient, and a line, A, is marked ⅛ inch buccal to the teeth (Fig. 13-1*a*). Then the form is trimmed to the line (*b*). The marginal half inch of the form is then dipped repeatedly into water which is kept at a temperature of 118°F. This portion should be soft enough so that the teeth may penetrate the wax easily. The palatal portion will remain hard so that the wax form will be rigid under biting stress.

Using the palmar surfaces of the forefingers of both hands, press the upper or shiny surface of the Aluwax form against the occlusal surfaces of the upper teeth—especially the central incisors—so that an index of all the occlusal surfaces may be obtained; this is the Aluwax index bite. With the thumbnail, nick the wax between the central incisors as a point of quick reference.

Training the Patient

A fundamental step in the process of preparing the centric-relation wax bite is training the patient to record correct centric relation. The patient must be trained to record an *unstrained* centric-relation wax bite. The dentist must be able to recognize immediately whether the patient is recording a correct centric-relation bite. When a patient is asked to close, usually he will go into his habitual convenience-occlusion bite. The dentist must be able to retrain the patient so that he will give a centric-relation bite. The following describes the procedure for training the patient and for securing an accurate centric-relation wax bite.

Tap quickly and lightly on the bracket table with an instrument handle to demonstrate the rate of speed at which the patient must tap his teeth together into the wax. Emphasize light and rapid mandibular movements because, as the patient opens and closes very quickly, usually he will close in a correct centric-relation arc rather than in any convenience relationship which he may have developed.

Seat the patient in a 45° reclining position (Fig. 13-2), and tell him to relax and to permit his jaw to hang loose. In this position, the forces of the antigravity muscles will be counteracted, and the mandible will tend to return to its proper position. Train the patient to give a correct centric-relation closure. He must open his mouth wide and move his jaw first to the right and then to the left. To relax all the muscles, this cycle of opening wide and moving the jaw to the right and to the left is repeated three times. Now place the ball of the thumb on the buccal surface of the upper right bicuspid and the ball of the forefinger on the upper left bicuspid (Fig. 13-3*a*). Place the ball of the right thumb on the incisal edge of the lower anterior incisors with the nail up (*b*). Direct the patient to tap lightly and rapidly on the thumbnail, then to stop tapping, to hold his teeth lightly against the thumbnail, and to push his upper jaw forward. This seems to be the best technique for causing the patient to retrude his lower jaw. Then, the dentist first having removed his thumb, the patient is told to close his jaws lightly. After this training the procedure has been completed. Tell the patient

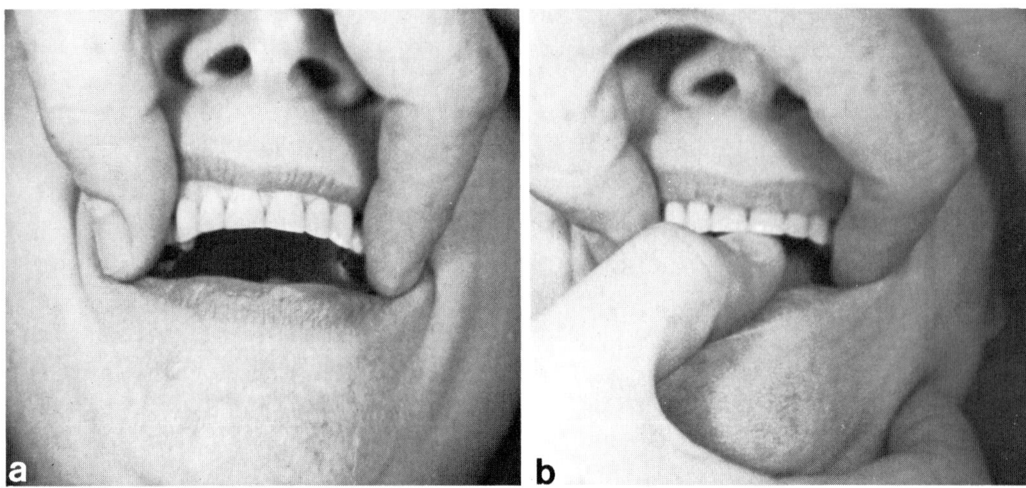

FIG. 13-3. Placement of the thumb and forefinger of the left hand on the upper bicuspids (*a*). Placement of the thumb of the right hand on the lower anteriors (*b*) during the training of the patient for a centric-relation registration. (Shore, N. A.: The equilibration of the occlusion of the natural dentition. JADA, *44:*414, 1952)

that the entire process will be repeated, this time using the Aluwax index bite which was made earlier.

Dip the half-inch marginal edge of the wax form into water at 118° F. and return to the patient's mouth, taking care to fit the teeth into their original imprints. Repeat the steps that were rehearsed during the training period but now with the wax form in the patient's mouth. In Figure 13-4*a* the Aluwax form is in place, and the patient is being trained to tap on the dentist's thumbnail, and in (*b*) the patient has closed in centric relation. This method of training the patient and taking the registration ensures a correct centric-relation bite because the forefinger and the thumb of the dentist's left hand at A

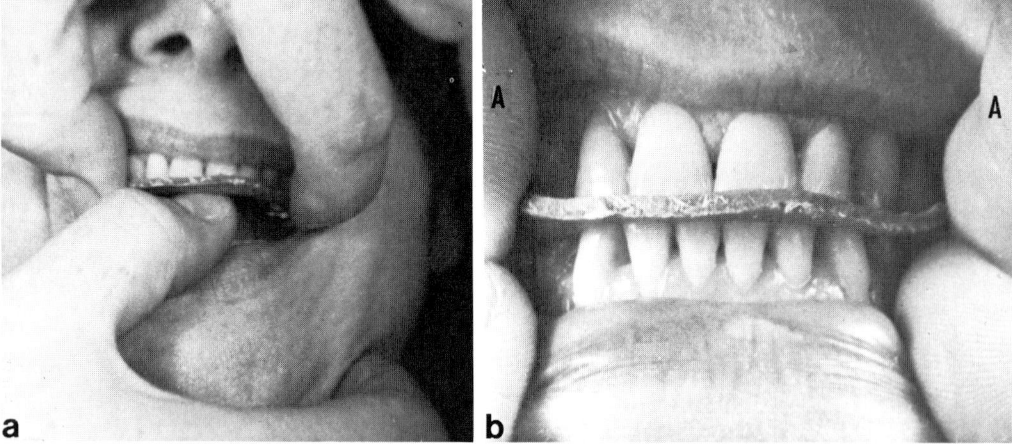

FIG. 13-4. Aluwax form against the upper teeth (*a*) and the patient being trained to tap on the operator's thumbnail. Patient closing in centric relation (*b*). (Shore, N. A.: The equilibration of the occlusion of the natural dentition. JADA, *44:*414, 1952)

(Fig. 13-4*b*) preclude eccentric movements in closure and immediately indicate when the patient is making other than centric movements. The patient should close lightly and repeatedly into the wax in a centric-relation bite until a clear index is secured without perforating the wax. This procedure will give an unstrained centric-relation bite. The wax must not be perforated, because a hole would indicate that closure has taken place to the degree that the cuspal inclines have taken over. This changes the relationship of the mandible to the maxilla.

An unperforated wax bite (Fig. 13-5) indicates that a correct relationship of the mandibular to the maxillary teeth has been recorded. Furthermore, the wax index will immediately reveal erratic eccentric closure because a blurred or tracked-up appearance of the wax bite will have been produced. As a matter of fact, the sharpness and clearness of the tooth indentations in the Aluwax form should be noted even though the patient has closed twenty or thirty times into the form.

It should be emphasized that the resultant wax bite is a record of an unstrained centric-relation bite which the patient voluntarily gave the dentist rather than a bite that was guided by the pressure of the operator's hand against the patient's lower jaw. If, because of the inexperience of the operator or the uncooperativeness of the patient, the mandible closed in different positions during the many opening and closing movements that are involved in this procedure, the Aluwax form will lack sharpness and definition.

Because of nervousness, anxiety to help or general tenseness, about 1 per cent of patients will find it extremely difficult to learn how to record the wax bite properly. However, calmness and patience on the part of the dentist will help the patient to cooperate so that the centric-relation bite may be recorded.

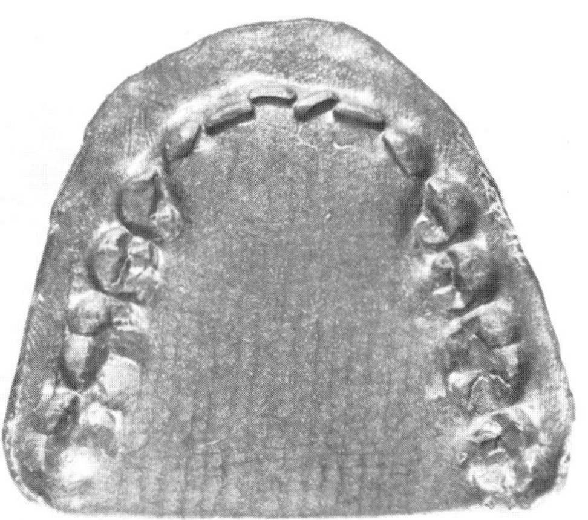

FIG. 13-5. A centric-relation wax bite. Note lack of perforations. (Shore, N. A.: The equilibration of the occlusion of the natural dentition. JADA, *44:*414, 1952)

When the patient is especially tense or nervous, the following procedure is helpful. Seat the patient in a 45° reclining position and place a Hickok retruder upon his head (Fig. 13-6). This device consists of an aluminum chin plate and a heavy rubber form that fits around the head. The rubber form has holes in the temporal region so that the entire device may be adjusted to the individual patient. For the patient's comfort, place some compound in the chin cup and tightly fit

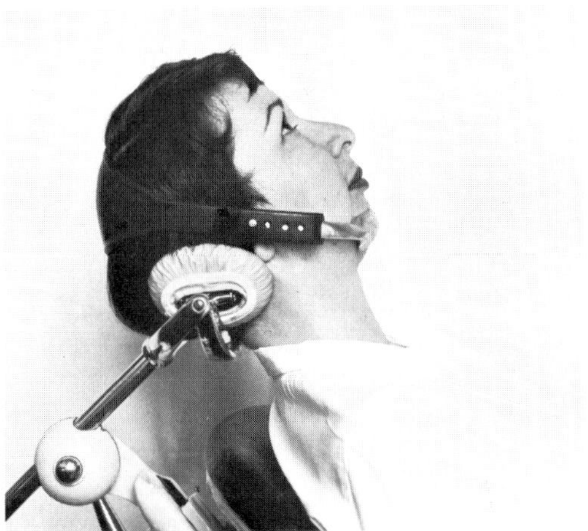

FIG. 13-6. Hickok retruder in position.

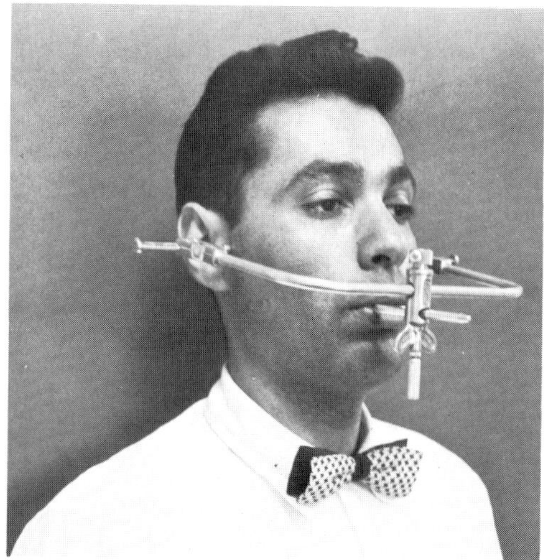

FIG. 13-7. Face-bow registration being taken with compound "lollipop" bite.

it to the patient. Then instruct him to open and close repeatedly. After 5 minutes, remove the retruder. By this time the patient should be ready to give a correct centric-relation bite, and the regular procedure that has been outlined can be carried out.

Mounting the Study Casts

A set of study casts should be made from accurate alginate or hydrocolloid impressions. Using a bite fork, take a compound "lollipop" bite of the case. Adjust the face-bow to the patient (Fig. 13-7); after the registration is made, remove the face-bow. As the patient's teeth are just touching in centric relation, draw two lines on the upper and the lower centrals along the long axis of the teeth (Fig. 13-8*a*). After the patient lowers his mandible in centric relation (*b*), extend the lines to the incisal edges (*c*). Instruct the patient to protrude his mandible until both lines are directly under each other (Fig. 13-9). This provides a protrusive position in which both condyles have come forward equally and in which the incisal guidance or angulation did not determine the protrusive movement. Give the patient a hand mirror and tell him that this end position is the one he is to assume when the pieces of wax are placed on the right and the left lower posterior teeth. Place two pieces of rolled, softened baseplate wax, A and A in Figure 13-9, on the lower teeth from the cuspids back to the last molar. Guided by the lines on the upper and the lower centrals as well as by the operator, the patient assumes the protrusive position. The incisal edges of the upper and the lower centrals must not touch; there should be a clearance of about ½ mm. and never exceeding 2 mm. Chill the wax and remove it.

If the incisal edges of the upper and the lower centrals touch under heavy muscular pressure in protrusive position, the result will be a steeper registration of the

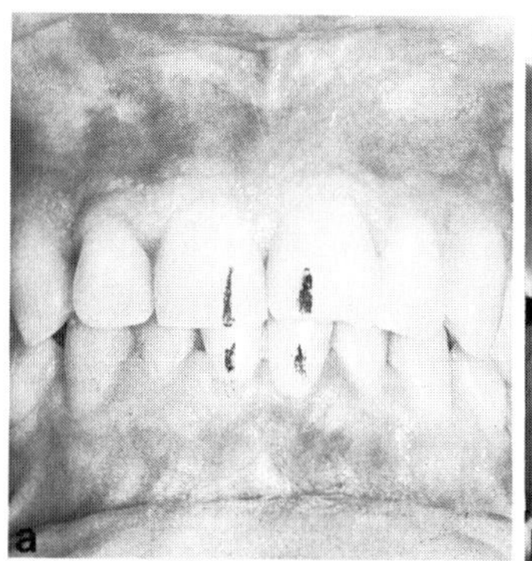

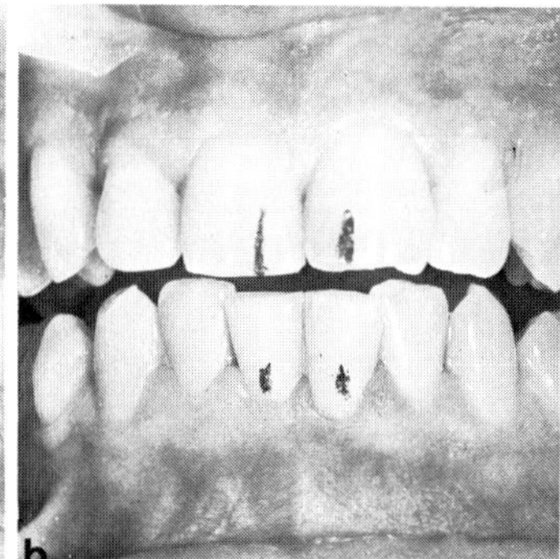

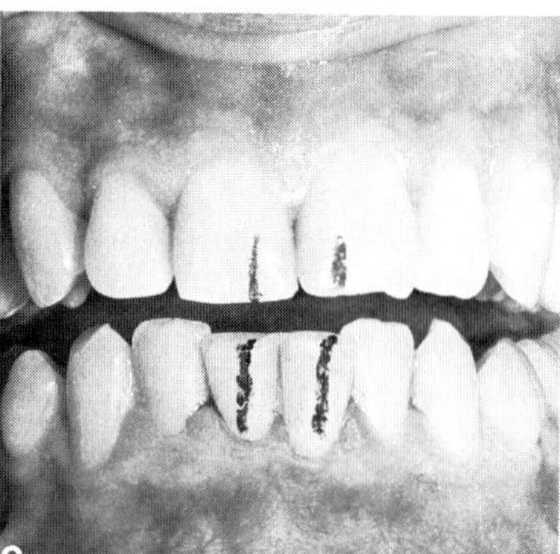

FIG. 13-8. The teeth to be used in protrusive bite registration are marked.

condylar inclination on the articulator than actually exists in the mouth. The dentist can become familiar with this procedure by experimenting with it in his own mouth. Protrude the mandible without making anterior tooth contact, then permit the anterior teeth to make contact. Notice how the musculature takes over. As the muscles change the position of the mandible, they also change the relationship in protrusive position. If the practitioner understands this action in his own mouth as well as on the articulator, he will have a good concept of what occurs in the temporomandibular joint. Always take two or three protrusive check bites before setting the condylar angulation on the articulator. Sometimes an elongated tooth will prevent an accurate protrusive registration. In such a case, the dentist must deal with the elongated tooth before carrying out the rest of the procedure.

After all the patient records have been taken, mount the casts on an adjustable articulator. Mount the upper casts on the articulator with the face-bow (Fig. 13-10) and mount the casts with dental stone. Using the accurate Aluwax centric-relation bite, mount the lower model (*a*) in proper relation to the upper model (Fig. 13-11*b*) with the condylar guide slots, A, in a vertical position.

The importance of the proper use of the face-bow is explained by the following line of reasoning. The jaw opens from centric-relation occlusion to a point before translation occurs, and closes from this point to a centric-relation occlusion in a hinge-axis movement. The face-bow orients the maxilla to the hinge-axis movement of the condyle which is a precise point in relation to the skull. This axis, if correctly transferred to the articulator, becomes the axis of the articulator. If casts are mounted on an articulator without the use of a face-bow, they may be incorrectly positioned anteroposteriorly, superoinferiorly, to the left, to the right, or in a combination of these errors. A hinge-axis face-bow may be used to secure the most accurate possible face-bow articulator mounting in centric relation. Mount the casts on an articulator that is designed to accept this type of face-bow. If properly mounted, the models will demonstrate the same centric-relation interfering contacts as are present in the mouth. The next step in the procedure is to transfer the protrusive readings to the articulator by using the protrusive wax records that have been taken.

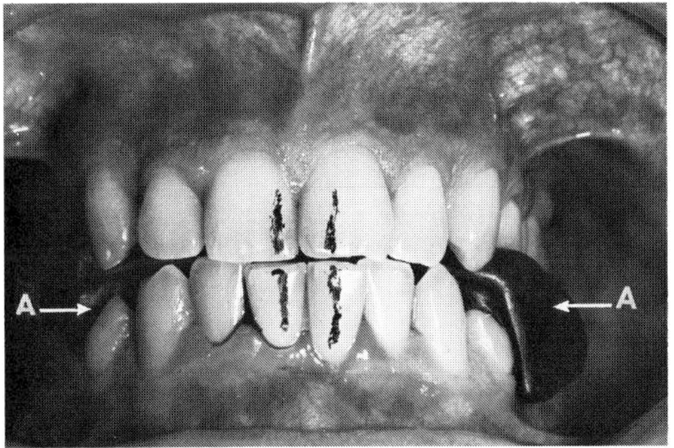

FIG. 13-9. Protrusive position registration with wax bites at A.

Figure 13-12 shows the two pieces of wax at A that make up the protrusive bite as well as the method used in setting up the wax bites to adjust the condylar

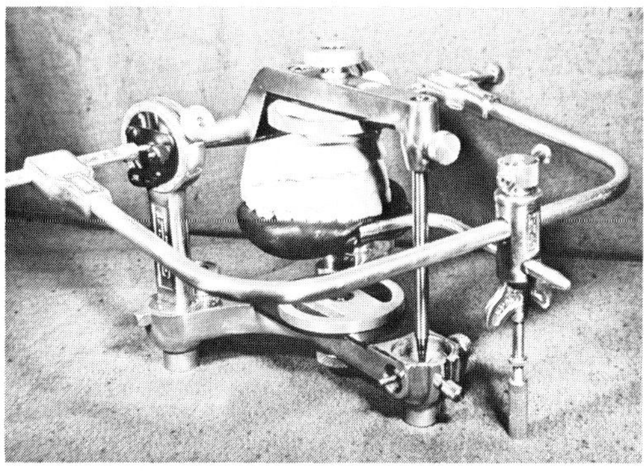
FIG. 13-10. Mounting the upper cast on an articulator using the face-bow, "lollipop" bite registration.

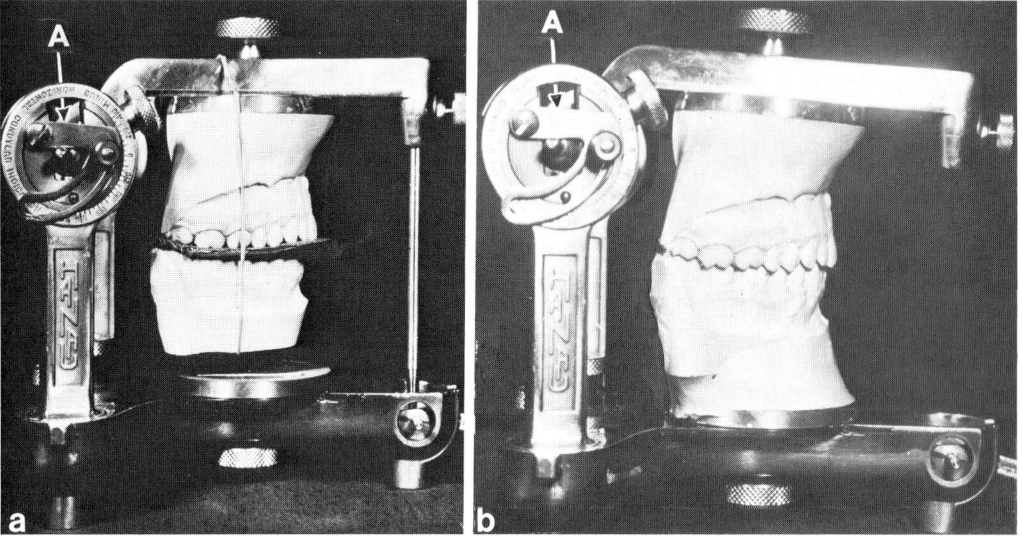

FIG. 13-11. The lower cast is related to the upper cast, using the Aluwax centric registration (*a*). The completed mounting of the models in centric relation (*b*).

readings on the articulator. It is wise to take two or three protrusive wax bites to check the accuracy of the registration. Even this, of course, is only an approximation, but it will enable the dentist to study and analyze the case in the functioning, nonfunctioning and protrusive ranges of articulation and to analyze on

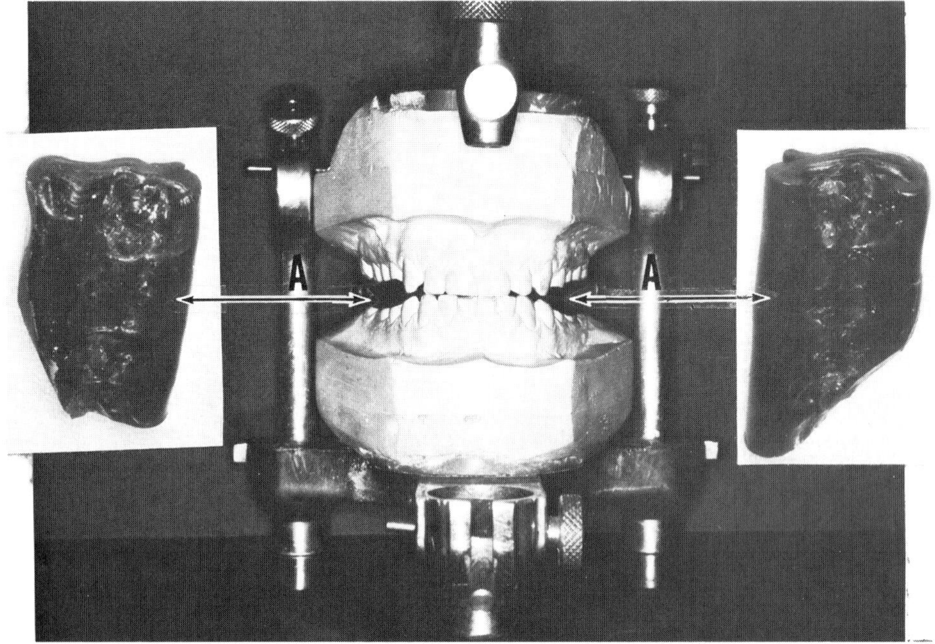

FIG. 13-12. The protrusive record A, as taken in Figure 13-9, set on the articulator.

the articulator the interfering occlusal contacts in all of these ranges. In this manner, study the pattern of all gliding movements of the mandible, especially those on the nonfunctioning side. Such a study cannot be conducted by holding study casts in the hands or by direct observation in the patient's mouth.

Figure 13-13 presents a full dentition as it appears to the practitioner when he holds the models in his hands; the occlusion seems to be fine. This case was mounted on an articulator. An interfering occlusal contact is indicated by the hole in the wax, A, Figure 13-14. This interfering contact is evident in the left second molar region at B. Note that none of the other teeth make contact. As the arms of the articulator are pressed together to cause the models to occlude, a space de-

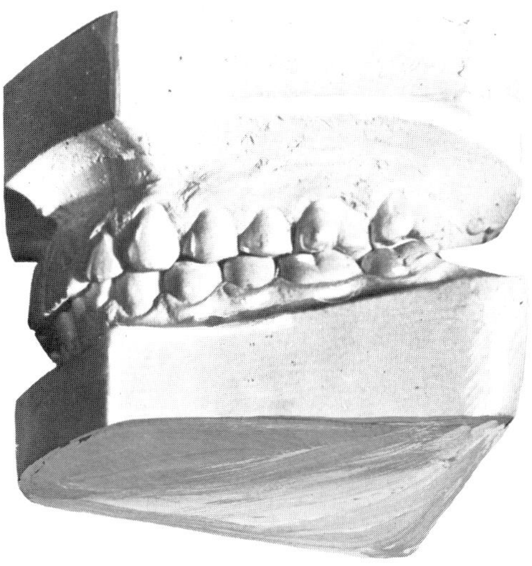

FIG. 13-13. Practitioner's view of a full dentition in occlusion as he holds the casts in his hand. (Compare with Fig. 13-14)

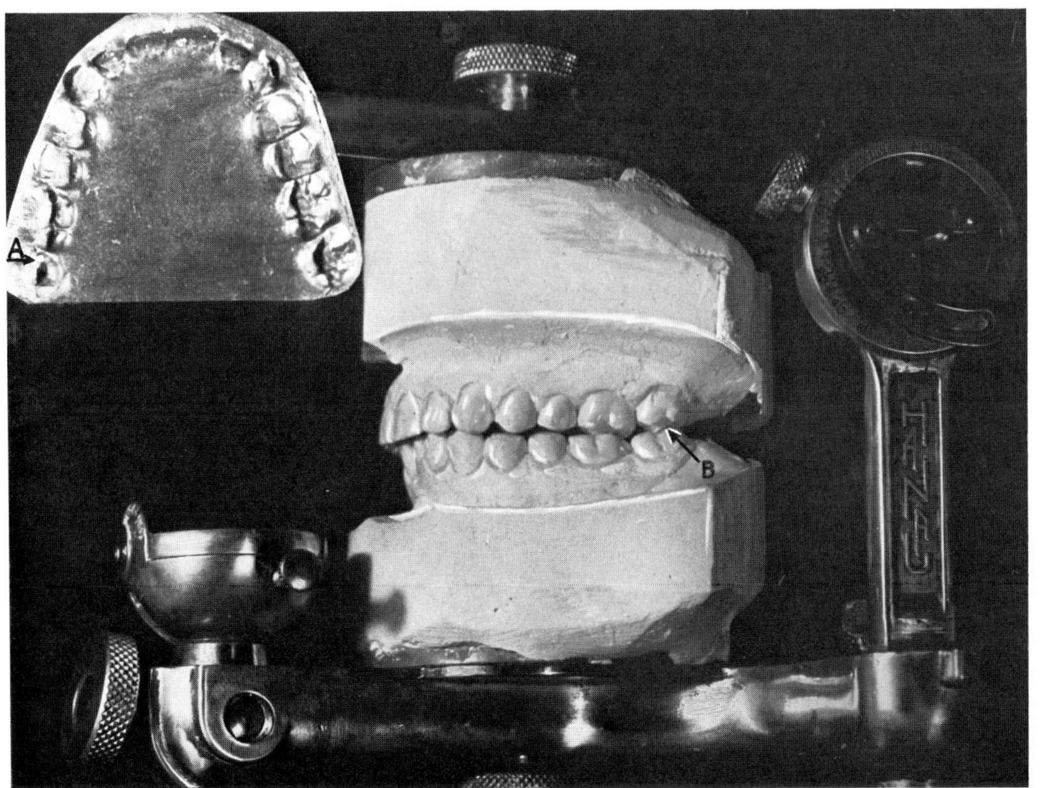

FIG. 13-14. Casts of Figure 13-13 mounted with a centric-relation wax bite. Note variation of the position of the teeth in centric relation with that seen when the casts are held in the hand. The contact at B appears as the hole A in a contact wax bite.

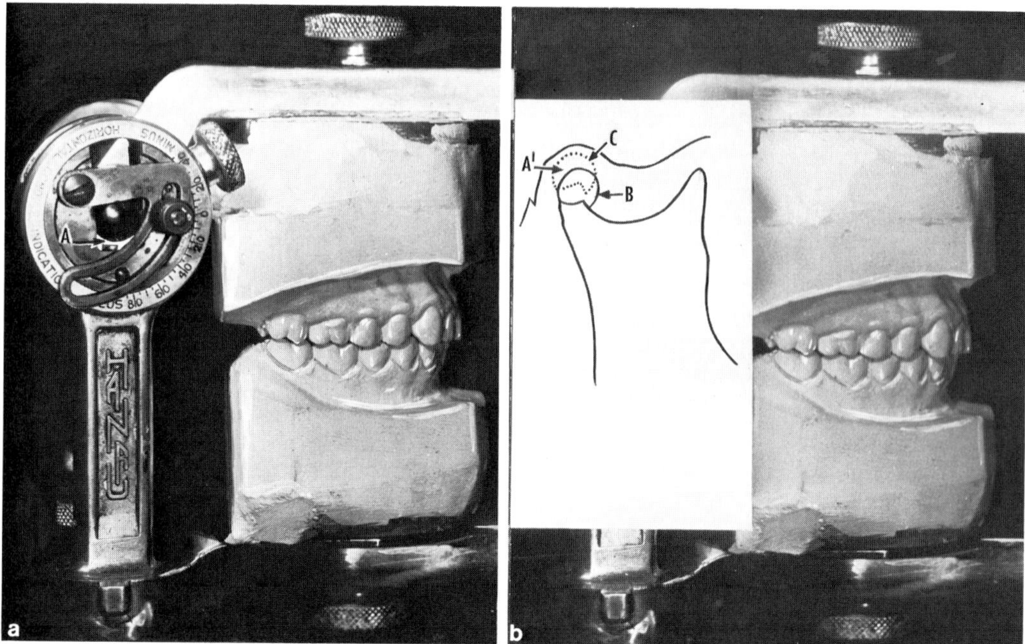

FIG. 13-15. Convenience occlusion of the teeth (*a*) producing a space between the ball and the base of the guide slot at A. A temporomandibular joint superimposed on the articulator (*b*) assuming the conditions depicted in (*a*).

velops between the ball and the base of the condylar guide slot at A, Figure 13-15*a*. The dotted line C, in (*b*), represents the normal position for the condyle. However, movement of the condyle has occurred, and the solid line, B, shows that the condyle is in an inferior and anterior position. The space at A in (*a*) is represented by A′ in (*b*). This movement of the condyle can be a combination of anterior, inferior and lateral displacement combined with corresponding movements of the opposite condyle. These displacements from normal position are at the root of temporomandibular joint symptoms. The interfering occlusal contact at B in Figure 13-14 displaced the mandible anteriorly and caused the labial surfaces of the lower anterior teeth to jam up against the lingual surfaces of the upper anterior teeth, thus gouging them out.

It is interesting to observe that the centric-relation bite and mounting approximately reproduce the hinge-axis movements of the condyle, and that the protrusive registration approximately reproduces the gliding movements of the condyle in the temporomandibular joint. When studying the articulator movements, bear in mind the fact that the mandible does not move of its own accord but rather is moved by the neuromuscular system. Remember that the articulator is limited by the absence of muscles and nerves, and a joint that only remotely resembles the human temporomandibular joint. It cannot reproduce the mobility of the individual teeth that is caused by function. In cases of vertical and horizontal overbites, it is sometimes found that the mandibular anterior teeth strike the gingiva and move mobile teeth. However, the articulator does offer the next best thing—an approximation of the mandibular movements.

Materials and Instruments Used in Occlusal Equilibration

The materials and instruments used in the procedures involved in the equilibration of the occlusion are:

1. Aluwax wax-cloth forms
2. Aluwax denture wax
3. Green casting wax, 30-gauge (¾″ × 3″ strips)
4. Green casting wax, 22-gauge (¾″ × 3″ strips)
5. Thick articulating paper book (remove outer cover and cut in half, ¾″ × 3″)
6. Miller articulating paper holders (2)
7. Red cotton adding machine ribbon (¾″ wide, one spool, medium inking, cut into 3″ strips)
8. Carbide 12-bladed fluted burs
9. Contra-angle carborundum stones, Chayes No. 32, 33, 34
10. Beauty pink wax, hard (cut into ¾″ × 3″ strips)
11. Any heater that will accurately maintain a water temperature of 118° F.
12. Anatomic articulator or Galetti articulator
13. Face-bow
14. Scissors

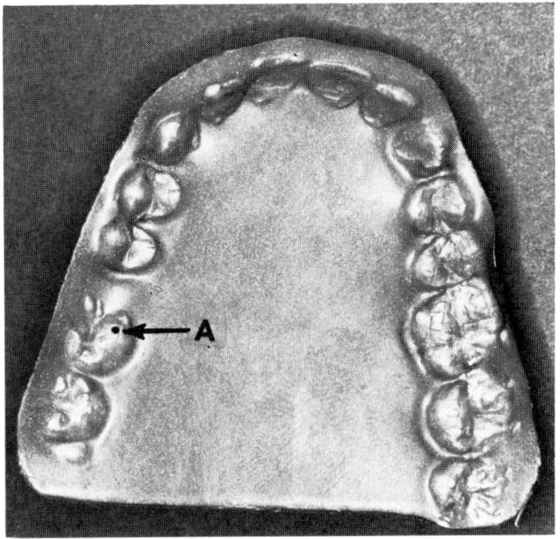

FIG. 13-16. An Aluwax centric-relation interfering contact wax bite showing hole at A, the point of interference.

LOCATING THE INTERFERING CONTACT SURFACES OF A PAIR OF OPPOSING TEETH

Obtaining a Centric-Relation Interfering Occlusal Contact Bite

The next step in the procedure is to obtain a centric-relation interfering occlusal contact bite. Trim another Aluwax form marginally as was done for taking the centric-relation bite. With the patient now seated in a 45°-reclining position, carry the same training procedure as was described in connection with the preparation of the centric-relation bite. The patient is instructed to open and close on the operator's thumbnail. When the patient is properly trained, dip the marginal half inch of the Aluwax form in the 118° F. waterbath and place it against the patient's upper teeth. Then ask the patient to open and close lightly and rapidly many times until the first sign of an interfering occlusal contact—a hole in the wax—appears. The letter A in Figure 13-16 indicates the hole which results from an interfering occlusal contact. If there is any doubt as to the accuracy of the interfering contact as shown in the wax form, fill the hole on the underside of the form with Aluwax denture wax, replace it in the patient's mouth and instruct him to open and close his jaws in centric relation. If the bite was accurate, the hole will reappear in the same position.

This is an accurate method for checking an interfering occlusal contact. Its accuracy is proved by the fact that two or three operators working on the same patient will obtain the same record repeatedly. It is clear, then, that one of the great advantages of this wax-form method is that it can be tested, verified and duplicated by various operators. Another advantage lies in the fact that the same piece of wax is used not only to find the first interfering occlusal contact in centric relation but also to locate new interfering contacts as they appear in sequence. There are obvious advantages in being able to use the same wax form to locate all interfering contacts as they are revealed and to check continually for the accuracy of the operating procedure.

It is important to understand the significance of the hole in the wax form. The first hole is the visual evidence of the first centric-relation interfering contact. It indicates the contacting or interfering surfaces of the offending teeth. This method of determining the interfering contact is so delicate that it will clearly reveal contacts that cannot be discovered in any other way. Once the first centric-relation interfering contact has been detected and accurately located, the relationships of the offending cusps can be studied in the wax, in the patient's mouth and on the articulated models. The location of the centric-relation interfering contact is basic to an analysis of habitual convenience movements of the mandible. A knowledge of the ideal centric-relation occlusion and the ranges of articulation will help to determine what discrepancies exist and, if restorations are to be made, how to plan and build them so that they may function to best advantage.

DECIDING WHICH TOOTH TO RESHAPE

Determining Which Surface of Posterior Teeth to Reshape

The decision as to which centric-relation interfering contact surface to reshape depends upon the relationships of these contacting surfaces in the eccentric ranges of articulation. The basic principle to remember is: *The centric-relation interfering contact surface that is least useful in the eccentric ranges of articulation is the surface that should be reshaped.* In determining which centric-relation interfering contact is to be reshaped, the following conditions must be satisfied:

1. Consider only the centric-relation interfering contact surfaces.
2. Consider only whether these surfaces are necessary in the eccentric ranges.
3. Do not consider the problem, at this time, that may arise if one of the centric-relation interfering contacts becomes a functioning or a nonfunctioning interfering occlusal contact. This problem will be resolved during the reshaping of the teeth in those ranges of articulation.

There are three primary types of interfering occlusal contacts in centric relation: cusp-to-fossa or cusp-to-plane, cusp-to-cusp and plane-to-plane. The cusp-to-fossa type includes the cusp-to-plane type, since the plane is considered part of a fossa and is treated accordingly. If the interfering occlusal contact is a cusp-to-fossa interference, the fossa is reshaped. In the usual, near-normal posterior occlusal relationship, the upper lingual cusps rest in the lower fossae, and the lower buccal cusps rest in the fossae of the upper teeth. In the functioning and nonfunctioning ranges, the cusps are used, but the fossae are not used. According to the principle of reshaping the least necessary surface, the fossa is reshaped.

Actual study of the articulated casts combined with careful study of the Centric Reshaping Determination Chart will provide a rapid and accurate guide for understanding the problem of where to grind and which surface to reshape. This chart is a simple device for recording on paper the centric-relation interfering contacts as well as the relationships of these contacting surfaces in the functioning and the nonfunctioning ranges of articulation. *The principle to follow is that the contacting surfaces to reshape in centric relation are those which are least used in the centric, functioning and nonfunctioning ranges.*

A completed chart for the determination of centric reshaping is illustrated in Figure 13-17. Above each column of the chart is illustrated the actual tooth position for that relationship. Assume that the centric-relation interfering contact exists between lingual cusp A of the

FIG. 13-17. The chart is filled out to determine the areas to reshape in cases of cusp-to-fossa, centric-relation interference.

CENTRIC RESHAPING DETERMINATION CHART

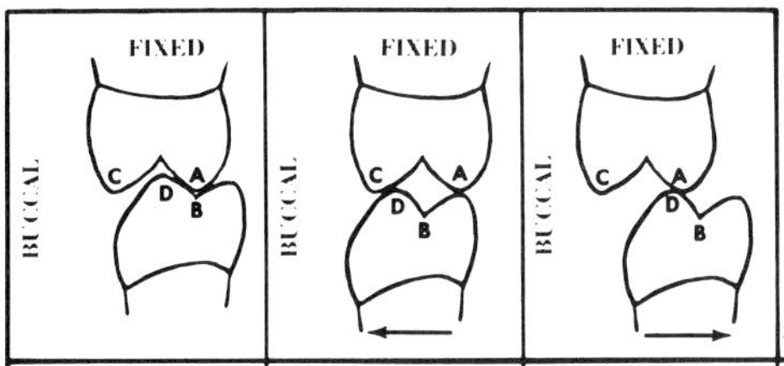

	FIXED / BUCCAL (C, A, D, B)	FIXED / BUCCAL (C, A, D, B)	FIXED / BUCCAL (C, A, D, B)	
	CENTRIC CONTACT	FUNCTIONING CONTACT	NONFUNCTIONING CONTACT	TOTAL NUMBER OF CONTACTS
UPPER	First Molar Lingual Cusp 1	1	1	= 3
LOWER	First Molar Central Fossa 1	0	0	= 1

upper right first molar and central fossa B of the lower right first molar. The upper interfering contact surface is recorded, and the numeral 1 is placed in the first square under *centric* next to *upper;* the lower interfering contact surface and the numeral 1 are recorded under *centric* next to *lower*. The articulated casts are moved into the right functioning position. The positional relationship of the teeth that were in interfering contact is now similar to the illustration above the functioning-contact column. The upper cusp A is needed to glide along the buccal plane of the lingual cusp of the lower molar; therefore, the numeral 1 is placed in the functioning-contact column for the upper contact. Fossa B is not used in this functioning movement. A zero is placed in the functioning-contact column for the lower contact. The articulated models are moved into the right nonfunctioning position, as illustrated by the diagram above the nonfunctioning-contact column. The upper cusp A is needed to glide along the lingual plane of the buccal cusp of the lower molar; therefore, the numeral 1 is placed in the nonfunctioning-contact column for the upper contact. Fossa B is not used in this movement; therefore, a zero is placed in the nonfunctioning-contact column for the lower contact.

In the column marked "Total Number of Contacts," add the number of contacts achieved by the upper cusp and the lower fossa. The chart shows that there are three uses for the lingual cusp of the upper right first molar and only one use for the lower central fossa of the lower right first molar. Therefore, the area to reshape is the central fossa of the lower molar. Should the centric-relation interfering contact exist between the buccal cusp of a lower molar and the central fossa of an upper molar, the principles and procedures for determining where to reshape the teeth would be the same as those described above.

It has been claimed that if a cusp and a fossa are in interfering contact in centric relation (Fig. 13-17), and the cusp also makes an interfering contact in the functioning and the nonfunctioning ranges, the cusp should be reshaped. This procedure will lead to difficulties for the following reasons:

1. The relationships of the upper cusps to the lower cusps in the functioning and the nonfunctioning ranges *cannot* be predicted until the case has been completely equilibrated in centric-relation occlusion.

2. By reshaping a cusp, there is chance for error produced by overgrinding the cusp with subsequent lack of cusp contact in another range when needed.

Figure 13-18 illustrates the relation-

CENTRIC RESHAPING DETERMINATION CHART

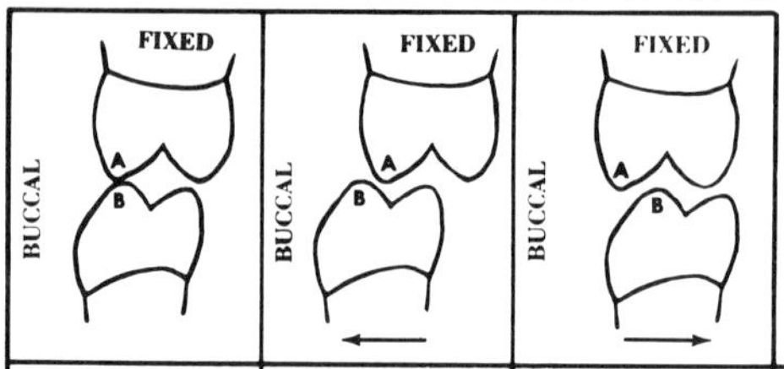

		CENTRIC CONTACT	FUNCTIONING CONTACT	NONFUNCTIONING CONTACT		TOTAL NUMBER OF CONTACTS
UPPER	First Molar Buccal Cusp	1	0	0	=	1
LOWER	First Molar Buccal Cusp	1	0	0	=	1

FIG. 13-18. The chart is filled out to determine the areas to reshape in cases of cusp-to-cusp, centric-relation interference.

ship that exists when a cusp-to-cusp interfering contact is found and how the situation is recorded on the chart. Guided by the procedure outlined above, the chart was completed. The total number of useful contacts is one for each of the upper and the lower cusps. Since the number of useful contacts is the same for both teeth, the procedure is to reshape both cusps equally. In the plane-to-plane, centric-relation interfering contact, the tooth relationship appears (Fig. 13-19) above the centric-contact column. When the chart was completed according to the procedure outlined, the total number of useful contacts was found to be two for each of the upper and lower planes. Under these conditions, too, the procedure is to grind both planes equally. If there is ever any doubt as to where to reshape the centric-relation interfering occlusal contact, study the articulated casts and fill out a Centric Reshaping Determination Chart. This procedure will locate the surface to be reshaped.

Determining Which Surface of the Anterior Teeth to Reshape

Three types of centric-relation interfering occlusal contacts may exist between the maxillary and the mandibular anterior

CENTRIC RESHAPING DETERMINATION CHART

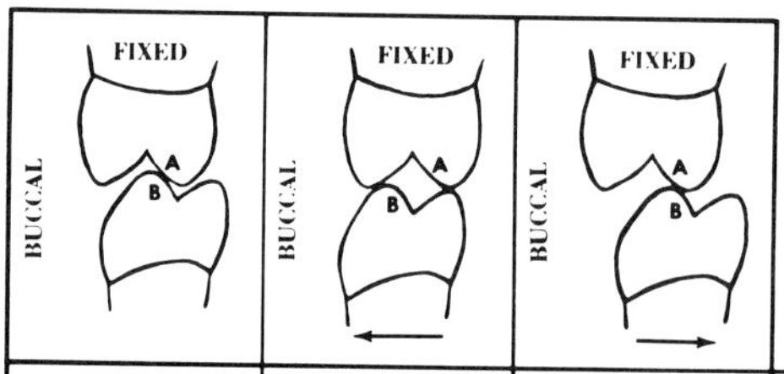

		CENTRIC CONTACT	FUNCTIONING CONTACT	NONFUNCTIONING CONTACT		TOTAL NUMBER OF CONTACTS
UPPER	First Molar Lingual Cusp Buccal Plane	1	0	1	=	2
LOWER	First Molar Buccal Cusp Lingual Plane	1	0	1	=	2

FIG. 13-19. The chart is filled out to determine the areas to reshape in cases of plane-to-plane, centric-relation interference.

teeth. In Figure 13-20*a* the centric-relation interfering contact exists between the incisal edge of a mandibular anterior tooth and the lingual plane of a maxillary anterior tooth. In this case, the lower tooth is reshaped for the following reasons:

1. It does not increase the incisal incline. If the maxillary tooth were to be ground, the incisal incline would be made greater and would cause difficulty during the reshaping of the teeth in the protrusive range.

2. Esthetics are easier to maintain when reshaping the teeth in the other ranges.

In Figure 13-20*b*, the centric-relation interfering occlusal contact exists between the lingual plane of a maxillary anterior tooth and the labial plane of a mandibular anterior tooth. In this case, the teeth should be reshaped by minimal grinding from the lingual plane of the maxillary tooth and the labial plane of the mandibular tooth.

In Figure 13-20*c*, the centric-relation interfering occlusal contact exists between the incisal edges of the maxillary and the mandibular teeth. In this case, the teeth should be reshaped by minimal grinding from each incisal edge. The amount of tooth structure removed is slight and will depend upon the esthetic requirements of the involved teeth.

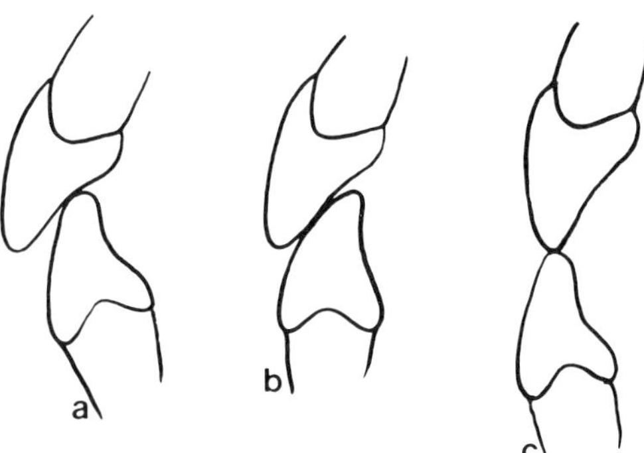

FIG. 13-20. The various types of interfering contacts of anterior teeth.

ACTUAL RESHAPING OF THE TEETH

Formulation of the Blueprint or Master Plan

The blueprint or master plan on which the dentist will approximate his actual treatment is formulated and modified during the equilibration of the occlusion of the articulated study casts. This is done before any reshaping is performed on the dentition of the patient. Two sets of casts should be utilized: one to act as study models, the second actually to be ground and used as the master plan or blueprint. This master plan technique has many advantages. It allows the dentist to show the patient the casts on the articulator and to explain to him approximately what will be done to his teeth, why it must be done and what results are anticipated. This is a valuable aid to patient education.

The casts also aid the dentist by enabling him to make a "practice run" so that he will have a good idea of the procedures that he will follow in the patient's mouth. Errors made in reshaping the teeth on the models may be corrected with wax, and thus the correct steps of operative procedure may be carefully determined. The master plan on articulated casts also permits ease in visualization of the plan as a whole as well as visualization of inaccessible areas of the mouth. Such previews of these areas will enable the dentist to operate more efficiently in the patient's mouth.

A list of the areas reshaped on the casts should be kept and used as a guide to the procedures that will be used in the actual operational equilibration of the occlusion in the patient's mouth. Of course, when it is applied to the actual mouth, this list may occasionally be incorrect; nevertheless, it will serve as a general approximate visualization of each step as it is accomplished. This chart will give an idea of the amount of tooth structure that will

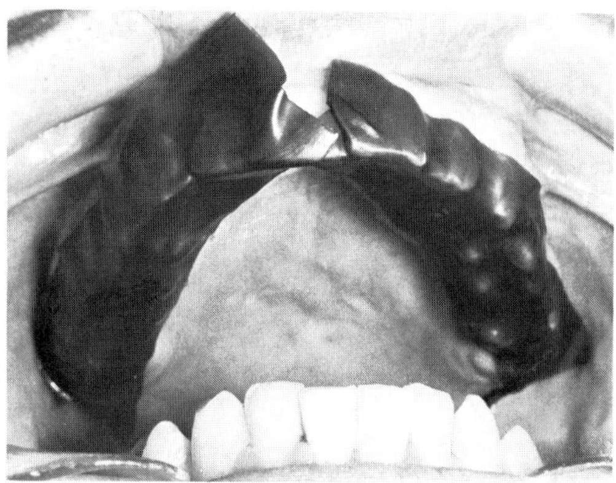

FIG. 13-21. Two strips of 30-gauge casting wax in position on the upper teeth, used to register occlusal interferences when making fine adjustments.

have to be removed. This reduces the possibilities of error during the actual reshaping in the patient's mouth. After the teeth are reshaped on the articulator, the dentist may decide that some occlusal rehabilitation or orthodontia should be done concomitantly for best results, or that restoration of vertical dimension is necessary. He may study the case, try out various plans in combination with occlusal equilibration and see results before initiating treatment.

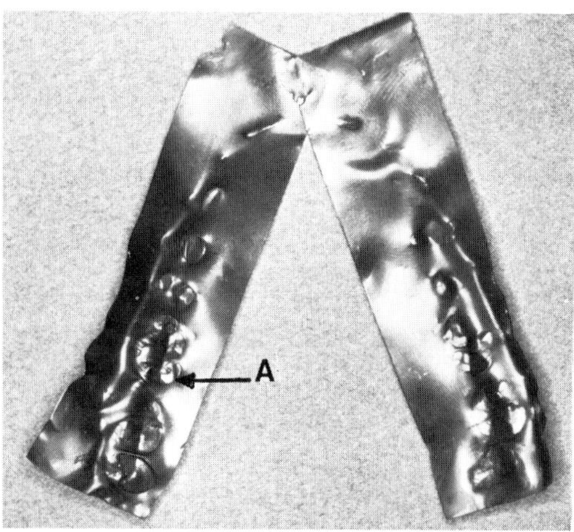

FIG. 13-22. Thirty-gauge casting wax strips showing the hole at A caused by the interfering occlusal contact of the articulated models.

After he has set up the condylar inclinations with the protrusive wax records, the dentist will be able to close the articulator without the centric-relation bite between the teeth and he will be able to see the first interfering occlusal contact of the stone teeth. Upon pressure of the upper bow of the articulator in the incisal pin region, the upper model will slide into the patient's convenience relationship, and the ball will move in the condylar guide slot. The convenience relationship of the mounted casts should be identical with that in the patient's mouth. The hole found in the Aluwax interfering contact bite should agree with the centric-relation interfering contact bite found on the study casts.

Aluwax is not used to locate interfering occlusal contacts on the casts, because it is too thick, and the force necessary to locate an interfering contact may fracture the stone teeth. Use the following procedure to locate interfering contacts on the casts. Position two green casting wax strips that have been dipped into water at 118° F. on the upper cast in the manner shown on the natural dentition in Figure 13-21. Bring the casts together lightly, and one hole should appear in the wax as A in Figure 13-22. In some cases it may be advantageous to lay the wax against the maxillary teeth of the cast and to mark them through the hole in the wax with a sharp pencil. Repeat this procedure on the lower cast.

A more accurate method of marking the teeth is through the use of articulating paper and red adding-machine ribbon. Blue articulating paper, in the holder (Fig. 13-23), is interposed between the teeth of the casts while they are lightly tapped together. Repeat the same procedure with the red ribbon. This method will now clearly indicate the interfering contact as a red spot on a blue background. After careful study of the formulated Centric Reshaping Determination Chart, lightly reshape the tooth surface with a carborundum stone, and again use green casting wax to check whether the interfering contact has been removed. If a hole appears in the wax in a new area, this indicates a new interfering contact and is evidence that the first interfering contact has been eliminated. Record the first interfering contact on the blueprint list, and repeat the entire procedure for the second interfering contact. Continue this procedure in centric relation until the maximum number of centric-relation occlusal contacts have been achieved without altering the vertical dimension.

It is important to remember that the blueprint procedure and the blueprint list are only *guides* to what must be done in the actual reshaping of the teeth in the patient's mouth. The primary function of the blueprint plan is to serve as a practice or trial run. In some cases it will be noted that a tooth or a cusp of a tooth in one jaw is extruded. In such a case, it is advisable to cut down the tooth on the cast and to build up the opposing tooth in wax to the correct occlusal plane. This procedure should also be recorded on the blueprint list. This blueprint list can be prepared in the form of the Centric-Relation Reshaping Guide List (Fig. 13-24). By listing on this chart all the reshaping that has been done on the stone casts, as well as all other pertinent facts, the practitioner will have an approximate step-by-step blueprint to follow when he starts to equilibrate the occlusion in the patient's mouth. Many of the steps carried out on the casts will be incorrect, and the final decision as to where to reshape the teeth will have to be made from the Aluwax interfering-contact records that were actually made in the patient's mouth.

Experience in a large number of cases has shown that the interfering occlusal

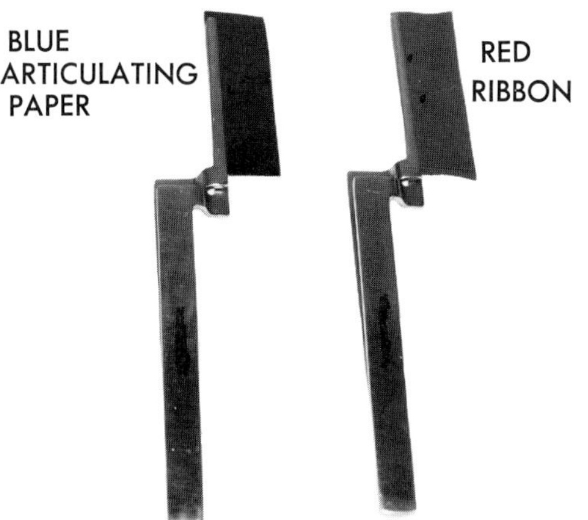

FIG. 13-23. Blue articulating paper and red adding-machine ribbon in Miller holders.

CENTRIC RELATION RESHAPING GUIDE LIST

STEPS	LOCATION	REMARKS
1	Distolingual plane of the distobuccal cusp 7|	Remove very little
2	Mesiolingual plane of the buccal cusp of |5	Grind near fossa
3	Mesiobuccal plane of the lingual cusp of |4	Grind center of plane
4	Central fossa 7|	
5	Proceed similarly	
6		

FIG. 13-24. This list is made as the articulated casts are ground, and is used as a guide for reshaping the patient's dentition in centric relation.

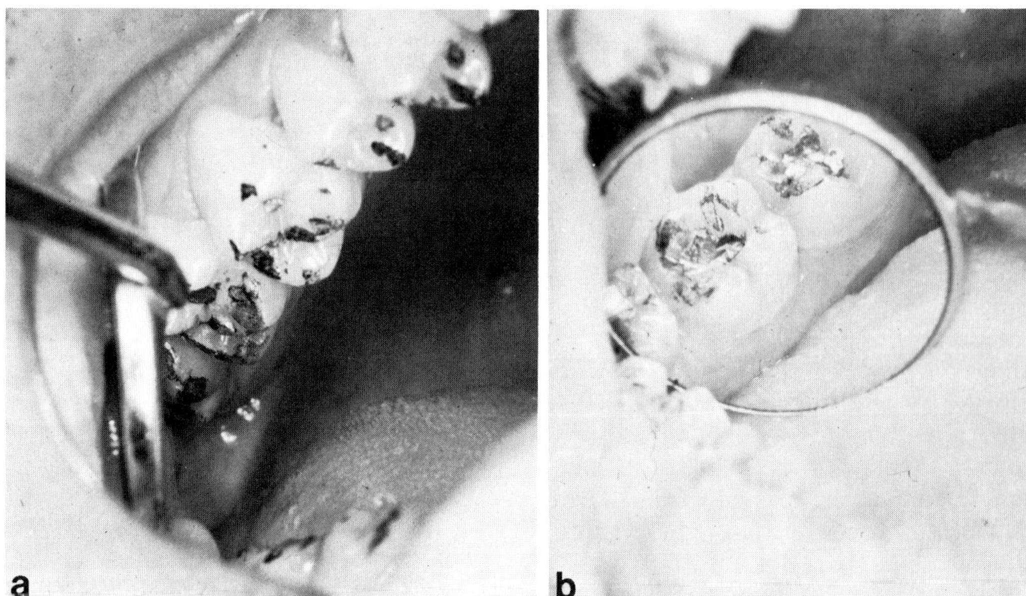

FIG. 13-25. The dentist makes blue and red marks (*a,b*) which confirm a hole that is seen in wax form.

contacts that are reshaped are found in the following locations: central fossae (planes) of the lower molars; central fossae (planes) of the upper molars; mesiobuccal plane of the lingual cusp of the upper first bicuspids (found in about 15 per cent of cases, probably because of the erratically formed anatomy and position of the lower first bicuspids); distal marginal ridge of extruded lower teeth; mesial marginal ridge of extruded upper teeth.

In Figure 13-25, there are many blue and red marks and the question arises whether to grind the upper or lower teeth. Actually the blue and red marks confirm the hole in the wax. It is the holes in the wax (Aluwax) that determine the contacting surfaces. When a cusp strikes a fossa in centric relation, always grind the fossa.

After equilibrating the models in centric relation on the articulator, they must also be equilibrated in right functioning range, left nonfunctioning range, left functioning range, right nonfunctioning range, and the protrusive range of articulation, and finally in the protrusive position. The principles behind the procedure for equilibrating the eccentric ranges of articulation on the mounted casts are identical with those used to equilibrate the corresponding ranges in the mouth. In the succeeding chapters the procedures of reshaping the teeth in the eccentric ranges of articulation and the use of waxes and other materials are clearly described. These chapters should be consulted for the methods of marking and reshaping the teeth in the eccentric ranges of articulation on the casts. It is advisable to correct several cases of mounted study models before undertaking any reshaping of the natural dentition.

EQUILIBRATION OF THE OCCLUSION OF THE NATURAL DENTITION IN CENTRIC RELATION

After all preliminary studies have been completed, proceed with the selective reshaping of the patient's natural dentition. Seat the patient in a 45° reclining position and train him to give a centric-relation bite in the manner that was described previously. In using Aluwax to secure the centric-relation bite, remember that the shiny, deep-green side is the upper side. Placing this shiny surface against the upper teeth, go through the procedure of taking a centric-relation interfering-contact bite. Figure 13-16 shows a wax bite with an interfering occlusal contact at A. To avoid errors in the placement of the wax form after refilling holes, develop the habit of always placing the shiny, deep-green surface of the Aluwax against the occlusal surfaces of the upper teeth. Then check the interfering-contact bite that was taken in the mouth against the interfering-contact bite that was located on the articulated study casts. They should agree.

Instruct the patient to tap the teeth together rapidly and lightly again and again in centric relation. As the patient is doing this, place flamed, thick articulating paper followed by red-cotton, adding-machine ribbon between the teeth on the side of the interfering contact as the teeth are tapped together. The interfering contacts will show up as clear red marks against a blue background. Then fill out the Centric Reshaping Determination Chart and decide where to reshape the teeth. The procedure for filling out this chart and for deciding which surfaces to reshape is explained in connection with Figure 13-19. If, in centric relation, an upper lingual cusp of a posterior tooth makes an interfering contact in a lower fossa, the fossa must be deepened. The point of the upper lingual cusp must not be ground. It is also wise to widen the groove slightly to allow lateral play to prevent locking during the Bennett movement.

In reshaping the surfaces, perform only enough grinding to remove the color marking before the surfaces are rechecked. *Very little of the tooth structure should be removed.* Use the carbide 12-bladed fluted bur (Fig. 13-26) in a high-speed handpiece. The value of this bur is that in addition to removing the enamel and gold, it polishes these surfaces.

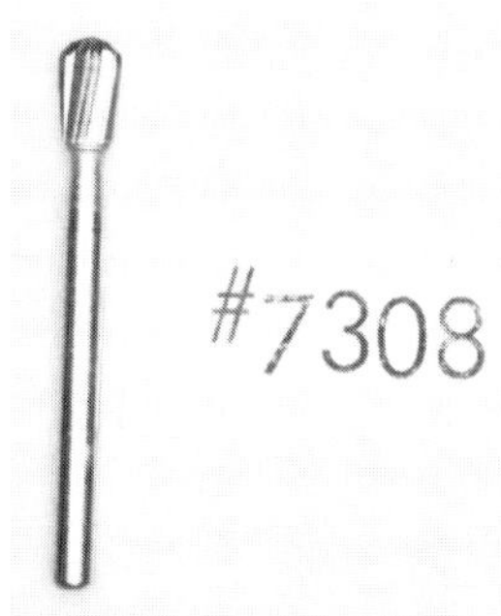

FIG. 13-26. This pear-shaped, No. 7308 Midwest carbide bur, is used for reshaping the teeth.

The next step in the procedure is to dip a sheet of denture Aluwax into water at 118° F. and to roll it into a cylinder. Melt Aluwax from this cylinder into the undersurface of the hole in the Aluwax form (Fig. 13-27). If wax were added to the upper surface, it would be difficult to position the form against the upper teeth. With this form, take another centric-relation interfering-contact registration. Again examine the form for a hole which indicates a new interfering contact. In

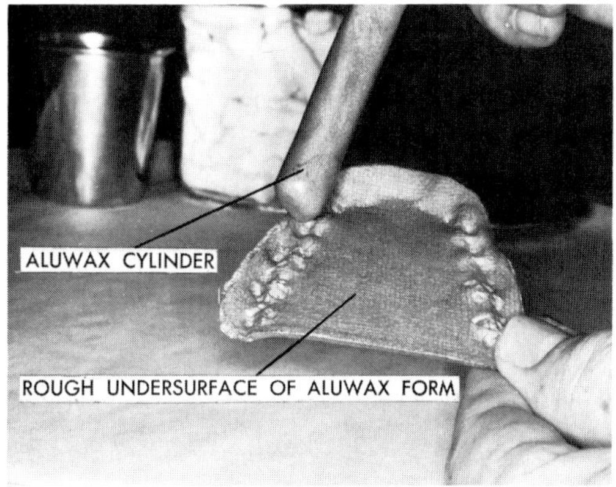

FIG. 13-27. Filling in an interfering occlusal contact hole on the undersurface of the Aluwax form.

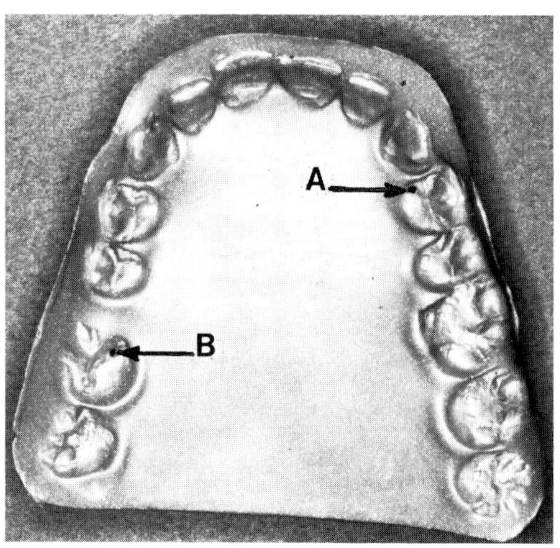

FIG. 13-28. Wax bite revealing two occlusal contacts that occurred at the same time.

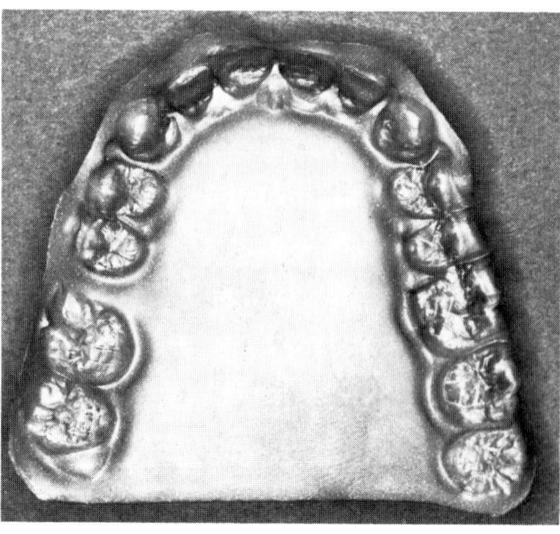

FIG. 13-29. Equilibration of a case in centric relation to the point where holes do not appear in the Aluwax bite form.

many cases the hole is extremely small; consequently, it is essential to hold the form toward daylight and examine it, using loupes. It is frequently helpful to run a dull explorer lightly over the wax to locate such extremely small holes. If more than one hole is discovered, refill the holes in the form with wax as before, and instruct the patient to tap lightly and repeatedly once again. Carefully reinspect the form. There should be only one hole. However, if, after several repetitions of the procedure, two holes still appear, like A and B in Figure 13-28, consider the more posterior of the two, B, the interfering contact. Record the new interfering contact on the centric reshaping determination chart so that a decision as to which surface to reshape may be made.

The procedure of biting into the wax, marking the teeth and carefully reshaping the interfering contact surfaces should be continued, theoretically, until there is a hole for each contact in centric-relation occlusion, or 16 holes for 32 teeth in contact. The purpose of this procedure is to achieve the greatest possible number of contacts in centric-relation occlusion without shortening the vertical dimension unintentionally. However, in actual practice abnormal tooth position and anatomy may limit the possible total number of occlusal contacts that may be achieved.

In most instances, as the case proceeds to a stage that is closer to an equal distribution of forces in centric relation throughout the mouth, holes will not appear in the Aluwax form, thus indicating that the equally distributed forces are insufficient to penetrate the wax (Fig. 13-29). In this case, although the cusp marks are quite transparent, no actual holes or perforations are present. When this stage is reached, it becomes necessary to make finer adjustments. Place two strips of 30-gauge green wax, that have been softened in the 118° F. water, over the occlusal and buccal surfaces of the upper teeth (Fig. 13-21). Instruct the patient to open and close lightly in centric relation a few times. Remove the wax and examine for holes. Use loupes to examine the wax. Check the holes with the Centric-Relation Reshaping Guide List and reshape the teeth accordingly. Repeat the biting, marking and reshaping procedures until the wax strips no longer show holes (Fig. 13-30).

After centric-relation occlusion has

been achieved, test the anterior teeth for trauma. The existence of trauma to the upper anterior teeth can be determined by placing the ball of the forefinger on an upper anterior tooth and feeling for movement while the patient closes his jaws in centric relation. If trauma is present, reshape the incisal edge of the lower anterior tooth, where the interfering contact is found. Removing tooth structure at the lingual area of the upper contact would make the incisal guidance even sharper. These contacts are located with articulating paper and ribbon.

Polishing Reshaped Surfaces

Check the patient's teeth for sharp edges, and instruct the patient to check each tooth with his tongue for rough areas. Such areas will irritate the soft tissues and form points of departure for initial changes in mandibular movements. *This polishing and checking procedure should be carried out after each visit in which any reshaping has been performed.*

IMPORTANCE OF MINIMAL REMOVAL OF TOOTH STRUCTURE

It is important to stress the fact that in reshaping a tooth, very little removal of tooth structure need be done. A good rule is to remove only enough tooth structure to eliminate the color marking from the interfering occlusal contact before retesting the tooth. The patient may be told that the amount of tooth structure removed is analogous to removing the dust from a mirror, and this analogy is a good one for the operator to bear in mind as well.

Very little tooth structure is removed in reshaping. The angles of inclination of the cusps are reduced. The cusps are not eliminated or flattened to zero; they are merely made less steep.

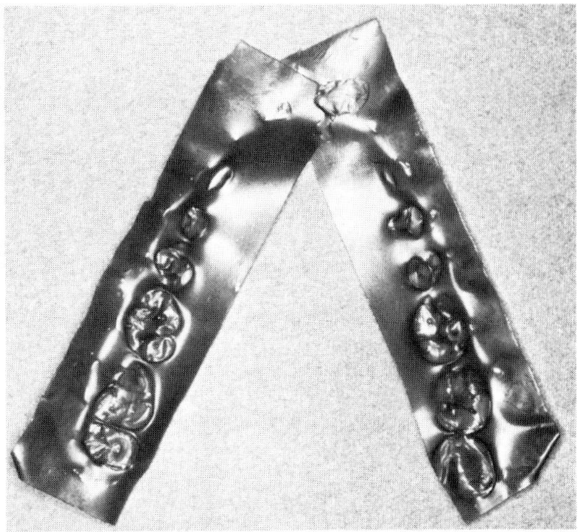

FIG. 13-30. Equilibration of a case in centric relation to the point where holes do not appear in the thin casting wax.

The beginner in the procedure of occlusal equilibration is usually surprised to find how small an amount of tooth structure need be removed to reduce an interfering contact. This is one advantage of first working on the cast. The reason for minimal removal of tooth structure becomes clear if the temporomandibular joint is visualized as a hinge joint on a door. The slightest amount of interference or the slightest change of position at the hinge of the door will be enormously magnified at the far edge of the door. For example, if a pencil is inserted close to the hinge, the door will remain ajar more than a foot at the far edge. Similarly in the mouth, a centric-relation interfering contact in the molar region is multiplied about three times in the incisor region. Every practitioner has had an experience that illustrates this point when he has ground down a slightly high molar inlay. Because much of the removal of tooth structure involved in reducing an interfering contact is done on angles rather than on flat surfaces, most dentists and their patients are amazed that such slight grinding can produce such remarkable results. Mathematically stated, the dentist is reducing the degree of angulation of the inclined planes because the interfering contact hits the inclined plane and skids. If this grinding is done properly, there is no danger of closing the vertical dimension.

Discussion

The purpose of using the 30- or 22-gauge casting wax after the Aluwax has been used is best explained as follows. The teeth are suspended by periodontal fibers and, therefore, have a slight degree of mobility. Teeth which are in improper occlusion are actually in supra- or infraocclusion and consequently are capable of more than normal mobility. As the Aluwax form is used repeatedly, and as more and more interfering contacts are removed, more and more teeth are brought into occlusal contact in centric relation. Since the same piece of Aluwax has been used for many closures in centric relation and, therefore, is transparently thin in the occlusal portions, the gauze which separates the two sheets of wax is exposed. Sometimes the threads of the gauze provide enough resistance to move or depress the teeth and to give an inaccurate reading. There may be additional factors leading to inaccuracy in the repeated heating and filling of the Aluwax form. Therefore, the 30- or 22-gauge wax strips are of great value in the final adjustment, and clinical experience has shown that they work effectively.

As he uses the various waxes, it is important for the practitioner to remember that not all patients use the same force in biting. One patient may perforate the Aluwax form with a single closure of his jaws. Such a patient usually has prominent masseter muscles that give evidence of heavy usage and also frequently exhibits the square type of face. The opposite type of patient is the indolent chewer with a thin face and flaccid musculature. He cannot muster much force in centric closure, and it may take a great deal of time and patience on the part of the dentist before the first interfering contact is revealed as a hole in the wax. With this type of person it is important to be calm and patient. There are also those patients who are perfectly willing to cooperate in closing in centric relation but cannot do so because of poor muscular habits and involved mandibular placement. The operator must exercise considerable tact and patience.

The operator must use his judgment in determining how best to stabilize mobile teeth while taking wax bites and reshaping the teeth. Finger support, wire, grassline ligatures and compound or plaster blocks are a few of the possible means of immobilizing the teeth.

After equilibration in centric relation has been finished, note from the roentgenograms those teeth that show bone loss, and from the clinical analysis those teeth that demonstrate mobility. The mobile teeth may have failed to register in the green wax. Recheck these with 30-gauge wax for interfering occlusal contacts while they are stabilized and reshape if necessary.

Stillman and McCall[4] suggested the use of sound as a diagnostic test in the equilibration of the occlusion. Before the dentition is equilibrated in centric relation, the teeth will make a dull, discordant, hollow sound when they are tapped together rapidly and lightly. After equilibration in centric relation has been completed, the sound of the teeth as they are tapped together is very revealing to the experienced operator. In a case that has been finely equilibrated, the sound that the teeth make in centric closure will be sharp, high, solid and definite, as if two solid blocks of hardwood had been tapped solidly together.

In some cases, it is possible to show the patient actual blanching of the gingiva as the tooth that makes the interfering contact is intruded or tipped when the teeth are brought together. This condition is usually found in the anterior region because, in contrast with the posterior teeth, the anterior teeth have single roots set at an angle which can be tipped. The blanching of the tissue, if it is chronic, will result in disturbed function. The distance traveled by the depressed tooth and the effects of the depression on the periodontal ligament and the lamina dura can be compared with the effects of pressure on a fingernail. When a fingernail is depressed, the bed of the nail blanches. The distance traveled by the nail is the approximate width of the periodontal ligament, and similar movement causes pressure on the lamina dura.

PRECAUTIONS TO BE OBSERVED

The following precautions must be observed by the operator in equilibrating the occlusion in centric relation:

1. To assure accurate registration, bring the Aluwax to proper malleability by dipping it into water that is exactly 118° F.
2. If a great amount of reshaping is anticipated, use local anesthesia, but not mandibular block, to prevent pain and apprehension. If mandibular block is used, the mandibular neuromuscular relationships will be disturbed.
3. Use true-running handpieces, contra-angles and diamond stones to prevent patient discomfort.
4. Place the finger of the left hand on the tooth that is being reshaped to minimize vibration.
5. Take great care to avoid removing too much tooth structure; remove only a small amount at a time. A good guide is to remove only the colors that mark the interfering contact.
6. Reshape the tooth so that the basic general anatomy is preserved.
7. After reshaping, polish the teeth.
8. If it is necessary to remove a large amount of tooth structure, provide metal veneers to cover the occlusal surfaces.
9. To obtain clear markings, dry the occlusal surfaces of the teeth with cotton before using the articulating paper or adding machine ribbon.
10. If possible, do not grind the mesiolingual cusp of the upper molar.
11. After equilibration, test the teeth for mobility induced by minute interfering contacts. This may be done by placing a finger on the tooth and in the buccal sulcus while the patient taps his teeth together in centric relation.
12. Warn the patient that after his teeth have been equilibrated, there may be some pain when he eats, owing to the fact that teeth which were not previously functioning are now bearing some of the masticatory forces. This pain will disappear. Also warn the patient not to test his teeth immediately by eating hard foods.
13. As the teeth are equilibrated in the eccentric ranges of articulation, constantly check centric-relation occlusion.
14. If restorations are made after occlusal equilibration has been completed, check in both centric and eccentric ranges to ensure their harmony with the established equilibrated occlusion.
15. Frequently, an interfering contact in centric relation occurs on the transverse ridge of a maxillary molar. This can be reshaped without too much loss of efficiency in the protrusive range.
16. If posterior teeth are to be removed for any reason, perform occlusal equilibration after the extraction.
17. If the interfering contact in centric relation is on the anterior teeth, reshape the mandibular teeth. This procedure will not eliminate the necessary contacts of the maxillary teeth in the eccentric ranges of articulation.
18. Carefully plan every step involved in equilibration, and do not remove tooth structure unless the rationale for the selective reshaping of the teeth has been firmly established.

A case can be considered to have been equilibrated in centric-relation occlusion when the following conditons have been satisfied.

1. The test with the green 30- or 22-gauge wax does not demonstrate any tears in centric-relation closure.

2. Rapid closure in centric-relation occlusion produces the characteristic high sound that is similar to that produced when two blocks of wood are tapped together.

3. The patient feels simultaneous contact of all the teeth in centric-relation closure.

4. The single place where the closure of the mandible is comfortable to the patient coincides with centric-relation occlusion.

It is interesting to note how quickly the patient abandons his former habitual convenience relationship closure when the interferences to centric-relation closure have been eliminated.

Other methods for detecting centric-relation interfering contacts have been suggested, but none meets the scientific requirements as accurately as does the Aluwax method that has been described. In one method, the patient helps the dentist to find the interfering contact by pointing to it. Obviously, this depends upon subjective impressions by an inexperienced and untrained patient. In another method, the dentist relaxes the patient with drugs, hypnosis or other methods. It has been found impossible for a second operator to reproduce results obtained with this technique. In still another method, the dentist forces the patient's jaws into centric relation. Here, the centric-relation impression depends largely upon the operator's skill and strength and cannot be readily duplicated by another operator. There are other methods that depend largely or wholly upon the use of such materials as rubber triangles, metal castings, grit, etc. Here, there is still too much dependence upon the unique skill of the operator in handling these materials.

The Aluwax method will enable the careful practitioner to discover the interfering occlusal contacts that are at the root of occlusal dysfunction and to determine a course of treatment and operative procedure that will remove the causes rather than merely alleviate the symptoms. The postulates of the scientific method stipulate procedures that are reproducible by any individual in similar circumstances and that are susceptible to the same conclusions.

REFERENCES

1. Alkory: *In* Ackermann, F.: Le Mecanisme des Machoires, Paris, Masson, 1953.
2. Hutchinson, J. A. F.: Occlusion. JADA, *14:*335, 1927.
3. Karolyi, M.: Beobachtungen uber pyorrhea alveolaris (Observations concerning the theory of pyorrhea alveolaris). O.U.V.f.Z., *17:*279, 1901.

   ———: Beobachtungen uber pyorrhea alveolaris und caries dentium (Observations concerning pyorrhea alveolaris and caries dentium). O.U.V.f.Z., *18:*520, 1902.

   ———: Über alveolar pyorrhea (Alveolar pyorrhea). O.U.V.f.Z., *21:*85, 1905.

   ———: Behandlung der alveolar pyorrhea (Treatment of alveolar pyorrhea). O.U.V.f.Z., *22:*193, 1906.

   ———: Zur therapie der erkrankungen der mundschleimhaut (Therapy of gingivitis), O.U.V.f.Z., *22:*226, 1906.
4. Stillman, P. R., and McCall, J. O.: Textbook of Clinical Periodontia. ed. 2. New York, Macmillan, 1939.
5. Warnekros, L.: Über die ursachen des fruhzeitigen verlustes der zahne (The causes of early loss of teeth). Berl. klin. Wchnschr., 25, 1906.

Additional Basic References

Ackermann, F.: Le meulage d'equilibration occluso-articulaire doit-il être automatique ou selectif? Rev. Mens. Suisse Odont., *53:*649, 1943.

———: Equilibre-desequilibre. Rev. Mens. Suisse Odont., *62:*49, 1952.

Anderson, J.: Seminar at L. D. Pankey Institute, Miami, Florida, October, 1973.

Bricker, F. A.: Diagnosis and correction of traumatic occlusion. JADA, *11:*697, 1924.

Brown, S. W.: Disharmony between centric

relation and centric occlusion as a factor in producing improper tooth wear and trauma. D. Digest, *52:*434, 1946.

Cripps, S.: Occlusal equilibration of the natural dentition. Br. D. J., *88:*90, 1950.

Eberle, W. R.: A study of centric relation as recorded in a supine rest position. JADA, *42:*15, 1951.

Graham, C. H.: Occlusal correction. D. J. Australia, *25:*181, 1953.

Grewcock, R. J. G.: A short survey of the principles involved in the establishment of balanced occlusion. D. Pract., *1:*234, 1951.

Guichet, N. F.: Procedures for Occlusal Treatment, a Teaching Atlas. Anaheim, Calif., Denar Corp., 1969.

Lauritzen, A. G.: Function, prime object of restorative dentistry: a definite procedure to obtain. JADA, *42:*423, 1951.

Lazarus, A. H.: Remedying dental pathology by restoring centric occlusion. New York State D. J., *17:*107, 1951.

Maunsbach, O., and Posselt, U.: Bettslipning som funktionskorrigerande hjalpmedel (Selective grinding as an aid in functional therapy). Odont. Rev., *6:*163, 1955.

Muller, M.: Grundlagen und aufbau des artikulationsproblemes im naturlichen und kunstlichen gebisse (Fundamentals and construction of the articulation problem in the natural and artificial teeth). Leipzig, Verlag, Dr. Werner Klinkhardt, 1925.

Radusch, D. F.: Grinding for relief of occlusal trauma associated with periodontoclasia. JADA, *30:*384, 1943.

Schuyler, C. H.: The use of baseplate wax in occlusal disharmony. New York J. Dent., *13:*461, 1947.

Scott, W. R.: Selective spot grinding. J. Can. D. A., *21:*18, 1954.

Shore, N. A.: The equilibration of the occlusion of the natural dentition. JADA, *44:*414, 1952.

———: Occlusal Equilibration. Film Library. ADA, Chicago, 1953.

Sorrin, S.: The equilibration of occlusion. Dentistry, *3:*6, 1943.

Stallard, H., and Stuart, C. E.: Concept of occlusion: what kind of occlusion should recusped teeth be given? D. Clin. North Am., *7:*591, 1963.

Stuart, C. E.: Why dental restorations should have cusps. J. Pros. Dent., *10:*553, 1960.

Thielemann, K.: Systematische umgestaltung der naturlichen kauflachen durch beschleifen als prophylax und therapie der paradentose (Changes of the natural surfaces of the teeth by grinding as a prophylactic measure). Korresp. Zahn., *4:*3, 1937.

Thomas, P. K.: Syllabus on Full Mouth Waxing Technique. ed. 2. San Diego, Instant Printing Services, 1967.

Vauthier, U.: Functional equilibration and analysis of occlusal-articular relationship by waxbites. Parodontologie, *10:*54, 1956.

Weinberg, L. A.: A visualized technique of occlusal equilibration. J. D. Med., *7:*9, 1952.

Westbrook, J. C.: A pattern of centric occlusion. JADA, *39:*407, 1949.

14 *Equilibration of the Occlusion in the Eccentric Ranges of Articulation*

THE FUNCTIONING RANGE

The lateral ranges of articulation consist of a functioning or working side and a nonfunctioning or nonworking side which is sometimes called the balancing side. *The functioning side is that side of the dentition that actually performs the act of mastication in the masticatory cycle, and the nonmasticating side is referred to as the nonfunctioning or nonworking side.* The term "balancing side" is a misnomer adopted from the prosthetic theory of three-point contact and should be avoided when referring to the natural dentition. When the dentition moves through the right functioning range of articulation, the left side automatically traverses the left nonfunctioning range. Conversely, when the left side moves through the functioning range, the right side automatically traverses the right nonfunctioning range of articulation.

Because of the masticatory habits of modern Western civilization, man does little incising or crushing of his food. The primary function of the teeth is grinding of food. Cuspal interferences to lateral excursions of the mandible on both the right and the left sides will force a patient to masticate in a choppy up-and-down manner that is both inefficient in preparing food for deglutition and digestion and injurious to the masticatory organ itself. Head[1] reported that approximately five times as much force is necessary to triturate food with a vertical stroke as is necessary with a lateral shearing action of the cusps. Since only one-fifth as much force is necessary in lateral trituration of food, the importance of freeing the occlusion for these movements is self-evident.

In many cases, cuspal inclines on one side of the mouth are so steep that the patient never learns to chew on that side because the effort involved is too great. However, as soon as propitious conditions of the masticatory organ are restored by means of occlusal equilibration, the muscles return to proper masticatory function, even though they have not been used properly for years. The problem is to make these restored eccentric movements an unconscious and habitual part of the patient's masticatory pattern. The patient who habitually chews on one side of his mouth must be retrained by demonstration and practice. At each session after equilibration and at each recall visit, check to see whether he has maintained a proper pattern of mastication. Uncorrected and unilateral chewing initiates a chain of events that results in tooth movement, poor periodontal tone and ultimate periodontal degeneration on the unused side.

Mandibular Movement in the Functioning Range

As the mandible moves in the functioning range of articulation, it moves downward and laterally in the masticatory cycle until the buccal cusps of the mandibular molars are under the buccal cusps of the maxillary molars. This is the functioning position. Completing the masticatory cycle, the mandible moves upward, and the buccal planes of the buccal cusps of the lower molars move against the lingual planes of the buccal cusps of the upper molars. At the same time, the buccal planes of the lingual cusps of the lower molars move against the lingual planes of the lingual cusps of the upper molars. As the mandible moves upward and laterally, it passes through a definite range and angulation of movement. Each cusp has its own prescribed path, and any deviation from this path renders the teeth unable to perform their masticatory functions properly. Improper corrective procedures will not restore function and may even exacerbate the poor conditons. The greatest importance must be placed on the last 2 to 3 mm. of gliding contact between the teeth during the lateral masticatory stroke. The masticatory organ starts from centric-relation occlusion and ends in centric-relation occlusion. The only tooth contact to take place during the intermediary cycle should be the 2 to 3 mm. of lateral gliding contact.

An interfering occlusal contact in the functioning range of articulation is called a horizontal or lateral interfering contact. In the functioning range of articulation, the forces exerted laterally against the teeth are vastly multiplied because of the factors of leverage that are involved. These forces are extremely destructive because the bony structure and the teeth are not designed to withstand such forces on one or two pairs of articulating teeth. As many cusps of the articulating teeth and as many articulating teeth as possible should share the load of mastication. This optimal situation can be provided by removing all interfering occlusal contacts in the functioning range of articulation.

The three objectives in equilibrating the occlusion in the functioning range of articulation are:

1. To reduce the lateral forces on individual teeth to tolerances within the range of the supporting tissues
2. To distribute the forces of mastication in the functioning ranges of articulation to as many teeth as possible
3. To harmonize the cuspal guiding inclines of the teeth with the mandibular movements so as to effect free gliding movements of the teeth. The last objective does not imply leveling all cusps in the eccentric ranges of articulation to provide a flat occlusal table. It is important to visualize the operation of the lateral masticatory cycle and to bear in mind the objectives of equilibrating the occlusion in the eccentric ranges of articulation.

As illustrated in Figure 5-25, the plane AB of the upper tooth and the plane AB of the masticatory cycle are identical. This results in a smooth closure which, at the same time, is harmonious with the movements of the head of the condyle within the temporomandibular joint. Correct distribution of the stresses and of the free gliding movements will help to promote and maintain proper physiological development. Also, it must be remembered that occlusal changes caused by wear and by change of position are going on constantly.[5]

Theoretical Principles of Equilibrating a Single Pair of Posterior Teeth

In the natural dentition, all the cusps of pairs of occluding bicuspids and molars should work in harmony in the functioning range of articulation. Figure 14-1 illustrates the theoretical basis for equilibrating a single pair of occluding molars so that the buccal and the lingual

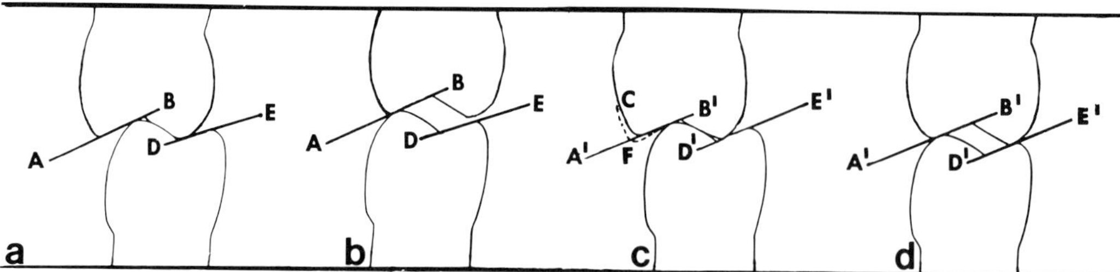

FIG. 14-1. The principle of equilibrating a single pair of opposing teeth in the functioning range of articulation. (Shore, N. A.: Equilibration of the occlusion of the natural dentition. JADA, *44*:414, 1952)

cusps will work in harmony in the functioning range of articulation. Drawing (*a*) represents an upper and a lower molar in centric-relation occlusion. Lines AB and DE, which represent the extension of the gliding planes of the cusps, are not parallel. In drawing (*b*), the molars are in the functioning position; in (*c*) the buccal cusps, represented by lines A′B′ and D′E′, are now parallel. Tooth structure was removed at line CFB′. If the tooth structure is removed to the dotted line, two important mechanical changes are accomplished: lines A′B′ and D′E′ are rendered parallel so that both cusps will work together in the functioning range; and as the occlusal area is reduced by rounding off the cusp to the dotted line, the line of force is brought closer to the long axis of the tooth. Drawing (*d*) shows that both cusps now make contact in the functioning range with A′B′ and D′E′.[5]

Theoretical Principles of Reshaping the Posterior Teeth in the Functioning Range

The theoretical ideal to be achieved in occlusal equilibration is the production of buccal and lingual cuspal contacts of all opposing teeth in the functioning range of articulation. However, this ideal cannot always be attained, and the dentist may have to be content to achieve two, three or four cuspal contacts of opposing teeth in the functioning range.

When the mandible moves into the functioning range of articulation, the condyle on the functioning side pivots and moves laterally. It is useful to think of the condyle on the functioning side as a pivot. Because of the varying distances of the occlusal planes of each tooth from the condyle pivot, the angle of each occlusal plane varies slightly. This slight variation is caused by the various radii of action from the pivot to the occlusal planes and is necessary to permit the occlusal planes to function harmoniously during this articulatory movement. For purposes of simplification, these planes will be considered as parallel.

It is helpful to visualize the approximating teeth of both arches during mandibular movement in the functioning range. Since it is difficult to do this in the patient's mouth, it will be necessary to do it schematically by turning the approximating teeth aside and by removing every other tooth. This is seen in Figure 14-2*a*, which depicts the proximating teeth on the right side of the jaw, showing cuspids, bicuspids and molars in centric-relation occlusion. Although there is cusp and fossa contact, the lines AB, CD, EF, GH and IJ are not parallel. In (*b*), the teeth are in functioning position. Only the cuspid makes contact, and there are spaces between the bicuspids and the molars. In (*c*) all the inclined planes, represented by lines A′B′, C′D′, E′F′, G′H′ and I′J′, have been made parallel. It also shows reduction of excess tooth surface at LMB′ on the cuspid, OSD′ and E′UF′

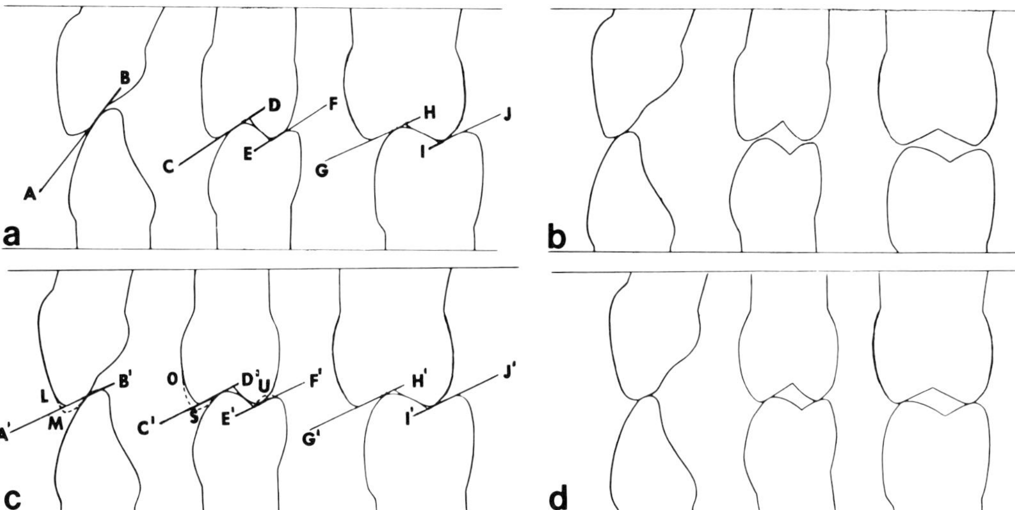

FIG. 14-2. The principles of equilibration of the proximating cuspid, bicuspids and molars in the functioning range of articulation. (Shore, N. A.: Equilibration of the occlusion of the natural dentition. JADA, *44:*414, 1952)

on the bicuspids, and slight reduction on the molars at G′H′ and I′J′. Only the inclined planes were reshaped. The centric-relation contacts of the cusps and the fossae were not altered. In (*d*) the teeth are shown in the functioning position as all the cusps make contact.

Reshaping the Cuspid Interfering Contacts

Frequently, the cuspids make the only interfering contact in the functioning range. This type of contact must be studied carefully. The upper cuspids are considered to be anterior teeth, but they also function like posterior teeth. Because of this dual relationship, they play a vital role in the protrusive and the functioning ranges of articulation. Because of hereditary factors, time of eruption, stress and masticatory habits, the cuspid assumes a wide variety of positions and angulations in the dental arch. The upper cuspid, which is the extension of the anterior pillar of bone in the maxilla, is probably one of the strongest teeth in the arch and is designed to withstand great stress. As a posterior tooth, it is single cusped and makes a plane-to-plane rather than a cusp-to-fossa contact with its opposing teeth. Therefore, it is at the mercy of excessive horizontal force factors. In many cases the cuspids shift laterally and posteriorly because they form the only functioning contact in the lateral range. This is a form of auto-orthodontia which is attempting to create a physiologic occlusion. In other cases, the cuspids do not shift but lock the occlusion. If such cases are followed, it will be observed that the vertical chopping stroke of mastication falls mainly on the bicuspids and not on the cuspids. In time, the bicuspids become mobile, and the periodontal tissues degenerate. If the dentition is equilibrated in the functioning range, the mobility of the teeth decreases, and the tissue tone improves.

In many cases it may seem that too much tooth structure would have to be removed from the upper cuspids to bring the other teeth into the functioning range of articulation, and that the resulting esthetics of the cuspids would be poor.

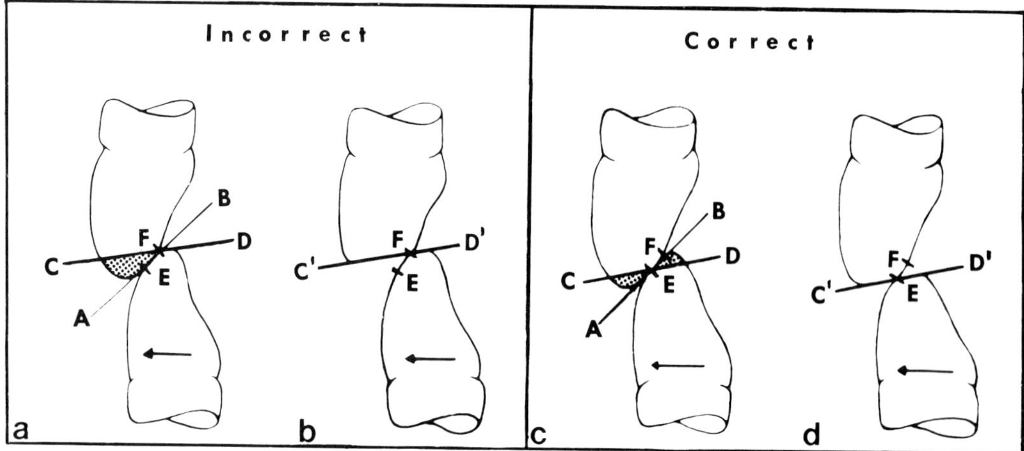

FIG. 14-3. The incorrect method (*a*) and (*b*), and the correct method (*c*) and (*d*), for removing interfering contacts, in cases of deep vertical overbite, in the functioning ranges of articulation. The esthetics of the teeth are maintained in (*c*) and (*d*).

However, there are many cases of this type in which the lower cuspid can be reshaped to decrease the amount of tooth structure that must be removed from the upper cuspid, thus giving an esthetic result.

In Figure 14-3*a* it should be noted that the centric-relation contact at EF is broad. If the patient moves into the functioning range of articulation, the lower tooth must travel along the steep incline, AB. If the rule of reshaping only the buccal cusps of the upper teeth were applied in this case, the cuspid would be disfigured in the attempt to achieve more tooth contacts in the functioning range; the results of this reshaping are illustrated in (*b*).

The correct method of establishing a less steep incline in the functioning range without disfiguring the upper cuspid is to find the contact, EF (Fig. 14-3*c*), and then to select the most gingival marking on the lower cuspid as the point to maintain centric-relation occlusion. In this case, the point is E. By reshaping the lower cuspid along the line ED from E upward, without removing E, the point of centric contact, a new and less steep inclination of the lower cuspid is provided. Now, by reshaping the lower cuspid along the path CE without touching the point of centric contact, E, less tooth structure will have to be removed from the upper cuspid. The incisal edges should be reshaped as in (*d*). Compare the results of reshaping by the correct method as in (*d*) with the results achieved by the incorrect method illustrated in (*b*). In this manner greater functional harmony can be attained with minimal removal of tooth structure. In Figure 14-4*a*, an actual case is presented. Note the large, broad, functioning-range contact on the labial of the lower cuspid. In (*b*), the tooth was reshaped according to the principles illustrated in Figure 14-3*c* and *d*. Thus, greater functional harmony was achieved with a minimal removal of tooth structure. This principle can be applied to other teeth, provided that a broad functioning-range contact exists on the buccal planes of the buccal cusps of the lower teeth.

The distal lobes of the lingual planes of the maxillary incisors perform during the functioning range of articulation. The anterior teeth should not interfere with the functioning range of articulation. If they do, the effects of trauma upon the anterior teeth will be so severe

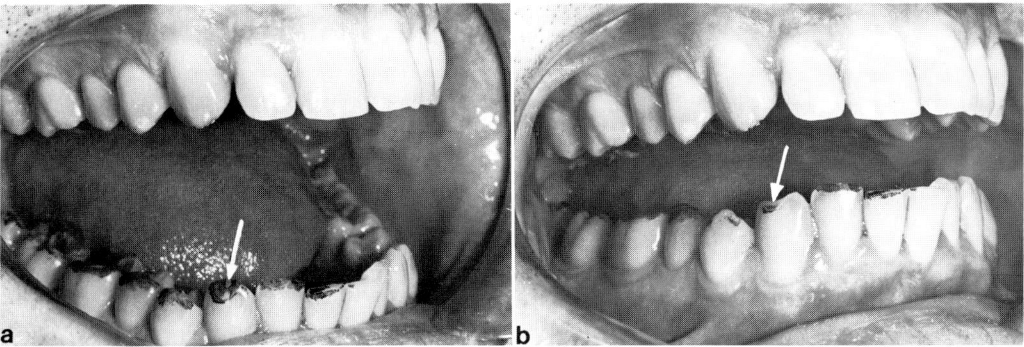

FIG. 14-4. A broad functioning-range contact (*a*) and its reduction in the lower arch (*b*) before reshaping the upper tooth, as in Figure 14-3 (*c* and *d*).

as to cause degeneration of the periodontal tissues.

At this point it would be well to review the normal articulation of the cusps of the teeth (Chap. 5). The normal articulation of the cusps of the teeth forms the basis for the study of the patient to determine whether there is any deviation from the normal in the functioning ranges of articulation.

In a normal or nearly normal occlusion, the rule for equilibrating the teeth in the functioning range of articulation is to reshape the lingual planes of the buccal cusps of the upper teeth and the buccal planes of the lingual cusps of the lower teeth. This is a simple rule, but it is important to adapt it to each individual case. It cannot serve as a blanket rule indiscriminately. *However, a rule that must be applied universally is to determine the location of the point of centric-relation occlusion contact, and then to grind from that point forward. If the centric-relation occlusion is ground, the vertical dimension will be shortened.*

Demonstration of Masticatory Pattern

Ask the patient to demonstrate his pattern of functioning-range gliding movements. Observe carefully while he is masticating some chewing gum or some soft baseplate wax. Note the limit and the amount of excursive movements in the functioning ranges. Note also whether the patient is limited by a horizontal or a vertical overbite and observe any unusual habit patterns. Each patient will demonstrate a unique pattern of movements that is related to the inclined planes and the interfering contacts of the cusps of his teeth. Some investigators have stated that left-handed people tend to masticate on the left side. The pattern of mastication depends upon the occlusal topography rather than on the handedness of the individual.

It is a good idea to demonstrate to the patient how to move his mandible laterally. Give the patient a hand mirror, and place the ball of your forefinger on the upper right cuspid, parallel with its axial inclination. Ask the patient to move or to rub his teeth upward toward his right ear, to stop as soon as he touches your forefinger and then to open his mouth quickly. The lateral movement will extend about 2 or 3 mm. It will be a revelation to most patients that they can make this movement only with great difficulty. It may actually be necessary to move the patient's jaw laterally in the direction desired to demonstrate the functioning range. Usually, the patient will tend to move his jaw in the direction opposite to the one in which the dentist in-

STEPS	ARTICULATORY MOVEMENT	LOCATION	REMARKS
1	Right functioning	Lingual plane of 3⌋	Remove very little
2	Same	Buccal plane of distolingual cusp 6⌋	Grind near tip
3	Left nonfunctioning	Lingual plane of the distobuccal cusp ⌈7	Center of plane
4	Proceed similarly in all the eccentric ranges.		
5			

FIG. 14-5. This list is made as the articulated casts are ground and used as a guide for reshaping the patient's dentition in the eccentric ranges of articulation.

structs him. To save time and to make things easier for patient and dentist alike, it is good practice to instruct the patient to perform these lateral jaw movements for a minute each morning after brushing his teeth, before he returns for the visit during which the occlusion is to be equilibrated in right or left functioning range.

Operative Procedure

The second step in the occlusal-equilibration procedure is the reshaping of the dentition in the functioning range of articulation. It makes no difference in the final results whether the right or the left functioning range of articulation is reshaped first. The important thing is that each step be done at successive visits spaced about a week apart to allow for slight tooth movement and adjustment. Check the previously completed selective reshaping in centric-relation occlusion to make certain that no shifting or movement of the teeth has taken place.

The only rules for reshaping the teeth that can be established definitely and categorically are those that will apply to teeth in normal or nearly normal position. Such a favorable situation is seldom found. Rules apply to identical or similar circumstances, and since there seldom are identical or even similar mouths, definite rules to cover all circumstances cannot be established. Therefore, it is extremely important to understand the general principles involved in deciding which surface is to be reshaped and which surface must be let alone. Then a plan of operation to suit each individual case can be developed. Such a procedure is obviously better than blindly following rules which may not apply to the individual case under treatment.

Study the models of the patient's teeth on the anatomical articulator. For the inexperienced operator, it is advisable to make a blueprint for the operative procedure (Fig. 14-5) which is based on the actual reshaping of the teeth of the casts in the lateral ranges. Of course, this blueprint or grinding list will not reflect accurately the actual dentition, but it will give an approximate idea of what must be done to the patient's dentition, and it will aid in carrying out the procedures involved in the occlusal reshaping.

At this point it is very important to check the casts for interfering occlusal contact on the nonfunctioning side. An

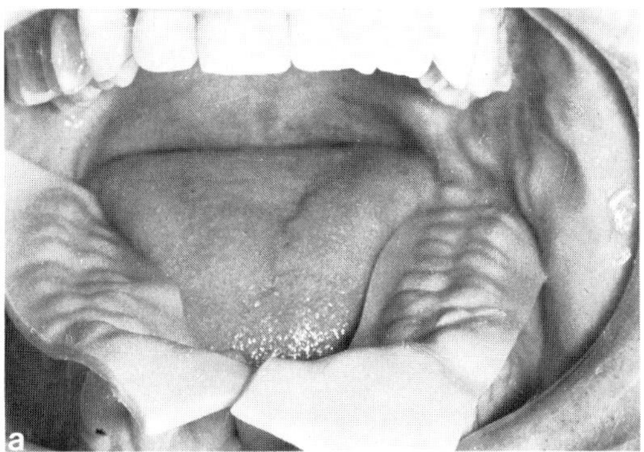

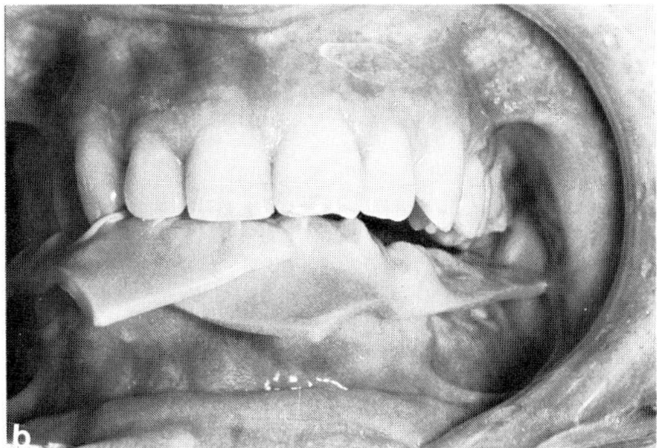

FIG. 14-6. Pink wax strips placed over lower teeth (*a*) and mandibular movement into the right functioning range of articulation (*b*).

interfering occlusal contact on that side will prevent the teeth on the functioning side from articulating properly. The explanation and the details of procedure for treating the nonfunctioning-side interfering contacts will be discussed in the next section of this chapter. *If an interfering contact is found on the nonfunctioning side, it must be removed before proceeding with the equilibration of the occlusion in the functioning range of articulation.*

The relationships of the articulating surfaces that maintain centric-relation occlusion for the individual patient must be borne in mind. When reshaping the teeth in the lateral ranges, be careful to maintain this centric-relation occlusion.

Instruct the patient to move his jaw to the right or to the left, observing himself in a hand mirror as he makes these movements. He should move his mandible laterally until the cuspids are in an almost edge-to-edge relation. Usually, one or two pairs of teeth will make contact in the functioning range of articulation. Dip two strips of Moyco beauty pink wax into 118° F. water and place over the entire lower arch (Fig. 14-6*a*). Tell the patient to bite lightly in centric-relation occlusion and then to move his mandible forcefully into the right functioning range of articulation (b). Note the contact at A made by the upper and the lower right cuspids (Fig. 14-7). There are no interfering contacts on the nonfunctioning side, as evidenced by lack of holes in the wax on that side. For future reference, record on the patient's chart the original tooth contacts in the lateral ranges of articulation before beginning selective reshaping of the teeth.

Decide which areas of the lateral interfering contacts to reshape to bring more teeth into contact. By reviewing the guide

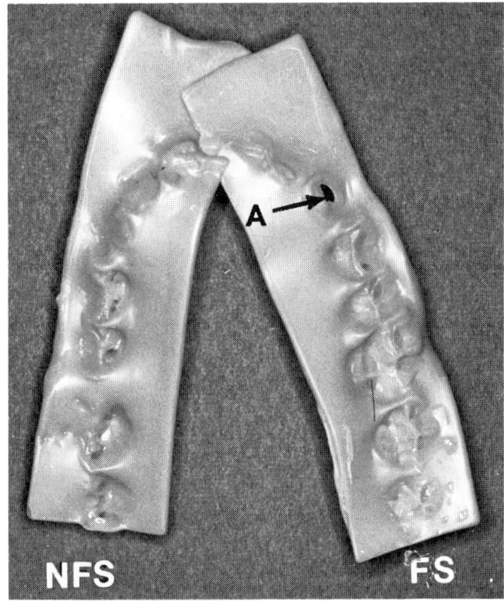

FIG. 14-7. An interfering contact, at A, in the right functioning range of articulation.

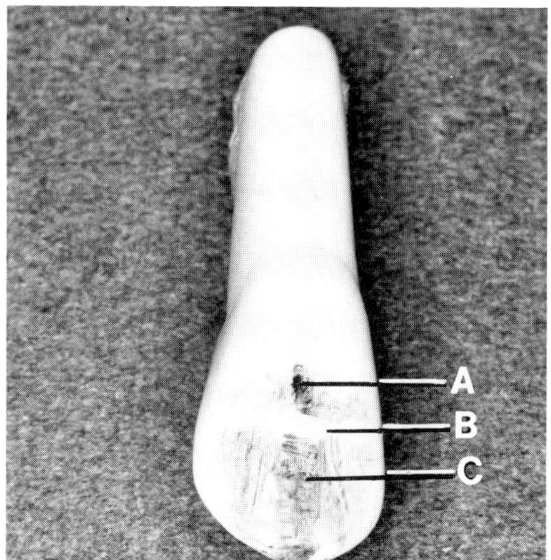

FIG. 14-8. Method of reshaping the lingual planes of buccal cusps of upper teeth.

list that was prepared during the reshaping of the teeth of the stone casts in the lateral ranges, the inexperienced practitioner will avoid errors when he works in the patient's mouth.

In this technique, a hard baseplate wax strip is used to demonstrate the interfering occlusal contacts and check on the markings made by the blue articulating paper and the red adding-machine ribbon. Properly used, wax yields the most accurate registrations. Marking papers and ribbons may color everything in sight and force the operator to place too much reliance on his subjective judgment in deciding which are the true and which are the false markings. However, wax demonstrates accurately the interfering occlusal contacting surfaces by a hole through the strip. Furthermore, these occlusal contacts can be registered repeatedly by different operators. If the teeth are mobile, the operator must interpret the holes in the wax carefully. To prevent false readings, it is advisable to stabilize the teeth by means of finger pressure, compound or ligation, before using the wax.

After the functioning-side wax bite has been taken, instruct the patient to close in centric relation, then to bite on a piece of flamed articulating paper and move his

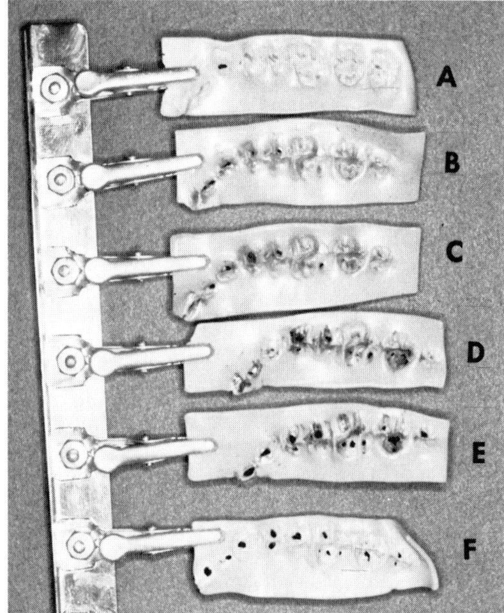

FIG. 14-9. Right functioning-side pink wax strips mounted in order, demonstrating the increase in the number of tooth contacts as the reshaping is performed.

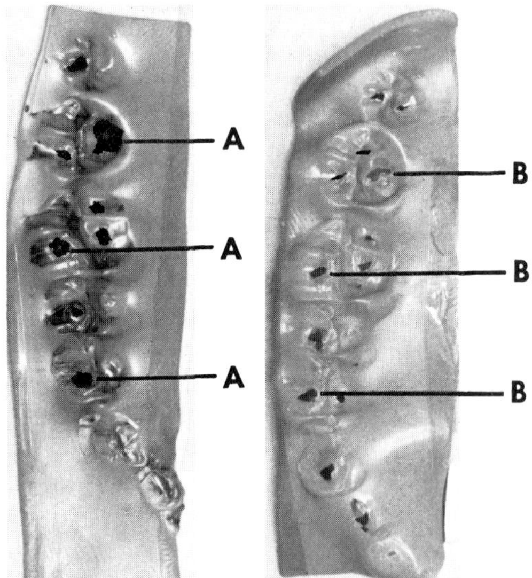

FIG. 14-10. Pink wax bite with large holes denoting broad contacts at A, and after the reduction of the broad contacts, the slight tears in the wax at B.

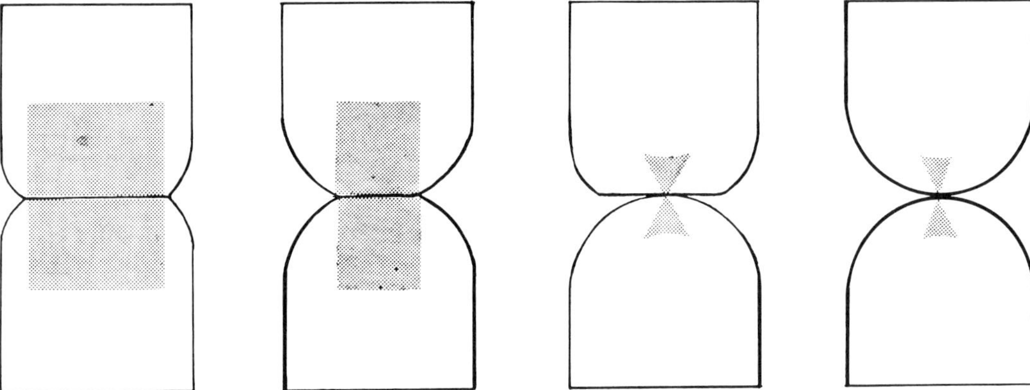

FIG. 14-11. The narrowing of occlusal contacts does not reduce the height of teeth.

mandible to the right. He is to move into the right functioning range while first articulating paper and then red ribbon are held between his teeth. Markings will be found on the lingual surface of the upper cuspid and the labial surface of the lower cuspid. Point A (Fig. 14-8) is the centric-relation occlusion contact on the lingual of the upper cuspid. An imaginary line, B, is drawn. The tooth is reshaped in the area C, from B to the incisal. The centric-relation occlusion point, A, is not touched. Selective reshaping is continued until as many teeth as possible are brought into contact (Fig. 14-2*c*). The procedure of taking pink wax bites, marking the teeth with articulating paper and red ribbon and reshaping the teeth is repeated until as many contacts are achieved in the functioning range of articulation as are feasible.

Point A (Fig. 14-9) illustrates a strip of wax on a holder showing a single hole or lateral interfering tooth contact before reshaping the teeth. Following this is a series of strips which were taken after each tooth reshaping step. The holes in the wax, B to E, illustrate the progressive increase in the number of tooth contacts made; F illustrates the final number of functioning contacts attained. It is very instructive to patient and dentist to mount each successive strip of pink wax on a metal bar with clips (Fig. 14-9). Thus, the patient and the dentist can observe the progressive improvement from one contact to many as shown by the increasing number of holes in the strips of wax.[5]

After the removal of a few interfering contacts on the functioning side, make a check of both the functioning and the nonfunctioning sides (Fig. 14-6). This procedure will reveal quickly whether an interfering contact on the nonfunctioning side is interfering with registrations given by the patient on the functioning side. If this is the case, halt all occlusal reshaping on the functioning side until the interferences on the nonfunctioning side have been removed. Then complete the reshaping of the teeth on the functioning side.

Reduction of Flat Contacts and Facets

After the reshaping of the teeth in the lateral range of articulation has been completed, use a pink wax strip to check areas of the occlusal contacts in the functioning range. The holes in the wax should not be large and circular like the ones illustrated by those marked A in Figure 14-10. Such holes are made when two large, flat surfaces rub against each other. The final tests should show diag-

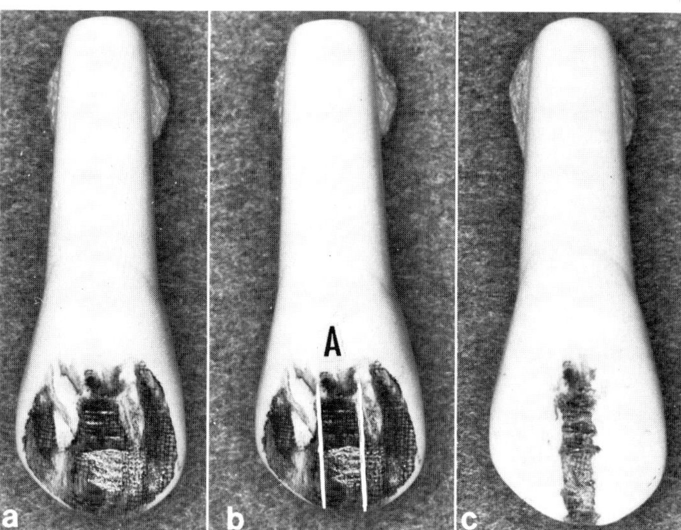

FIG. 14-12. The reduction of broad contacts in the functioning range of articulation brings the forces closer to the long axis of the teeth.

onal tears such as are illustrated by those marked B. These are produced by point-to-plane contacts. Since more force is required to cause broad surfaces to penetrate food than is required by narrow surfaces, the ideal condition is a point-to-plane contact of the cusps; therefore, facets should be eliminated. In Figure 14-11, the schematic representation shows that the narrowing of the contact does not change the height of the tooth.

Bringing the forces closer to the central axes of the teeth is accomplished by reducing the width of the contact. For purposes of demonstration, Figure 14-12*a* shows this type of contact on the lingual of an upper cuspid. The contact has been marked with blue articulating paper and red ribbon. Two lines are drawn on the teeth, such as those on each side of the area A in *b*. Tooth structure should be removed (the white areas, as in *c*), leaving the center path to maintain centric-relation occlusion and to provide a smooth, uninterrupted glide in the functioning range of articulation. The anatomy of the teeth should be preserved as much as possible during reshaping.

At the completion of occlusal equilibration in the right and the left functioning ranges of articulation record on the patient's chart, for future reference and comparison, the number and the location of the contacts that have been achieved in these ranges. Check the teeth for mobility by placing a forefinger on the buccal surface of each upper tooth in turn, as the patient performs the functioning range of articulation. If forces are excessive, movement of the teeth will be felt. The gliding of the teeth during the functioning range should be smooth and regular; there should be no grating noise. As the final step, highly polish all surfaces that have been ground.

OCCLUSAL EQUILIBRATION IN THE NONFUNCTIONING RANGE OF ARTICULATION

As the teeth on one side of the arch move through the functioning range of articulation, the lingual planes of the buccal cusps of the mandibular teeth on the other side of the arch move against the buccal planes of the lingual cusps of the maxillary teeth. *This movement constitutes the nonfunctioning range of articulation, and the position of the teeth at the termination of this movement is the nonfunctioning position.* If the right side is performing in the functioning range of articulation, the left side is the nonfunctioning side; conversely, if the left side is performing in the functioning range, the right side is the nonfunctioning side. In the nonfunctioning position, the buccal cusps of the mandibular posterior teeth contact the lingual cusps of the maxillary posterior teeth while the teeth on the other side of the arch are in the functioning position. The anterior teeth may be out of contact.

Theoretical Principles

A nonfunctioning-side interfering occlusal contact is one that occurs between an upper and a lower tooth on the nonfunctioning side as the teeth on the other side are attempting to pass through the functioning range of articulation. During the analysis of the case on the articulator, there should be a careful check for possible interfering contacts on the nonfunctioning side. The important and serious effects that interfering contacts on the nonfunctioning side can have on the components of the temporomandibular joint have been clearly demonstrated in Figure 8-22. The force in the masticating cycle is exerted on the functioning side of the arch from the lateral range toward centric occlusion. This force brings the jaw to centric occlusion and a bit (the Bennett movement) past centric. The condyle on the functioning side of the arch is set well into the fossa. In this position, only the Bennett movement is present, and the muscles that close the jaw pull upward. This is the power movement.

On the nonfunctioning side of the arch, the condyle must travel quite a distance backward and sideways to get the mandible back into its place in centric occlusion. The condyle on the functioning side acts almost as a pivot about which the condyle on the nonfunctioning side makes its movements. Actually, the condyle on the nonfunctioning side is in free movement during traverse, and any interfering contact of the teeth on the nonfunctioning side will act as a fulcrum, producing a lever of the first class, which forces the condyle on the nonfunctioning side forward. This effect will produce strain and torque on both joints and on the mandible.

Which areas of the teeth should be reshaped depends upon the relationship of these teeth in the other ranges of articulation and in centric-relation occlusion. The general principle to follow for nearly normal occlusions is to reshape either the lingual inclines of the buccal cusps of the lower teeth or the buccal inclines of the lingual cusps of the upper teeth or to reshape each area slightly, depending upon the height and the angulation of the teeth involved. All reshaping is done up to, but not including, the points of centric contact, thus preserving the centric-relation occlusion contacts whenever possible. Facets that occur because of nonfunctioning interfering contacts are evidence of nature's attempts to reshape the teeth into function.

Because of the large number of possible abnormal tooth relations, stringent rules for reshaping the teeth cannot be established. The principles behind reshaping the teeth must be thoroughly understood, and the guide to the removal of tooth structure in each case must be these principles tempered by reason and common sense.

In the natural dentition, it is usual to find cuspal contact only on the functioning side, without any cuspal contact evident on the nonfunctioning side. Ideally, cuspal contacts on the nonfunctioning side that occur simultaneously with cuspal contacts on the functioning side are desirable, but they are not necessary. These simultaneous contacts are desirable only if they can be secured

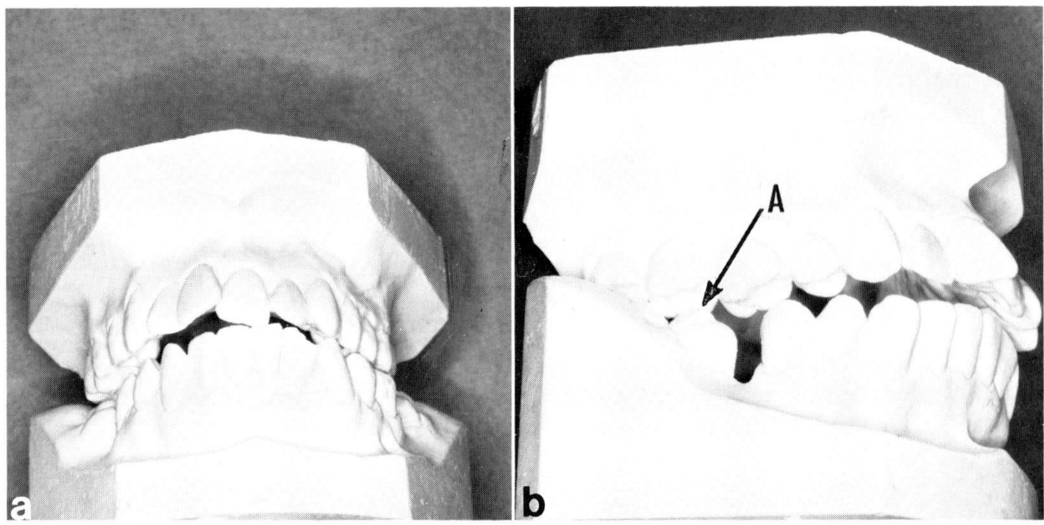

FIG. 14-13. The casts are in the LEFT functioning range of articulation (*a*). A RIGHT nonfunctioning-side interfering contact is present at A (*b*).

without removing too much tooth structure on the functioning side.

It is important to be particularly careful when inserting occlusal amalgam restorations in the lower first molars of children, because if the amalgam is placed in infraocclusion—a procedure that sometimes occurs when overcarving to prevent amalgam fractures—the lingual cusp of the upper molar will descend to the new occlusal level. This occlusal contact will seem passable in centric relation, but it will become an interfering occlusal contact when that side acts as the nonfunctioning side. Because of interference on the nonfunctioning side (side with the amalgam restoration), a whole chain of pathological sequelae may be initiated. These will lead to maldevelopment as well as malfunction of the temporomandibular joint on the nonfunctioning side, caused by interfering contacts and disuse atrophy on the opposite or functioning side of the arch.

This same cause-and-effect relationship should be considered when examination of the nonfunctioning range of articulation of the natural dentition reveals that the only missing tooth on one side is a lower first molar. What usually happens is that the second and the third molars drift anteriorly and incline mesially (Fig.

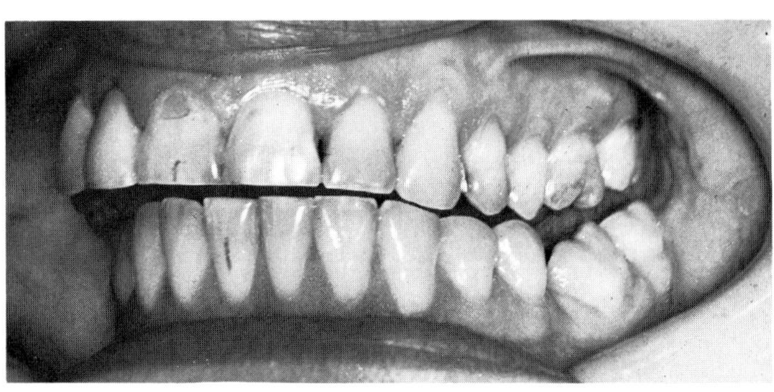

FIG. 14-14. Lack of LEFT functioning-side contact due to a RIGHT nonfunctioning-side interference.

14-13). The upper molars elongate and the contacting inclined planes of the upper and the lower molars develop a steeper relationship. The usual result of this situation is the development of an interfering contact in the nonfunctioning range of articulation. Figure 14-14 illustrates lack of occlusal contact on the left functioning side owing to an interfering occlusal contact on the right nonfunctioning side. This case is similar to the one illustrated in Figure 14-13.

The existence of an interfering occlusal contact on the nonfunctioning side means that the guiding lingual planes of the lower buccal cusps are striking the cusp tips or the buccal planes of the upper lingual cusps. At this point it might be advisable to review the normal cuspal contacts on the nonfunctioning side as they are discussed in the section on the articulation of the teeth on the nonfunctioning side.

In many cases calling for restorative procedures, large restorations or full crowns are placed on the molars and usually are checked in centric occlusion and in the functioning range of articulation but hardly ever for nonfunctioning-side contacts. All restorations should be checked for nonfunctioning-side contacts as a matter of routine procedure.

The objective of occlusal equilibration on the nonfunctioning side is to remove interfering contacts which interfere with or prevent cuspal contacts on the functioning side and, if possible, to do this without injuring the nonfunctioning side when that side becomes the functioning side. Another objective is to create simultaneous cuspal contacts, if possible, on the nonfunctioning and the functioning sides during eccentric ranges of articulation.

Operative Procedure

The inexperienced operator should practice the removal of nonfunctioning-side interfering contacts on the articulated models before he attempts any selective reshaping of the patient's dentition. Using 22-gauge green casting wax strips, blue articulating paper and red adding-machine ribbon, locate the interfering contacts on the articulated models and remove them by careful reshaping. During this procedure carefully prepare a guide list for reference when operating on the patient's dentition. In equilibrating the natural dentition, substitute pink wax for green wax. Place the strips of warmed pink wax on the occlusal surfaces of the entire lower arch, and instruct the patient to move laterally (Fig. 14-6). An interfering contact on the nonfunctioning side similar to the hole A in Figure 14-15 will appear in the wax. In this case, the wax shows that the lingual planes of the buccal cusps of the lower first molar and the buccal planes of the lingual cusp of the upper first molar on the nonfunctioning side are the surfaces that are in interfering contact. Record on the patient's chart, for future reference, the interfering contacts in the nonfunctioning range before occlusal equilibration has been started.

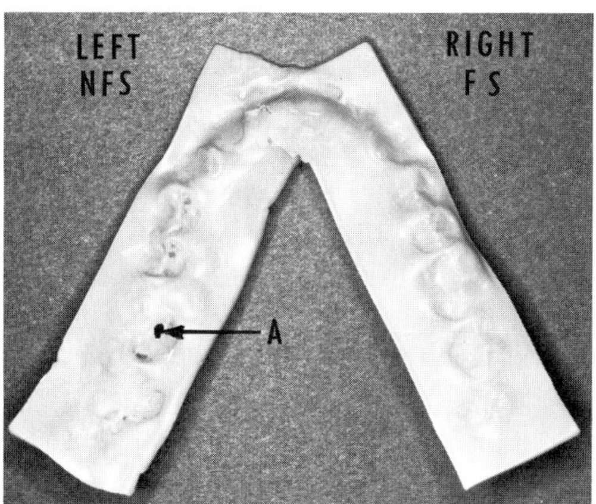

FIG. 14-15. Left nonfunctioning-side (NFS) contact at A, and lack of right functioning-side (FS) contact.

If there are any interfering contacts on the nonfunctioning side, decide which

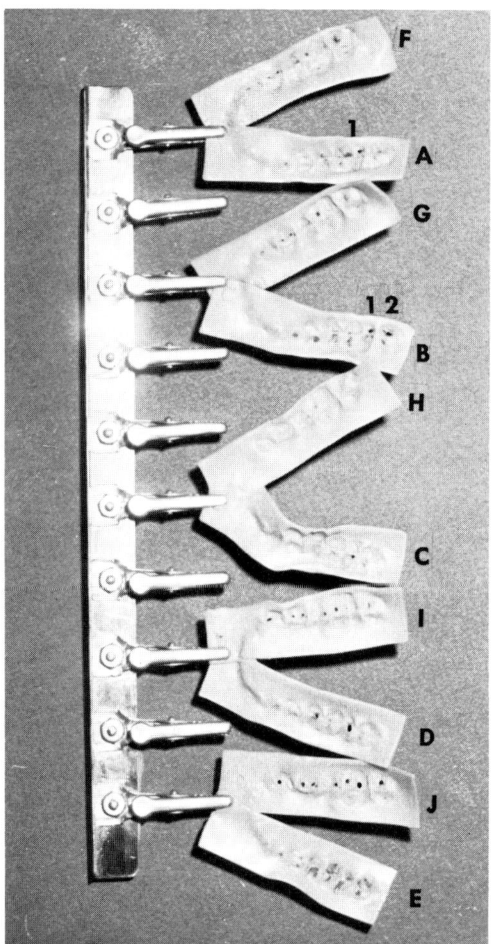

FIG. 14-16. A series of full-mouth wax bites in which nonfunctioning-side reshaping increased the number of functioning-side contacts. A–E are nonfunctioning-side contacts, and F–J are functioning-side contacts.

spot to reshape without taking the tooth out of centric-relation occlusion. *Reshaping the teeth on the nonfunctioning side will bring the teeth together on the functioning side so that they can be equilibrated.* This is illustrated in Figure 14-16, which shows a series of wax bites taken as the teeth were reshaped on the nonfunctioning side. Wax strip A illustrates one nonfunctioning-side interfering occlusal contact (hole in the wax marked 1) before occlusal equilibration. Wax strip B demonstrates two holes after the first interfering contacts have been reshaped. The hole marked 1 in B is identical with the hole marked 1 in A, but the other hole at 2 is the result of a new contact. The reshaping of the teeth was continued, based on the wax strips C and D, until a wax strip evidencing no hole resulted, as at E. Note the increase of functioning-side contacts in the wax strips F, G, H, I and J as the reshaping of the nonfunctioning side progressed. Figure 14-17*a* illustrates a case in centric-relation occlusion. In (*b*), the functioning side is not in contact because of an interfering occlusal contact on the nonfunctioning side. In such a situation, the question of which tooth to reshape arises. The purpose of reshaping the teeth is to make the nonfunctioning-side glide plane, CD, parallel with the functioning-side glide plane, EF, and also to reduce the height of the interfering glide plane, CD, so that contact is achieved on the functioning side. This has been achieved

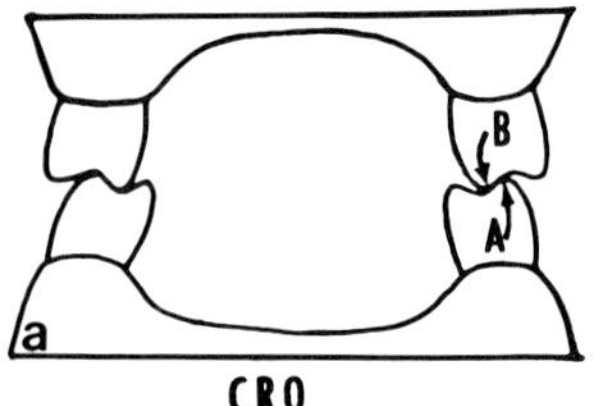

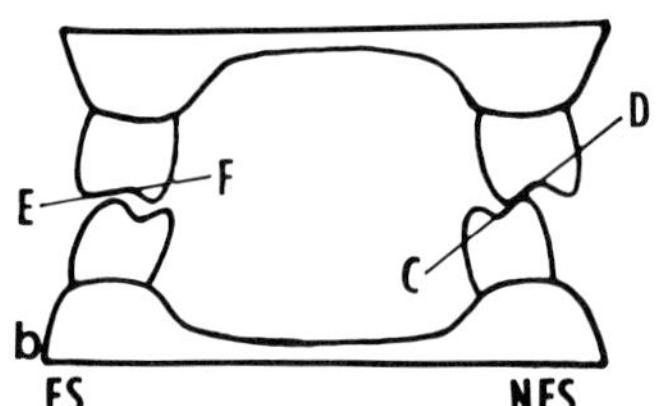

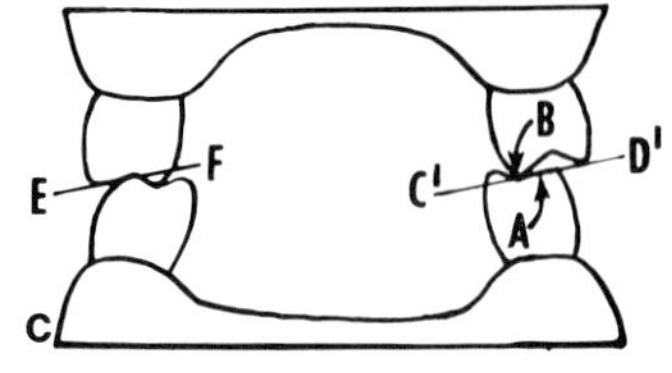

FIG. 14-17. Reduction of a nonfunctioning-side (NFS) interference to gain functioning-side (FS) contact. In this case, cusps A and B maintain centric-relation occlusion (CRO) on the nonfunctioning side.

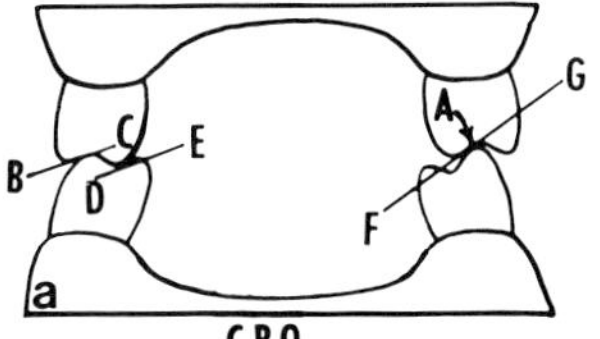

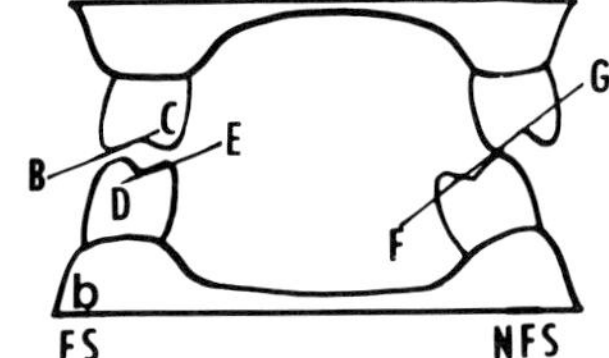

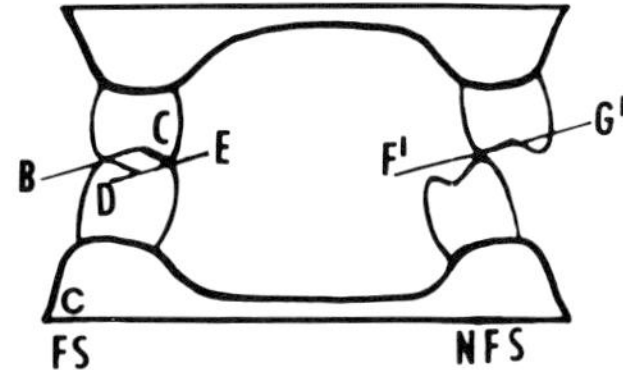

FIG. 14-18. Reduction of a nonfunctioning-side (NFS) interference to gain functioning-side (FS) contact. In this case only cusp A maintains centric-relation occlusion (CRO) on the nonfunctioning side.

in (*c*) by reshaping to the plane C′D′. The fossa at A and the remaining cusp, B, maintain centric-relation occlusion. If the removal of the tooth structure is insufficient to provide contact on the functioning side, one of the static centric-relation contacts must be sacrificed.

In centric-relation occlusion, the upper molars have a large mesiolingual cusp and a small distolingual cusp, and these cusps contact the fossae of the lower molars. There are two buccal cusps to maintain centric-relation occlusion in both the upper and the lower molars. Therefore, in deciding which tooth of an interfering occlusal contact to reshape on the nonfunctioning side when that contact is the mesiolingual cusp of the upper molar and a buccal plane of the lower molar, tend to favor the upper lingual cusp and reshape the lingual plane of the lower buccal cusp if possible. This is done because there are two lower buccal cusps present to maintain centric-relation occlusion. As a rule, do not touch the tips of the contacting cusps, but confine the removal of tooth structure to the ridges or planes of the cusps. If it is necessary to remove the tip of a cusp, reshape only the one cusp that is least needed in the functioning positions. In this regard, the maxillary lingual cusps are most important in maintaining centric-relation occlusion.

Figure 14-18*a* illustrates a case in which there is a single cusp-to-fossa relationship in centric-relation occlusion on one side at A—the buccal cusp of the mandibular molar and a fossa of the maxillary molar. Note that the lingual cusp of the maxillary molar does not contact the fossa of the mandibular molar and that the dissimilarity of the slope of the lines BC and DE to the slope of the line FG is much steeper. As the patient moves into the left functioning range (*b*), a space becomes evident on the functioning side, and an interfering occlusal contact reveals itself on the nonfunctioning side. If the inclination of the line FG is reduced by reshaping the maxillary lingual cusp, no contact that is necessary for centric-relation occlusion is touched, and there is no loss in vertical dimension. The upper lingual cusp is reshaped, plane FG is altered to angulation F′G′ (*c*) and is reduced in size so that, as the patient moves into the functioning range, contact is evident on both the functioning and the nonfunctioning sides. If an incorrect decision is made to reshape the mandibular buccal cusp X in Figure 14-19, the inter-

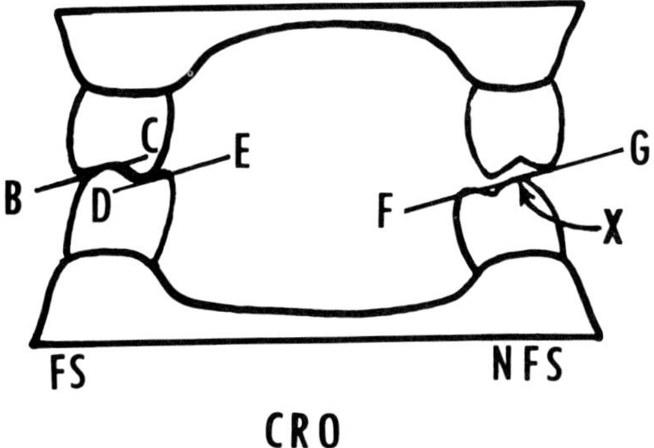

FIG. 14-19. Incorrect reshaping of a nonfunctioning-side contact, as related to Figure 14-18, resulting in the loss of centric-relation occlusion on the nonfunctioning side.

fering occlusal contact on the nonfunctioning side will be relieved, but both molars will be removed from centric contact.

At this time note on the patient's treatment chart that it will be necessary to build up the occlusal surface of the mandibular molar that does not make contact in centric-relation occlusion.

In some cases of occlusal interference on the nonfunctioning side, the mesiolingual cusp of the upper molar contacts the distobuccal groove of the lower molar. In such a situation, establish the centric point at the base of the groove and remove tooth structure from that point buccally to remove the interfering contact without disturbing the relationship of cusp to fossa in centric. This procedure should first be practiced and checked on the articulated casts.

Interfering occlusal contacts on the nonfunctioning side are usually found on the third, the second and the first molars, in that order. In some cases interfering contacts are found on the bicuspids. The adult with a complete dentition, high cusps, deep grooves, long cuspids and a large vertical overbite usually shows bilateral interfering occlusal contacts on both sides of the arch as each in turn becomes the nonfunctioning side. In such cases, as the practitioner proceeds to equilibrate the occlusion, he will note that a great deal of reshaping will need to be done on previously restored teeth. This is because few restorations in the lower molar regions are checked for an interfering occlusal contact when that side of the arch becomes the nonfunctioning side.

The objective of equilibration of the occlusion on the nonfunctioning side is to have smooth, uninterrupted and uninterfered-with movement by the occlusal surfaces of the teeth in the nonfunctioning range of articulation. If occlusal contacts are not present in the nonfunctioning range, nothing should be done. However, if there are such contacts, they must be in harmonious articulation with the occlusal contacts on the functioning side. There may be fewer than 100 per cent contacts in the nonfunctioning range of articulation, but none of the existing nonfunctioning side contacts should be an interfering contact.

After the reshaping of the teeth in the nonfunctioning range of articulation has been completed, instruct the patient to close in centric-relation occlusion. Place the palmar surface of your forefinger in the buccal sulcus above each maxillary tooth in turn as the patient's mandible goes into the nonfunctioning range of articulation. If movement of the teeth is detected, further reshaping is necessary.

After the reshaping of the teeth in the nonfunctioning range of articulation has been completed, the teeth must be reshaped buccolingually to bring the stresses close to the central axes of the teeth, but be careful not to remove necessary contact areas. As the final step, all surfaces that have been reshaped should be highly polished.

OCCLUSAL EQUILIBRATION IN THE PROTRUSIVE RANGE OF ARTICULATION

A distinction must be made between protrusive position, *which is the edge-to-edge bite in protrusion,* and the protrusive range of articulation, *which is the entire range of movement,* as the incisal edges of the mandibular anterior teeth move against the lingual surfaces of the maxillary anterior teeth from protrusive position to centric-relation occlusion. This range is used in shearing, tearing and biting through food that is otherwise too large to be accepted into the buccal cavity.

Figure 14-20 illustrates the protrusive action of the mandible, which is motivated primarily by the external pterygoid muscles acting in conjunction with the other muscles of the stomatognathic system. These muscles should contract evenly, steadily and simultaneously to produce a smooth, forward movement. During the protrusive movement of the mandible, both condyles should move downward and forward an equal distance toward the articular eminences. The shape of each glenoid fossa, the inclination of the anterior wall, the shape of the meniscus and the shape of the condyle and the neuromusculature determine the direction and the path of each condyle. The condyle path is also known as the condylar guidance. If the incisal and occlusal guidances are correct, the mandible will move straight forward until the anterior teeth reach protrusive position. For incision, the mandible moves downward, forward and upward. The incisal edges of the lower anterior teeth then contact the incisal edges of the upper anterior teeth and, in a quick, scissorslike action, shear the food. During this scissorslike action, the mandibular incisors glide on the lingual planes of the anterior maxillary teeth. At the same time the mesial planes of the mandibular posterior teeth glide on the distal planes of the posterior maxillary teeth, and the head of the condyle is guided along the anterior wall of the glenoid fossa.

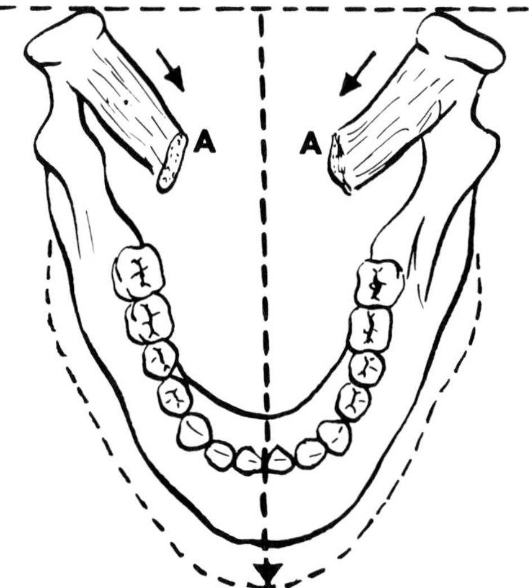

FIG. 14-20. The movement of the mandible into the protrusive range of articulation as caused by the contraction of the external pterygoid muscles, A. (After Massler and Schour: Atlas of the Mouth, Chicago, ADA, 1958)

Ideally, the anterior incisal guidance (*a*), the posterior occlusal guidance (*b*), and the condylar guidance (*c*), should all have harmonious angles of inclination, as demonstrated in Figure 14-21. The joint space at (*c*) is taken up by the meniscus. Although they are so depicted, it is erroneous to consider the inclines in (*a, b* and *c*) as parallel, because the protrusive movement of the mandible is a sliding movement tangential to a large curve.

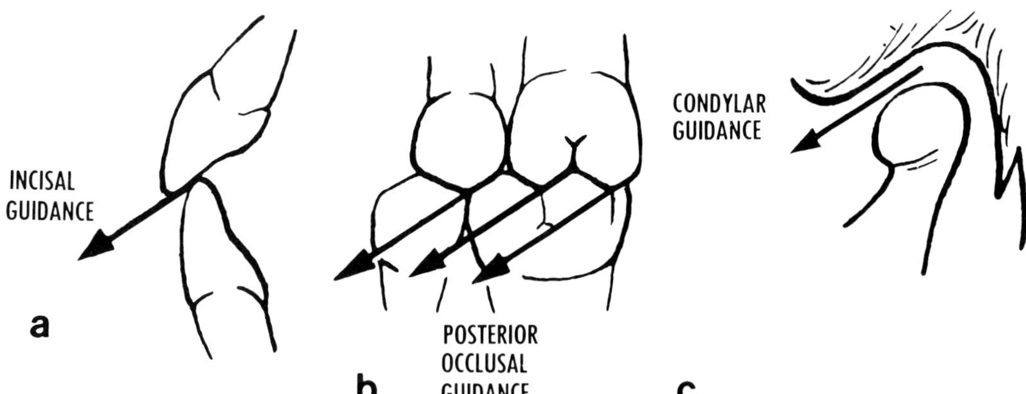

FIG. 14-21. The ideal protrusive range of articulation occurs when the incisal guidance (*a*), posterior occlusal guidance (*b*), and the condylar guidance (*c*), are harmonious, as illustrated by the parallelism of inclines.

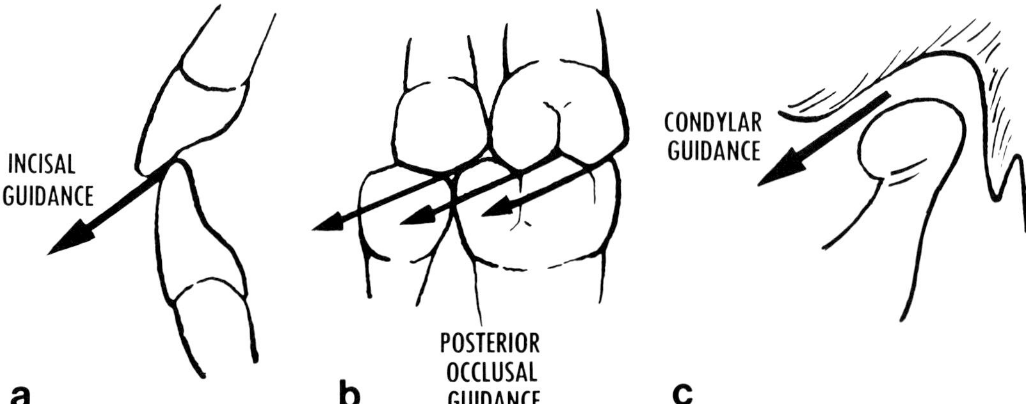

FIG. 14-22. The usual condition that is presented by dental patients. The steepness of the anterior incisal guidance (*a*), precludes contact at (*b*), the posterior occlusal guidance during the protrusive range of articulation.

However, for purposes of explanation, it is easier to consider the incisal guidance, posterior occlusal guidance and the condylar guidance as parallel, although in reality they are in harmony with one another.

In the dentition that is usually encountered in office practice, the protrusive range of articulation exhibits only incisal and condylar guidance due to steepness of the angles at *a* and *c* and the shallowness of the angles at *b* as in Figure 14-22. The steepest inclines followed by the incisors will guide the mandible, and the posterior teeth will not be used in the protrusive range. Occlusal equilibration of the natural dentition in the protrusive range of articulation usually involves the reshaping of the upper anterior teeth so that a harmonious relation is created between the planes of the lingual surfaces of the upper anterior teeth and the articulating surfaces of the lower anterior teeth. This harmonious relationship will provide more contacting teeth during the protrusive range as they are guided by the new incisal guidance.

In a few cases, posterior protrusive con-

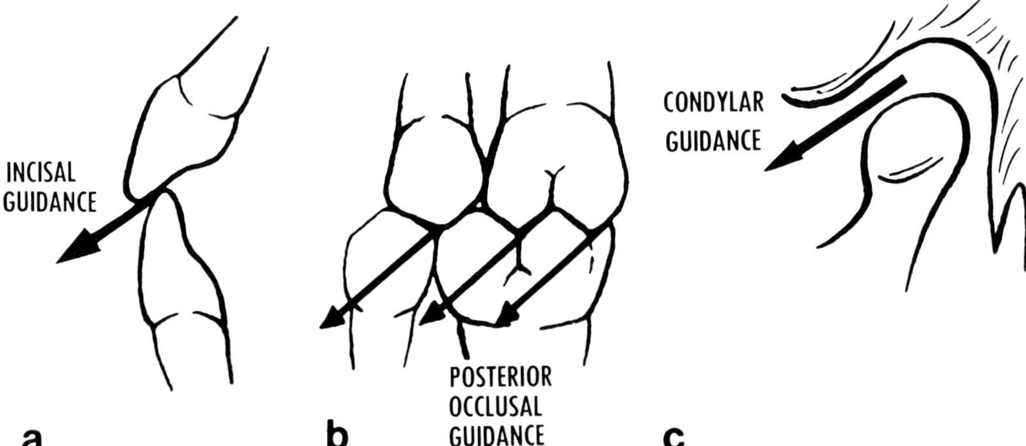

FIG. 14-23. The steepness of the posterior occlusal guidance (*b*), precludes contact at (*a*), the anterior incisal guidance during the protrusive range of articulation.

tacts may have to be reshaped before anterior incisal guidance contact can be effected. The practitioner must be careful to locate and correct any posterior interfering occlusal contacts in the protrusive range of articulation. In Figure 14-23, which represents a case in centric-relation occlusion, note the angulation of guidances *a*, *b* and *c*. *B* is the steepest incline; thus, as the mandible moves forward into the protrusive range, there are bicuspid and molar-interfering occlusal contacts at *b*. As a result, the maxillary and the mandibular incisors do not make contact, and the guidance of the mandible is directed by the posterior teeth. The points of the lingual cusps of the upper bicuspids and molars should not be removed. Sufficient closure may be provided by reshaping the planes of the cusps. Closure may be provided by reshaping the distal planes of the maxillary cusps and the mesial planes of the mandibular cusps of the posteriors. Any reshaping must be done carefully to avoid disturbing centric-relation occlusion.

An exaggerated case of interfering occlusal contact in the protrusive range is illustrated in Figure 14-24. As the patient moves into the protrusive range and attempts to incise food with a protrusive-position bite, the extruded lower molar, K, which is above the occlusal plane, prevents the completion of the cycle of incision. The protrusive interfering occlusal contact, K, acts as a fulcrum. As incision is attempted by the incisors, the condyle is displaced from L, its normal protrusive position, to M, the displaced position. This condition is usually accompanied by symptoms of temporomandibular joint arthrosis. This type of case must be studied carefully before any correction is attempted.

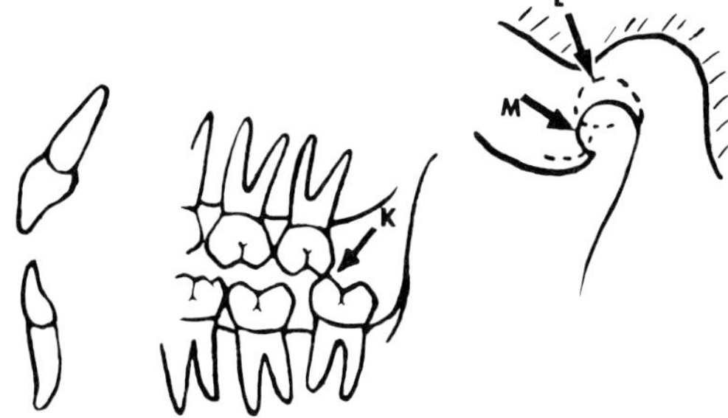

FIG. 14-24. As the patient attempts to bring the incisors into protrusive position, the posterior contact, K, becomes a fulcrum. Dotted line, L, indicates the normal position of the condyle in the protrusive range of articulation. The solid-line condyle, M, indicates the displacement caused by the rocking of the mandible on point K.

In most cases, only one or two pairs of teeth make contact in the protrusive range of articulation. If only one pair of teeth is in contact during the protrusive range, for example an upper and a lower central (Fig. 14-25), 100 per cent of the load of incision is carried by these two teeth. If only one additional pair of upper and lower anteriors is brought into contact, the load will be reduced 50 per cent. If four contacts are achieved, each pair of teeth bears 25 per cent of the load. The 100 per cent load on a single pair of contacting teeth will cause degeneration of both the teeth and the periodontium, because these structures are neither physiologically nor anatomically capable of withstanding such abnormal stress. A 25 per cent load is more tenable. If, through slight additional reshaping, the cuspids and some of the posterior teeth can be brought into contact and thus share the load, this slight additional removal of tooth structure is worthwhile.[5]

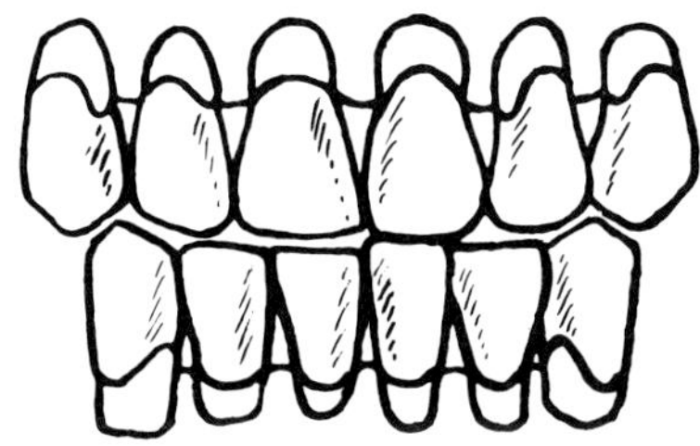

FIG. 14-25. Only one pair of incisor teeth in contact in the protrusive range of articulation.

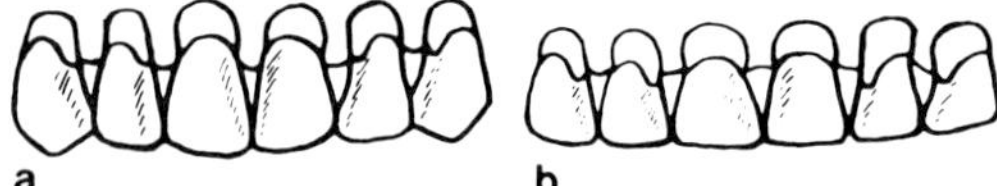

FIG. 14-26. The case as initially presented (*a*), and (*b*) the marring of the anterior teeth due to excess reshaping in order to bring the posterior teeth into contact (*b*).

There is a limit or a law of diminishing returns applicable to the results or values that can be achieved by reshaping the anterior teeth. Figure 14-26*a* illustrates a case as it was presented initially. It is undesirable, for example, to mar the appearance of the anterior teeth to obtain posterior contact, as was done in (*b*). If it is possible to improve the stress factor by removing the load from one pair of teeth and distributing it among four or five pairs of contacting teeth, a great mechanical advantage leading to a physiologic occlusion has been obtained.

By shifting the force closer to the central axis of the tooth, it is possible to reduce stress on the periodontium. This can be clarified by a mathematical demonstration. Figure 14-27*a* illustrates an upper and a lower anterior tooth in protrusive position. The point of centric contact is located at D. This point should not be touched. Line BC indicates the steep incisal guidance of the upper tooth. If a force is applied on this plane, it will be concentrated by the lower incisor during the phase of contact for the distance DE. This force will act along the inclined plane DE in the direction of the perpendicular line G. Torque will be produced about A, the center of torque, through the distance S. The same tooth is seen in (*b*) after reshaping has been completed in the protrusive range of articulation. It is important to note that D, the point of centric contact, has not been touched; reshaping was done from this point forward. Line B′C′ indicates the new, less steep angle of inclination. E′G′, the new direction of force, approaches nearer the long axis of the tooth, thus diminishing the torque distance to S′. The total mathematical result is a diminution of torque.

The theory of reshaping the anterior teeth to bring more teeth into contact

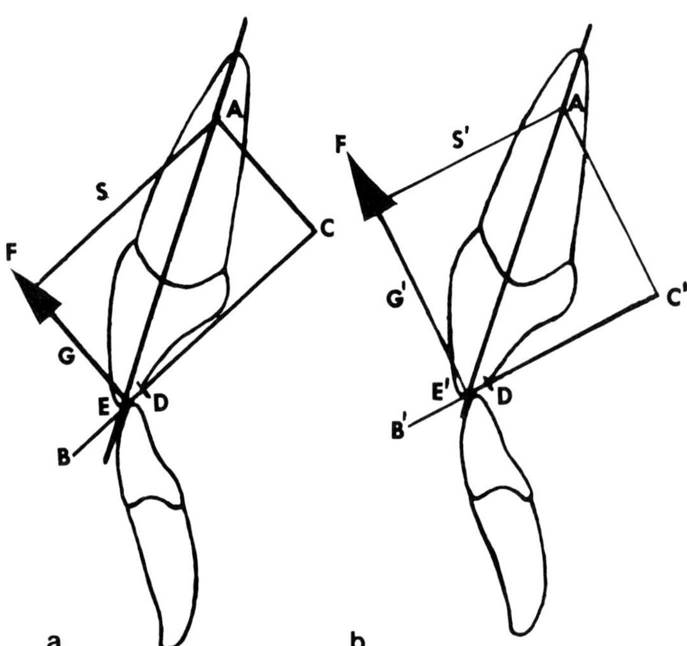

FIG. 14-27. The diminution of torque from (*a*), before reshaping, to (*b*), after reshaping, by changing the incline of BC to B′C′.

during the protrusive range of articulation is presented in Figure 14-28. A is the point of centric-relation occlusion contact. By removing tooth structure from B to C, leaving A untouched, the incisal guidance has been made less steep, and other teeth have been brought into contact in the protrusive range. The upper anterior teeth may be thought of as having buccal and lingual cusps. Utilizing this concept, apply the rule to reshape the lingual plane of the upper buccal cusps in the protrusive range and never touch the incisal of the lower anterior, because it maintains centric-relation occlusion. However, like all rules in occlusal equilibration, this one is not unalterable. There are many conditions in which it is necessary to reshape the lower anterior teeth. For example, when the protrusive path produces a broad labial mark on the incisal of the lower anteriors, it is possible to remove tooth structure from the incisal of the lower anteriors and thus to achieve great mechanical advantage (Fig. 14-3). Improper reshaping will result in the loss of centric contact and in extrusion of the anterior teeth.

The objectives of occlusal equilibration in the protrusive range of articulation are:

1. To achieve as much simultaneous incisal contact as possible between the mandibular anterior teeth and the lingual planes of the maxillary teeth, and between the distal planes of the maxillary posterior teeth and the mandibular posterior teeth as the mandible moves in the protrusive range of articulation from protrusive position to centric-relation occlusion
2. To create a harmonious path of protrusion of the mandible
3. To decrease torque on the teeth, thereby decreasing stress on the periodontium
4. To provide proper incisal guidance without marring the esthetics

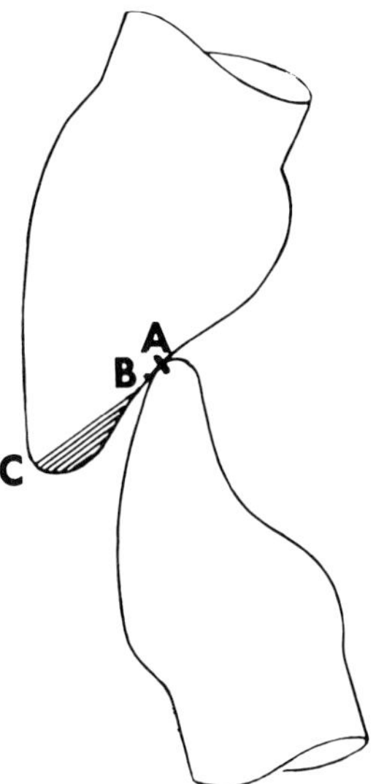

FIG. 14-28. Centric-occlusion contact at A must remain untouched, and by removing tooth structure from B to C the incisal guidance is changed, and more teeth will share in the protrusive range of articulation.

Operative Procedure

The casts should be studied to determine whether there are any interfering cusps in the protrusive range; then whether any bicuspid or molar interferences are present; and to search for anterior interferences. Note on the patient's chart, for future reference, all interfering occlusal contacts in the protrusive range of articulation. It is almost essential for the inexperienced operator to go through a practice run on the articulated casts, reshaping the anterior teeth in the protrusive range of articulation. This will give the practitioner an approximate plan of procedure to be followed in the patient's mouth. Use green wax strips, blue articulating paper and red ribbon to locate and mark the contacting surfaces in the protrusive range. Correct the protrusive range on the articulated casts, and while working on them prepare a guide list for reference as the actual work is performed in the patient's mouth.

Many patients will deny that they use

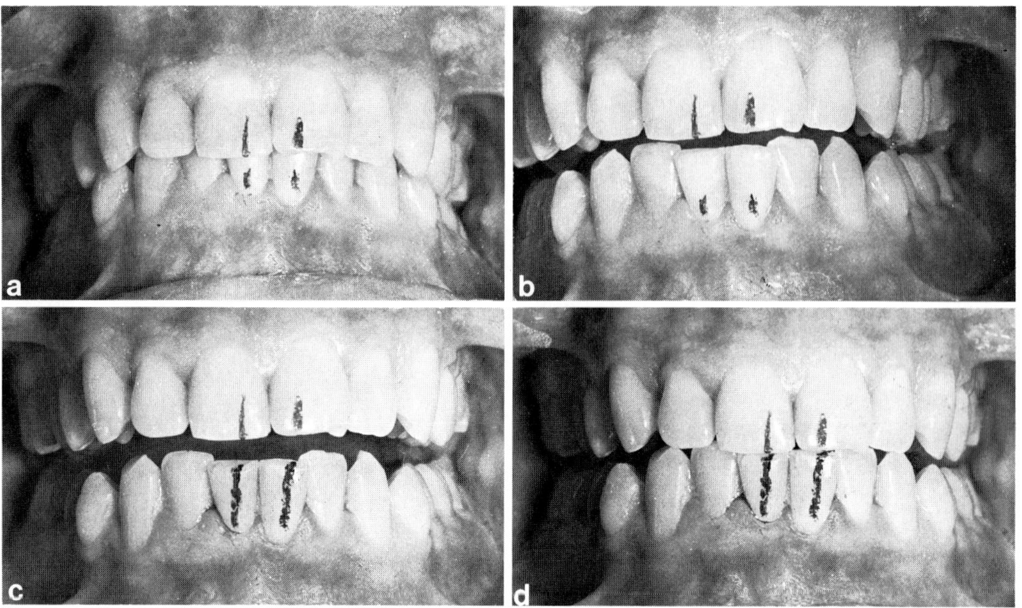

FIG. 14-29. The technique of marking the teeth to help the patient attain the correct protrusive range of articulation is illustrated in steps.

the edge-to-edge bite of protrusive position. To demonstrate this position in the patient's mouth, warm a piece of wax and hold it about an inch away from the patient's lips. Instruct the patient to bite the wax quickly and to keep his jaw in that bite position. He will invariably move his jaw into a protrusive position as he bites the wax. Use a handmirror so that the patient can observe this position as well as the rest of the demonstration. Explain that the first step in the cycle is incision, or the edge-to-edge bite. After this, the incisal edges of the mandibular incisors travel backward and upward on the lingual planes of the maxillary incisors. For the sake both of convenience in operative procedure and of ease in explaining this unconscious movement, reverse the direction of the path of incision as protrusive pink wax registrations are taken.

The technique of marking the teeth to help the patient attain the correct protrusive range of articulation is an important one to master. As the patient is in centric-relation occlusion, draw a line with an eyebrow pencil on the labial surfaces, parallel with the central axis of each upper central (Fig. 14-29*a*). Continue the lines downward onto the labial surfaces of the lower centrals. Train the patient to open in a centric-relation arc, opening and closing the jaws about 10 mm. As he opens about 5 mm. and separates his lips, continue the markings on the labial surfaces of the lower centrals to the incisal edges as in (*b*) and (*c*). Give him a hand mirror and instruct him to keep the marks on the labial surfaces of the lower anteriors under the marks on the labial surfaces of the upper anteriors and then to bring his mandible forward, still maintaining the positions of the marked lines. He should stop the motion of his mandible when the lines are under each other and the teeth are in edge-to-edge relation as in (*d*). This is protrusive position. This procedure must be undertaken slowly and patiently, because it may be quite difficult for the patient to protrude his mandible evenly.

Figure 14-30 illustrates the habitual convenience-protrusive relationship of the patient. Note the relationship of the

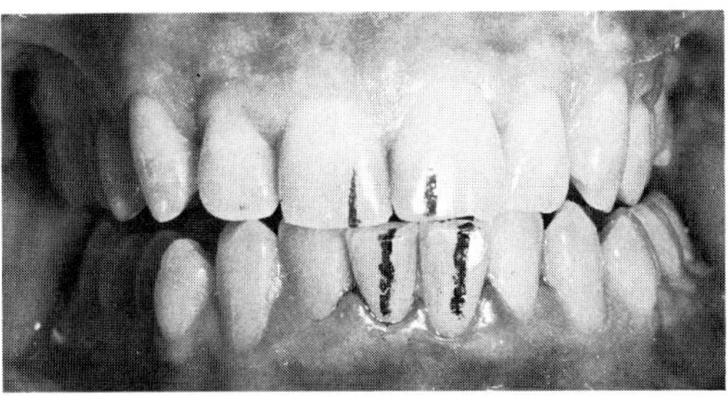

FIG. 14-30. Habitual convenience relationship markings, now in protrusive position, illustrating the deviation of the markings on the mandibular incisors that were in line with the markings on the maxillary incisors in centric-relation occlusion.

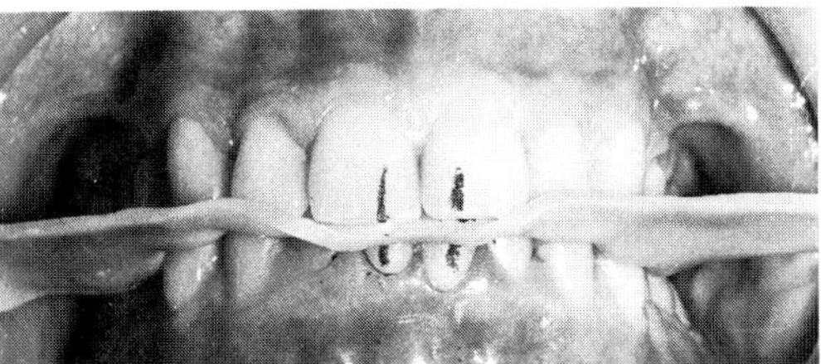

FIG. 14-31. The patient is biting into pink wax in centric-relation occlusion before moving into the protrusive range.

lines on the maxillary and the mandibular incisors which demonstrate the degree of mandibular shift caused by protrusive interferences. Usually, the lingual surfaces of the anterior teeth are worn and irregular; consequently the mandible is guided laterally along a wavering path as it moves forward.

It may be necessary to guide the patient's jaw as he tries to protrude his mandible properly. Once the patient has accomplished this procedure, he should practice it as he observes himself in a hand mirror.

The next step is to locate the exact contacting surfaces as the mandibular teeth move from centric-relation occlusion to protrusive position. With a strip of warmed pink wax placed under the incisal surfaces of his upper anterior teeth, the patient should close in centric-relation occlusion (Fig. 14-31) and then move through the protrusive range of articulation to protrusive position while maintaining the proper relationship of the penciled guide lines on the labial tooth surfaces as in Figure 14-29*d*. Then he separates his jaws. This procedure must take place, of course, while the patient is observing himself in a hand mirror. Usually the wax shows a single tear, as in A of Figure 14-32. To mark the contacting surfaces that made the tear in the pink wax, repeat the same marking procedures, first with blue paper and then with red ribbon. Then reshape the patient's dentition, using the theoretical principles that have been outlined previously and the guide list that was prepared during the equilibration of the protrusive range. Continue the marking and the reshaping of the teeth until as many teeth as possible are brought into function during the protrusive range of articulation. Figure 14-32 depicts the progression of contacts from one in A to six in F.

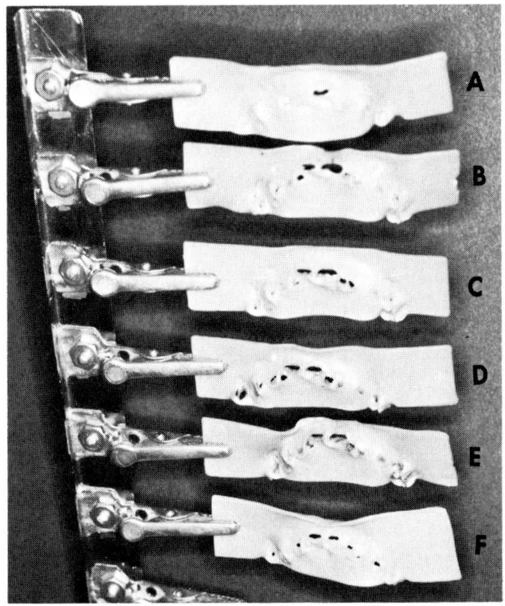

FIG. 14-32. Pink wax strips in the order of their use during the procedure of equilibration to illustrate the increase in the number of contacts in the protrusive range of articulation.

In reshaping these teeth, always hold a finger on the labial while reshaping a maxillary anterior tooth. Thus, less vibration is produced by the action of the diamond stone on the tooth, and the removal of tooth structure is less annoying to the patient.

Theoretically, all the teeth should be in contact during the protrusive range. Practically, however, the achievement of six pairs of contacting teeth during this range is considered a good result. Posterior contact is desirable but not necessary. Originally, the lateral deviation from the normal protrusive range (Fig. 14-30) was considerable because the mandible had been guided by malposed or worn teeth. However, after occlusal equilibration in the protrusive range, the patient can move his mandible into the proper protrusive range without difficulty and without guiding himself in a hand mirror.

Individual tooth movement in the protrusive range of articulation should be checked carefully. After the teeth have been reshaped in the protrusive range, instruct the patient to close in centric-relation occlusion. Place the ball of your forefinger in the buccal sulcus above each maxillary tooth in turn as the patient moves his mandible into the protrusive range of articulation. Tooth movement will be made apparent by a definite thrust. If such tooth movement is present, it will be necessary to reshape the tooth further.[5]

LATERAL PROTRUSIVE FUNCTIONING RANGE OF ARTICULATION

The lateral protrusive functioning range of articulation is within the area of mandibular movements between the lateral range and the straight protrusive range. It is an intermediate area. When a piece of food is incised in the cuspid region, the momentarily static relationship of the teeth is called the lateral protrusive functioning position. The principles for reshaping the teeth in the lateral protrusive functioning range and the protrusive functioning position are the same as those which underlie the reshaping of the teeth in the straight protrusive range of articulation and the straight protrusive position.

LATERAL PROTRUSIVE NONFUNCTIONING RANGE OF ARTICULATION

During the lateral protrusive functioning range of articulation, the opposite central, lateral and cuspid are out of contact, and there is now an in-between contact of the posterior teeth on that side. This falls between the straight nonfunctioning range of articulation and the straight protrusive range of articulation. Interfering occlusal contacts in the protrusive nonfunctioning range of articulation must be removed. The guiding principles for their removal are identical with those that were utilized in the removal of interfering occlusal contacts in the nonfunctioning range of articulation and in the protrusive range of articulation. At the completion of occlusal equilibration in the protrusive range of articulation, record on the patient's chart, for future reference and comparison, the contacts achieved in this range.

When the reshaping of the teeth in the protrusive range of articulation has been completed polish all areas that have been reshaped. Check all teeth for sharp edges, and instruct the patient to check each tooth with his tongue for rough areas. If such areas are not polished, they will irritate the soft tissues and may form points of departure for initial changes in mandibular movements.

OCCLUSAL EQUILIBRATION IN PROTRUSIVE POSITION

The term "protrusive position" is applied to the relationship that exists when both condyles are brought forward equidistant in the glenoid fossa, when the maxillary and the mandibular incisors are in edge-to-edge contact, and when the buccal and the lingual cusps of the maxillary teeth are respectively in contact with the buccal and the lingual cusps of the mandibular teeth. Incision of food takes place between the protrusive position and the beginning of the protrusive range of articulation. It is worthwhile demonstrating the protrusive position to the patient who maintains that he never bites in that position by utilizing the method described in the previous section.

Theoretical Principles

The function of the protrusive position in the total scheme of the masticatory organ may be compared with the function of the starter in an automobile. Stepping on the starter, or activating it, turns over the engine which then maintains itself in motion while the starter itself is disengaged, its function completed. Similarly, the protrusive position operates only during that moment of incision when the incisal edges of the mandibular incisors touch and pass to the lingual planes of the maxillary incisors. This incisal contact is used only seldom compared with the use of other tooth contacts in a functioning occlusion, but, like the action of the starter in an automobile, the action of the protrusive position is highly important in the total functioning of the masticatory organ. Therefore, it is important that the protrusive position be in proper working order so that its function can be carried out efficiently and effectively.

There are two reasons for making the reshaping of the dentition in the protrusive range of articulation and in the protrusive position the last step in the complete procedure of equilibrating the occlusion. First, in esthetically reshaping the maxillary and the mandibular incisors, it is possible inadvertently to take a tooth out of a contacting relationship that may be needed later. Second, the protrusive range of articulation and the protrusive position are the least frequently used of the mandibular movements and tooth contacts.

The following precautions should be observed in reshaping the teeth in protrusive position.

1. Provide as much simultaneous contact of the anterior teeth as possible without removing the functional contacting surfaces in the other ranges of articulation.
2. It is desirable, but not necessary, to attain posterior contact.
3. Reshape the maxillary and the mandibular teeth carefully.

The objectives of occlusal equilibration in protrusive position are the following:

1. To distribute the stresses in this position to as many teeth as possible
2. To bring the forces of articulation as close as possible to the central axes of the individual teeth and so to decrease leverage on them
3. To prevent and to correct abnormal incisal tooth contact habits
4. To aid in curing speech defects that are caused by abnormal incisal tooth contacts
5. To create and maintain better esthetics of the anterior teeth

In connection with the cure or the prevention of speech defects, it has been observed that an elongated tooth may interfere with the production of certain sounds. Another mechanism which can create a speech defect occurs as a patient attempts to hide a distorted tooth by contorting his lips. In the same fashion, elongated teeth frequently lead to the development of insidious habits which are responsible for periodontal diseases about these teeth.

Operative Procedure

Before any reshaping of the teeth is done in the patient's mouth, study the re-

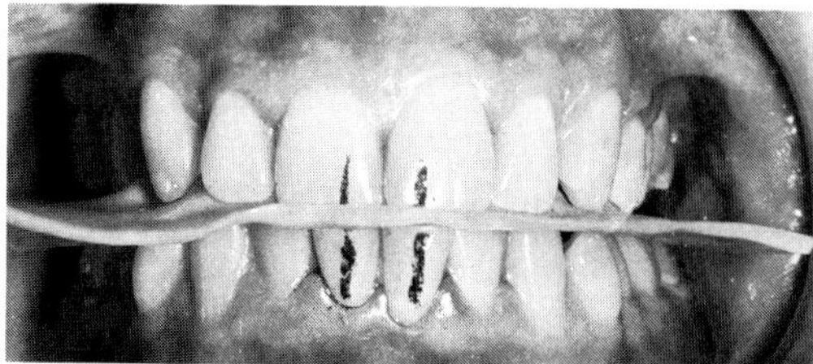

FIG. 14-33. Using the lines marked on the incisors as the guide, the patient bites into the pink wax in protrusive position.

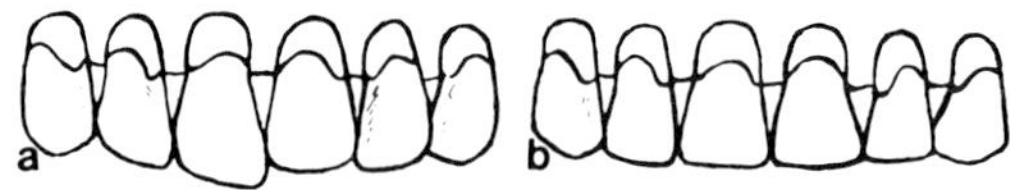

FIG. 14-34. The elongation of incisal edges of upper right central, lateral and cuspid (*a*). The reshaping of these teeth after the determination that the elongated portions are functionally unnecessary (*b*).

lationships of the anterior teeth in protrusive position on the articulated casts. As in the other ranges and positions, a practice or trial run on the casts is highly advisable for the inexperienced operator. It will also make possible an approximate plan of procedure. The results of the removal of tooth structure can be seen before a single tooth in the patient's mouth is touched. Women are especially apprehensive about their anterior teeth. Reshaping the casts will help to assure them that the procedure of equilibration will do nothing to harm their appearance and, as a matter of fact, will usually improve it.

To identify the actual contacting surfaces that must be reshaped, repeat the procedure of placing lines on the labial surfaces of the maxillary and the mandibular teeth, which was described earlier. Instruct the patient to tap lightly in an edge-to-edge bite into a softened strip of pink wax with the lines on the teeth opposing each other (Fig. 14-33). Mark the teeth with articulating paper and red ribbon. The hole in the wax will identify the pair of teeth that must be considered for reshaping. Decide where to remove tooth structure so that the tooth will not be removed from any of the other functional contacts. Usually, reshaping will be confined to the incisal edges of the maxillary incisors, and this will not disturb any of the functional contacts. Repeat the biting, marking, reshaping sequence until this phase of the reshaping has been completed by bringing as many teeth into contact as is practical and possible.

In reshaping the teeth for the protrusive position and for the improvement of esthetics, it is of paramount importance to maintain the contacts of centric-relation occlusion and of the protrusive range of articulation. The centric point of contact, A in Figure 14-28 and the reshaped surface from B to C in the same figure must not be touched. This figure is not meant to depict one tooth but is a schematic plan of all four upper incisors. The cuspids have a different relationship and must be considered separately. The only area that can be shortened is point C. The reshaping of the area, C, on all four incisors does not alter the centric-relation occlusion which is still maintained by point A, nor does it change the protrusive range of articulation which is maintained by the incline, BC, on all four incisors.

In Figure 14-34*a*, note that the incisal edges of the upper right central, lateral and cuspid are elongated. If these portions of the teeth are functionally unnecessary, reshape them to achieve the result that is illustrated in (*b*). In some cases it will be practical to reshape lower anterior teeth instead of upper anterior teeth to achieve better esthetics.

Figure 14-35*a* presents this type of case in which the centric-relation occlusion contact lies below the incisal edge of the lower anterior tooth. The point of contact on the lower incisor at A maintains both the centric-relation occlusion contact and the protrusive range of articulation contact and, therefore, must not be disturbed. The shaded area, B, is not used in any functional movement. Therefore, any part of this area may be removed to achieve uniform and equal contact in protrusive position, as in (*b*). In these cases it is possible both to attain optimal protrusive position and to preserve the length of the maxillary incisors and optimal esthetics. In Figure 14-36 a finished case of protrusive position is illustrated on a patient (*a*), and is shown diagrammatically in (*b*).

When equilibration is completed, retest the anterior teeth by placing the ball of your forefinger against the labial surfaces of each of the patient's upper anterior teeth and instruct him to bite in centric-relation occlusion. If movement is detected in a maxillary tooth, mark the lower occluding incisor with articulating paper and red ribbon, and remove only the colored marking from the incisal edge of the lower incisor. Test the maxillary tooth again with the forefinger, and remove more tooth structure if movement is still evident. Sometimes it may be advisable to give the traumatized maxillary incisor a period of rest while additional reshaping of the mandibular incisor is done.

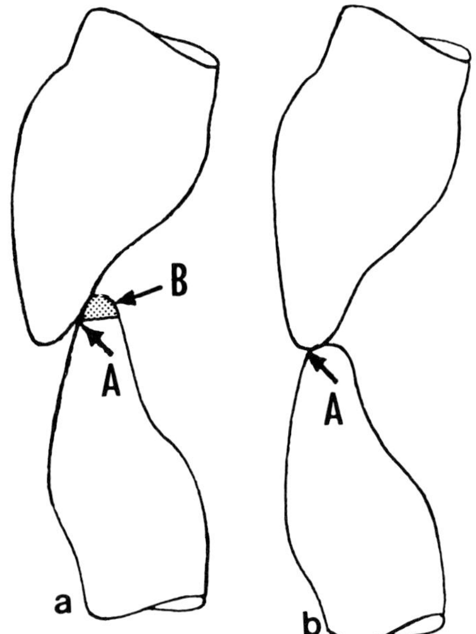

FIG. 14-35. Point A maintains the centric-relation occlusion contact and must not be disturbed (*a*). The shaded area B is functionally unnecessary and may be removed to achieve uniform contact in protrusive position as in (*b*).

CHECKUP AND COMPLETION OF THE CASE IN CENTRIC-RELATION OCCLUSION AND IN ALL THE RANGES OF ARTICULATION

The next step in the overall procedure of occlusal equilibration—both in centric-relation occlusion and in all the ranges of articulation and position—is careful rechecking.

Since each phase of occlusal equilibration was done at a separate weekly visit, by the time of this checkup visit, from 4 to 6 weeks will have elapsed since the equilibration was initiated. If the concept of the teeth as being suspended by periodontal fibers is recalled, it must be realized that now, for the first time, many

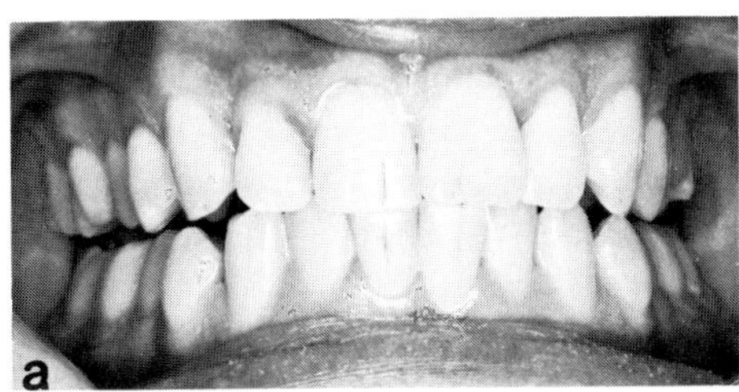

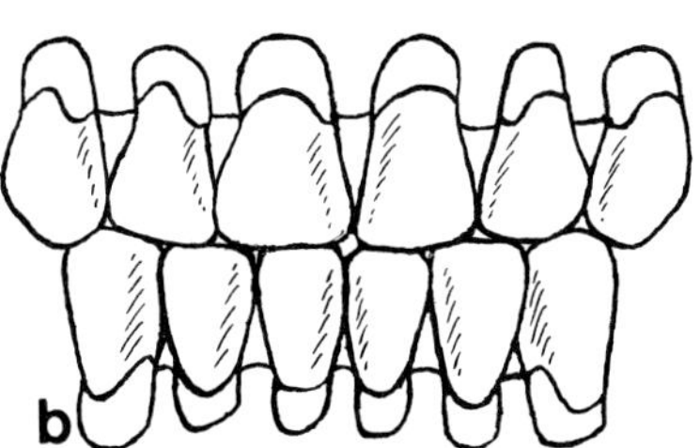

FIG. 14-36. Demonstration of the attainment of optimal protrusive position without sacrificing esthetics, on a patient (*a*) and in a diagram (*b*), using the principle illustrated in Figure 14-35.

teeth that had carried no load at all are bearing a physiological load. On the other hand, some teeth that had been carrying excessive loads are now bearing only a small portion of the load they were bearing when the patient first presented himself. All teeth, or as many teeth as possible, are now sharing the stresses and the strains of function. In an effort to adjust to these new stresses and strains, the teeth may actually move. This should not cause any surprise, because the teeth are suspended by periodontal fibers attached to the bone and bone builds up and breaks down according to the functional demands that are placed upon it and in the direction of the stresses and strains applied to it. Since form is determined by function, the teeth move slightly under their new functional demands.

Since centric-relation occlusion is the basic position, check it first. Again train the patient to close in centric relation. Dip two strips of 30- or 22-gauge green wax in water at 118° F. Mold them over the occlusal surfaces of the maxillary teeth, as described in the section on centric relation. Instruct the patient to tap his mandibular teeth lightly into the wax about four or five times. This time it is probable that an interfering occlusal contact will be found. Test the teeth and correct them again and again until the wax shows the imprints of all the occlusal surfaces clearly but does not show any perforations that indicate an interfering occlusal contact. At this time place the ball of your forefinger into the buccal sulcus of each tooth in turn, both maxillary and mandibular, and try to detect tooth movement as the patient closes in centric occlusion. If tooth movement is detected, hold the tooth in position by pressure of the fingernail in the buccal-cervical area and mark with blue paper and red ribbon. Reshape the offending tooth according to centric-relation principles until no further movement can be detected.

Next, warm two pink wax strips evenly over the Bunsen burner or in the 118° F. water and lay them over the occlusal surfaces of the mandibular teeth to cover the entire arch. The patient should close in centric relation and move into the right functioning range of articulation. Remove the wax strips and examine the nonfunctioning-side registration for interfering occlusal contacts. If any exist, remove them according to the principles of reshaping interfering contacts on the nonfunctioning side. If none is found or if all the teeth make contact, attention should be turned to the pink wax strip registering the functioning side. As many teeth as possible should make contact. Compare the number of contacts with those that were created when the case was first equilibrated in the right functioning range of articulation. There should be the same number of contacts. Repeat the procedure in the left functioning range of articulation, both on the functioning and the nonfunctioning sides. If any of the holes in the wax is quite large, reduce the size of the contacts by the method that was described in the section on equilibration in the lateral ranges of articulation.

The next step is to retest the number of contacts in the protrusive range of articulation and in the protrusive position. With a warmed pink wax strip, test the patient in the protrusive range of articulation. Compare the number of contacts now present with the number that were achieved when the protrusive range was first equilibrated. If the numbers do not correspond, undertake further equilibration in the protrusive range of articulation. Perform the same test in protrusive position that was performed when this position was corrected initially. Check the number of contacts against the number achieved initially, and correct any discrepancies.

ESTHETIC CONSIDERATIONS

Finally, check the esthetics of the anterior teeth, and make any minor adjust-

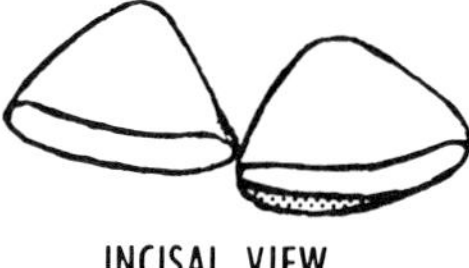

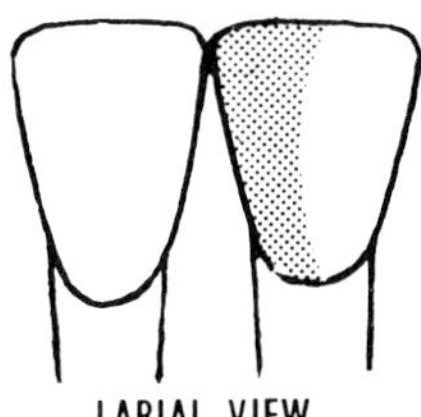

FIG. 14-37. Esthetic improvement of a tooth in labioversion by reshaping the shaded areas.

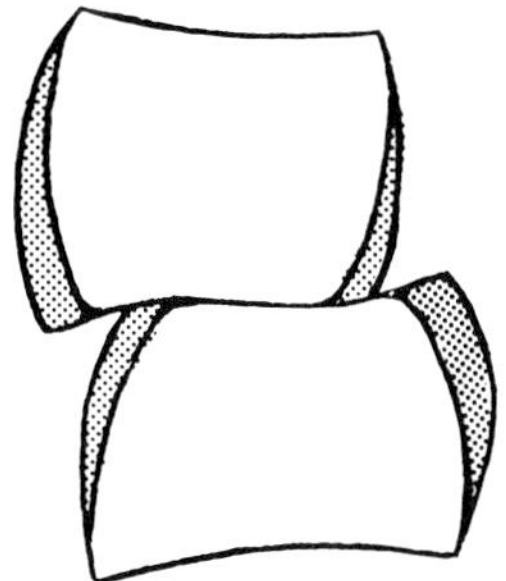

FIG. 14-38. Buccolingual reshaping of the teeth to reduce forces of mastication necessary to triturate food.

ments or changes necessary. Esthetics or proper tooth form in relation to all the other teeth and to the entire arch form is a highly important consideration in dentistry. As a matter of fact, appearance is probably one of the greatest of all motivating factors in the public's desire for dentistry. The ingenuity and the ability of the operator will aid him greatly in the reshaping of the anterior teeth. The drastic changes in the general appearance of the dentition made by a few minute alterations are amazing. Patients are almost extravagant in their appreciation and praise for these improvements in appearance, for here are results of dentistry that can be seen clearly and readily.

The appearance of the maxillary and the mandibular teeth, especially in the anterior region, can usually be greatly improved through esthetic reshaping, but this must not be achieved at the cost of proper tooth function. Square, boxlike teeth give the appearance of age. Corners of the maxillary teeth should be carefully rounded mesially, distally and labially. Such reshaping of a tooth gives it personality. Irregular incisal surfaces and chipped or worn edges are rounded and smoothed into curves, using sandpaper discs coated with cocoa butter. For the esthetic reshaping of teeth, diamond stones or fast-cutting discs should not be used because they may cut too much or too quickly. Fine sandpaper discs coated with cocoa butter will cut slowly and smoothly and will not overheat the teeth.

Much can be done to improve appearance of a malpositioned tooth by removing a bit of the enamel and thus establishing a new tooth form. By planing the distolabial or mesiolabial surface as shown by the shaded area (Fig. 14-37), not only can esthetics be improved, but also food impaction can be prevented. Of course, the enamel should be highly polished after it has been reshaped.

ACCESSORY CORRECTIONS

It may be necessary to make certain accessory corrections in occlusal equilibration; although not applicable in all cases, they are extremely important when they do apply. The following are some of these accessory changes but they should not be performed at the expense of good tooth relationships. Before performing the necessary accessory corrections on the patient, make a "trial run" on the casts as follows.

1. To reduce vertical leverage of the teeth, narrow the buccolingual table and slightly round the sharp cusp edges. Extreme or excessive occlusal wear produces flat surfaces which should be reshaped. Figure 14-38 illustrates a pair of teeth that have been worn flat. The stip-

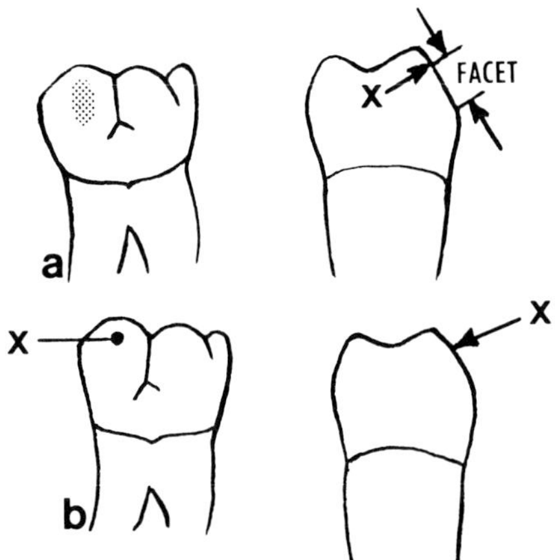

FIG. 14-39. Reduction of facets. The facet in buccal and cross-sectional views before reduction, with X the point of centric and lateral contact (*a*). The reshaped tooth in which point X has been maintained (*b*).

pled areas denote the parts to be reshaped to reduce the occlusal table without disturbing centric-relation occlusion.

2. If facets and grooves are found on the surfaces of the teeth study them carefully because they are an indication of how the patient has been trying to reshape his teeth into occlusion. A facet is an area of excessive wear. Such cuspal topography calls for the creation of a point contact. Because of their larger areas, facets increase the pressure that is required to triturate food, and thus masticatory efficiency is impaired. Remove facets on all surfaces by careful reshaping of the teeth. Mark them with blue paper and red ribbon, and note the centric and functioning points of contact. Figure 14-39*a* illustrates a broad-facet contact. Leaving point X to maintain centric and functioning contact, the remaining portion of the facet is rounded off; note the result of such reshaping in (*b*).

3. It is claimed that a plunger cusp produces a wedging action by forcing teeth apart and, therefore, it should be removed. This hypothesis needs reexamination. If the teeth are forced apart by a plunger cusp, this would mean that the plunger cusp is actually part of an interfering occlusal contact. If this is so, reshaping of the occlusal surfaces in centric relation would remove the interfering contact. Therefore, in this procedure of occlusal equilibration, plunger cusps are not treated as such. Finally, plunger cusps cease to exist because the occlusal surfaces of the teeth have been reshaped to function in centric relation and in all the eccentric ranges of articulation.

4. The marginal ridges of all adjacent posterior teeth should be approximately on the same level, and the mesiodistal grooves, or central fossae, should be in a straight line. Keep this in mind when restoring a tooth with a crown or an inlay. This is important because the lower fossae will glide forward in a straight line along the upper lingual cusps as the patient protrudes his mandible. If one ridge is superior to another, the upper lingual cusp will be an interfering occlusal contact as it strikes the higher marginal ridge as the mandible goes into protrusion. In Figure 14-40*a*, arrow XY depicts the

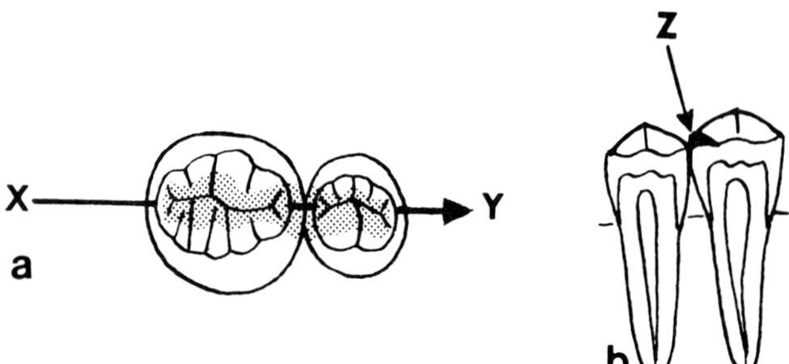

FIG. 14-40. Reshaping of marginal ridges of teeth so that they are aligned correctly with the mesiodistal groove (*a*), and at a harmonious level with the adjacent teeth (*b*).

average direction of the mesiodistal groove. In (*b*), Z points to a marginal ridge that has been aligned by reshaping to harmonize with the ridge level of the adjacent tooth. It may be necessary to correct marginal ridges of approximating teeth that are in labioversion or linguoversion or that are rotated.

5. Reshape sharp, flat planes of the cusps to parabolic curves, if possible. Carefully polish all surfaces.

6. Restore the proper anatomy harmonious with the anatomy of the other teeth by reshaping the occlusal surfaces to provide spillways, grooves and sluiceways, and to provide for greater efficiency of teeth as cutting and triturating instruments.

7. Reduce surface-to-surface contacts of the lower anterior teeth to point-to-plane contacts in function. Place blue paper on the incisal surfaces of the lower anterior teeth, and have the patient close in centric relation and then go into the protrusive range of articulation. Repeat this procedure using red ribbon. Note that the marking covers the entire incisal edge (Fig. 14-41*a*). By lightly taking off the colors at X and Y, a bit on each side of the long axis of the tooth has been removed. The only remaining contact is now in the center of the tooth, so that any force that is brought to bear on this tooth in centric relation or in the protrusive range of articulation is brought to bear along the long axis of the tooth.

8. Check the lingual incisal edges of the lower anterior teeth for sharp angles, and remove such angles. The lingual edge is not used in normal functional movements, the incisal-labial areas being the contacting surfaces. It is well to remember that the upper functional contact is usually on the lingual and incisal and that labial reshaping is relatively safe.

SPECIAL SUGGESTIONS

Since judgment comes with experience, it is important for the beginner in occlusal equilibration to follow a set, tested procedure, as listed below, which will prevent many errors caused by mistaken judgment.

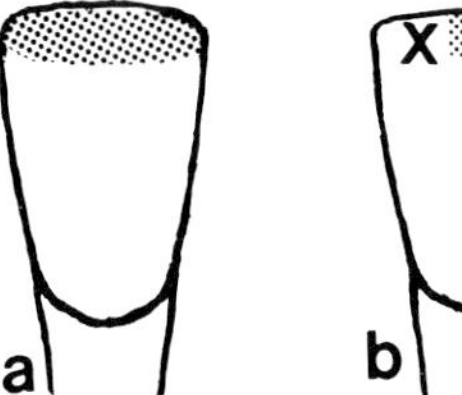

FIG. 14-41. Reduction of large facets on the incisal areas of the lower anterior teeth. The complete marking of the area. Removal of a small amount of tooth structure at X and Y maintains the contact of the tooth in the long axis (*b*).

One of the cardinal rules of occlusal equilibration is that it is better to remove too little tooth structure than too much. Careful study and trial reshaping of the articulated casts will prevent the necessity for rectifying mistakes. Know exactly what you are going to do and why, and be absolutely certain that what you are to do is correct.

1. Care and precision are necessary in all phases of occlusal equilibration; otherwise errors are inevitable.

2. For all removal of tooth structure, use true diamond stones under a water spray to keep the tooth moist and cool.

3. Use light pressure on the diamond instrument.

4. By finger pressure, support the tooth that is being reshaped to prevent excessive vibration.

5. The reshaping of a mobile tooth is a very exacting procedure. Support such a tooth by your finger, a splint of wire, or by plaster or compound. Whichever supporting device is used, do the reshaping carefully.

6. During reshaping, keep in mind constantly the ideal form of the tooth because the anatomy of the tooth must be preserved.

7. Remove the tips of the mesiolingual cusps of the upper molars only as a last

resort because they are the pillars of the dentition. The long axes of the molars pass through these cusps.

8. In cases in which there has been a great amount of occlusal wear on a tooth that should be reshaped, it is wise to examine the roentgenograms immediately before further removal of tooth structure. It is important to know the precise location of the pulp.

9. A characteristic place of interfering occlusal contact in about 15 per cent of cases will be the mesiobuccal plane of the lingual cusp of the upper first bicuspid.

10. Never use abrasive pastes to mill-in the teeth. The use of such pastes produces the effects of excessive tooth wear by removing the points of contact that maintain vertical dimension. Abrasive pastes will grind the tips of the cusps, cause loss of vertical dimension and will do very little to the rest of the occlusal surface.

11. The importance of producing a high polish on all areas of a tooth after reshaping cannot be overemphasized. High polishing decreases the coefficient of friction. The inclined planes of the teeth must be free from irregularities and rough margins of fillings. As the point of a cusp passes over the cusps of the opposing teeth, it should glide in the same way that a rocking chair makes contact with the floor. Any slight elevation on the floor causes a jar throughout the rocking chair. The same jarring effect takes place when a tooth is slightly irregular.

12. After occlusal equilibration, it is important to retrain those patients who habitually chewed on only one side of the mouth. They must be trained to use both sides during masticatory function. If necessary, these patients may be given some warmed baseplate wax and actually taught how to function properly.

13. Esthetics are important, but if too much tooth structure is destroyed for the sake of appearance, degeneration will eventually be the result.

14. To secure a good marking with blue paper and red ribbon, the tooth should be absolutely dry and the articulating paper should be flamed. Marking highly glazed porcelain or highly polished gold is facilitated if the occlusal surfaces are first cleaned with acetone.

15. Set the thermostatically controlled water heater accurately at 118° F. for proper softening of the waxes.

16. Sound in centric-relation closure can be used as a diagnostic guide. If the patient whose teeth have been equilibrated properly taps his teeth together lightly and rapidly, a characteristic solid sound will result. If there are any interfering occlusal contacts, there will be a chattering kind of sound. Experience will enable you to identify a finished case by the solid sound that results from rapid centric-relation closure.

17. When all marking and reshaping phases have been completed, remove all markings with a pledget of cotton saturated with acetone.

18. Sometimes it may be desirable to mark a centric-relation interfering occlusal contact by a method other than that of using blue paper and red ribbon. This can be done by placing a piece of pencil lead in a porte-polisher, placing the Aluwax centric-relation interfering contact bite against the teeth and marking the tooth through the hole in the wax.

19. Some practitioners feel that they can dispense with the step of preparing articulated casts. This is a serious mistake. The time spent in mounting the casts on the articulator, studying them and reshaping them experimentally is time well spent, because it enables you to discover many important things about a case before you work on the natural dentition, and because it helps you to avoid errors in technique or judgment.

20. Because of age and inadequate tissue support, sometimes it is necessary to reduce the inclines of the planes of the

upper buccal and the lower lingual cusps of all the teeth in the functioning range of articulation. However, before this is done, make certain that you have maintained an equal distribution of stresses by equilibrating all the teeth in all the functioning ranges of articulation. Observe the case over a period of time to be sure that the equalization of stresses is maintained, and only then reduce the inclines of the contacts in the functioning ranges if the periodontal condition does not improve.

EDUCATION FOR RECALL VISITS

Prepare the patient psychologically for what will happen during his recall visit. Because of wear, mesial drift of the teeth and general degeneration, there will be slight changes in the occlusal relationships of the teeth as time goes on. Make the patient aware of this fact and of the fact that slight amounts of reshaping may be necessary from time to time. If he is not thus prepared, the patient may resent the fact that additional reshaping must be done at various intervals after the entire occlusal equilibration has been completed. He will feel that the original work was not completed. At each recall visit, check the patient's ability to function on each side of his mouth by asking him to chew on a piece of warmed baseplate wax. Observe all mandibular movements carefully. If the patient cannot function properly on one side, or if he has not broken his habit of unilateral function, give him additional instruction and impress him with the importance of bilateral functional stimulation.

The actual occlusal equilibration of the natural dentition by the selective reshaping of the teeth should be done in a systematic and orderly manner. It is best to perform the operative steps involved in at least five to seven visits. Before starting each new step, carefully check the stage completed during the previous visit.

Visit 1. Equilibration of the occlusion in centric-relation occlusion

Visit 2. Equilibration of the right functioning range of articulation and of the left nonfunctioning range, if necessary

Visit 3. Equilibration of the left functioning range of articulation and of the right nonfunctioning range, if necessary

Visit 4. Equilibration of the protrusive range of articulation and of the protrusive position

Visit 5. Correction of abnormal occlusal anatomy; checking of centric-relation occlusion and all ranges and positions

THE EFFECTS OF OCCLUSAL EQUILIBRATION

The procedure of occlusal equilibration does artificially what nature intended the dentition to do naturally. The teeth were not designed to retain all their enamel throughout life. By natural wearing of the enamel at a normal rate, the occlusion should compensate for various changes in the condition of the dental organ so that it will continue to function properly. Actually, if it were left completely to natural causes to establish proper compensation, the result would be a functional malocclusion concomitant with the following possibilities:

1. The teeth will wear, move or fracture.
2. The periodontium will resist or degenerate.
3. The temporomandibular joint will resist or be traumatized.
4. Imbalance of the neuromuscular system will occur.
5. Any combination of the four possibilities mentioned above will occur.

These possibilities represent the self-adjusting or compensating mechanisms of the stomatognathic system. If the compensating adjustments of the teeth, the supporting structures, the temporomandibular joint and other parts of the stomatognathic system are slight, the occlusion may be said to be physiologic.

A tooth that is in physiological equilibrium permits the osseous, ligamentous and tissue elements of the periodontium to attain optimal development and growth. The associated structures will be affected similarly by the normal functioning of the masticatory organ and the stomatognathic system. Physiological tissue change is induced only by functional stimulation. Equilibration of the occlusion produces physiological tissue changes by adding new physiological forces and by reducing the effects of old pathological forces. Actually, the dentist is providing functional therapy when he equilibrates the occlusion.

Tooth Response to Occlusal Equilibration

Definite visual effects of occlusal equilibration, including those listed, may be observed in the dentition:

1. The teeth operate more efficiently, both individually and collectively, because they are in proper form and function.
2. Tooth mobility is decreased.
3. Food impaction is decreased.
4. The likelihood of tooth and restoration fracture is reduced.
5. Bruxism is relieved and its recurrence prevented.
6. Mucous plaques and debris tend to disappear because of proper physiological function.
7. The teeth are no longer sensitive to thermal changes.
8. Further attrition is retarded.
9. Stresses are distributed to as many teeth as possible.
10. Stresses are brought as close as possible to the central axis of each tooth.
11. There is retardation in the development of cervical caries.
12. There is a diminution of pain in the cervical areas of the teeth.
13. Wandering anterior teeth show evidence of a cessation of motion and tend to return to their original positions.
14. Restorations are aided by the distribution of stress.
15. Because of the distribution of the stresses of function, the investing structures of the abutments of fixed bridgework and partial dentures are subject to less stress.

Periodontal Response to Occlusal Equilibration

Soft Tissue Response

After occlusal equilibration and thorough periodontal prophylaxis, the soft tissues will *usually* show the following changes:

1. Reversion of the pathological interproximal papillae to normal color
2. Reversion of the edematous and hypertrophied marginal gingiva to normal color, tone and contour
3. Reduction of edematous and hypertrophied gingival tissues, but not quite to normal size
4. Disappearance of gingival clefts
5. Return of tissue color to the characteristic pale pink of the healthy gingiva
6. Replacement of the reddish sheen of inflamed tissue by the characteristic stippled appearance of healthy tissue
7. Restoration of the gingival tissues to a condition of firmness and turgidity
8. Reduction of general inflammation
9. Reversion of spongy, bleeding gums to normal or nearly normal condition
10. Arrest of buccal and palatal gingival recessions
11. Disappearance of parietal abscess, if due to trauma
12. Elimination of thermal sensitivity of the gingiva
13. Improvement of pregnancy gingivitis
14. Removal of causes that predispose to Vincent's gingivitis

15. Reduction of distended veins in the palatal or mucobuccal fold
16. Relief of tissue pain caused by abnormal function
17. Relief of muscle and tissue fatigue caused by abnormal function

The distribution of stresses to as many teeth as possible causes marked improvement in the periodontal ligaments of individual teeth and gives them physiological stimulation. Even though periodontal tissue fatigue is undemonstrable, tooth mobility is evidence of its existence. Occlusal equilibration aids and maintains the physiological stimulation of the periodontal ligament.

Bone Response

After occlusal equilibration, the osseous tissues usually show evidence of the following changes:

1. Anterior alveolar bone loss is arrested, because the mandible does not go into the habitual convenience relationship.
2. A thin lamina dura around teeth previously in hypofunction is now seen roentgenographically as a thickened lamina dura due to normal function.
3. Interproximal bone height may be maintained.
4. A general recontouring and trabecularization of the alveolar bone takes place and supports the teeth in physiological function.
5. In cases of bone fatigue or low resistive capacity the rate of bone resorption is decreased.

The proof that occlusal equilibration satisfies nature's plan is demonstrated by the dentition of the Eskimos. According to Williams,[7] Eskimos who are on a local, hard diet unadulterated by the white man's food evidence the following conditions:

1. The occlusal load is distributed among all the teeth.
2. Oblique cusps are worn, and horizontal forces are converted to axial loading.
3. The extra-alveolar arm is shortened.
4. Over many years of hard wear, the effective height of the teeth is only slightly reduced.
5. Even though the teeth are worn, they present a good appearance.
6. The gingival margin is at the cementoenamel junction.
7. The teeth are usually in an end-to-end relationship.

In the light of these facts, it is justifiable to assume that occlusal equilibration will repair the effects of the deterioration of the stomatognathic system, and proper function will prevent recurrence of deterioration. Therefore, it follows that the diet of children should serve as a stimulus to functional growth of the entire stomatognathic system, and, according to Moyer's studies,[4] the dentition of the child should be equilibrated. Adequate metabolism is insufficient for masticatory development; there must also be adequate stimulus and function. Williams' studies[6] demonstrated that the jaws of hard-diet people are larger by weight and volume than the jaws of soft-diet people. The thickness of the alveolar plate in the former averages 0.094 mm., while in the latter it averages only 0.088 mm. The result of inadequate functional stimulus is inadequate, thin, buccal bone covering the roots of the teeth. It is also interesting to note that the gingival tissues of the hard-diet people are denser, neater and stronger than those of the soft-diet people.

The research of Korkhaus[2] on self-corrections of occlusal anomalies indicates that stimulation of the dentition by strenuous activity encourages the mandible to find its correct position and also causes a physiological raising of the bite in children until correct vertical dimension is attained.

J. J. Martini's studies[3] of radiogenicity of bone, that is, the measurement of the density of bone by its ability to withstand roentgen-rays, show the effects of function on basal bone. Martini says:

> So long as these people adhere to their native, sturdy diets of tough foods that have not been overcooked, the stresses exerted by a well-developed and well-exercised musculature during masticatory processes produce a type of bone which is heavy and dense.

Detergent, coarse foods or good artificial hygiene increases the protective keratohyaline layer of the gingival mucosa. Civilization is responsible for the locked overbite, lack of attrition and deep, high, locked cusps. Everything modern man eats is refined; he has become the victim of his own diet.

Occlusal equilibration is not a panacea for all ills and disturbances of the stomatognathic system. However, it is a vitally important adjunct to every other procedure in dental practice. It does not stand alone but is the integrating and interrelating factor between the procedures of dentistry and physiological function.

REFERENCES

1. Head, J.: The human skull used as a gnathodynamometer to determine the value of trituration in the mastication of food. D. Cosmos., *49:*1189, 1907.
2. Korkhaus, G.: The forces involved in self-correcting occlusal anomalies. Int. D. J., *5:*3, 1955.
3. Martini, J. J.: Personal communication.
4. Moyers, R. E.: An electromyographic analysis of certain muscles involved in temporomandibular movement. Am. J. Orth., *36:*481, 1950.
5. Shore, N. A.: Occlusal Equilibration. Film Library, ADA, Chicago, 1953.
6. Williams, C. H. M.: Correction of abnormalities of occlusion. JADA, *44:*749, 1952.
7. Williams, C. H. M.: Lecture to the Society of Oral Physiology, 1955.

Additional Basic References

Goldman, H. M., Schluger, S., Fox, L.: Periodontal Therapy. p. 387. St. Louis, C. V. Mosby, 1956.

Goldstein, R. E.: Esthetics in Dentistry. Philadelphia, J. B. Lippincott, 1976.

Müller, M.: Gründlagen und Aufban des Artikulationsproblems (Basis of Problems in Articulation). Leipzig, Klinkhardt, 1925.

Orban, B., Wentz, F. M., Everett, F. G., Grant, D. A.: Periodontics. p. 379. St. Louis, C. V. Mosby, 1958.

Thielemann, K.: Biomechanik der Paradontose. p. 116. Munich, Barth, 1956.

Wild, W.: Funktionelle Prosthetics (Functional Prosthetics). Basel, Schwabe, 1950.

15 *The Equilibration of the Occlusion of Malposed Teeth and Abnormal Arch Segments*

One of the first factors to be considered in the correction of malposed teeth or abnormal arch segments is the possibility of resorting to orthodontic movement. If this has been discarded as the therapy of choice, then occlusal equilibration can serve as a palliative measure. However, occlusal equilibration may help the case and may slow down the degenerative process, but it cannot altogether prevent such degeneration.

In considering the occlusal equilibration of malposed teeth, it is imperative that the articulated casts be studied carefully in centric relation and in all the eccentric ranges and positions of articulation. A résumé of the findings in all these positions should be carefully prepared, for it will serve as the basis for planning the entire procedure or any necessary modifications and adaptations.

The maxillary and mandibular centrals and laterals may be situated in a wide variety of deviations from their normal positions. They may be in mesioversion, distoversion, buccoversion or linguoversion or in rotation, extrusion or intrusion. Therefore, treatment procedure must be outlined in general terms, because it is impossible to provide for the many contingencies that may exist in individual cases. It is of paramount importance to maintain or to establish centric-relation occlusion. The principles of reshaping the teeth in centric relation must be adapted to suit the conditions of the individual case as it presents itself. The same problem of adapting principles to meet specific cases exists in the equilibration of the eccentric ranges of articulation. The order of importance of the articulatory ranges is lateral and protrusive, and protrusive position. The guiding principle is to retain equilibration in the most important range, even if it is necessary to sacrifice it in a less important one.

TEETH IN LINGUOVERSION

Teeth that are in linguoversion may produce a locked bite which may result in one or more of the following types of conditions:

Type 1—a straight vertical mandibular movement on the centric-relation arc

Type 2—unilateral mandibular movement to one side

Type 3—a shift of the mandible into habitual protrusive relationship

In these conditions the initial step is to equilibrate the occlusion in centric relation. The second step is to restore the functioning ranges of articulation. This must be done with great care after study of the mandibular movements both in the mouth and on the articulator. In the Type 1 case of an upper central or lateral that is in linguoversion, the initial step is the establishment of the centric-relation occlusion contact, as in A of Figure 15-1. In

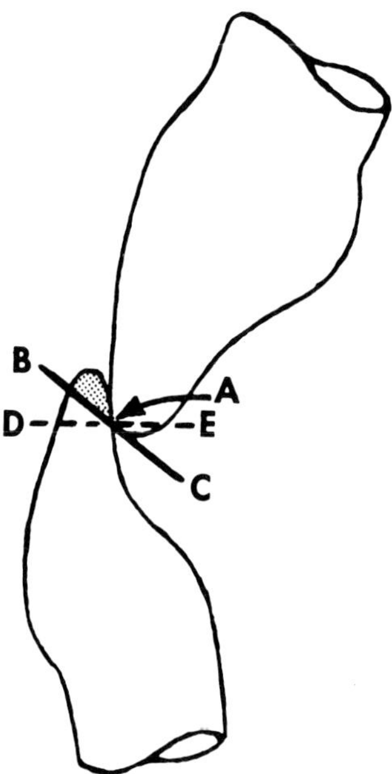

FIG. 15-1. Reshaping of the anterior teeth in cases of linguoversion of the maxillary incisors or in cases of false Class III (Angle) malocclusions.

equilibrating to free the eccentric ranges of articulation, the lower incisor should be reshaped from the point of centric contact, A, forward and upward in the line BC. The centric point should not be touched. This procedure makes it possible for the mandible to function bilaterally. If the lower incisor is cut to the dotted line DE, no advantage to mandibular movement would accrue and the lower tooth would be disfigured.

In a Type 2 case that consists of unilateral mandibular movement to one side, the removal of the centric-relation interference is the first step, and the function in the eccentric ranges must be established.

The Type 3 case is the functional or false Class III (Angle) malocclusion. It has two divisions:

1. Vertical dimension is maintained by posterior teeth, and the mandible is in protrusive convenience relationship in which maxillary incisors are lingual to mandibular incisors.

2. Vertical dimension is shortened, owing to loss of posterior teeth, and the mandible is in protrusive relationship in which maxillary incisors are lingual to mandibular incisors.

In false Class III malocclusions, the condyles are in a protrusive position in the glenoid fossa, and strain and stress are produced within the tissues of the temporomandibular joint. This is a difficult type of case to treat and must be approached slowly. The great problem is to secure a centric-relation Aluwax registration that is correct for the patient rather than a habitual convenience-relation bite, which is actually a habitual protrusive registration.

The treatment for cases in which vertical dimension has not been lost (Division 1) follows this procedure. Study of the articulated casts will make evident the interfering contact, which acts as the trigger mechanism that shifts the entire mandible into a protrusive convenience relationship. Centric-relation occlusion cannot be established until the mandible is free to assume its normal position. This can be accomplished by removal of tooth structure along a horizontal path to allow the interfering teeth to glide past one another. If Figure 15-1 is considered a false Class III relationship, tooth structure is removed along the path DE. This will remove the impediment and will allow the mandible to assume its normal position. When the mandible has assumed its centric-relation position, the usual procedure for equilibrating in centric relation and in all ranges is followed. In Division 2 cases with lost vertical dimension, occlusal equilibration cannot be initiated until the mandible is placed in centric relation. To maintain this position, a splint on the posterior teeth is necessary.

The treatment for cases in which vertical dimension has been lost (Division 2) depends upon the patient's symptoms. If the patient presents a Division 2 relationship, shortened anterior teeth and is free of temporomandibular joint symptoms, it is advisable to proceed in a similar manner as in the treatment of a Class V case. The dentition and the splints are equilibrated in centric-relation occlusion and in all the ranges of articulation. If a partial denture is used as the restoration of choice, the occlusion is similarly equilibrated.

In the case just described, the patient presented a false Class III, Division 2, with shortened anterior teeth and without any temporomandibular joint symptoms. The object of the treatment was to restore only enough vertical dimension to allow the mandible to return to centric relation. The age of the patient is a factor that must be considered in restoring vertical dimension. If the patient presents a false Class III, Division 2, as above, concomitant with the temporomandibular joint syndrome, it is advisable to restore the full vertical dimension. The splints should be shaped until comfort is attained, and only then should the occlusion be equilibrated.

In the true Class III malocclusion, the mandible is not in a habitual protrusive relationship and cannot be retruded. This class of malocclusion can be aided by occlusal equilibration only in proportion to the number of tooth contacts that can be achieved in centric-relation occlusion and in the eccentric ranges of articulation.

If it is found possible to equilibrate the occlusion only in one range of articulation and not in centric, such equilibration should be performed so that the best results under the circumstances may be achieved. Patience and ingenuity will help to achieve the best possible solution to any of the infinite variations of position to be found in malposed teeth. A trial run on the articulated casts and the establishment of an orderly and logical procedure will help to avoid many errors.

Because of its position at the turn of the arch, the cuspid may be found in 45° rotation from normal or in any other deviation from normal. In the 45° rotation, the mesial surface of the tooth may be in linguoversion while the distal surface may be in some semblance of normal relationship. In this type of case, the procedure is to treat each surface individually as though it were a separate tooth. The principles of reshaping the teeth that were outlined in the discussion of malposed centrals and laterals should be applied. Again, use discretion, skill and ingenuity to solve the infinite number of dilemmas that will appear.

In cases of malposed bicuspids, the upper teeth are usually found to have one cusp in linguoversion, while the lower teeth are found to have one cusp in buccoversion. In many cases, this means unilateral function and interference or blockage of mandibular movement to the other side. To study such a case, turn the articulator upside down so that the lower bicuspid may be treated as though it were an upper bicuspid, and the upper bicuspid as though it were a lower bicuspid. Before treating such a case in the mouth, correct it on the articulated casts both in centric relation and in the eccentric ranges of articulation. As the work is being done on the articulated casts, prepare a careful guide list. Using the completed articulated casts and the reshaping guide list, correct the interferences in the dentition.

A malposed molar presents a greater variety of problems than do other malposed teeth since there are more molars, because of their position in the mouth, and because each of them has more cusps than other teeth. If occlusal rehabilitation, extraction and orthodontia have been ruled out as possible procedures, do the best you can under the circumstances. The important principle is to maintain centric, lateral and protrusive relationships, in that order.

After the malposed teeth have been

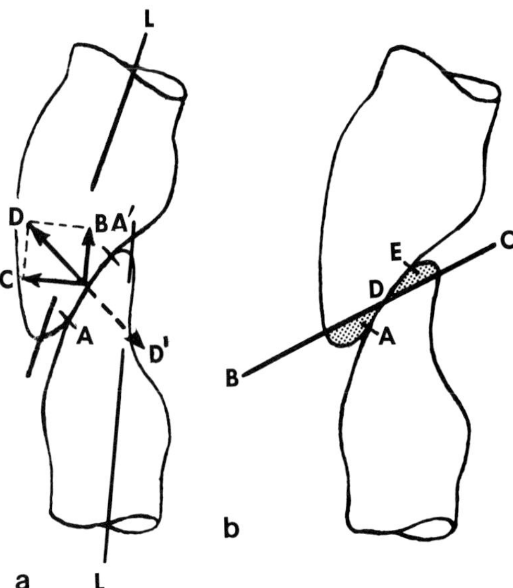

FIG. 15-2. Forces on the teeth that must be considered in deep overbite cases (*a*). Equilibration in the protrusive range of articulation in deep overbite cases (*b*).

equilibrated, perform the maximum esthetic reshaping of the malposed teeth. Finally, complete the case and polish the teeth in the routine manner described earlier.

DEEP VERTICAL OVERBITE

In many cases, the deep vertical overbite may be normal for the individual patient and not at all due to loss of vertical dimension. This may be verified by roentgenograms of the temporomandibular joint. The patient usually displays a vertical closure in centric relation with little or no movement in the eccentric ranges of articulation. The lower anteriors may be inclined lingually. In this type of case, mandibular movement is determined by the incisal guidance of the anterior teeth and by the movement of the condyle on the inclines of the glenoid fossa. This type of occlusion tends to produce buckling of the arch, abnormal functional habits and directional stresses which the teeth were not designed to bear.

If orthodontics and occlusal rehabilitation have been ruled out, the patient can still be helped considerably through application of the principles of occlusal equilibration. Once more, articulator studies and analysis as well as correction of the articulated casts will provide clues to actual operative procedures. In these cases, it is of the utmost importance to establish centric-relation occlusion. If any posterior interfering occlusal contact is present, the mandible will skid forward and the labial surfaces of the lower anteriors will be forced against the lingual surfaces of the upper anteriors with resultant wear or tooth movement. This contact is usually not a point of contact but a very large-surface facet contact, like A′ in Figure 15-2*a*. Such a contact initiates force directed at approximately 70° to the physiological load-bearing axis, L in this figure. The force of mandibular closure movement is represented by vector B. Because of the posterior interfering contact, the mandible moves anteriorly at the same time with force C. The result of forces B and C is force D acting on the upper tooth and force D′ acting on the lower tooth in the area of contact, A′, at approximately 70° to the load-bearing axis of the teeth, causing a large torque on the anterior teeth. Usually the upper anterior teeth are mobile, and the removal of the posterior interfering occlusal contact will allow the upper anterior teeth to go back to their normal position, reestablishing the contact A′. A similar condition of mobility and movement of the lower teeth may occur. Removal of the centric-relation interfering contact that exists in the posterior region will remove some of the force of vector C.

After centric-relation occlusion has been established, the next step is to consider the protrusive range of articulation. This is a change from the customary procedure in which the step that follows the establishment of centric-relation occlusion is the equilibration of the functioning ranges of articulation. The deep overbite causes this change in procedure to be desirable. The patient cannot move into the functioning ranges. In this type of case it will be easier to correct the functioning ranges of articulation after the protrusive range has been equilibrated. Reshaping the teeth in the usual manner for equilibrating the protrusive range of articulation would result in excessive removal of tooth structure from the upper anterior teeth.

In this case, the facet AE (Fig. 15-2*b*) is quite large and cannot be treated by the usual method of reshaping faceted teeth because too much of the lower tooth would be removed (refer to reshaping of facets in Chap. 14). Therefore, point D, a position halfway between, should be chosen to maintain centric-relation occlusion. The shaded areas are not necessary for centric-relation occlusion, which is maintained by D. As the shaded areas are removed along the line BC, a decreased incisal guidance results. Point D itself must not be touched. Actually, only a very small amount of tooth structure is removed, yet the general plan for locating the area to be reshaped and testing it must be followed. After this has been accomplished, follow the usual procedure for equilibrating the occlusion in the protrusive range. Next return to the equilibration of the occlusion in the functioning ranges of articulation. Shortening the lower anterior teeth makes possible a wider lateral excursion. Utilizing the principles of equilibration in the functioning ranges of articulation, as many teeth as possible are brought into function. It may be possible to bring 1, 2, 3, 4, or more pairs of teeth into function. Any improvement in the original condition of the locked vertical chop-bite will greatly improve the functional efficiency.

Figure 15-3 illustrates an extreme case; yet the principles of occlusal equilibration can be applied, and the results will be of inestimable value to the patient from the point of view of function. The finished case may have only a millimeter or two of lateral motion, but this is better than having no lateral motion at all. In completing the case, esthetics should not be neglected. The reshaping of the anterior teeth can be of great benefit to the patient esthetically as well as physiologically.

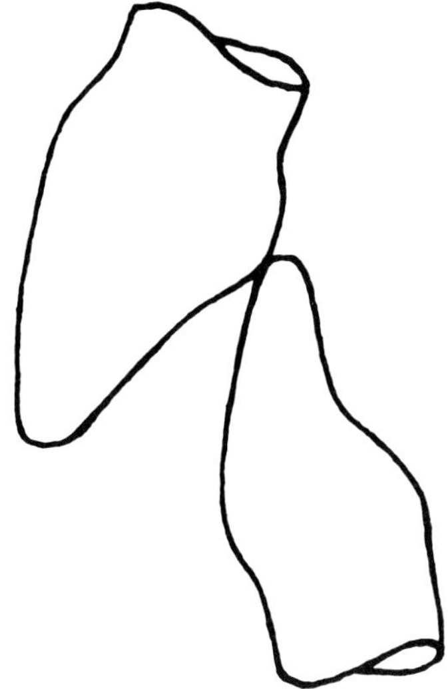

FIG. 15-3. An extreme case of deep vertical overbite.

EDGE-TO-EDGE BITE

The number of possible variations of position in the edge-to-edge bite are impossible to compute, but they must be dealt with; otherwise, changes in tooth position will take place. This type of case must be studied carefully on the articulator, the articulated casts corrected, and a complete reshaping guide list prepared. This type of case is treated as a normal one except that the problem of the individual tooth in edge-to-edge position must be considered. The decision as to which surface to reshape in centric relation must be made after study of the tooth relationships in the eccentric range of

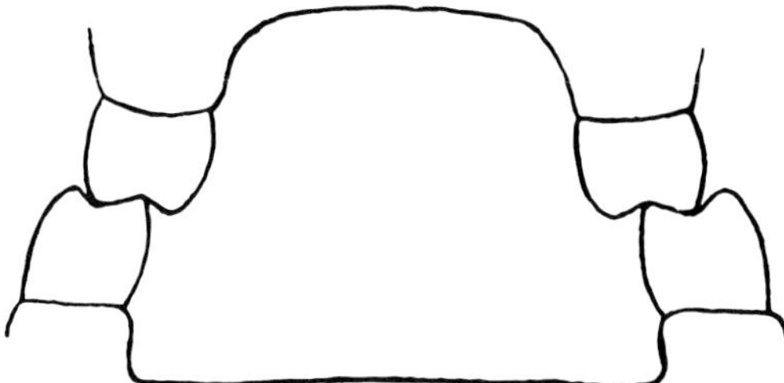

FIG. 15-4. A case of double crossbite. Note that the buccal cusps of the maxillary teeth and the lingual cusps of the mandibular teeth maintain vertical dimension and must not be disturbed.

articulation. Actually, in a true edge-to-edge relationship, it does not matter whether a bit is taken off the lower or the upper anterior teeth. To be absolutely safe, go through a trial run on the articulated casts before working on the teeth themselves.

The equilibration of posterior segments of the arch that are in crossbite or inverted tooth relationships must be approached very cautiously. In such a relationship, the buccal cusps of the maxillary teeth and the lingual cusps of the mandibular teeth maintain vertical dimension (Fig. 15-4). Study the articulated casts carefully and equilibrate in centric relation before doing any work in the patient's mouth. In many cases the crossbite is accompanied by lateral mandibular displacement. Correction in centric relation is of paramount importance. It is also important to note the unusual necessity of reshaping the upper lingual cusps and the lower buccal cusps in the functioning ranges of articulation. The problem is to distribute the stresses of function to as many teeth as possible in the eccentric ranges of articulation. However, take care that, in achieving this aim, the vertical dimension is not shortened. The correction of malposed teeth presents special problems in diagnosis, plan of treatment and therapy.

16 Occlusal Equilibration and Dental Restorations

Unless the maxillary and the mandibular teeth are equilibrated before any restorations are made, existing defects will be exacerbated. Teeth that are out of normal relation or that are extruded may have to be altered, shortened, covered or removed entirely. The quality of the replacements themselves is of paramount importance. Teeth and parts of teeth should be replaced with well-planned, well-constructed and properly functioning restorations. Many otherwise fine restorations are doomed to ultimate failure because they have become the interfering occlusal contacts that prevent proper terminal closure of the mandible.

RESTORATIONS AS DENTAL REMEDIES

If dentists were to think of restorations as dental remedies for pathological conditions in the same way that physicians think of drugs as remedies for illness, they would realize that it is the disease, the pathological condition, that is of utmost importance, not the restoration.[2] This would preclude the danger of becoming preoccupied with the mechanics of the fabrication of restorations and would place the emphasis of restorative dentistry where it properly belongs—on the cure and the correction of pathological conditions. With this line of reasoning, an important question is, "Why did the pathological condition arise?" If the disease is caries, it may have arisen as a result of food packing between proximal surfaces because of an open proximal contact. This open proximal contact may be caused by a cusp in interfering occlusal contact or by some other factor. If the pathological condition is loss of alveolar bone and consequent mobility of the teeth, mere splinting will not suffice. The causes of the pathological condition must be sought. One possible cause may be excessive force, which can be corrected by distributing the forces of function to more teeth. Restorations that are in infraocclusion should be replaced. In short, the remedy or restoration should not only restore the lost tooth structure and return the tooth to proper function but also attempt to prevent recurrence of the pathological condition by removing the underlying cause of the disease. A restoration should satisfy three basic requirements:

1. It should restore the form of the dentition.
2. It should restore the function of the dentition.
3. It should be designed to prevent a recurrence of the pathological condition that it is correcting. In many cases, the equilibration of the occlusion after a restoration has been placed will prevent the repetition of the pathological condition that the restoration is correcting.

Since each tooth functions both individually and as a part of the entire masticatory organ, it follows that a restoration placed in a tooth should function physiologically. The plan of treatment should include the following procedures:

1. Equilibration of the existing occlusion in centric relation and in all the ranges of articulation
2. Concomitant prophylaxis or periodontal treatment
3. Restoration of teeth
4. Equilibration of the occlusion, including the new restorations in centric-relation occlusion and in all the ranges of articulation

COORDINATING SINGLE RESTORATIONS WITH THE EQUILIBRATED OCCLUSION

The first step in coordinating single restorations is to equilibrate the occlusion of the existing dentition so that a foundation or base is established upon which the rest of the dental structure may be rebuilt. The patient will have definite points of reference in centric-relation closure and in the eccentric ranges of articulation. Thus, each tooth can be restored to a corrected occlusion. The wax bridge bite that is used to fabricate the restoration will be a true centric-relation occlusion bite rather than a habitual convenience bite.

As each restoration is placed in the mouth, it is carefully equilibrated so that when all of the restorative work has been completed, it is not a great task to equilibrate the entire occlusion. However, it must be borne in mind that no matter how carefully each restoration is equilibrated, minor adjustments and corrections will have to be made after all the restorative work has been completed. On the other hand, if restorations are fabricated in conformity with the patient's habitual convenience relationship, the malrelationships of the occlusal contacts in habitual convenience relation and in the eccentric ranges of articulation will be accentuated and perpetuated.

If all the restorations are placed before the occlusion has been equilibrated, there is danger that margins of inlays will be exposed, that holes will be ground through the occlusal surfaces of crowns, and in some cases that restorations will be placed in infraocclusion. Such restorations may restore the forms of teeth, but they will not restore function.

The task in restorative dentistry is to place restorations correctly and to coordinate the angulation of the cusps of the restorations with their opposing articulating surfaces. Occlusal equilibration makes it possible to aid this principle if the restorations have been shaped properly. Each restoration should be checked in centric-relation occlusion, in the functioning and the nonfunctioning ranges, and in the protrusive range of articulation. Because of the difficulty of obtaining proper functioning range contacts when fabricating cast crown and inlay restorations on the articulator, the upper buccal cusps are elongated for upper restorations and the lower lingual cusps for lower restorations. When these restorations are placed in the mouth, the cusps can be reshaped to conform to the existing occlusal pattern in the functioning and the nonfunctioning ranges by occlusal equilibration.

In restoring the crown of a tooth that is in malrelation (Fig. 16-1), the tooth should be restored to its correct position, as indicated by the dotted line. The cuspal inclines should be coordinated with those of the maxillary teeth.

THE FIXED BRIDGE

What has been pointed out previously in regard to all restorative dentistry must be emphasized particularly in the field of fixed bridgework. The articulated study casts should be studied carefully before

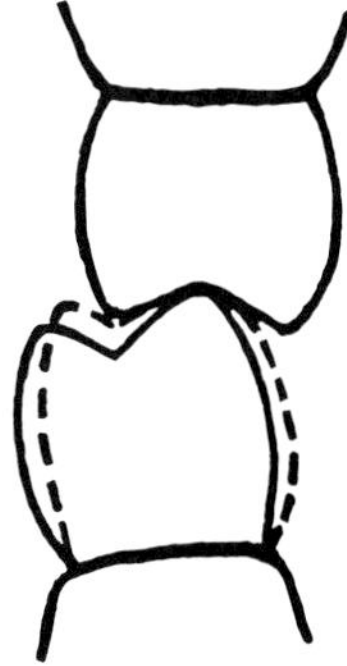

FIG. 16-1. The restoration of the crown of a tooth in linguoversion. The tooth is restored to its correct position as indicated by the dotted line.

any actual restorative work in the mouth is attempted, and the occlusion must be equilibrated in centric relation and in all the ranges of articulation. This will result in the best possible cuspal relationship without restorations. However, examination of the plane of occlusion may show that elongated or shifted teeth may need alteration to provide for better physiological function. Examination of the functioning and the nonfunctioning side movements, each in turn, may show that the restoration can be planned to provide additional cuspal contacts. By checking the articulating movements both on the anatomical articulator and during actual mandibular movements in the mouth, a restoration can be planned which will function in all the ranges of articulation as well as in centric-relation occlusion.

Loss of a tooth without replacement will result in a malocclusion of the dentition. Figure 16-2 illustrates the loss of a lower first molar. The lower second and third molars have drifted mesially and in turn caused movement of the upper molars. The upper first molar has extruded, and the bicuspids have changed their cuspal relationships. This figure demonstrates only centric-relation occlusion and not the eccentric ranges of articulation. A bridge constructed to this "roller coaster" occlusion will replace the missing tooth but will not restore the functioning contacts in the eccentric ranges. By removing parts of the upper

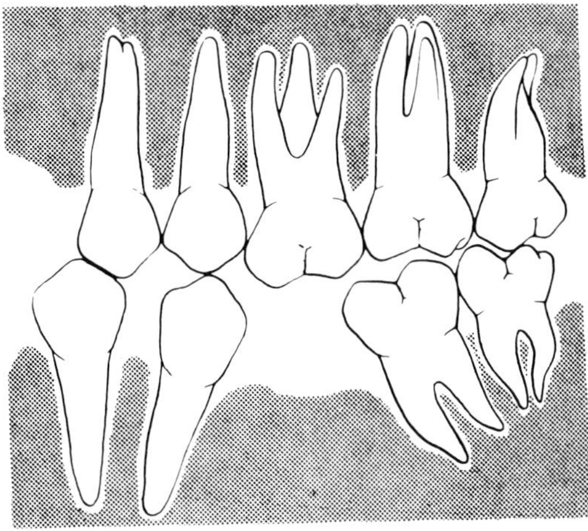

FIG. 16-2. The effect on the occlusion by the loss of the lower first molar.

first molar on the stone cast, and by adding wax on the lower teeth of the cast wherever necessary, a better physiologic occlusion can be achieved for study. Figure 16-3*a* demonstrates an actual case before restoration. Note the plane of occlusion and the upper first molar. The case after the restorations have been placed is seen in (*b*). The upper first molar was adjusted to the new occlusal curve, and a mesio-occlusodistal inlay was placed to protect the exposed dentin and to restore the carious mesial and distal surfaces. A lower fixed bridge was constructed from the second bicuspid to the second molar. The creation of a proper occlusal curve facilitated mandibular movement in centric-relation occlusion and the eccentric ranges and thus made possible an equilibrated functional occlusion.

Many of the failures of bridgework can be attributed to a failure to recognize that tremendous forces are generated by the muscles during function and that these forces are expended through the occlusal surfaces of the teeth. Some of the many situations that result from a lack of proper cuspal relationship of a fixed bridge in centric-relation occlusion and all the ranges of articulation are inefficient function; mobility of the abutment teeth; painful abutment teeth; irritation of the

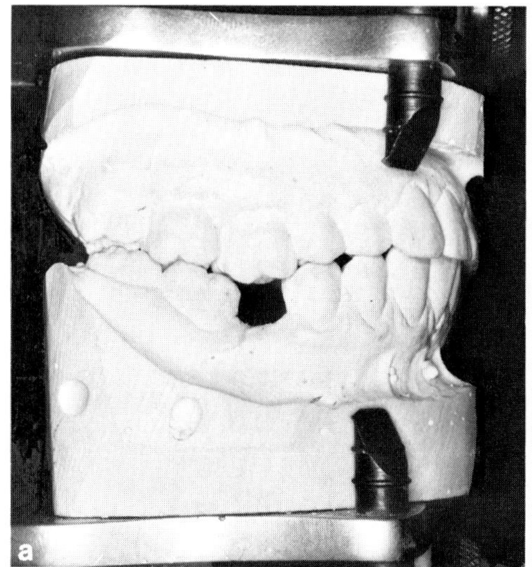

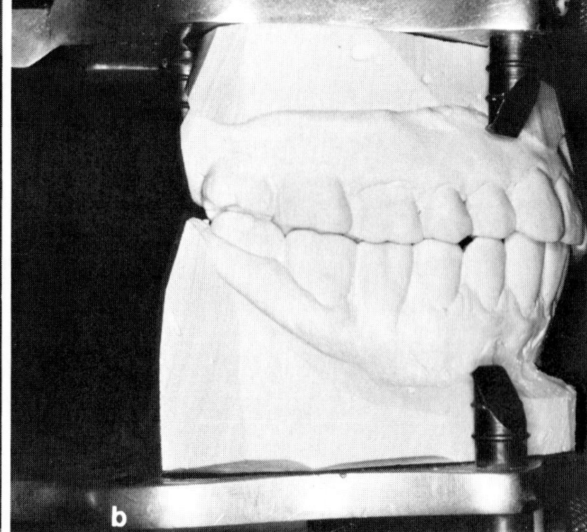

FIG. 16-3. The "roller-coaster" occlusion caused by the loss of a lower first molar and the resultant extrusion of the opposite tooth (*a*). The same case after the restorations have been placed (*b*).

soft tissues; and fracture or loosening of the pontics.

In many cases of fixed bridgework, the occlusal surfaces have been shaped by the excursive movements of the teeth. In some cases the gold that overlays the porcelain or acrylic pontic is stretched or finned out because the functioning-side articulation was not considered in the fabrication of the bridge. This finning out or flattening of the bridge cusp actually creates new leverage problems by delivering the forces of occlusion farther away from the long axes of the teeth. The addition of a pontic to the bridge abutment in proper relationship introduces an increased load and multiplies the forces acting upon the abutment. E. S. Smyd,[5] who has done important work in the field of dental engineering, states:

> Prodigious pressures develop if only one or a few cusps of the lower teeth bear the full brunt of the working bite against the buccal cusps of the upper bridge. As an illustration of the order of values that might take place under the circumstances, the pressure under the needle point of an ordinary phonograph pickup arm weighing less than an ounce is about *10 tons* [*per square inch*]. Pressures of this magnitude permanently deform the buccal cusps by stretching them as surely as if the gold went through rollers. This means that the stretched buccal cusps are longer than they were when the pontic was cast.

In the fabrication of a maxillary or a mandibular posterior fixed bridge, there are a few principles that aid in establishing a physiologic occlusion. A thorough understanding of the role of the articulator will prevent blind slavery to its possible fallacies. The articulator is merely a jig which approximates jaw relationships. The only true relationship that can be registered is a centric relation.

If a maxillary tooth is to be replaced, the following procedure should be used.

1. Using the bridge articulator as a straight-line articulator, build the bridge with the lingual cusps in centric-relation occlusion. Make no attempt to secure lateral cuspal contacts on the articulator.
2. Slightly elongate the buccal cusps.
3. Place the framework of the bridge on the patient's teeth.
4. Reshape the bridge as the patient moves his mandible into the functioning range and then into all the other ranges of articulation.
5. If a mandibular posterior tooth is to be replaced, build it with buccal cusps in

centric-relation occlusion and with high lingual cusps. Do not attempt to obtain lateral cuspal contacts on the articulator.

6. After the mandibular framework has been finished, place it on the abutment teeth; then reshape it in all the ranges of articulation.

7. After the bridge is in proper function, complete the porcelain or acrylic facings. Of course, proper occlusal anatomy must be maintained throughout this procedure.

8. After all the restorations have been placed, adjust any further discrepancies of the articulation by careful checking and equilibration in all the ranges of articulation.

In summary, the following steps must be followed if a fixed bridge is to be fabricated properly:

1. Plan on the study casts for the restoration of a normal occlusion on the side of the arch where the bridge is to be placed.
2. Equilibrate the occlusion of the natural dentition.
3. Fabricate the fixed bridge.
4. Equilibrate the occlusion in centric-relation occlusion and in all ranges of articulation with the fixed bridge on the patient's teeth.

A more detailed consideration of the fabrication of extensive bridgework properly belongs in a treatise on oral rehabilitation rather than in one on occlusal equilibration.

THE PARTIAL DENTURE

The natural dentition must be equilibrated before a partial denture is constructed for a patient. Follow the same procedure as in dealing with a full complement of teeth. Again, the aim is to bring as many cuspal surfaces as possible into contact in centric-relation occlusion, as well as in all the ranges of articulation. This procedure will also remove any interferences in these positions.

There are many forces that act upon a single tooth when it is in its correct position in the masticatory organ. When such a tooth becomes an abutment for a partial denture, the load that it must then bear is frequently physiologically untenable, and its retention in the arch will depend upon the resistive capacity of the bone. Therefore, it becomes vital to the supporting structures of the teeth that the functional stresses produced upon them be shared among as many teeth as possible. Occlusal equilibration will contribute toward satisfying this objective. Experience has shown that proper distribution of all the stresses to the partial dentures and the natural dentition can keep forces within physiological limits.

The teeth that serve as abutments carry enormous loads and vertical torques in centric-relation occlusion closure because of the pump-handle action of the partial denture (Fig. 9-3*a*). Figure 9-3*b* shows that there is also a horizontal torque action, which is produced by the lateral movement of the partial denture saddle, illustrated by the dotted line, as the patient functions in the eccentric ranges. Usually it is a combination of these forces that bears upon the abutment teeth. Before proceeding, mount the casts on an anatomical articulator and carefully plan and design the work on the articulated cast. Elongated teeth may have to be altered to achieve a proper plane of occlusion. If necessary, build teeth by veneering with metal onlays to provide advantageous modification of cusp height and form, which will assure harmonious relationships and freedom in all the ranges of articulation.

In summary, the procedure for making a partial denture should embrace the following steps:

1. Plan on the study casts for the restoration of a normal occlusion.
2. Equilibrate the occlusion of the natural dentition in centric relation and in all ranges of articulation.
3. Make a trial fit of the metal framework of the partial dentures and equili-

brate the occlusion with the framework in place.

4. Take a centric-relation occlusion Aluwax bite and remount the upper cast on the articulator to set up the partial-denture teeth properly.

5. Make a trial fitting of the framework of the partial denture with the denture teeth set in wax so that they may be moved about if necessary.

6. Place the finished denture in the patient's mouth and equilibrate the occlusion in centric-relation occlusion and in all ranges of articulation.

One advantage of fabrication according to the method described is that the teeth of the finished partial denture will not present occlusal interferences during function and, therefore, will not produce excessive torque and loads on the supporting teeth and their investing structures. Another advantage of this method is that the teeth of the partial denture will function in the eccentric ranges of articulation. Many partial dentures function only in centric-relation occlusion, permitting the patient to function only in that position. The result is a short, choppy bite with great vertical pressures on the abutment teeth and consequent excessive strain beyond the physiological capacity of the tissues to withstand or compensate.

LOST VERTICAL DIMENSION

In true cases of lost vertical dimension (Chap. 8, Class V malocclusion), the patient will have a freeway space of 8 to 10 mm. He will also show missing or badly worn teeth. The first step in correcting this condition is to equilibrate the occlusion in centric relation in order to establish a correct centric-relation closure and to permit the mandible to open and close in a centric-relation arc rather than in a motion that is deflected by cuspal interferences. The patient will feel more comfortable and will be ready to cooperate in carrying out the further prosthetic procedures. Regardless of whether fixed bridgework or partial dentures are used to restore the vertical dimension, the following procedures must be observed:

1. Plan on the study casts for the restoration of normal occlusion and vertical dimension.

2. Equilibrate the occlusion in centric relation.

3. Use temporary occlusal guide splints to restore vertical dimension according to the method of choice of determining lost dimension; equilibrate the splints both in centric relation and in the eccentric ranges of articulation, and reduce the vertical dimension if the patient shows any untoward symptoms. (Note that the purpose of the treatment is *not* to raise the bite but to restore lost vertical dimension if it has been shortened.)

4. Restore the vertical dimension with the appliance of choice and equilibrate the occlusion both in centric relation and in the eccentric ranges of articulation.

DYNAMIC CONCEPT OF ORTHODONTICS AND PEDODONTICS

A set of casts illustrating ideal occlusion actually demonstrates static occlusion only. Function must be illustrated with the teeth in function. A complete concept of orthodontics must include an evaluation of the dentition in function. The orthodontist treats a developing organ which is responding to and integrating with the entire stomatognathic system. The chief functioning parts of this system are the teeth, the periodontium, the bone, the neuromuscular system and the temporomandibular joint. Of these, the orthodontist attempts to control only one part of a pathologically developing system—the teeth.

The placement of the teeth must be evaluated in terms of their total integration with the masticatory organ which, in turn, functions as part of the stomatognathic system. Function is the purpose of all organs, and as the organ functions, its form develops. No single part of the masticatory organ can assume total responsibility for the occlusion of the teeth. The problem of the orthodontist is the correct placement of the dentition in the skull. However, this is merely the static phase of the entire problem. The dynamic phase is the correct maintenance of the cuspal inclines of the teeth as they function.

A child, in the mixed-dentition state, should have lateral articulatory movements to enable him to chew the coarse foods which exercise the masticatory organ and aid in its development. The cuspid is usually the greatest offender in preventing such movements. Careful equilibration in the eccentric ranges of articulation will usually free the locked bite and enable the masticatory organ to function and develop properly.

The establishment of a harmonious relationship between the inclined planes of the teeth, the neuromusculature and the temporomandibular joint in function is the purpose of occlusal equilibration. Actually, occlusal equilibration may be considered a form of orthodontic therapy.

Figure 16-4*a* shows the position and the axis of a true standing tooth. Note the angle of the cusp at 1. In (*b*), the tooth, as it presents itself, illustrates that the cuspal incline at 2 interferes with function. In (*c*), by reshaping the incline at 3, a situation almost similar to that at 1 is produced without moving the tooth. In this manner, occlusal equilibration created the same inclined plane that would have been created if the tooth at (*b*) had been uprighted. Many occlusal deviations can be corrected readily in this manner.

One of the basic reflex patterns established before birth is the neuromuscular control of the mandible which governs suckling, swallowing, breathing, coughing, etc. The neuromuscular system has a tremendous influence on the growth and the development of the facial bones and influences bone growth before any teeth have erupted. At birth, the neuromuscular-system reflex control of the mandible is the most highly developed reflex in the entire body. It is a deep, unlearned reflex. Simply stated, when the anterior teeth appear in an infant's mouth, each incisor has a periodontal ligament containing proprioceptors. As the incisors touch each other, an afferent signal runs up the mesencephalic root of the 5th nerve and finally creates a synapse with the motor center. The latter then instructs the muscles that they had better move the mandible a bit or the teeth will come into violent collision. Under the control of the nerves, the muscles learn to move the mandible, and thus there is the beginning of the postural position of the mandible.

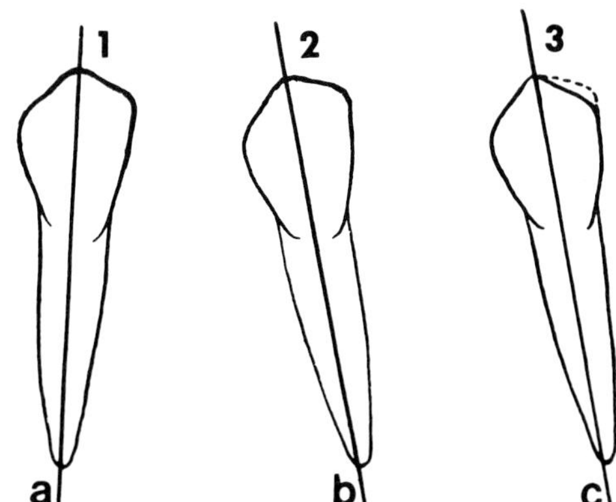

FIG. 16-4. An effect similar to moving a tooth orthodontically can be produced by reshaping. The tooth in ideal position (*a*). The tooth as presented clinically (*b*). By reshaping along the dotted line (*c*) the same effect is achieved as presented (*a*).

Moyers[3] feels that when the 6-year molars erupt into an end-to-end bite, the primary dentition should be reshaped to allow orthodontic Class I interdigitation of the 6-year molars instead of permitting them to retain a teeter-totter action for 5 or 6 years or until the primary teeth are lost. If normal wear does not take place, Moyers believes that it should be provided artificially. Malocclusions in children are a combination of abnormal bone growth, abnormal positions of the teeth and abnormal function. This investigator proved by means of extensive electromyographic recordings the hypothesis behind the equilibration of the occlusion of adults. His researches in this field are fully described in the literature.

If function is accepted as the aim of orthodontic therapy, the movements of the teeth through the various ranges of articulation are of great importance. The following factors are a few over which orthodontic appliances have no control:

1. Discrepancies of tooth sizes and shapes
2. Lack of wear owing to variable hardness of the enamel or to malposition or a tooth plane
3. Poorly restored teeth in which the anatomical portions are not restored to proper form causing excessive tooth contact
4. Temporomandibular joint syndrome caused by deflection of the mandible from the centric-relation arc
5. Vertical and/or horizontal overloading of one or two pairs of teeth

Actually, the course of cuspal interferences can be considered to follow this pattern:

1. The teeth move to protect themselves from overloading, as though an orthodontic appliance were being used.
2. If the teeth do not move, the head of the condyle will shift in the glenoid fossa and will develop minor or major pathological conditions.
3. Interfering contacts in centric-relation occlusion between an upper and a lower cuspid will cause crowding and buckling of lower anteriors.

There are many finished cases in orthodontic therapy which are actually compromise solutions. Occlusal equilibration will keep such cases at their optimal state and will prevent them from collapsing. Ponitz[4] states:

> By banding only the molars, the forces of occlusion and the pressure of the tongue, lip, and cheek muscles are given the greatest latitude to mold and move the dentition into a position of balance. If all the teeth are banded, such forces are not active until the retainer stage. At the retainer stage, these forces may be less beneficial to the corrected occlusion but more effective in producing relapse, because the arches were expanded during treatment without the guiding and controlling pressure of the surrounding musculature. Halderson[1] and coworkers stated: "Relapse of any case is nothing more than a failure to place the teeth into a stable position of equilibrium among the forces acting on the denture. Until a great deal more work is done, we shall continue to see a few perfectly treated cases fail to retain well."

The orthodontist should inform the patient of the need for occlusal equilibration when the patient presents himself initially; otherwise, the necessity for this work will come as a surprise. The procedure of occlusal equilibration during orthodontic therapy should embrace these steps:

1. Remove interfering occlusal contacts in centric relation during the first month of the retention period
2. Recheck centric relation about a month later to compensate for the slight movement that may have taken place; do preliminary reshaping in the eccentric ranges of articulation by removing only gross cuspal interferences
3. Complete equilibration of the occlusion in centric relation and in all ranges of articulation from 4 to 6 months after the bands have been removed
4. Introduce exercises designed to teach the patient how to function in all ranges of articulation

As an adjunct to orthodontic therapy, occlusal equilibration will prevent occlusal trauma and a traumatogenic occlusion. It can also prevent or alleviate temporomandibular joint disorders and do much to stabilize the teeth during the development of the masticatory organ.

REFERENCES

1. Halderson, H., Johns, E. E., and Moyers, R. E.: Selection of forces for tooth movement. Am. J. Ortho., *39:*25, 1953.
2. McCollum, B. B., and Stuart, C. E.: A research report, fundamentals involved in prescribing restorative remedies, D. Items Int., *61:522,* 641, 724, 852, 942, 1939.
3. Moyers, R. E.: Personal communication.
4. Ponitz, P. V.: The relative importance of appliances in orthodontic therapy. J.A.D.A. *55:*488, 1957.
5. Smyd, E. S.: Dental engineering. J. D. Res., *27:*649, 1948.

Additional Basic References

Applegate, D. C., and Nissle, R. O.: Keeping the partial denture in harmony with biologic limitations. JADA, *43:*409, 1951.

Bignell, K. A.: Diagnosis and reconstruction technic for the treatment of interarticular and peridental trauma and disuse atrophy. JADA, *24:*256, 1937.

Bronstein, B. R.: An evaluation of basic concepts in mouth rehabilitation. J. Pros. Dent., *1:*560, 1951.

Doxtater, L.: The importance of occlusal coordination in bridgework. JADA, *18:*2343, 1931.

Goldstein, M. C.: Orthodontics in crown and bridge and periodontal therapy. D. Clin. North Am., *8:*449, 1964.

Graber, T. M.: Orthodontics, Principles and Practice. ed. 2. Philadelphia, W. B. Saunders, 1966.

Granger, E. R.: Mechanical principles applied to partial denture construction. JADA, *28:*1943, 1941.

Klaffenbach, A. O.: Gnathodynamics. JADA, *23:*371, 1936.

Moyers, R. E.: Tongue problems and malocclusion. D. Clin. North Am., *8:*529, 1964.

Osborne, J., Brills, N., and Lammie, G. A.: Partial dentures. Internat. D. J., *7:*26, 1957.

Rothner, J. T.: Occlusal equilibration—correction of occlusal factors as a part of orthodontic treatment. Am. J. Ortho., *38:*521, 1952.

Schuyler, C. H.: Partial denture design giving thought of the maintenance of balanced occlusal relations. D. Cosmos, *72:*272, 1930.

———: Occlusal harmony as a basic requisite in orthodontics. New York J. Dent., *24:*386, 1954.

Woodruff, H. S.: Fixed bridge construction. New York J. Dent., *14:*287, 1944.

17 Instructions to Patients

The average patient with temporomandibular joint dysfunction is referred to various medical specialists—often an internist, otolaryngologist, neurologist and psychiatrist—before an accurate diagnosis is rendered. This chain of referrals, combined with unrelenting, unidentified head pain, often reinforces the patient's self-drawn conclusion that he or she has a brain tumor. In addition, although patients may have agonizing head pain, many are told that they are psychosomatically ill. The aforementioned factors, compounded by the stresses of today's society, point up the importance of obtaining the patient's confidence and establishing good rapport.

THE FIRST APPOINTMENT

During the first appointment the patient completes medical and dental history forms, then discusses his or her symptoms, in depth, with the dentist. In my office, such interviews average an hour. Since patients may become tense and inhibited while seated in dental chairs, interviews should be conducted in consultation rooms. With a relaxed patient, open, two-way communication is much more likely than with a tense patient.

The interview is followed by a clinical examination (see Chap. 6), during which visual aids are used to help give the patient a thorough understanding of the problem. For example, a plastic skull is used to help explain the structure and function of the temporomandibular joints and the rationale for the various procedures that must be undertaken. With the plastic skull as an aid, it is relatively easy to explain the relationship between the condyles, discs and fossae of the temporomandibular joints, as well as the relationship of the teeth to jaw movement. Illustrations such as Figure 17-1 help to further correlate the malposition of teeth with the malposed mandible.

Since clicking and muscle spasms occur in about 90 per cent of all patients with temporomandibular joint dysfunction, it is advantageous to give the patients etiological explanations.

PATIENT EDUCATION PROGRAM

An educational program for patients with temporomandibular joint dysfunction can be developed from the material presented in Chapter 10.

For example, patients who experience clicking noises must learn to open their mouths in a restricted manner. Illustrations can help explain to them the "why" and "wherefore." For example, Figure 17-2, which depicts the temporomandibular joint, and Figure 17-3, which shows the normal function of the joint complex

Fɪɢ. 17-1. As the mandible passes through the centric-relation arc (CRA) toward terminal closure, the interfering occlusal contact at E (*arrow*) prevents closure to K. The mandible has described the arc, JE′, and is deflected into the habitual convenience relationship at H; it follows the path of E′H. The condyle has rotated on X. The joint gap, F, is unevenly spaced in the glenoid fossa, B.

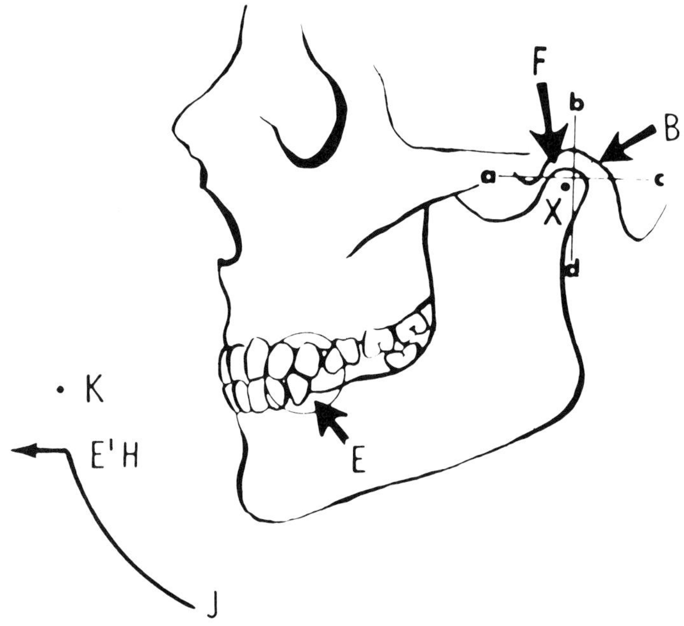

during mouth opening and closing, have proved extremely helpful. Figures 17-4 and 17-5, demonstrating why some joints click, also have been useful in explaining joint problems and exercise regimens. As an extra "cosmetic dividend" resulting from prescribed exercises, patients can be told that their suprahyoid muscles (Fig. 17-6) will become more firm, thereby providing an improved appearance.

Much of the information on the temporomandibular joint can be presented to patients who, once they realize that the ligaments are bruised and stretched, will understand the rationale for dietary restrictions. As noted in Chapter 10, rehabilitation of the ligaments, and thus restoration of normal function, are aided by avoiding hard and "chewy" foods.

Most patients with temporomandibular joint dysfunction are instructed "Never open your mouth wider than the thickness of your thumb." Some of these patients, however, are barely able to open their mouths. For these patients, a "finger-thumb" exercise is prescribed.

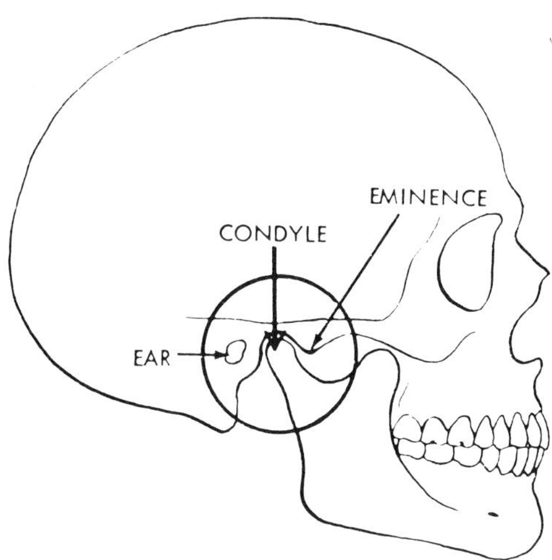

Fɪɢ. 17-2. The right side of the skull shows the condyle within the temporomandibular joint (area within circle).

Finger-Thumb Exercise

Place the thumb on the biting edge of the upper central teeth and the forefinger on the biting edge of the lower central teeth.

With slight pressure, force the teeth and jaws apart until *slight* pain is encountered.

Do this for 30 seconds every 2 hours.

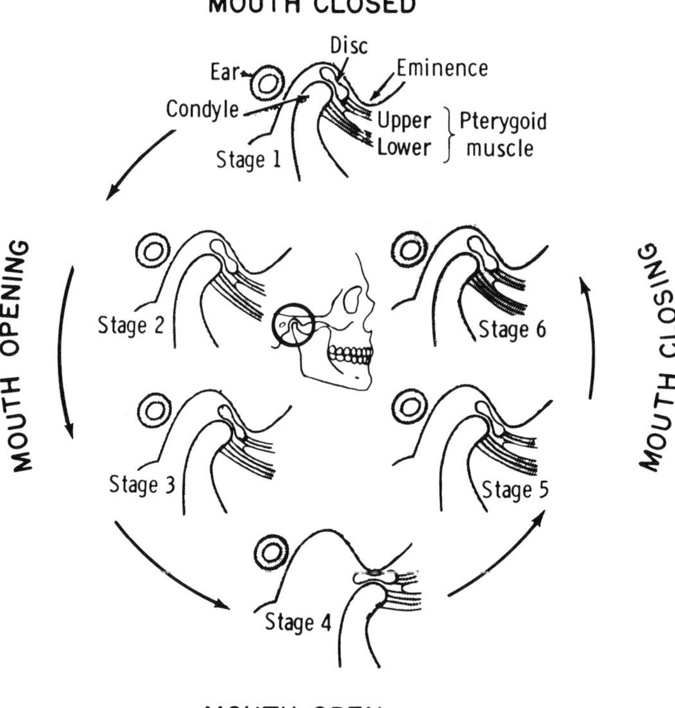

FIG. 17-3. Various stages of a normal right temporomandibular joint (area within the circle of center drawing of skull) as the jaw opens and closes the mouth.

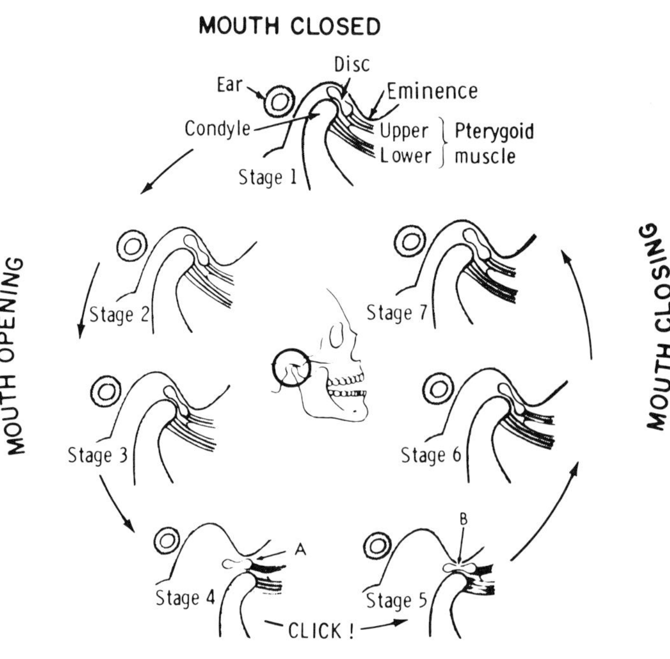

FIG. 17-4. Various stages of an abnormal (spastic) right temporomandibular joint as the jaw opens and closes the mouth. The upper and lower parts of the external pterygoid muscles are functioning incoordinately.

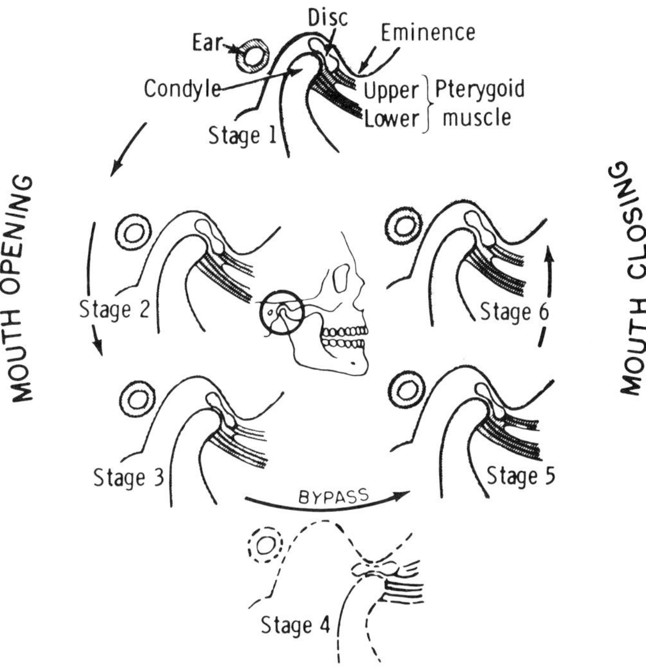

FIG. 17-5. Modified stages of opening and closing the mouth to avoid clicking.

> ***Cork Exercise***
>
> Gradually insert the small end of a tapered cork into your mouth until your jaws are separated and you begin to feel pain in the jaw joints and muscles.
>
> Leave the cork in place for 30 seconds before removing it. Repeat this procedure every 2 hours.

The extent of jaw opening gradually increases if finger-thumb exercises are done regularly. When the patient can open his mouth 12 mm. without experiencing pain, the following cork exercise is prescribed.

The latter routine, properly followed, will increase the jaw opening capacity to 35 mm. For further details on the cork

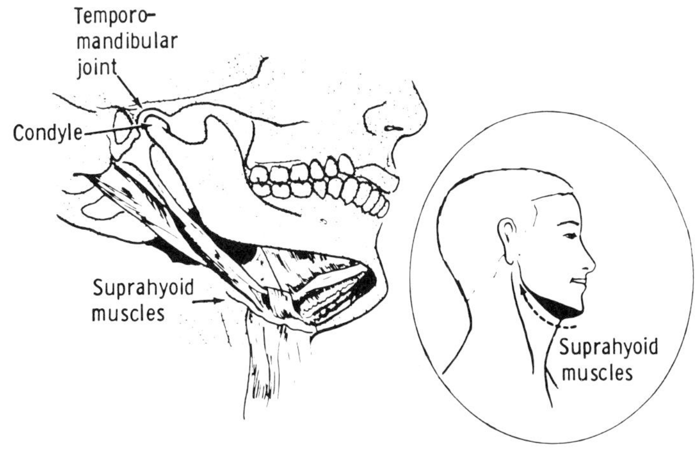

FIG. 17-6. The suprahyoid muscles, located under the chin, are seen in their relationship to the temporomandibular joint.

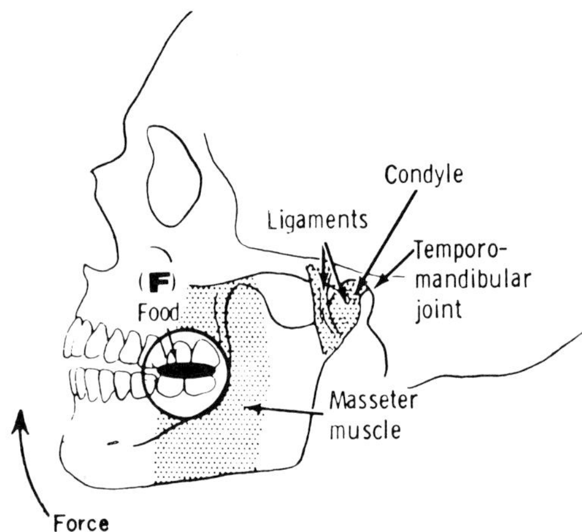

FIG. 17-7. Left side of skull is depicted with jaws slightly open. Note the temporomandibular joint and its components, and relationship of the joint to the masseter muscle. Large arrow indicates direction in which masseter muscle pulls upward when chewing food (F).

exercise, see Chapter 10 (Figs. 10-16 and 10-17).

In explaining the need for chewing restrictions and a semi-soft diet for 4 to 6 months, or until there is a remission of symptoms, illustrations again are helpful. Figure 17-7, for example, shows a temporomandibular joint with the jaws slightly open. In order to chew hard food (F), it can be explained, the masseter muscle pulls upward (*arrow*). But when there is dysfunction and a weakened joint, the hard food acts as a fulcrum and temporary disjointing results, producing intense head and facial pain.

The temporomandibular joint may be compared to a nutcracker (Fig. 17-8) to explain normal joint function (*a*) as contrasted to a weak complex (*b*). The temporomandibular joint also can be likened to a computer system and its components. The existing dysfunction is like a computer program that contains inaccuracies. In order to make corrections, the entire computer program must be shut down completely and the problems analyzed, followed by reprogramming, testing and reanalyzing. This is done until a fully operational, efficient system exists. Similarly with temporomandibular joint dysfunction: In order to eliminate muscle spasms and pain caused by malocclusion (and engrams—bad habits) soft foods and medication are prescribed, and the patient is fitted with a Shore Mandibular Autorepositioning Appliance. After the mandible has properly repositioned itself, occlusal equilibration can be accurately accomplished and normal function restored. Figure 17-9 summarizes the aforementioned analogy.

As an aid to defining ligaments as dense bands of tissue that connect and support bone, reference can be made to Figure 17-10. In discussing stretched ligaments, Figure 17-11 may facilitate the patient's understanding of his problem.

When a person with normal jaw ligaments bites hard food with the anterior

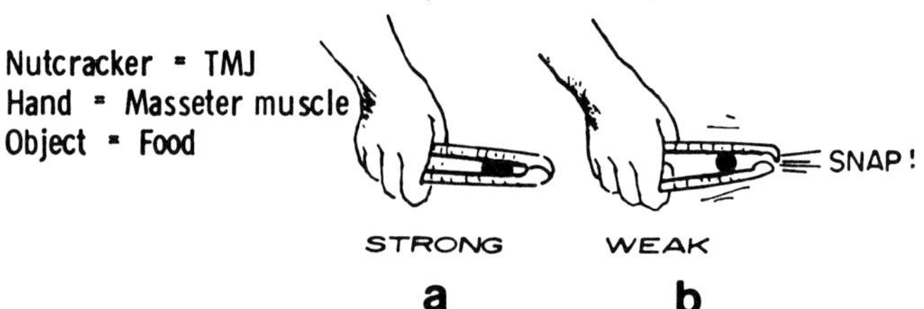

FIG. 17-8. The way in which the temporomandibular joint works when chewing hard food can best be illustrated by its comparison with a nutcracker. The nutcracker is strong and crushes the nut (*a*). The mechanism (nutcracker) is weak (*b*). Instead of cracking the nut, the nutcracker itself comes apart.

TMJ		COMPUTER
Muscle spasm, pain, malocclusion, etc.	⟷	Program errors, nonoperational system
Soft foods—medication	⟷	Shut down system
Appliance	⟷	Analyze errors, reprogram and test
Equilibration	⟷	System reprogrammed
Normal temporomandibular joint	⟷	System operational

FIG. 17-9. Computerized comparative analysis of the temporomandibular joint.

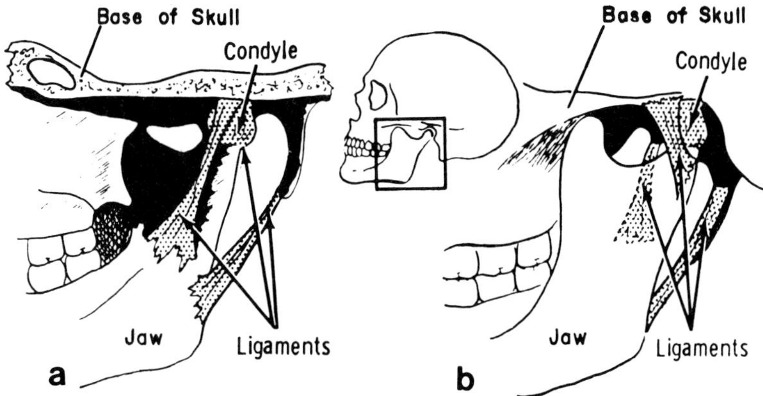

FIG. 17-10. Detailed inner surface of the temporomandibular joint shows inner set of ligaments, which hold the jaw to the base of the skull (*a*). Outer surface of the temporomandibular joint and the outer set of ligaments that hold the jaw to the base of the skull also are depicted (*b*).

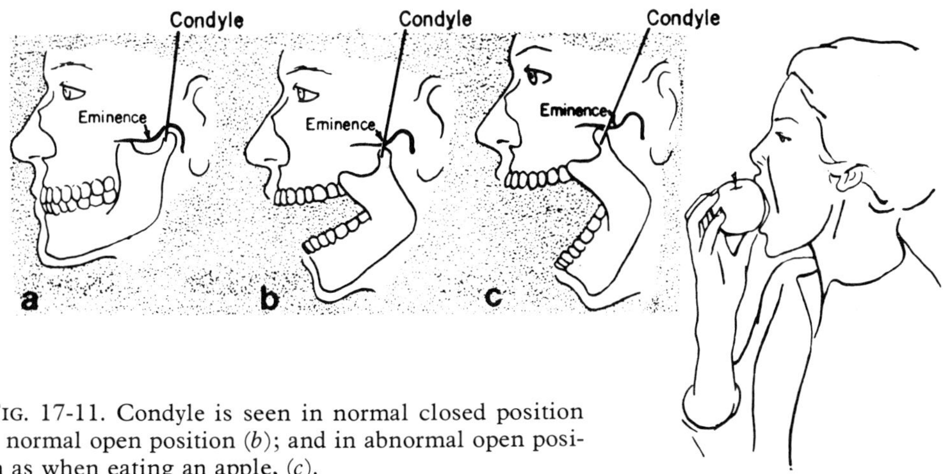

FIG. 17-11. Condyle is seen in normal closed position (*a*); normal open position (*b*); and in abnormal open position as when eating an apple, (*c*).

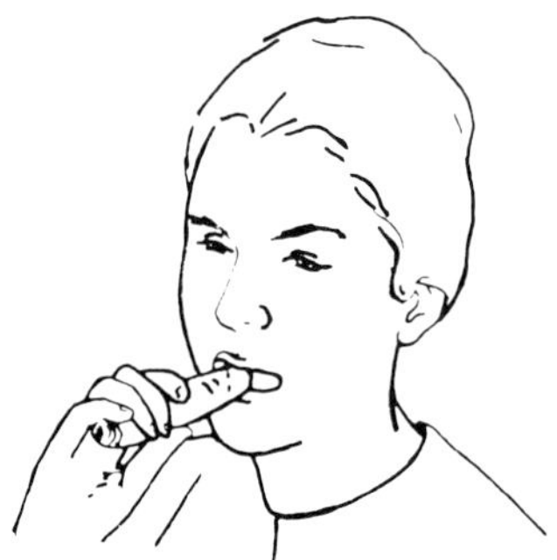

FIG. 17-12. A person with normal ligaments bites a carrot with the anterior teeth, without any problems.

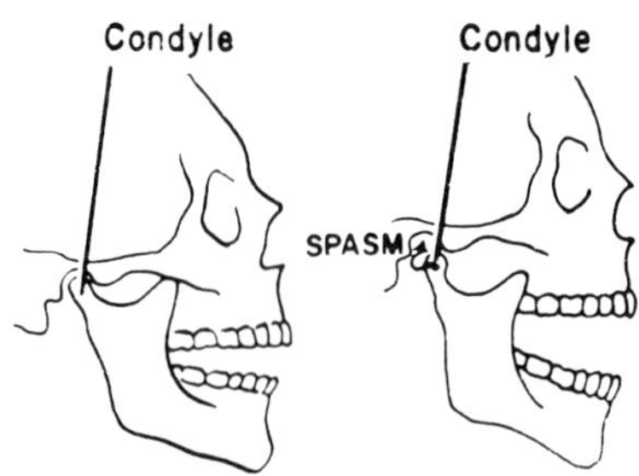

FIG. 17-13. Muscle spasm is initiated when a person with stretched (abnormal) jaw ligaments bites food with the anterior teeth. The condyle, as noted, is brought to the front of the eminence. Because of uncoordinated contraction, the external pterygoid muscles go into spasm.

teeth (Fig. 17-12), no problems are encountered. Strong, elastic ligaments help guide the condyle in a smooth, coordinated fashion. However, as Figure 17-13 demonstrates, when the jaw ligaments are stretched, biting food with the anterior teeth results in muscle spasm, clicking and pain. Instruct patients with temporomandibular joint dysfunction to cut food into small, bite-size pieces and chew them deliberately with the posterior teeth—never with the anterior teeth. Additionally, caution them against having long conversations, especially on the telephone, to avoid further stretching and pressures on the ligaments.

Following the interview of a new patient during the first office visit, conduct a clinical examination (see Form I, p. 107). Obtain a study cast of the dentition and

NATHAN ALLEN SHORE, D.D.S.

210 CENTRAL PARK SOUTH

NEW YORK, N. Y. 10019

To supplement the questionnaire you were good enough to fill out in my office, I should like you to write out, in as great detail as you can remember, the complete story of your dental difficulties. If possible, put your account in chronological order starting with the first dental symptoms you experienced, the first doctor you visited for the problem, the first treatment and the results (good or bad). Be sure to list the area where you experienced pain or any other abnormal sensation.

In other words, although the questionnaire you completed may seem to cover much of the same subject matter, I want an account in your own words of your dental experiences until the time you came to my office. It will help me to help you.

FIG. 17-14. After the first visit, the patient is given a request form.

LIPS TOGETHER AND TEETH APART

One of the most important steps in breaking the habit of clenching and grinding the teeth is to become self-conscious when it occurs and, of course, to cease the habit. One excellent way to avoid clenching is to learn to keep the lips together and the teeth apart. This simple step will not only make it impossible to clench the teeth, but, even more important, it will relax the very muscles that become tense and taut. Keeping the lips together and the teeth apart also permits normal positioning of the various components of the temporomandibular joints.

The more self-conscious you are about this very basic procedure of relaxing the jaw muscles, the faster you will master a new and beneficial way of overcoming a harmful habit. Gradually, you will find yourself waking up in the morning without your teeth clenched. But you must persevere. Remember that you have had the bad habit for a long time, and it won't vanish overnight. You must make a conscious effort to separate your teeth, while at the same time keeping your lips closed. Repeat to yourself several times a day: "Lips together and teeth apart." An extra dividend: You'll find this facial posture will improve your expression and appearance!

FIG. 17-15. Instructions for breaking the habit of clenching and grinding the teeth are given to the patient.

full-mouth radiographs. At the end of the first visit give the patient instructions (Fig. 17-14) that request a written summarization of his or her dental problems. The summary supplements the history forms (see p. 104) completed earlier by the patient.

THE SECOND OFFICE VISIT

The new patient's second office visit is primarily to communicate findings based upon the clinical examination, radiographs, and medical and dental histories. Both the patient's radiographs and study cast (mounted on an articulator) are useful in presenting findings, outlining the therapeutic regimen, and giving assurance that surgery is not necessary for this clinically reversible condition. Assuming that the patient accepts the recommended therapy, a Shore Mandibular Autorepositioning Appliance (see Chap. 11) is fabricated after the second visit.

THE THIRD APPOINTMENT

The Shore Mandibular Autorepositioning Appliance is fitted to the upper arch during the patient's third office visit.

Various instructions are given to the patient during the third appointment—verbally and in writing.

A number of pressure-sensitive, amber labels with the phrase LIPS TOGETHER —TEETH APART are given to the patient, to be affixed to telephones, refrigerators and bathroom mirrors. The stickers will remind the patient of this effective way to break the habit of clenching and grinding the teeth. The patient is given a written explanation (Fig. 17-15).

Dear

Now that we have begun treating your temporomandibular joint dysfunction, I want to outline the diet you will be following for the next few months. And I also want to list some general instructions.

1. Cut all food into small, bite-size pieces, and DO NOT open your mouth any wider than the thickness of your thumb.
2. DO NOT eat hard crusts of bread, tough meat, raw vegetables, gum, or any other food that requires prolonged chewing.
3. DO NOT bite any food with your front teeth. Don't protrude your jaw, as you must do when biting off a piece of thread. Also, when putting on lipstick don't bring your jaw forward. Try to avoid long telephone conversations, which may strain your joint ligaments. Don't protrude your jaw when smoking. If you find yourself clenching your teeth, remember: "Lips Together and Teeth Apart."

I'm sure you will agree that these instructions are easy to follow. I have had a food list printed separately so that you can carry it with you, or keep it posted in the kitchen for handy reference. After awhile you will find yourself automatically rejecting the foods you should avoid.

Sincerely,

FIG. 17-16. A personalized letter is given to the patient summarizing DO's and DON'T's.

A personalized letter summarizing several DO's and DON'Ts (Fig. 17-16) is given to the patient when therapy is initiated, as a reminder of dietary and nutritional restrictions, and other limitations aimed at optimizing rehabilitation of the joint ligaments. In addition, a list of foods that are permitted and prohibited (Fig. 17-17), is provided to those undergoing treatment.

Since patients who have had injections into the temporomandibular joints are likely to be curious about the effect, a written explanation is provided (Fig. 17-18). And those who are suffering from especially painful joints will find in their packet of information, instructions for applying moist heat to obtain prompt pain relief (Fig. 17-19).

THE FOURTH APPOINTMENT

Prescriptions for muscle relaxants, vitamins and other medications (see Chap. 10) are given to patients during the fourth office visit. In addition, if the patient has unrelenting pain, Xylocaine without epinephrine may be injected into the temporomandibular joints or external pterygoids to relieve muscle spasm.

USING THE SHORE MANDIBULAR AUTOREPOSITIONING APPLIANCE

Instructions in using the Shore Mandibular Autorepositioning Appliance are explained, in detail, to patients as follows:

DIET FOR ALL PATIENTS WITH TEMPOROMANDIBULAR JOINT DYSFUNCTION			
PERMITTED		PROHIBITED	
Meats:	Any ground meat (hamburgers, meatballs, or meat loaf made with beef, pork or veal, tongue and boiled chicken	Meats:	No steak, fried chicken or roasts of any kind
Potatoes:	Mashed, baked or boiled potatoes, well-cooked spaghetti	Potatoes:	No fried potatoes
Vegetables:	Any cooked or canned vegetable such as peas, beets, beans or cauliflower	Vegetables:	No raw vegetables or salads, no corn-on-the-cob
Fish:	Any boiled or baked fish	Fish:	No shellfish of any kind, no fried fish
Dairy Foods:	Eggs, cottage cheese, sour cream, milk, ice cream		
Bread:	Only white bread (crusts removed) and soft rolls	Bread:	No sandwiches, except open-faced on one slice of crustless white bread. No bagels, hard rolls, rye bread or toast
Junior Baby Foods:	All kinds		
Fruits:	Any canned or stewed fruit. Melon, bananas, apples or peaches but only if cut into thin slices	Fruits:	No whole raw fruits or berries
Desserts:	All soft puddings, custards and gelatins		
Liquids:	All beverages; fortified "liquid meals" are recommended		
Miscellaneous:	Any of the variety of nourishing mixtures that can be mixed in a blender (milk shakes, frosteds, fruit or vegetable blends)	Miscellaneous:	No hard or chewy candies, no gum, no dried fruits

FIG. 17-17. A diet list of foods permitted and prohibited is given to the patient.

Purpose. The appliance is intended to reposition the various components of the chewing apparatus into a harmonious, smoothly functioning system. When malocclusion of the teeth exists, as in your case, the teeth control the jaw. The jaw muscles are then twisted, and this causes muscle spasm and pain and forces the jaw into malposition. The continued use of the appliance allows the jaw to find its proper position—by eliminating the teeth as the dominant factor and letting the jaw function correctly. In order to break up the harmful habits of jaw malposition, the appliance *must be worn* day and night. Learn to eat with it, laugh with it, and speak with it.

Usage. After 3 days you should have no difficulty speaking while wearing the appliance. To speed up the process of getting accustomed to the appliance, practice reading very slowly before a mirror for 15 minutes at a time, three times a day for the first 3 days.

The appliance must be worn at all times, except when eating. You will notice an excessive flow of saliva for the first 2 days because the salivary glands will be "fooled" by the presence of the appliance, and will react as if it were food. Do not be concerned about this; excess salivary flow will disappear in a few days.

When the appliance is removed for cleaning, you will notice that only one or two teeth meet one another. This is to be expected. Actually, what has happened is that the appliance is allowing the jaw to find its proper position.

Adjustment. The biting surfaces of the appliance will be changed whenever you come to the office. Do not be alarmed if you notice that one side is thick while the other side is thin. This difference is due to the malposition of your jaw. When the appliance is adjusted in the office, thin areas may appear in it and tiny particles may even break off. This is nothing to worry about, and is in fact an indication that the jaw is finding its proper position. Between office visits if a thin area should wear through or snap off, remove the appliance and smooth off rough edges of the broken area with an emery board, before reinserting it. One last word of reassurance: When small pieces of the appliance break off, do not be alarmed. It is a good sign and means that the jaw is finding its proper position.

Care of Appliance and Teeth. Brush both sides of the appliance carefully with toothpaste every time you brush your teeth, then rinse the device thoroughly in an antiseptic mouthwash solution. When brushing the teeth, pay special attention to the inner surface of the *upper teeth.* Brush them very carefully; then proceed to the other surfaces. Whenever you come to the office, the appliance will be highly polished and sterilized in an ultrasonic apparatus.

Possible Inconveniences. Because the tongue has not yet become accustomed to the appliance, food may become lodged under it in the roof of the mouth. This will occur only for the first few days; the tongue soon will accustom itself to the presence of the appliance.

If you feel any pain from pressure of the appliance on the gums or pressure of clasps on the teeth, please call the office so that we can decide whether a special visit is necessary.

Duration of Treatment. The usual length of time for wearing the appliance is 3 to 4 months. At the end of that period, it will become merely a crutch to be used while the teeth are being reshaped. Once reshaping is accomplished, the jaw will be in correct position—in harmony with the other components of the chewing apparatus—and the appliance will not be needed under normal circumstances. However, situations of severe emotional strain, illness, or overwork can bring about muscle spasm. If this happens, insert the appliance and contact our office.

AFTER AN INJECTION

After receiving a temporomandibular joint injection, it is quite natural to exhibit curiosity about its effect. However, DON'T test the results by opening the jaw to see if there is more motion than before the injection. You MUST refrain from opening the jaws to the point of causing the slightest pain. For this reason, it has been found advisable to adhere to a liquid or soft diet for at least 24 hours following the injection.

Avoid any food that requires prolonged chewing, including meats; crusts of bread, toast, or rolls; uncooked fruits, raw vegetables, and salads; chewy candies.

You may have junior baby foods; soft pudding and Jello; soft, rare hamburgers; milk shakes, including any one of the variety of nourishing drinks that can be mixed in an electric blender; cottage cheese; eggs.

You won't starve—and you'll make much faster progress if you REFRAIN from putting your jaws through any kind of test. Be especially careful when you feel like yawning, for yawning can get you in trouble. Here's a good way to stop the impulse. Make a fist and put it under your chin. Then, with the other hand, cup the elbow of your supporting arm. When your fist is placed beneath your chin, the force of the yawn is taken up by facial muscles. Otherwise, the force is taken up by the temporomandibular joint ligaments.

FIG. 17-18. A printed form is given to the patient explaining the effect of injections into the temporomandibular joint.

APPLICATION OF MOIST HEAT

Moist heat applied to the area around a painful joint usually provides prompt pain relief. The following procedure should be followed carefully:

Soak two large turkish towels in HOT water. Wring out one towel and apply it to the painful area. When the first towel cools, remove it and wring out and apply the second hot towel.

Keeping the water as hot as is bearable, this procedure should be carried out for 5 minutes every half hour, for a total of 2 hours (in other words, 4 times in 2 hours). After an interval of 4 hours, repeat, if necessary.

FIG. 17-19. Instructions for applying moist heat are given the patient.

WEANING THE PATIENT FROM THE SMAA

1. From now on you will not be wearing the Shore appliance during the day. You will be weaned away from the appliance at night. This is the procedure:

> Wear the appliance tonight when you go to sleep but don't wear it the next night.
> Wear it for a night then don't wear it for two nights.
> Wear it for a night then don't wear it for three nights.
> Wear it for a night then don't wear it for four nights.

Follow this procedure until seven nights have elapsed without wearing the appliance. The best idea is to mark on a calendar when you are to wear the SMAA. After that time of weaning from the appliance, only wear it if necessary. Bring the appliance with you each time you have an office visit, so the bite can be checked and the appliance can be cleaned and sterilized ultrasonically.

2. Stay on a soft food diet for approximately another month. At that time, if you feel able, you may start eating firmer foods. But remember to open you mouth no wider than the thickness of your thumb; don't protrude the lower jaw; lips together—teeth apart; and cut food into small, bite-size pieces.

3. When having dental work done, a slightly longer appointment must be made since you should not keep your mouth open for long periods of time. Have the dentist work on your teeth for a few minutes, then have him let you close your mouth a few seconds to relax the jaw muscles. This procedure will help prevent the straining and spasm of the muscles. When you are having a large biting surface restored (filling) you should have either gold inlays or crowns placed (as needed) for a much stronger biting retention surface.

4. When not wearing the SMAA keep it wrapped in moist tissue, inside a plastic container, and keep it refrigerated. This will prevent bacteria from growing on the appliance or the tissue. Change the tissue approximately once a week.

5. Even though your jaw is in the correct position and your ligaments are in the process of healing, you can easily strain or stretch the ligaments again if you do not adhere to these instructions for at least the following year. Don't worry if, under stress, you have occasional sensitivity. Insert the appliance for a day or two and take a muscle relaxant if necessary. If the condition persists, contact us to ask if an office visit is warranted.

6. Continue on the prescribed medication until your next office visit.

FIG. 17-20. Instructions are given the patient to help wean him from the SMAA.

Miss Jane Doe
2701 Grand Concourse
Bronx 55, New York

Dear Miss Doe:

Perhaps the greatest satisfaction we in the dental profession can derive from our work is the realization that we have been able to restore a patient to health. The entire staff joins me in thanking you for the confidence and cooperation you have shown during treatment. You have made it possible for us to enjoy a sense of satisfaction and achievement. And we hope you will accept our sincerest wishes for the very best of health and comfort in the years ahead.

It goes without saying, I hope that our professional relationship in the future may be limited to routine periodic check-ups.

The importance of check-ups, I might add, can hardly be overemphasized. To prevent possible relapses of your condition, it will be necessary for you to adhere rigidly to the check-up schedule I spoke to you about at the beginning of treatment. In case it has slipped your mind, let me remind you of it:

1. The first year following completion of treatment, I will have to see you at 4-month intervals.

2. The second year, I must see you at 6-month intervals.

3. From then on, only one visit a year will be necessary.

There is, of course, no charge for check-ups until one year following the date of the original confirmation letter—that is to say, until after (date, year). After that, a modest fee will be charged for each visit.

I urge you, however, not to hesitate to telephone us if you feel discomfort between check-up visits. As you know, some small imbalance can create great pain. Let us decide if the trouble demands immediate correction. Please be assured we are always ready to help you in any way that we can.

With warmest personal regards,

Cordially,

FIG. 17-21. After successful therapy, the patient is sent an informative letter.

After several months of therapy with the Shore Mandibular Autorepositioning Appliance, spasm and pain patterns caused by engrams are broken up and, with the patient symptom-free, the occlusion is equilibrated accurately. Subsequently, the patient must be weaned from the appliance, in accord with the instructions detailed in Figure 17-20.

Finally, at the completion of successful therapy, the patient is sent a letter (Fig. 17-21), that includes a schedule of follow-up appointments. Also included are comments about the effectiveness of maintenance visits in preventing imbalances and potential relapses into dysfunction.

Prior to and for the duration of treatment, it should be borne in mind that knowledgeable patients are usually cooperative and likely to follow prescribed regimens—an obvious benefit to both the practitioner and the patient undergoing therapy.

BASIC REFERENCES

L. D. Pankey Institute for Advanced Dental Education. Seminar, 1972.

Shapiro, M.: The vital art of patient communication. D. Survey, *48:*55, 1972.

Shore, N.A.: Educational program for patients with temporomandibular joint dysfunction, J. Prosthet. Dent., *23:*6, 1972.

18 *Conclusion*

By maintaining control over the teeth (correcting the occlusion), control can be exerted and maintained over the periodontium, the alveolar bone, the neuromuscular system and the temporomandibular joints—over the entire stomatognathic system.

Because it embodies the establishment of physiological function, occlusal equilibration should be the final treatment of all cases of occlusal disharmony, regardless of their origin. The dentist may be dealing with temporomandibular joint dysfunction, arthrosis, periodontics, crown and bridgework or a simple occlusal amalgam, but the last procedure must be the correction of any existing pathologic occlusion.

If centric relation is regarded primarily as a skull-to-mandible relationship, with the traverse of the mandible through the centric-relation arc as the basic consideration for an evaluation of normal function, the rationale for this approach to the problem becomes crystal clear. An interfering occlusal contact is the trigger mechanism that deflects the mandible in centric-relation closure and consequently initiates the sequelae of degeneration in the tissues, the alveolar bone, the joints and the neuromuscular system. The interfering occlusal contact prevents terminal closure of the mandible on the centric-relation arc. When terminal closure of the mandible on the centric-relation arc exhibits intercuspation of the teeth, centric-relation occlusion occurs.

In modern dentistry, as in clinical medicine, the emphasis is—or should be—on prevention of disease. In the course of this book, the author has been consciously dogmatic in his insistence on the importance of a comprehensive examination and clinical analysis of the patient prior to the initiation of treatment. Such an examination has the double merit of establishing a precise diagnosis and of uncovering minute signs of degeneration, thereby preventing gross pathological dysfunction.

Discussions of temporomandibular joint dysfunction and occlusal equilibration are usually included in specialty texts on periodontics and prosthodontics. The credo of this volume, as in the first edition, is that these two entities should be part and parcel of basic treatment by the general practitioner, rather than by the specialist. Throughout this second edition, in the detailed explanations of the recommended procedures, an attempt has been made to present each step of the diagnostic and clinical regimen in a logical, sequential manner. It is hoped that this deliberate style will enhance the testing and evaluation of all the steps in every technique described herein.

One of the new features of this second edition is a description of the Shore Mandibular Autorepositioning Appliance, an appliance which has value both as a diagnostic and a therapeutic measure.

Another new feature is the emphasis on patient education and the reproduction of routinely used examination forms and instructions to patients. Use of the examination forms helps pinpoint an accurate diagnosis, and the instructions to patients forestall their most often repeated queries.

The author has attempted to define temporomandibular joint problems precisely, with specific, well-delineated etiological manifestations. In outlining the general plan of treatment, he has tried to make a contribution to the ever-increasing acumen and discernment of the dental profession. If he has succeeded only in some small measure, the aims and purposes of this book will have been realized.

Index

Numbers in *italics* indicate illustrations.